Fluid, Electrolyte, and Acid-Base Imbalances

CONTENT REVIEW PLUS PRACTICE QUESTIONS

Allison Hale, MSN, BA, RN
Author, Educator, Consultant

Mary Jo Hovey, MSN, RN, CNE
ADN Instructor

F.A. Davis Company • Philadelphia

F. A. Davis Company
1915 Arch Street
Philadelphia, PA 19103
www.fadavis.com

Printed in the United States of America
Last digit indicates print number: 10 9 8 7 6 5 4 3 2 1

Publisher, Nursing: Robert G. Martone
Director of Content Development: Darlene D. Pedersen
Senior Developmental Editor: William Welsh
Project Editor: Victoria White
Design and Illustration Manager: Carolyn O'Brien

Library of Congress Cataloging-in-Publication Data
Hale, Allison.
Fluid, electrolyte, and acid-base imbalances : content review plus practice questions / Allison Hale, Mary Jo Hovey.
p. ; cm. — (Davis's need to know series)
Includes bibliographical references and index.
ISBN 978-0-8036-2261-6
I. Hovey, Mary Jo. II. Title. III. Series: Davis's need to know series.
[DNLM: 1. Water-Electrolyte Imbalance—nursing—Examination Questions. 2. Water-Electrolyte Imbalance—nursing—Nurses' Instruction. 3. Acid-Base Imbalance—nursing—Examination Questions. 4. Acid-Base Imbalance—nursing—Nurses' Instruction. 5. Body Fluids—physiology—Examination Questions. 6. Body Fluids—physiology—Nurses' Instruction. WD 220]

616.3'992—dc23

2011044890

Allison Hale: *To the memory of my beloved aunt, Kathy Woodcock Grant, who lost her battle with cancer during the development of this book. I will miss her hilarity, her passion for life, and, most of all, her love and friendship. Godspeed. —AH*

Mary Jo Hovey: *To my wonderful family, husband Tom, son Joey, and daughter Katie with many thanks for all the love, encouragement, and extra work they've done while Mom worked on "the Project."*
To my parents, Joseph T. and Mary Lou (also a Registered Nurse) White, for their lifetime of love and support.
And to my talented students, who hopefully will benefit from this endeavor. You have chosen one of the most challenging yet rewarding professions in the world.

Contributors/Reviewers

Barbara Barry, MSN, RN, CNE
ADN Instructor
Cape Fear Community College
Wilmington, North Carolina

Patricia H. White, MSN, RNC
Faculty Lecturer
University of North Carolina at Wilmington
Wilmington, North Carolina

Nell Britton, MSN, RN, CNE, NHA
Nursing Division New Student Coordinator/Nursing Instructor
Trident Technical College
Charleston, South Carolina

Dae Bugl, MSN, MS, MA
Professor
Capital Community College
Hartford, Connecticut

Rene R. Corbett, RN, MSN, APRN-BC, NP
Gerontological Nurse Practitioner
Lower Cape Fear Hospice and Life Care Center
Wilmington, North Carolina

Margaret M. Gingrich, RN, MSN
Professor
Harrisburg Area Community College
Harrisburg, Pennsylvania

Mary M. Goetteman, RN, EdD
Professor
Daytona State College
Daytona Beach, Florida

Linda Kapinos, RN-BC, MSN, MEd
Professor
Capital Community College
Hartford, Connecticut

Elaine B. Kennedy, EdD, RN
Professor
Wor-Wic Community College
Salisbury, Maryland

Susan J. Lamanna, RN, MA, ANP, CNE
Professor
Onondaga Community College
Syracuse, New York

Stephanie Turner, EdD, MSN
Nursing Faculty
Wallace State Community College
Hanceville, Alabama

Susan J. Waltz, RN, DNP
Professor and Nursing Department Chair
Ivy Tech Community College of Indiana
Columbus, Indiana

Preface

Almost every illness can threaten the delicate homeostasis the body must maintain to function and survive. *Fluid, Electrolyte, and Acid-Base Imbalances: Content Review Plus Practice Questions*, the first book in Davis's Need to Know series, is designed to help you gain a thorough understanding of the body's regulation of fluids and solutes.

This text presents critical nursing concepts related to fluid and electrolyte and acid-base balance in an easy-to-understand format to assist you during your course work, while simultaneously preparing you for the NCLEX-RN examination. The text covers such concepts as:

- Normal function, distribution, movement, and regulation of fluid and electrolytes in the body
- Regulation of acid-base balance in the body, including the role of the lungs, kidneys, and natural buffers
- Factors affecting normal fluid, electrolyte, and acid-base balance
- Signs and symptoms of common imbalances
- Nursing interventions to correct specific imbalances
- Medications used when treating imbalances

Nursing Alert Icons Throughout the book, these icons focus your attention on critical, life-saving information that you should commit to memory.

The **Did You Know?** feature provides information and facts that will help you remember important concepts related to specific fluid, electrolyte, and acid-base imbalances.

The **Making the Connection** feature clearly explains the relationship between common pathological disorders and the fluid, electrolyte, or acid-base imbalances that accompany them.

Real-life case studies are provided at the end of each chapter to help you put it all together. These real-life scenarios are intended to encourage you to develop the habit of thinking critically about your clients. The questions following each case study allow you to use the **nursing process** to:

1. Differentiate between *subjective* and *objective* client **assessment** data
2. Identify common fluid, electrolyte, and acid-base imbalances through data **analysis**
3. Provide rationales for the **planning** and **implementation** of client care
4. Develop client outcomes to **evaluate** the effectiveness of collaborative care

Complete answers to all case study questions are located in Appendix A at the back of the book to keep you on track.

End-of-chapter tests, two 100-item comprehensive tests in the book, and a 100-item final examination on a **bonus CD-ROM** help you develop your test-taking skills and master these difficult concepts. In all, **600 practice questions** are provided to reinforce these challenging concepts and help you identify areas of strength and weakness as you progress in your nursing program and prepare for the increasingly difficult **NCLEX-RN** examination. All practice questions are based on the latest NCLEX-RN Test Plan and include a variety of formats, such as multiple-response, fill-in-the-blank, prioritization, hot spot, chart/exhibit, and new graphic test items.

The NCLEX-RN Examination

The National Council Licensure Examination for Registered Nurses (NCLEX-RN) is a required examination that measures the competencies needed to perform safely and effectively as an entry-level registered nurse in the United States. The test is based on a framework of four major **Client Needs** categories (Table P.1):

- Safe and Effective Care Environment
- Health Promotion and Maintenance
- Psychosocial Integrity
- Physiological Integrity

Table P.1 Distribution of NCLEX-RN Test Content

Client Needs	Percentage of Test Items From Each Category/Subcategory
Safe and Effective Care Environment	
• Management of Care	17–23
• Safety and Infection Control	9–15
Health Promotion and Maintenance	6–12
Psychosocial Integrity	6–12
Physiological Integrity	
• Basic Care and Comfort	6–12
• Pharmacological and Parenteral Therapies	12–18
• Reduction of Risk Potential	9–15
• Physiological Adaptation	11–17

The concepts included in all four major client need categories of the NCLEX-RN® Test Plan may be tested on the NCLEX-RN® examination. Examples of how these concepts may be encountered on the examination include the following:

Safe and Effective Care Environment

- Clients with fluid, electrolyte, and acid-base imbalances are at risk for falls and seizures.
- Nurses should ensure client safety when administering IV fluid replacement therapy.
- Improper administration of potassium-containing solutions can cause injury or death.
- Registered nurses are responsible for the delegation of responsibilities to and supervision of unlicensed personnel, who are often assigned to measure and record intake and output.

Health Promotion and Maintenance

- Registered nurses teach clients how to prevent dehydration and how to avoid electrolyte imbalances.
- Many commonly prescribed medications may cause fluid and electrolyte imbalances.
- Registered nurses teach clients about their specific medical conditions; their medications and possible side effects; and the signs and symptoms of fluid, electrolyte and acid-base imbalances that should be reported to a health-care provider.

Psychosocial Integrity

- The actions of many commonly prescribed psychotropic medications may be affected by fluid and electrolyte imbalances.
- Registered nurses should observe for altered levels of consciousness, which may indicate the presence of a fluid, electrolyte, or acid-base imbalance.

Physiological Integrity

- Registered nurses should be able to identify clients who are at risk for imbalances.
- Assessment of fluid, electrolyte, and acid-base imbalances requires the application of knowledge about the anatomical and physiological responses of the body.
- Registered nurses must interpret laboratory data and observe for clinical signs to identify the presence of fluid, electrolyte, and acid-base imbalances.
- Nursing care must be prioritized and coordinated for clients diagnosed with imbalances.
- Clients receiving IV fluid replacement can quickly develop fluid volume excess, life-threatening electrolyte imbalances, or both.

One of the most important strategies you can use to prepare for the NCLEX-RN examination is to become familiar with the NCLEX-RN Test Plan, available online at https://www.ncsbn.org/2010_NCLEX_RN_Detailed_Test_Plan_Candidate.pdf. For more information on the NCLEX-RN examination, contact:

The National Council of State Boards of Nursing, Inc.
111 East Wacker Drive, Suite 2900
Chicago, IL 60601-4277
Phone: (312) 525-3600
When calling from outside the United States:
011 312 525 3600
www.ncsbn.org

Contents

Review of Fluid, Electrolyte, and Acid-Base Balance

I. Fluid Balance

Water is the primary component of the body, accounting for approximately 60% of the total body weight of an adult. Total body water varies with age, gender, and body type; it decreases from birth to old age, with most of the loss occurring during the first 10 years of life (Table I.1.). Fat contains very little water; therefore, an individual with a high percentage of body fat has a lower amount of total body water, and an individual with a high percentage of lean muscle mass has a higher amount of total body water. The human body functions best when internal conditions, such as fluid volume and dissolved particles, are kept in balance (**homeostasis**).

DID YOU KNOW?

Total body water *decreases* with age, as body fat *increases* and thirst sensation *decreases*.

A. Body compartments. Water is needed to deliver dissolved nutrients, electrolytes, and other substances to all cells, organs, and tissues. Within the body, water is divided into two main compartments: extracellular and intracellular (Fig. I.1).

1. **Extracellular fluid (ECF)** is fluid outside the cells. It makes up about 40% of total body water and includes plasma, interstitial fluid (fluid between the cells, also called the *third space*), and transcellular fluid (fluids in special body spaces, such as cerebrospinal, peritoneal, pleural, and synovial fluids).
2. **Intracellular fluid (ICF)** is fluid inside the cells. It makes up about 60% of total body water.

Table I.1 Average Total Body Water in Humans

Infants	70%–80%
Men	65%
Women	55%
Lean muscular adults	Up to 75%
Obese adults	45%
Adults aged 60 and older	50%–55%

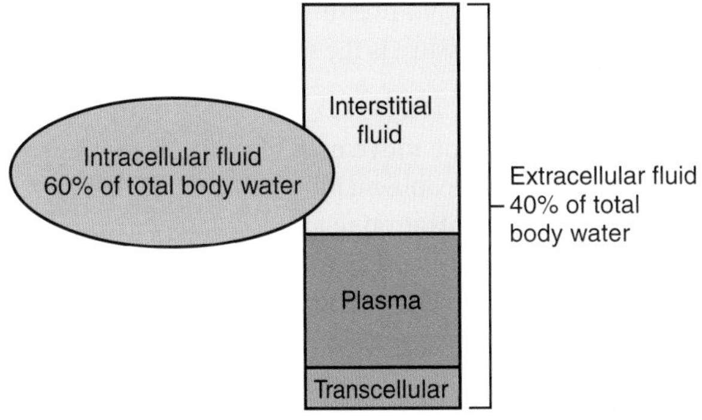

Fig I.1

B. How fluids move. Body fluids are composed of water (the solvent) and particles that are dissolved or suspended in water (the solutes). To maintain a stable internal environment, the body uses four processes: filtration, diffusion, osmosis, and active transport.

1. **Filtration** is the movement of fluid through a permeable cell membrane or blood vessel membrane because of differences in water volume (hydrostatic pressure) pressing against the confining walls of the space. Fluids that are more viscous than water, such as blood, have higher hydrostatic pressures because of their weight and volume (Fig. I.2). Examples of filtration are:
   a. **Blood pressure.** Whole blood is pumped by the heart to the capillaries, where filtration occurs to exchange water, nutrients, and waste products. The hydrostatic pressure of capillary blood is greater than that of the interstitial fluid, causing water to filter freely to an area of lower pressure (down a pressure gradient).
   b. **Edema.** In clients with right-sided heart failure, the volume of blood in the right side of the heart increases because the right ventricle is too weak to pump blood into the pulmonary vessels. Blood backs up into the venous system, and the venous hydrostatic pressure increases, causing the pressure in the capillaries to increase. Water filters from the capillaries into the interstitial tissue space, resulting in visible edema.

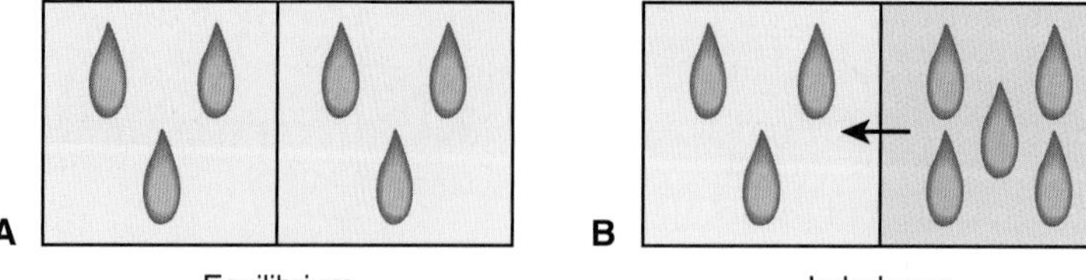

Fig I.2 Filtration. (A) No pressure difference between the two sides. (B) Higher pressure on the right side; filtration occurs until the pressure is the same in both spaces (equilibrium).

2. **Diffusion** is the movement of particles (solute) across a permeable membrane from an area of higher concentration to an area of lower concentration (down a concentration gradient) by random molecular motion. This movement continues until the particles are gradually "mixed" and equilibrium is achieved (Fig. I.3). Examples of diffusion are:
   a. **Respiration.** In the alveoli of the lungs, oxygen molecules diffuse into the blood, and carbon dioxide molecules diffuse out because of the differences in partial pressures across the alveolar-capillary membrane. Lungs have a large surface area to facilitate this gas exchange process. Capillary membranes permit the diffusion of these small-sized particles down a concentration gradient; cell membranes are selective, however, permitting the diffusion of some particles but not others.
   b. **Movement of glucose into the cells.** In some instances, diffusion across a cell membrane requires assistance (**facilitated diffusion**). The ECF contains a higher concentration of glucose than the ICF. Even though a steep concentration gradient exists, glucose requires the help of insulin to move across the cell membrane into the ICF. Insulin binds to the insulin receptor sites on the cell membrane, making the membrane more permeable to glucose. Glucose can then cross the cell membrane down the concentration gradient until equilibrium is achieved (Fig. I.4).

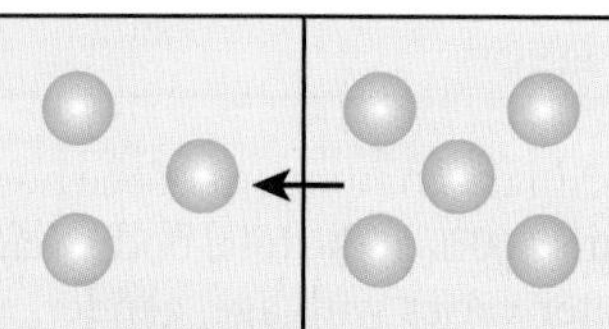

Fig I.3 Diffusion of particles continues as long as a concentration gradient exists.

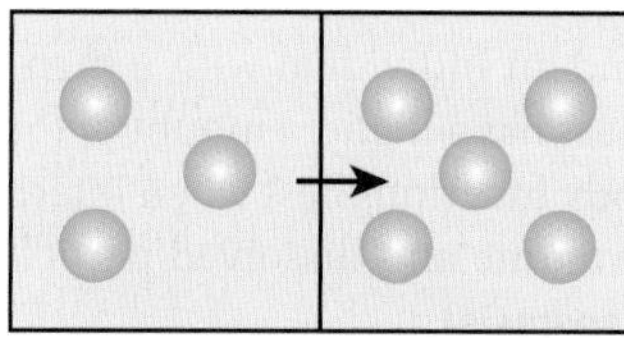

Fig I.4 Facilitated diffusion is the passive transport of molecules or ions across a biological membrane, assisted by transport proteins.

3. **Osmosis** is the movement of only water through a semipermeable membrane across a concentration gradient. Water moves from areas of lower particle concentration (hypotonic) to areas of higher particle concentration (hypertonic) until the concentration is the same on both sides of the membrane, even though the total number of particles and volume of water are different (Fig. I.5).
   a. The body functions best when the osmolarity of fluids is about 300 mOsm/L.
   b. When all body fluids have this particle concentration, the body fluids are **isosmotic** (equal osmotic pressure) or **isotonic** (same concentration of solutes as blood).
   c. Fluids with osmolarity greater than 300 mOsm/L are **hyperosmotic** or **hypertonic**. These fluids pull water from areas of low concentration to areas of high concentration until equilibrium is achieved.
   d. Fluids with osmolarity less than 270 mOsm/L are **hypo-osmotic** or **hypotonic**. These fluids, which have low osmotic pressures, are pulled into areas where the osmotic pressure is higher, until equilibrium is achieved.
   e. An example of osmosis occurs by means of the **thirst mechanism**. When body water is lost, such as through excessive sweating, the ECF volume is decreased and the ECF osmolarity is increased. Osmoreceptors in the brain respond

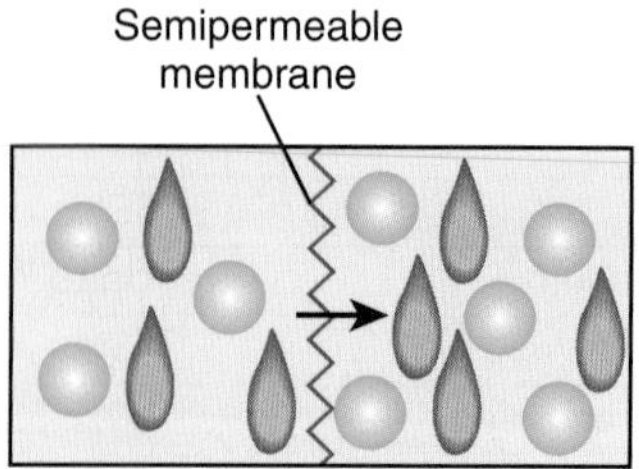

Fig I.5 Osmosis is the movement of water through a selectively permeable membrane from a hypotonic area of concentration to a hypertonic area of concentration.

to the increasing osmolarity and trigger the person's awareness of thirst, causing the person to drink. Drinking replaces the water lost and decreases the ECF osmolarity to normal.

4. **Active transport** is the movement of particles across a cell membrane, from areas of lower concentration to areas of higher concentration, by combining with a carrier on the outside of the cell membrane that then moves inside the cell. Once inside the cell, the particle and the carrier separate, and the particle is released inside the cell. This requires an expenditure of energy (Fig. I.6).
   a. An example of active transport occurs in the maintenance of **sodium and potassium balance.** The ECF has about 10 times more sodium ions than the ICF does. Even though a steep concentration gradient exists, sodium cannot diffuse across the cell membrane into the ICF because the membrane is impermeable to sodium. Special "sodium-potassium pumps" move excess sodium out of the cell (against the concentration gradient) and into the ECF, and they move potassium into the ICF (also against the concentration gradient), where potassium concentrations are higher, to maintain homeostasis.

C. **Why fluids move.** The kidneys, which are the primary regulators of fluids and electrolytes, balance body fluids by controlling water and electrolyte excretion. The body's endocrine system helps control fluid and electrolyte balance by acting on the kidneys with three primary hormones: aldosterone, antidiuretic hormone, and natriuretic peptides.

1. **Aldosterone** is a hormone secreted by the adrenal cortex whenever the ECF sodium level is decreased; it prevents sodium and water loss.
   a. Aldosterone acts on the kidney nephrons and triggers them to reabsorb sodium and water from the urine back into the blood, increasing blood osmolarity and blood volume.
   b. Aldosterone prevents the excessive excretion of sodium by the kidneys and prevents potassium levels from getting too high.
   c. The **renin-angiotensin-aldosterone mechanism** is activated when blood flow or pressure to the kidneys decreases. When this occurs, renin is released, causing angiotensin to be converted to angiotensin I, which is converted to angiotensin II by angiotensin-converting enzyme (ACE). Angiotensin II acts directly on the kidney nephrons, promoting sodium and water retention and the release of aldosterone. Aldosterone causes sodium and water to be retained, restoring blood volume and renal perfusion (Fig. I.7).
2. **Antidiuretic hormone (ADH)** regulates water. It is produced in the brain, stored in the posterior pituitary gland, and controlled by the hypothalamus.
   a. Osmoreceptors in the hypothalamus detect increases in blood osmolarity and decreases in blood pressure or blood volume, which causes

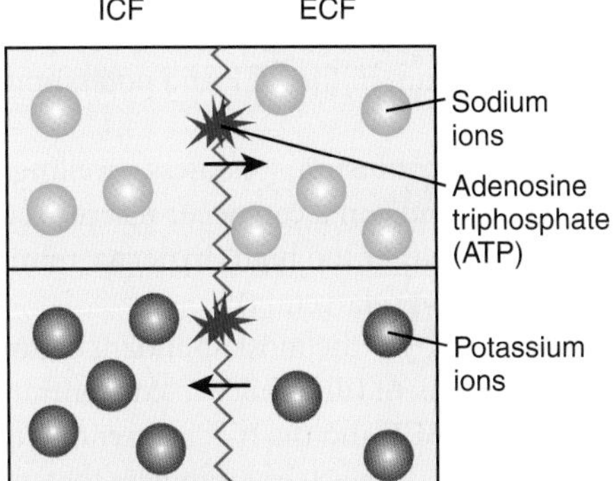

Fig I.6 Active transport moves particles, using enzymes and specific carriers, from areas of lower concentration to areas of higher concentration.

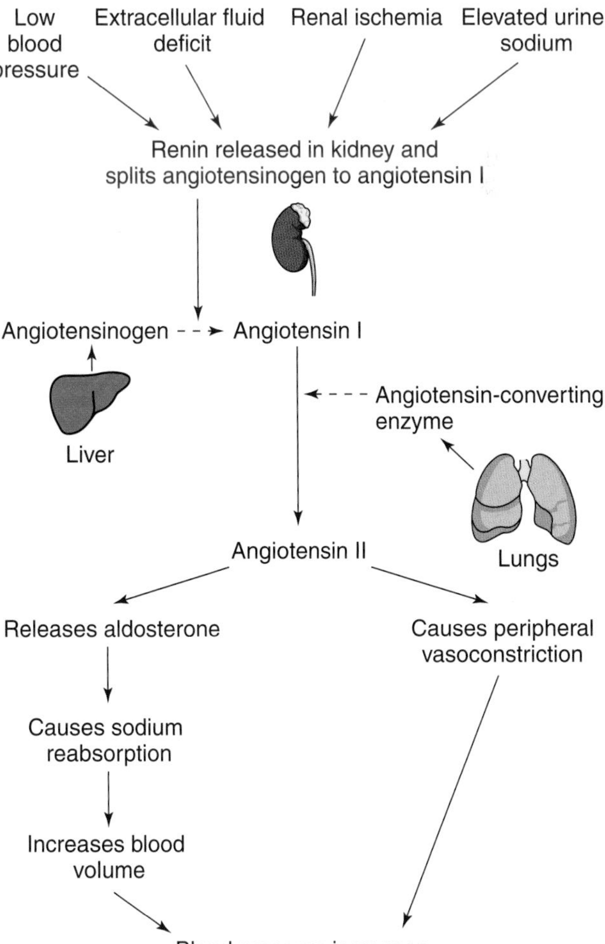

Fig I.7 The renin-angiotensin-aldosterone mechanism.

ADH (also called *vasopressin*) to be released from the posterior pituitary gland.

b. ADH acts directly on the kidney tubules and collecting ducts, making them more permeable and thus allowing water to be reabsorbed in the tubules and returned to the blood, which decreases blood osmolarity.

c. When blood pressure, blood volume, or plasma osmolarity (specifically, the serum sodium level) returns to normal, ADH is inhibited, and the absorption of water stops.

3. **Natriuretic peptides** are hormones secreted by the cells that line the atria (atrial natriuretic peptide [ANP]) and ventricles (brain natriuretic peptide [BNP]) of the heart. These hormones are secreted in response to increased blood volume and blood pressure, which stretch the heart tissue.

   a. Natriuretic peptides have the opposite effect of aldosterone: they inhibit the absorption of sodium and increase glomerular filtration, causing an increase in urine output. As a result, circulating blood volume and blood osmolarity are decreased.

D. **Intake and output.** Under normal conditions, body fluids (which are constantly filtered and replaced) are maintained through intake and output. Intake and output must be relatively equal to maintain normal fluid balance.

1. **Intake** includes all fluids that enter the body. This includes fluids that are consumed orally, such as water, ice chips, juice, milk, and coffee, and fluids administered by other routes, such as IV solutions via parenteral or central lines, feeding tubes, irrigation, lavage, and blood transfusions (Table I.2).

   a. If intake is greater than output, the volume of fluid in the blood increases (hypervolemia) and edema, electrolyte imbalances, or other complications may occur.

Table I.2 Fluid Intake and Output

Average Adult Intake	Average Adult Output
Sensible (measurable)	
Oral fluids: 1,500 mL/day	Urine: 1,400–1,500 mL/day
Parenteral fluids: variable	Emesis: variable
Enemas: variable	Feces (liquid form): variable
Irrigation fluids: variable	Drainage from body cavities: variable
Insensible (not measurable)	
Solid foods: 800 mL/day	Perspiration: 100 mL/day
By-product of metabolism: 300 mL/day	Insensible loss: 500–1,000 mL/day (via skin, lungs, and stool)

2. **Output** includes all fluids that leave the body, such as urine, diarrhea, vomiting, drainage from all tubes, blood loss, and fluids lost through perspiration, respiration, and loss of body heat (insensible fluid loss) (see Table I.2).

   a. If output is more than intake, the volume of fluid in the blood decreases (hypovolemia), and dehydration and electrolyte imbalances may occur.

DID YOU KNOW?

Insensible fluid loss can be significant—especially in older adults.

II. Electrolyte Balance

Electrolytes are substances that become ions in solution and acquire the capacity to conduct electricity. Many different electrolytes are present in the human body and are required for normal cell and organ function. Most electrolytes enter the body through dietary intake and are excreted in the urine and feces. The concentration of electrolytes in the body is controlled by different hormones. Specialized kidney cells monitor the amount of sodium, potassium, and water in the bloodstream. Hormones such as renin (made in the kidney), angiotensin (from the lung, brain, and heart), aldosterone (from the adrenal gland), and antidiuretic hormone (from the pituitary) maintain electrolyte balance. The two main types of electrolytes, cations and anions, must remain in balance for the body to maintain normal functioning (Table I.3).

A. **Cations** are ions that carry a positive charge due to a loss of electrons. Cations in the body include sodium, potassium, calcium, and magnesium.

1. **Sodium (Na^+)** is the most abundant cation in the ECF and is a significant part of water regulation in the body because water goes where sodium goes.

   a. Sodium is needed to generate electrical signals in the body, allowing the muscles to contract and the brain to work.

   b. Sodium is part of the sodium-potassium pump, located in all cell membranes, which keeps sodium in the ECF and potassium inside the cell.

   c. Lethargy, confusion, weakness, swelling, seizures, and coma can occur if serum sodium levels are either too high (**hypernatremia**) or too low (**hyponatremia**).

2. **Potassium (K^+)** is the most abundant cation in the ICF. The gradient (difference in concentration) between the ECF and the ICF is essential for the generation of the electrical impulses that allow the muscles and the brain to function.

   a. High serum potassium levels (**hyperkalemia**) can cause abnormal electrical conduction in the

Table I.3 Normal Serum Electrolyte Levels and Their Functions

Electrolyte	Normal Adult Serum Levels	Functions
Cations		
Sodium (Na^+)	135–145 mEq/L	• Maintaining blood volume • Regulating ECF volume and distribution • Transmitting nerve impulses • Contracting muscles
Potassium (K^+)	3.5–5.0 mEq/L	• Maintaining ICF osmolarity • Transmitting nerve impulses • Regulating cardiac impulse transmission • Skeletal and smooth muscle function • Regulating acid-base balance
Calcium (Ca^{2+})	8.2–10.2 mg/dL	• Forming bones and teeth • Transmitting nerve impulses • Regulating muscle contractions • Blood clotting • Activating enzymes
Magnesium (Mg^{2+})	1.6–2.6 mg/dL	• Maintaining intracellular metabolism • Operating sodium-potassium pump • Relaxing muscle contractions • Transmitting nerve impulses • Regulating cardiac function
Anions		
Chloride (Cl^-)	97–107 mEq/L	• Producing hydrochloric acid • Regulating acid-base balance • Regulating ECF balance and vascular volume • Acting as a buffer in oxygen–carbon dioxide exchange in red blood cells (RBCs)
Phosphate (PO_4^-)	2.5–4.5 mg/dL	• Forming bones and teeth • Muscle, nerve, and RBC function • Metabolism of carbohydrates, proteins, and fats • Regulating acid-base balance • Regulating calcium levels • Cellular metabolism (ATP and DNA)
Bicarbonate (HCO_3^-)	22–26 mmol/L (arterial) 24–28 mmol/L (venous)	• Major buffer in acid-base regulation

heart and potentially life-threatening abnormal heart rhythms (dysrhythmias).

b. Low serum potassium levels (**hypokalemia**) may not cause symptoms if the deficit is mild. Moderate or severe hypokalemia can cause dysrhythmias, especially in clients with heart disease; constipation; fatigue; muscle weakness or spasms; muscle damage (rhabdomyolysis); and paralysis.

3. **Calcium** (Ca^{2+}) is the most abundant cation in the body. More than 99% of calcium is stored in the bones and teeth. Calcium is needed to help the muscles and blood vessels contract and expand, to secrete hormones and enzymes, and for the transmission of nerve signals.
   a. High serum calcium levels (**hypercalcemia**) can cause kidney stones, abdominal pain, depression, and cardiac dysrhythmias.
   b. Low serum calcium levels (**hypocalcemia**) can cause weakness, muscle spasms, and cardiac dysrhythmias.
4. **Magnesium** (Mg^{2+}) is a cation that is required for a variety of metabolic activities, such as relaxation of smooth muscle, contraction of skeletal muscle, and stimulation of neurons in the brain.
   a. High serum magnesium levels (**hypermagnesemia**) can cause cardiac dysrhythmias, muscle weakness, nausea and vomiting, and breathing difficulties; hypermagnesemia is often associated with hypocalcemia (low calcium) and hyperkalemia (high potassium).
   b. Low serum magnesium levels (**hypomagnesemia**) can also cause dysrhythmias and muscle weakness but can also cause muscle cramping, confusion, hallucinations, and seizures; low magnesium levels are often associated with hypokalemia.

B. Anions are ions that carry a negative charge and are attracted to cations (e.g., Na^+ and Cl^- form NaCl, or table salt). The major anions in the body include chloride, phosphate, and bicarbonate (see Table I.3).

1. **Chloride (Cl^-)** is the most abundant anion in the ECF. Blood and other body fluids have almost the same concentration of chloride as seawater. Chloride balance is tightly regulated by the body.
   a. High serum chloride levels (**hyperchloremia**) are usually asymptomatic and may be associated with excess fluid loss via vomiting and diarrhea. Hyperchloremia can lead to an increase in blood glucose (hyperglycemia) in diabetic clients and, if severe, may result in Kussmaul respirations, weakness, and intense thirst.
   b. Low serum chloride levels (**hypochloremia**) cause the kidneys to retain bicarbonate and sodium ions to compensate for the chloride loss. As a result, bicarbonate accumulates in the ECF, raising the pH level and leading to hypochloremic metabolic alkalosis; hypochloremia is often associated with hypokalemia, hyponatremia, and metabolic acidosis. (See Acid-Base Balance, below.)
2. **Phosphate (PO_4^-)** is an anion that is found in every cell of the body, but it is stored mainly in the bones and teeth. Its primary function is the formation of bones and teeth, but it also assists in muscle contraction, kidney functioning, regulation of heart rate, and nerve conduction.
   a. High serum phosphate levels (**hyperphosphatemia**) result in low serum calcium levels because phosphate and calcium have an inverse relationship.
   b. Low serum phosphate levels (**hypophosphatemia**) result in high serum calcium levels; most of the signs and symptoms of phosphate imbalance are caused by associated calcium imbalances.
3. **Bicarbonate (HCO_3^-)** is an anion that helps buffer the acids that build up in the body as normal by-products of metabolism. Bicarbonate binds with free hydrogen ions released from the acid to form carbon dioxide and water.
   a. The amount of bicarbonate in the bloodstream indicates how severe an acid-base imbalance has become. (See Acid-Base Balance, below.)

III. Acid-Base Balance

The human body produces both acids and bases to maintain the pH level of body fluids. Hydrogen ions (H^+) cause the blood to be acidic. Thus, acid-base balance is influenced by the production and elimination of hydrogen ions. Acid-base imbalances impair the functioning of many organs by altering the response of excitable membranes, making the heart, nerves, muscles, and gastrointestinal tract either more or less active; reducing the function of hormones and enzymes; affecting the distribution of electrolytes; and decreasing the effectiveness of many drugs.

A. Acids are substances that release hydrogen ions when dissolved in water, increasing the concentration of hydrogen ions and lowering pH. Acids are substances with a pH below 7. Normal metabolic processes produce acids. The primary acids produced by the body are carbonic acid, sulfuric acid, and lactic acid.

1. **Carbonic acid** forms when carbon dioxide (CO_2) combines with water. It is one of the principal substances that affect pH and is a natural waste product of carbohydrate metabolism.
   a. Carbonic acid levels are normally controlled by the lungs through the retention or the excretion of CO_2; problems of regulation lead to respiratory acidosis or alkalosis.
   b. Blood pH is influenced by how much CO_2 is produced by the cells during metabolism versus how rapidly that CO_2 is removed by breathing.
2. **Sulfuric acid** forms as a by-product of protein metabolism, although the most common by-product of protein metabolism is nitrogen.
   a. Sulfuric acid is produced when sulfur-containing amino acids are broken down in the body.
   b. **Fatty acids** form when organic fatty acids, especially those found in animal and vegetable fats and oils, are broken down in the body.
   c. **Ketone bodies** are compounds produced as by-products when fatty acids are broken down for energy by the liver and kidneys. Some ketone bodies are used as a source of energy by the heart and brain, but one type is a waste product excreted from the body.
3. **Lactic acid** forms as a by-product of carbohydrate breakdown under anaerobic conditions (no oxygen).
   a. When the oxygen level in the body is normal, carbohydrates break down into water and carbon dioxide, and energy is produced.
   b. When the oxygen level in the body is low, carbohydrates break down incompletely, producing some energy and forming lactic acid.

B. Bases are substances that bind free hydrogen ions in water, reducing the concentration of hydrogen ions and increasing pH.

1. **Bicarbonate (HCO_3^-)** is an electrolyte and the principal alkaline substance (base) in the body. It responds slowly to changes in pH, but its effects are long lasting.
   a. Bicarbonate binds with free H^+ in the ECF and ICF to decrease hydrogen ion concentration.
   b. Bicarbonate and H^+ levels are controlled by the kidneys; problems of regulation lead to metabolic acidosis or alkalosis.

2. **Ammonia (NH_3)** is a weak base composed of nitrogen and hydrogen. In the presence of moisture, ammonia binds with acids to form salts that can be eliminated from the body.
   a. Ammonia is a colorless gas with a characteristic pungent odor.
   b. Ammonium is excreted in the urine, resulting in the loss of acid and increasing the serum pH.

C. **Buffers** are substances that bring body fluids back to the normal pH range of 7.35 to 7.45 by either releasing hydrogen ions (to make fluids more acidic) or binding with hydrogen ions (to make fluids more alkaline). It is important to note that a buffer may be either an acid or a base. If a fluid is basic, buffers release hydrogen ions to decrease pH. If a fluid is acidic, buffers act as a base by binding with free hydrogen ions. The primary buffers in the body are bicarbonate, phosphate, and protein buffers.
   1. **Bicarbonate (HCO_3^-)** is considered the major extracellular buffer in the body. This buffer binds with free hydrogen ions to increase the body's pH.
   2. **Phosphate** is an intracellular buffer that is active in the ICF. This buffer binds with free hydrogen ions to increase the body's pH; the bound hydrogen ions are excreted in the urine.
   3. **Protein buffers** are the most common buffers, these intracellular buffers can either bind or release free hydrogen ions, as needed, in the ECF and ICF, increasing or decreasing the pH of blood and body fluids. There are two main types of protein buffers, albumin/globulins and hemoglobin.
      a. **Albumin/globulins** are major protein buffers, making up 6% to 8% of the blood. These serum proteins bind or release free hydrogen ions to help regulate the blood pH.
      b. **Hemoglobin** is a major cell protein buffer that buffers hydrogen ions directly and buffers acids formed during the production of carbon dioxide.

DID YOU KNOW?

Buffers, such as bicarbonate and phosphate, are the first line of defense against changes in blood pH.

D. **Measuring acids and bases**
   1. The **pH scale** is used to measure how acidic or basic a body fluid is, based on the fluid's free hydrogen ion level. The pH has the narrowest normal range of all laboratory values. Even small changes in the pH of body fluids can impair the functioning of many organs (Table I.4).
      a. The pH scale ranges from 1 (extremely acidic) to 14 (extremely basic).
      b. Distilled water has a pH of 7, which is considered neutral.
      c. The normal body pH is slightly alkalotic.

Table I.4 The Range of Blood pH in the Human Body

Blood pH				
<6.8	<7.35	7.35–7.45	>7.45	>7.8
Death	Acidosis	Normal	Alkalosis	Death

      d. Maintaining pH within the normal reference range involves balancing acids and bases in the body.

The normal pH reference range of arterial blood is 7.35 to 7.45.

ALERT A blood pH less than 6.8 or greater than 7.8 is usually fatal.

   2. Laboratory tests measure the pH and the amount of gases, such as carbon dioxide, bicarbonate, and oxygen, in arterial and venous blood. Arterial blood gases provide the most information about acid-base balance (Table I.5).
      a. An **arterial blood gas (ABG)** is a laboratory test that measures the pH and levels of oxygen (Pao_2), carbon dioxide ($Paco_2$), and bicarbonate (HCO_3^-) in arterial blood. Drawing ABG specimens can be painful; complications, such as arterial bleeding and arterial blood clots, sometimes occur.
      b. A **venous blood gas (VBG)** is a laboratory test that measures the pH and levels of carbon dioxide (Pco_2) and bicarbonate (HCO_3^-) in venous blood. Although VBGs can provide the information needed to diagnose acid-base imbalances, they are usually not performed on clients who are critically ill or in cardiac arrest. VBG specimens are faster and easier to draw, less painful to the client, and less likely to cause bleeding or clots; it should be noted, however, that because venous blood has much less oxygen than arterial blood, VBG oxygen levels are not measured.

DID YOU KNOW?

The CO_2 level in venous blood is not the same measurement as the $Paco_2$ in arterial blood. These values are commonly confused.

E. **Compensation.** Compensation is the body's attempt to correct abnormal changes in blood pH. Acid-base imbalances that cannot be corrected by the buffer system can be compensated in the short term by changing the respiratory rate, which alters the concentration of carbon dioxide in the blood, thus changing its pH. The kidneys are slower to

Table I.5 Acid-Base Assessment: Normal Ranges for Adults

Test	Arterial	Venous
pH	7.35–7.45	7.31–7.41
Oxygen	Pao_2: younger than 90 years, 80–100 mm Hg; older than 90 years, 70–90 mm Hg	Not measured
Carbon dioxide	$Paco_2$: 35–45 mm Hg	Pco_2: 38–52 mm Hg
Bicarbonate (HCO_3^-)	22–26 mmol/L	24–28 mmol/L
Lactate	3–7 mg/dL	5–20 mg/dL

compensate but exert a long-lasting effect on serum pH by excreting excess acids or bases.

1. **Respiratory compensation** is an attempt by the lungs to correct acid-base imbalances caused by metabolic problems. For instance, if the blood pH drops too low, the body will compensate by increasing the respiratory rate and eliminating carbon dioxide, which increases serum pH. Conversely, if the blood pH rises too high, the body will compensate by decreasing the respiratory rate and retaining carbon dioxide, which decreases serum pH.
   a. The respiratory system is the second line of defense (after buffers) against pH changes, responding to such changes in seconds to minutes.
   b. The respiratory system is sensitive to acid-base changes and begins compensation efforts immediately, but these efforts are limited and short-lived.
2. **Renal compensation** is an attempt by the kidneys to correct pH imbalances caused by respiratory problems. Although the kidneys are less sensitive than the lungs and slower to compensate for serum pH imbalances, renal compensation lasts much longer than respiratory compensation. For instance, if the blood pH drops too low, the kidneys reabsorb and produce more bicarbonate, secrete more hydrogen ions, and convert ammonia to ammonium, which traps hydrogen ions for excretion in the urine and increases blood pH. Conversely, if the blood pH rises too high, the kidneys excrete more bicarbonate and secrete fewer hydrogen ions, lowering serum pH.
   a. The renal system is the third line of defense against pH changes and is activated when the respiratory system is overwhelmed or is not healthy.
   b. Because the renal system is less sensitive to pH changes, renal compensation is not triggered unless the blood pH has been abnormal for at least 24 to 48 hours.
   c. Although the renal system is slower to respond to pH changes, renal compensation is powerful and has a long-lasting effect on the blood pH.
3. **Partial compensation** occurs when the lungs or kidneys attempt to correct pH imbalances but the pH remains slightly outside the normal reference range; partial compensation prevents the acid-base imbalance from becoming severe or life threatening.
4. **Full compensation** occurs when the lungs or kidneys successfully correct the pH imbalance and the pH returns to the normal reference range, even though the carbon dioxide or bicarbonate level may remain abnormal.
5. If the body has not yet begun to compensate or is unable to make adjustments for changes in blood pH, the imbalance is said to be **uncompensated**.

UNIT I

Fluid Imbalances

Fluid Volume Excess

KEY TERMS

Edema—Swelling of soft tissues as a result of excess fluid accumulation; classified in the extremities as either "pitting" or "nonpitting"
Fluid volume excess—A clinical sign of a disorder in which fluid intake or retention is greater than the body's fluid needs; not a disease
Hypertonic overhydration—Sodium and fluid excess caused by excessive sodium intake; sodium intake exceeds water intake, making the blood hypertonic to normal body fluids
Hypervolemia—Abnormal increase in the volume of the bloodstream (intravascular space)
Hypotonic overhydration/water intoxication—Fluid excess caused by the overconsumption or excessive IV administration of salt-free solutions; water intake exceeds sodium intake, making the blood hypotonic to normal body fluids
Isotonic overhydration/hypervolemia—Plasma volume increases while plasma composition remains unchanged
Overhydration—Excess water in the extracellular fluid
Pulse pressure—Difference between the systolic and diastolic blood pressures; represents the force the heart generates each time it contracts

I. Description

Fluid volume excess (FVE) develops when there is more fluid than the body needs. Excess fluid, consisting primarily of water and sodium, builds up in the soft tissues of the body, resulting in an increase in body weight. This may be caused by excessive salt intake, diseases affecting the kidneys or liver, or poor pumping action of the heart. This excess fluid can disrupt the concentration (osmolarity) of substances in the blood, such as sodium, potassium, and chloride, causing electrolyte imbalances. Remember that overhydration is not the same as **hypervolemia,** which is an abnormal increase in the volume of the bloodstream. **Overhydration** means that there is excess water in the extracellular fluid (ECF), but it does not include the electrolyte changes that occur in hypervolemia.

DID YOU KNOW?

An increase in body weight is the most accurate indicator of FVE.

II. Types of Fluid Volume Excess

There are three main types of FVE. Each type of overhydration causes water to move into or out of the cells in a different way. It is important to understand how each type of FVE affects the fluid balance in the body.

A. Isotonic overhydration
  1. An excess of both water and sodium.
  2. The most common type of FVE.
  3. There is little or no change in the concentration of electrolytes and water in the bloodstream.
  4. Water is neither pulled from the cells into the circulation nor pulled from the circulation into the cells.
  5. The ECF volume becomes elevated, but the intracellular fluid (ICF) volume remains normal.
  6. The serum osmolarity (electrolyte concentration) of the blood remains normal: from 275 to 295 mOsm/kg.

B. Hypotonic overhydration (water intoxication)
  1. An excess of water causing a dilutional deficiency of sodium and other electrolytes (Fig. 1.1).
  2. Water dilutes the electrolytes in the bloodstream and causes fluid to shift *out of* the ECF and *into* the cells, causing them to swell and possibly burst (lysis).
  3. Cerebral cells absorb water more easily than other types of cells, making increased intracranial pressure a concern when hypotonic overhydration occurs.

Hypotonic Overhydration

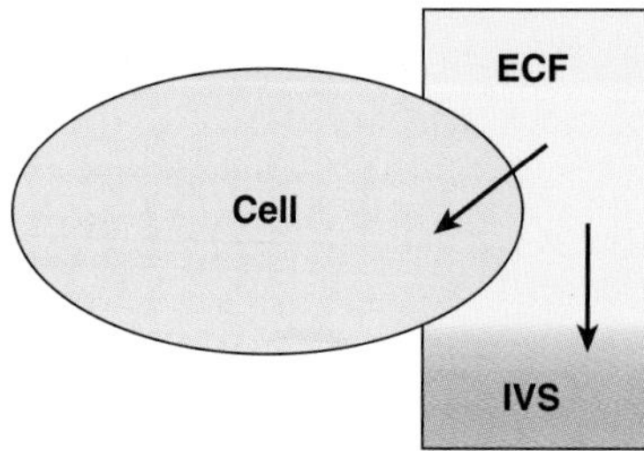

Hypotonic overhydration causes fluid to shift out of the ECF and into the cells, causing them to swell and possibly burst (lysis).

Fig 1.1 Hypotonic overhydration: excess water is administered or ingested, causing the ECF and ICF volumes to increase.

Hypertonic Overhydration

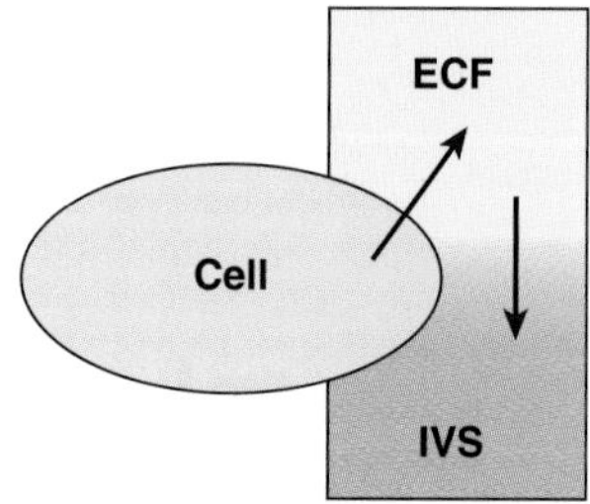

Too much sodium in the blood causes fluid to shift out of the cells and into the ECF to restore sodium balance.

Fig 1.2 Hypertonic overhydration: sodium and water are retained in the ECF; the osmotic pressure in the ECF increases, pulling fluid from the cells into the ECF.

4. The ECF and ICF volumes are both increased.
5. The serum osmolarity of the blood decreases (becomes diluted) to less than 250 mOsm/kg, causing electrolyte imbalances.

C. Hypertonic overhydration
1. An excess of fluid and sodium usually caused by excessive sodium intake (Fig. 1.2).
2. Too much sodium in the blood causes its osmolarity to increase to greater than 295 mOsm/kg, causing fluid to shift out of the cells and into the ECF to restore sodium balance.
3. The volume of the ICF then decreases, causing the cells to shrink and the electrolytes inside the cells to become more concentrated (increased osmolarity).
4. The increase dosmolarity of the ICF results in electrolyte imbalances.

MAKING THE CONNECTION

Edema

Edema, an abnormal accumulation of fluid in the organs, body cavities, or extremities, develops when (1) increased hydrostatic pressure (pushing pressure) forces fluid out of the arterial end of the capillaries into the tissues and (2) decreased oncotic pressure (pulling pressure) does not draw fluid back into the venous end of the capillaries. These pressure abnormalities result in mild to severe swelling in one or more parts of the body. Edema is the body's normal response to inflammation or injury and may be caused by FVE; heart, liver, or kidney diseases; low albumin levels in the blood (hypoalbuminemia); allergic reactions; obstruction of blood flow; pregnancy; burns; life-threatening infections; and other critical illnesses. Box 1.1 describes the different types of edema.

Box 1.1 Types of Edema

Anasarca—Severe generalized edema
Ascites—Accumulation of excess fluid in the peritoneal cavity (membrane lining the abdominal organs)
Cerebral edema—Accumulation of excess fluid in the brain
Cutaneous edema—Accumulation of fluid under the skin; often resulting from insect bites or contact with certain plants
Generalized edema—Swelling throughout the body, involving multiple organs and extremities
Lymphedema—Swelling caused by blockage of the lymph vessels that drain fluid from tissues throughout the body
Periorbital edema—Swelling around the eye
Peripheral edema—Swelling of the extremities, usually the legs
Pleural effusion—Accumulation of fluid in the pleural (lung) cavity
Pulmonary edema—Accumulation of fluid in the lungs

III. Causes of Fluid Volume Excess

Excessive fluid intake, abnormal retention of fluid caused by certain medical conditions or medications, long-term corticosteroid therapy, adrenal gland disorders, and excessive administration of sodium bicarbonate, may place a client at risk for FVE (Table 1.1).

A. Causes of isotonic overhydration
1. Excessive or rapid administration of isotonic IV solutions, such as 0.9% sodium chloride (normal saline), lactated Ringer's solution, and 5% dextrose in sterile water (D_5W), may cause isotonic overhydration.
   a. If the amount or rate of fluid administration exceeds the kidneys' ability to excrete fluid and sodium, hypervolemia results.
   b. This can easily occur when isotonic IV fluids are administered in the perioperative setting, so careful monitoring of IV fluid administration is

Table 1.1 Causes of Fluid Volume Excess

Type	Causes
Isotonic overhydration (hypervolemia)	Excessive administration of isotonic IV fluids Abnormal retention of water and sodium • Heart failure • Renal failure • Nephrotic syndrome • Acute glomerulonephritis • Liver cirrhosis Long-term corticosteroid therapy
Hypotonic overhydration (water intoxication)	Excessive intake of salt-free solutions, such as water In infants, ingestion of diluted formula or excess water Irrigation of wounds and body cavities with hypotonic fluids Liver failure Syndrome of inappropriate antidiuretic hormone secretion (SIADH)
Hypertonic overhydration	Excessive ingestion of sodium chloride, such as drinking seawater Excessive administration of hypertonic IV solutions Primary hyperaldosteronism Cushing's syndrome Excessive intake of sodium bicarbonate

required during the pre-, intra-, and postoperative periods.

c. Isotonic overhydration can also be caused by improper blood administration.

2. Abnormal retention of water and sodium causes the ECF volume to increase.
   a. Heart failure is a condition in which the heart is unable to pump a sufficient amount of blood to meet the needs of the body's tissues; circulation is diminished, causing a decrease in blood flow to the kidneys and resulting in fluid retention and edema.
      1) In right-sided heart failure, edema commonly starts in the ankles and may also occur in the abdominal cavity (ascites).
      2) In left-sided heart failure, edema can occur in the lungs (pulmonary edema), reducing gas exchange and causing shortness of breath, orthopnea (shortness of breath when lying down), and paroxysmal nocturnal dyspnea (respiratory distress that causes the client to awaken during the night).
      3) The most common causes of heart failure are coronary artery disease (CAD) and hypertension.

MAKING THE CONNECTION

Congestive Heart Failure

When a client experiences heart failure, the heart is unable to adequately pump blood and oxygen to the tissues. Reduced perfusion (blood flow) to the kidneys stimulates the release of aldosterone from the adrenal glands, which promotes salt and fluid retention by the kidneys (see Renin-angiotensin-aldosterone mechanism, p xv). The blood volume increases, and the heart becomes so congested with blood that the heart muscle cannot contract efficiently, resulting in a decrease in stroke volume (the volume of blood pumped from a ventricle with each beat). The heart rate increases in an attempt to maintain cardiac output, but this decreases ventricular filling time, further reducing stroke volume. Blood pressure increases, pulse pressure narrows, and increasing hydrostatic pressure forces fluid out of the capillaries and into the tissues, causing edema. Fluid builds up in the organs, abdominal cavity, or extremities, depending on whether the heart failure is right-sided, left-sided, or both.

   b. Acute renal failure is the sudden loss of the kidneys' ability to filter and remove fluid and waste and to concentrate urine, leading to fluid and waste product retention; also known as acute renal injury.
   c. Chronic kidney disease is a gradual loss of the kidneys' ability to filter and remove fluid and waste, leading to fluid and waste product retention.

DID YOU KNOW?

The most common cause of chronic kidney disease is damage to the kidney from high blood pressure and diabetes.

   d. Nephrotic syndrome, a nonspecific disorder in which the kidneys are damaged, and acute glomerulonephritis, a disorder of the small blood vessels in the kidneys, inhibit the kidneys' ability to filter and absorb fluid from the bloodstream.
   e. Liver cirrhosis, the replacement of liver tissue by scar tissue resulting from chronic liver disease, also causes the retention of fluid and sodium, especially in the peritoneal cavity (ascites).
3. Long-term corticosteroid therapy causes water and sodium retention.
   a. Corticosteroids, also called steroids, are man-made drugs that closely resemble cortisol, a hormone naturally produced by the adrenal glands.
   b. Corticosteroids are used to decrease inflammation and reduce the activity of the immune system.

c. Commonly prescribed corticosteroids are cortisone, prednisone, and dexamethasone.
d. Side effects of long-term corticosteroid therapy include sodium and water retention and excessive potassium loss.

B. Causes of hypotonic overhydration

1. Rapid, excessive intake of salt-free solutions, such as water, results in hypotonic overhydration.
   a. Athletes are at risk for hypotonic overhydration because they may lose significant amounts of sodium through perspiration and rapidly consume water to relieve thirst.
   b. Compulsive polydipsia (excessive thirst manifested by excessive water intake) can cause overconsumption of water.
   c. Psychogenic polydipsia occurs in clients with psychiatric disorders and is characterized by water-seeking and excessive drinking; it is often accompanied by hyponatremia and water intoxication.

DID YOU KNOW?

Water intoxication can be fatal if water is ingested more quickly than the kidneys can compensate for the lack of sodium.

2. Ingestion of diluted infant formula and ingestion of excess water are common causes of hypotonic hypervolemia in infants and young children.
   a. Parents who cannot afford to buy enough baby formula or are running low may add extra water to dilute the prepared formula and make it last longer, thus giving the infant excess free water.
   b. Using a bottle of water to calm or pacify an infant can also result in the ingestion of excess water.
   c. Remember that infants and children have a greater percentage of body water than adults and are more susceptible to fluid and electrolyte imbalances.
3. Irrigation of wounds and body cavities with hypotonic solutions, such as gastric lavage or bladder irrigation, causes the blood to become diluted as water is absorbed through the gastrointestinal tract, resulting in hypotonic overhydration. Frequent plain-water enemas can have the same effect.
4. Liver failure occurs when liver cells are significantly damaged and no longer able to function; this causes fluid retention and cerebral edema.
   a. Acute liver failure occurs over a period of days and may be caused by acetaminophen overdose, hepatitis, prescription drugs, herbal supplements, metabolic disease, or cancer.
   b. Chronic liver disease develops slowly over years and is caused primarily by alcohol abuse and other conditions such as hepatitis B and C, cytomegalovirus, and malnutrition.
   c. Liver cirrhosis, the replacement of liver tissue by scar tissue, is the end result of chronic liver disease; cirrhosis also causes the retention of fluid and sodium, especially in the peritoneal cavity (ascites).
5. Syndrome of inappropriate antidiuretic hormone secretion (SIADH) is an abnormal condition characterized by the excessive release of antidiuretic hormone (ADH), which alters the body's fluid and electrolyte balances. It results in various malfunctions, such as the inability to produce and secrete dilute urine, water retention, increased ECF volume, and hyponatremia (sodium deficit).
   a. ADH causes water to be retained, but sodium is lost, resulting in concentrated urine and hyponatremia.
   b. It is important to remember that in SIADH, hyponatremia results from an excess of water, not a deficiency of sodium.

MAKING THE CONNECTION

Liver Failure

When liver failure occurs, the liver does not produce enough albumin, the body's predominant serum-binding protein. Albumin and other proteins act like sponges that hold water in the blood. When albumin levels are low, the "pushing" pressure exerted by fluid in the blood vessels (hydrostatic pressure) exceeds the "pulling" pressure that draws water into the blood vessels (oncotic pressure), causing fluid to move out of the vascular space and into the ECF. This results in the accumulation of fluid in the tissues (edema).

C. Causes of hypertonic overhydration

1. Excessive or rapid administration of hypertonic IV solutions, such as 5% dextrose in 0.9% saline solution, 5% dextrose in lactated Ringer's solution, or 3% saline solution, is a common cause of hypertonic overhydration.
2. High intake of sodium also causes the body to retain water.
   a. Using excessive table salt or eating foods that contain significant amounts of sodium increases the amount of sodium in the body, resulting in fluid retention as the body attempts to dilute the sodium concentration and return the serum sodium level to normal.
   b. Drinking seawater can also cause hypertonic overhydration and other electrolyte imbalances that can be fatal.

3. Primary hyperaldosteronism is an overproduction of the hormone aldosterone by the adrenal glands.
   a. Aldosterone causes an increase in sodium and water retention and potassium excretion in the kidneys.
   b. Aldosterone causes sodium to be exchanged for potassium in the kidneys, so an increase in aldosterone leads to increased levels of serum sodium (hypernatremia) and decreased levels of serum potassium (hypokalemia).
   c. When increased aldosterone levels are caused by a benign tumor (adenoma) on one or both adrenal glands, this is known as Conn's syndrome.
4. Cushing's syndrome is a relatively rare hormonal disorder caused by prolonged exposure of the body's tissues to high levels of the hormone cortisol.
   a. Cortisol is naturally produced by the adrenal glands to control the stress response.
   b. Increased cortisol production may be caused by surgical stress, depression, alcoholism, malnutrition, panic disorders, and glucocorticoid hormone administration.
5. Excessive sodium bicarbonate therapy can cause hypertonic overhydration.
   a. The excessive oral intake of sodium bicarbonate, often used as an antacid, causes the body to retain fluid in an attempt to dilute excess sodium.
   b. The administration of IV sodium bicarbonate to treat metabolic acidosis and to replace bicarbonate lost through severe diarrhea may also cause hypertonic overhydration.

IV. Nursing Assessment for Fluid Volume Excess

The nurse should conduct a focused nursing assessment for FVE, beginning with a thorough nursing history. Interview the client or family members to reveal any risk factors or preexisting conditions that would contribute to FVE, such as chronic health problems or recent surgery, trauma, or burns. Include a current dietary history, and inquire about recent changes in appetite and sodium intake. The nursing history should also include lifestyle factors and current medication use. A thorough physical assessment is necessary because FVE affects many body systems; assess each body system, observing for signs and symptoms of FVE (Table 1.2).Measure and record the client's vital signs. Be sure to weigh the client, because weight is the most reliable indicator of FVE. Review the client's laboratory data to assess for the presence of FVE and any associated electrolyte imbalances.

Table 1.2 Signs and Symptoms of Fluid Volume Excess

Vital Signs	
Blood pressure	Increased
Heart rate	Increased
Pulse pressure (difference between systolic and diastolic pressures)	Decreased
Respiratory rate	Increased
Temperature	Within normal limits
Weight	Sudden weight gain (!) 1 kg (2.2 lb) gained equals 1 L retained! • Mild FVE: 2% of body weight gain • Moderate FVE: 5% of body weight gain • Severe FVE: 8% of body weight gain
Signs and Symptoms by Body System	
Cardiovascular	• Hypertension • Bounding pulse volume • Narrow pulse pressure • Jugular vein distention with head of bed elevated to 45 degrees or higher • Peripheral vein distention • Capillary refill less than 3 seconds • Tight or bulging fontanelles in infants younger than 18 months • Gallop heart rhythm in adults (S_3 heart sound)
Gastrointestinal	• Ascites • Hepatomegaly (enlarged liver) • Splenomegaly (enlarged spleen)
Integumentary	• Pale, cool, taut skin • Dependent, pitting edema • Generalized edema or anasarca
Musculoskeletal	• Muscle spasms
Neurological	• Headache • Confusion • Lethargy • Seizures • Coma secondary to cerebral edema
Renal	• Polyuria: excessive passage of urine and urinary frequency (with normal kidney function) • Oliguria: less than normal urination • Anuria: failure to form urine
Respiratory	• Excess fluid in and around the lungs • Dyspnea: shortness of breath • Crackles (rales) • Paroxysmal nocturnal dyspnea: waking in the middle of the night with shortness of breath • Dry cough that eventually becomes wet and productive • Infants: intracostal and substernal retractions, nasal flaring, expiratory grunting

Continued

Table 1.2 Signs and Symptoms of Fluid Volume Excess—cont'd

Laboratory Values	
Blood urea nitrogen	Decreased
Hematocrit	Decreased
Serum osmolarity	Decreased
Urine output	Normal, decreased, or increased, depending on the etiology of FVE
Urine specific gravity	Low

V. Nursing Interventions for a Client With Fluid Volume Excess

A. Weigh the client daily
  1. Evaluate the client's weight gain over 1 to 3 days.
  2. Weigh the client at the same time each day, preferably before breakfast, with the same amount of clothing on and using the same scale.

B. Assess for peripheral edema
  1. Assess the client's extremities for edema.
     a. Check for the presence of edema before the client rises in the morning or after the client has been seated with legs elevated for a period of time.
     b. Little or no peripheral edema before rising may indicate that subsequent edema is caused by stasis (a slowing or stoppage of the normal blood flow).
     c. The presence of edema before rising may indicate generalized edema related to heart, kidney, or liver disorders.
  2. Determine whether the edema is pitting or nonpitting.
     a. Edema is nonpitting if pressure applied to the skin does not result in a persistent indentation.
     b. Edema is pitting if pressure applied with the finger for 5 seconds causes persistent indentation.
  3. Measure or grade pitting peripheral edema and record it (Fig. 1.3).

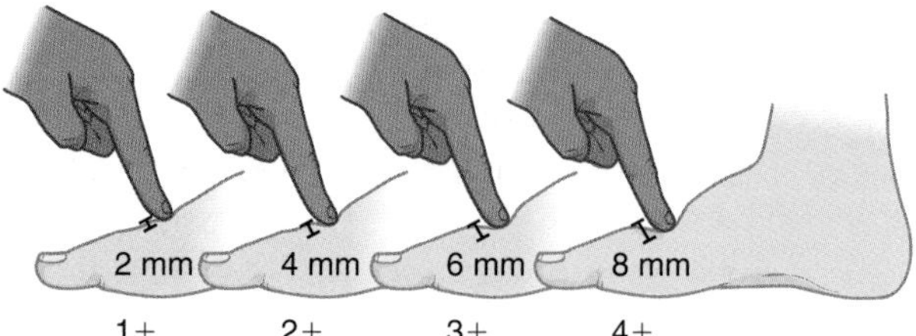

Fig 1.3 Grading of pitting edema: **1+, mild pitting**—slight indentation of 2 mm or less; no perceptible swelling of the leg. **2+, moderate pitting**—indentation greater than 2 mm and up to 4 mm; subsides rapidly. **3+, deep pitting**—indentation greater than 4 mm and up to 6 mm; remains for a short time; leg looks swollen. **4+, very deep pitting**—indentation greater than 6mm; lasts a long time, leg is very swollen.

DID YOU KNOW?

Measuring edema with a millimeter tape is more accurate than grading edema using a 1 to 4 scale.

C. Monitor the client
  1. Obtain the client's vital signs as prescribed and compare to baseline.
     a. Observe for changes in heart rate and blood pressure.
     b. Pulse oximetry values below 95% are considered "low" for a client with healthy lungs; normal baseline may be decreased in smokers and in clients with preexisting heart or lung disorders.
  2. Calculate the client's pulse pressure ("third blood pressure").
     a. The **pulse pressure** represents the force the heart generates each time it contracts and can be used as an indirect measure of cardiac output.
     b. It is calculated by using the following formula:

        Systolic blood pressure (top) – Diastolic blood pressure (bottom) = Pulse pressure

        For example, if the client has a blood pressure of 120/80 mm Hg, the pulse pressure would be 120 – 80 = 40 mm Hg.
     c. The resting pulse pressure in healthy adults, in a sitting position, is about 30 to 40 mmHg.
     d. Pulse pressure is considered low or "narrow" if it is less than 30 mm Hg, indicating a significant decrease in cardiac output.
     e. If the pulse pressure is extremely narrow, 25 mmHg or less, the cause may be a low stroke volume, indicating congestive heart failure, cardiac tamponade, or shock.
     f. Pulse pressure is considered high or "wide" if it is consistently greater than 40 mm Hg.
     g. A consistent resting pulse pressure greater than 60 mm Hg is harmful and accelerates the normal aging of the organs; it is an important risk factor for adverse cardiac events, especially in adults older than 50 years.
     h. It is normal for the pulse pressures of a healthy adult to be high (about 100 mm Hg) during or shortly after exercise.

DID YOU KNOW?

A high (wide) pulse pressure combined with bradycardia (a slow heart rate) and an irregular breathing pattern is known as the "Cushing triad." It is associated with increased intracranial pressure and is a medical emergency because it is an indication of intracranial hemorrhage or edema.

3. Monitor the client's respiratory status.
   a. Observe for signs of pulmonary edema: shortness of breath, coughing, labored breathing, rapid breathing (tachypnea), difficulty breathing when lying down (orthopnea), pale skin (pallor) or blue skin (cyanosis), and anxiety.
   b. Auscultate for abnormal heart sounds and moist crackles (rales) in the lungs; these usually begin in the bases and then move into the upper lung fields.
   c. Normal respiratory rate for an adult is 12 to 20 breaths per minute.
4. Obtain and evaluate laboratory values.
   a. Monitor for changes in hematocrit, blood urea nitrogen (BUN), serum sodium, serum potassium, and other electrolyte levels; FVE and treatments for it may cause electrolyte imbalances.
   b. Monitor arterial blood gas (ABG) or venous blood gas (VBG) values to determine oxygenation status or the presence of an acid-base imbalance (see Chapter 8, p 190).
   c. Observe for changes in level of consciousness (LOC).
   d. Be alert for signs of overcorrection (fluid volume deficit) (see Chapter 2, p 37).

D. Measure intake and output (Fig. 1.4)
   1. Measure intake.
      a. At least every 8 hours, record the type and amount of all fluids received and describe the route as oral, parenteral, rectal, or by enteric tube.
      b. Record ice chips as fluid at approximately one-half their volume.
      c. Compare the client's intake with the intake of an average adult.

DID YOU KNOW?

The average 24-hour intake value for an adult is 2,600 mL (1,300 mL oral fluids, 1,000 mL in food, 300 mL from oxidation of food). The average 24-hour output value for an adult is 2,400 to 2,700 mL (1,500 mL urine, 200 mL in stool, 400 to 600 mL through the skin, 300 to 400 mL through respiration).

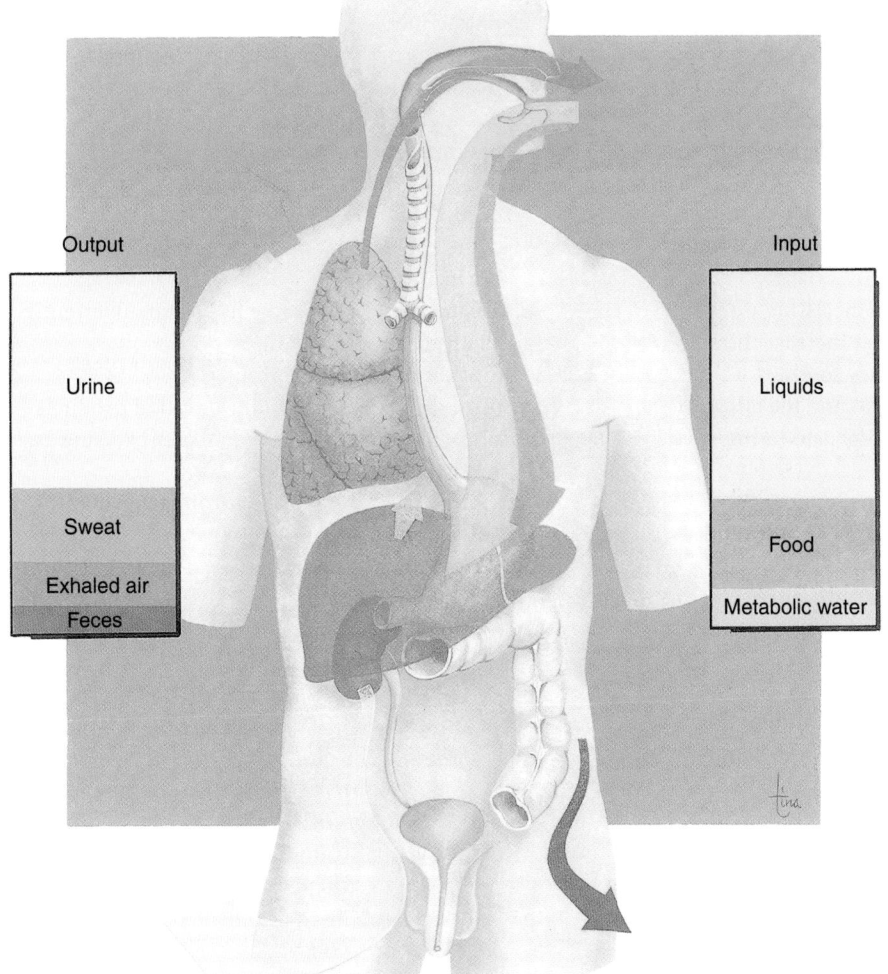

Fig 1.4 Intake and output.

2. Measure output.
   a. Record the type and amount of all fluids the client has lost, and indicate the route; describe output as urine, liquid stool, vomitus, tube drainage (including from chest, closed wound drainage, and nasogastric tubes), and any fluid aspirated from a body cavity.
   b. Measure the amount of irrigation fluid instilled; subtract it from the total output when irrigating a nasogastric or other tube or the bladder.
   c. Measure drainage in a calibrated container. Observe it at eye level, and record the reading at the bottom of the meniscus.
   d. Compare the client's output to that of an average adult; intake and output should be relatively equivalent.

E. Restrict fluids
1. Explain to the client and the family or caregivers the rationale for fluid restriction.
   a. Tell the client and family the exact amount of fluids allowed per day.
   b. Develop a plan with the client to divide the allotted fluids.
2. Determine whether the restriction includes IV fluids. Add IV fluid intake to fluids taken by mouth, nasogastric tube, or gastrostomy tube when caring for hospitalized clients.
3. Divide fluids across specific time periods, shifts, or medication administration times; do not limit fluids to meals only.
4. Use strategies to limit intake.
   a. Avoid offering liquids with meals, as food may quench thirst.
   b. Reserve liquids for between meals.
   c. Limit the intake of foods that increase thirst, including dry, salty, and spicy foods.
   d. Collaborate with the dietitian and the client to increase the client's knowledge and to improve control and compliance.
5. Offer ice chips.
   a. Record the amount of melted ice consumed.
   b. The volume of melted ice is one-half that of solid ice; therefore, a full 240-mL cup of ice equals only 120 mL of intake.

DID YOU KNOW?

It is important to provide frequent oral hygiene to fluid-restricted clients.

F. Control rates of intravenous infusions

Solutions that contain sodium should be administered with great care, if at all, in clients with congestive heart failure, severe renal insufficiency, or edema secondary to sodium retention.

1. Know the drop factor.
   a. Determine the manufacturer's drop factor for each IV administration set used; the larger the bore of the tubing, the faster the fluid flows.
   b. Drop factors range from 10 gtt/mL (largest diameter) to 60 gtt/mL (smallest diameter). Other drop factors are 12, 15, and 20 gtt/mL.
   c. When the drop factor is between 10 and 20, it is called macrodrip tubing; microdrip tubing has a drop factor of 60. You must know the drop factor of the tubing being used to calculate the drip rate.
2. Calculate the hourly rate, if it is not specified in the order. Divide the volume to be infused by the number of hours it is to be infused.

   Example: 1,000 mL ÷ 8 hours = 125 mL/hr

3. Calculate the drip rate.
   a. Multiply the volume to be infused by the drop factor (number of drops per milliliter).
   b. Divide the result by the time in minutes to obtain the drip rate.

   Example: 500 mL × 10 (drop factor) ÷ 60 minutes = 83.3 gtt/min

4. Begin the infusion, and monitor hourly.
   a. Follow the manufacturer's instructions for priming the tubing.
   b. Attach the tubing to the client's IV access site per institution policy.
   c. Regulate the speed of flow using the roller clamp; use a watch with a second hand, and count the number of drops entering the chamber in 1 minute.
   d. Ensure that the flow rate has not inadvertently changed.

G. Use intravenous infusion pumps
1. Control the flow rate of fluids or blood products administered through an IV catheter by using an IV pump.
2. Use microdrip tubing with a drop factor of 60 gtt/mL when using an IV pump.
   a. Simplify the calculations based on an infusion time of 60 minutes (1 hour), because pumps are routinely programmed in milliliters per hour rather than drops per minute.
   b. Follow the manufacturer's instructions for priming the tubing and loading the administration set into the pump.
3. Program the pump with the infusion rate and the volume to be infused.
   a. Enter the total volume of the IV bag minus 25 to 50 mL so the infusion does not "run dry."
   b. Attach the tubing to the client's IV access site per institution policy.

4. Start the infusion, and monitor hourly.
   a. Ensure that all alarms are turned on and are in working order.
   b. Ensure that the flow rate has not inadvertently changed.

The use of IV pumps DOES NOT relieve the nurse of responsibility for calculating and monitoring the flow rate.

H. Administer medications as ordered

Always double-check medication calculations.

1. Angiotensin II receptor blockers or antagonists: administered to block the vasoconstriction and aldosterone-producing effects of angiotensin II, resulting in dilation of blood vessels, reduction of blood pressure, and lessening of heart failure. The primary indication for use is hypertension.
   a. candesartan (Atacand)
   b. eprosartan (Teveten)
   c. losartan (Cozaar)
   d. valsartan (Diovan)
2. Angiotensin-converting enzyme (ACE) inhibitors: administered to block the conversion of angiotensin I to the vasoconstrictor angiotensin II, resulting in dilation of blood vessels, reduction of blood pressure, and lessening of heart failure. The primary indication for use is hypertension.
   a. captopril (Capoten)
   b. enalapril (Vasotec)
   c. fosinopril (Monopril)
   d. lisinopril (Prinivil, Zestril)
3. Cardiac glycosides: administered to increase the force of cardiac contraction by increasing the concentration of intracellular calcium; they also enhance vagal tone over the heart, increasing cardiac output and slowing the heart rate.
   a. digoxin (Lanoxin)
4. Loop diuretics: administered to inhibit sodium and chloride reabsorption from the ascending loop of Henle and distal renal tubule; they also increase the renal excretion of water, sodium, chloride, magnesium, potassium, and calcium; effectiveness persists in those with impaired renal function.
   a. bumetanide (Bumex)
   b. ethacrynic acid (Edecrin)
   c. furosemide (Lasix)
   d. torsemide (Demadex)
5. Potassium-sparing diuretics: administered to inhibit sodium reabsorption in the distal nephron and collecting duct, promoting the excretion of water and sodium.
   a. amiloride hydrochloride
   b. eplerenone (Inspra)
   c. spironolactone (Aldactone)
   d. triamterene (Dyrenium)
6. Thiazide and thiazide-like diuretics: administered to promote the excretion of sodium, chloride, potassium, and water by decreasing absorption in the distal tubule.
   a. chlorothiazide (Diuril)
   b. chlorthalidone (Hygroton)
   c. hydrochlorothiazide (HydroDIURIL, Oretic)
   d. metolazone (Zaroxolyn)

I. Assist the client in managing diet

1. Provide a sodium-restricted diet.
   a. Limit sodium intake to 500 to 2,400 mg per day for healthy adults.
   b. Americans typically consume more than 4 to 5 g of sodium daily.
2. Reduce sodium in the client's diet.
   a. Use fresh or frozen vegetables. If the client must use canned vegetables, use those labeled "no salt added."
   b. Avoid canned or processed foods.
   c. Cook without salt; use herbs, spices, and salt-free seasoning blends instead.
   d. Choose foods that are labeled "low sodium" or "reduced sodium."
   e. Rinse canned foods (tuna, beans) to remove some of the salt.
   f. Use herbs, spices, and salt-free seasoning blends in the salt shaker.

J. Educate the client

1. Teach the client or caregiver the causes of FVE.
2. Provide specific information regarding the client's medical diagnosis and related interventions and treatments.
3. Teach the client how to prevent sodium excess.
   a. Instruct the client to avoid high-sodium foods (Box 1.2).
   b. Advise the client to eat a low-sodium diet, which ranges from 400 to 2,000 mg per day.
   c. Familiarize the client with the specific definitions of reduced-sodium food products.
      1) Low sodium: less than 140 mg per serving
      2) Very low sodium: less than 35 mg per serving
      3) Salt or sodium free: less than 5 mg per serving
   d. Recommend the use of salt substitutes, if allowed by the primary health-care provider.
   e. Instruct the client and family how to read food labels, which list the amount of sodium contained in each serving and identify the presence of other sodium-containing compounds, such as the following.
      1) Monosodium glutamate (MSG)
      2) Baking soda

Box 1.2 Foods High in Sodium

Foods High in Added Sodium

Processed Meat and Fish
- Bacon
- Luncheon meat and other cold cuts
- Sausage
- Smoked fish

Selected Dairy Products
- Buttermilk
- Cheeses
- Cottage cheese
- Ice cream

Most Canned Goods
- Meats
- Soups
- Vegetables

Processed Grains
- Dry cereals (most)
- Graham crackers

Condiments and Food Additives
- Barbecue sauce
- Chili sauce
- Ketchup
- Margarine, salted
- Meat tenderizers
- Pickles
- Saccharin
- Salad dressings
- Soy sauce
- Worcestershire sauce

Snack Foods
- Gelatin desserts
- Nuts
- Popcorn, salted
- Potato chips
- Pretzels

Foods Naturally High in Sodium
- Brains
- Carrots
- Clams
- Crab
- Dried fruit
- Kidneys
- Lobster
- Oysters
- Shrimp
- Spinach

3) Baking powder
4) Disodium phosphate
5) Sodium alginate

4. Identify signs and symptoms of fluid volume excess.
   a. Instruct the client to monitor weight daily and to notify the primary health-care provider if weight increases by more than 2 lb in 3 days.
   b. Advise the client and family to notify the primary health-care provider if the client exhibits any signs or symptoms of FVE or if they have any other specific concerns.
5. Ensure that the client or caregiver understands the specifics, rationale, potential side effects, and desired effects of the treatment regimen.
   a. Include medication administration, nutrition, hydration, and dietary restrictions (foods high in sodium) in client teaching.
   b. Be aware that a client with FVE related to a chronic condition may be on long-term fluid and sodium restrictions (Box 1.2).

K. Evaluate and document
1. Document all interventions and the client's response to them, per institutional policy.
2. Evaluate and document the client's response to interventions and education.
   a. Vital signs and weight should return to baseline.
   b. Laboratory values should return to the normal reference range.
   c. Breathing should be unlabored; lungs should be clear on auscultation.
   d. Level of consciousness should return to baseline.
   e. Edema should resolve.
   f. Underlying cause of FVE should be resolved.

CASE STUDY: Putting It All Together

Subjective Data

A 68-year-old female presents to an urgent care clinic with shortness of breath and dyspnea on exertion. She reports swelling of the feet and ankles and a weight gain of 10 lb over the past week but denies pain. The patient has a history of myocardial infarction 3 years previously, a 30–pack year smoking history, and obesity. She has no known allergies, and her current medications are:

- metoprolol (Toprol-XL) 50 mg PO daily
- aspirin 81 mg PO daily

Objective Data

Nursing Assessment

1. Heart sounds S_1 and S_2 are loud and regular, with no murmur
2. No jugular vein distention noted
3. Respirations shallow and slightly labored at rest
4. Presence of moist crackles in anterior and posterior bilateral lower lobes
5. Occasional moist, nonproductive cough
6. 3+ pedal and ankle edema present bilaterally
7. Pedal and radial pulses regular, 4+, and bounding bilaterally
8. Skin of lower extremities is pale and taut bilaterally

Vital Signs	
Current weight:	256 lb (116 kg)
Temperature:	99°F (37.2°C) orally
Blood pressure:	188/96 mm Hg
Heart rate:	126 bpm, regular
Respiratory rate:	24 per minute
O_2 saturation:	88%

Laboratory Results	
Serum Na^+:	130 mEq/L
Serum K^+:	3.4 mEq/L
Blood glucose:	98 mg/dL
Serum creatinine:	1 mg/dL
Serum BUN:	18 mg/dL
Brain natriuretic peptide (BNP):	340 pg/mL

Health-Care Provider Orders

1. Administer O_2 at 6 L/min via mask until O_2 saturation (sat)is greater than 95%.
2. Administer furosemide (Lasix) 40 mg IV × 1 now.
3. Administer labetalol HCl 20 mg IV bolus over 2 minutes, then 20 mg IV bolus every 10 minutes until systolic blood pressure is less than 140 mm Hg. Do not exceed 300 mg.
4. Insert Foley catheter; monitor input and output (I & O).
5. Provide ice chips PO only; no fluids.
6. Record vital signs every 15 minutes × 1 hour, then every 30 minutes × 1 hour.
7. Reevaluate after 2 hours.

Case Study Questions

A. What *subjective* assessment findings indicate that the client is experiencing a health alteration?

1. ______________________
2. ______________________
3. ______________________
4. ______________________
5. ______________________
6. ______________________
7. ______________________

Continued

CASE STUDY: Putting It All Together *cont'd*

Case Study Questions

B. What *objective* assessment findings indicate that the client is experiencing a health alteration?

1. ___
2. ___
3. ___
4. ___
5. ___
6. ___
7. ___
8. ___
9. ___
10. ___
11. ___

C. After analyzing the data that have been collected, what **primary** nursing diagnosis should the nurse assign to this client?

___

D. What interventions should the nurse plan and/or implement to meet this client's needs?

1. ___
2. ___
3. ___
4. ___
5. ___
6. ___
7. ___
8. ___
9. ___

E. What client outcomes should the nurse use to evaluate the effectiveness of the nursing interventions?

1. ___
2. ___
3. ___
4. ___
5. ___
6. ___
7. ___

REVIEW QUESTIONS

1. A nurse preparing to assess pediatric clients on a step-down unit should know that, compared with an adult, an infant has which amount of fluid per total body weight?
   1. Less fluid per total body weight
   2. More fluid per total body weight
   3. Double the fluid per total body weight
   4. The same amount of fluid per total body weight

2. A client is diagnosed with hypernatremia secondary to primary hyperaldosteronism caused by an adrenal adenoma. A nurse, thinking critically about the client's diagnosis, knows that the primary function of aldosterone is the protection of sodium balance and the regulation of fluid balance by which mechanism?
   1. Increasing fluid excretion
   2. Suppressing the adrenal cortex
   3. Constricting the afferent arteriole
   4. Increasing sodium reabsorption from the renal tubules

3. A medical-surgical nurse attends an in-service presentation on fluid and electrolyte imbalances. The nurse should recall that the regulators of fluid balance include which substances? **Select all that apply.**
   1. Sodium
   2. Calcium
   3. Protein
   4. Albumin
   5. Adrenaline

4. A nurse administers captopril (Capoten) to a client with FVE. Which option is **decreased** by this medication?
   1. Renal blood flow
   2. Fluid overload
   3. Arterial dilation
   4. Renin production

5. Which meal option should a nurse choose for a client with FVE who is placed on a low-sodium diet?
   1. Bologna sandwich on whole wheat bread, potato chips, sliced cucumbers, and iced tea
   2. Spaghetti with meat sauce, salad, hard-crust bread, and milk
   3. Baked chicken breast, corn on the cob, dinner roll, and milk
   4. Steak, broccoli with cheese sauce, crackers, and hot tea

6. A nurse is caring for a client diagnosed with congestive heart failure secondary to FVE. Which factors, if exhibited by the client, should the nurse associate with FVE? **Select all that apply.**
   1. Increased cardiac output
   2. Decreased fluid output
   3. Decreased fluid intake
   4. Increased sodium intake
   5. Decreased sodium intake

7. An elderly client presents to a clinic complaining of fatigue, shortness of breath, and restlessness. A nurse assesses the client, suspecting FVE. Which manifestations identified during the assessment should the nurse associate with FVE? **Select all that apply.**
   1. Polyuria
   2. Weak pulse
   3. Weight gain
   4. Crackles in lungs
   5. Increased respirations

8. A pediatric nurse assesses a 1-year-old infant hospitalized for SIADH. Which finding should the nurse identify as the most reliable indicator of fluid retention in an infant?
   1. Peripheral edema
   2. Nocturnal dyspnea
   3. Sudden weight gain
   4. Increased respiratory rate

9. A client diagnosed with renal failure experiences a 2% increase in total body weight over a 48-hour period. How should a nurse classify this weight gain?
   1. No FVE
   2. Mild FVE
   3. Moderate FVE
   4. Severe FVE

10. A nurse is recording intake and output for an adult client. The client reports consuming a 600-mL soft drink out of a bottle, has received 500 mL of IV fluids, and has voided 350 mL of urine. Determine the client's intake in milliliters. Record your answer as a whole number.

    ____

11. A 185-lb male client with moderate FVE gains 5% of his total body weight over a 2-day period. How many kilograms of weight did the client gain? Record your answer using one decimal place.

    ____

12. A physician orders hydrochlorothiazide 3 mg/kg/day in two divided doses by mouth for a 46-lb child with edema secondary to congestive heart failure (CHF). How many milligrams of hydrochlorothiazide should a nurse administer to this child every 12 hours (twice daily)? Record your answer using one decimal place.

    ____

13. A physician orders hydrochlorothiazide oral solution 2 mg/kg/day in two divided doses for a 36-lb child with edema secondary to CHF. The dose on hand is 10 mg/mL. How many milliliters should a nurse administer to this child every 12 hours? Record your answer using one decimal place.

    ____

14. A physician orders spironolactone (Aldactone) 400 mg/day in two divided doses by mouth for a client diagnosed with primary hyperaldosteronism. The dose of spironolactone on hand is 50 mg/tablet. How many tablets should a nurse administer to the client every 12 hours? Record your answer as a whole number.

____

15. A nurse reviews the laboratory report of an adult client who has been taking furosemide (Lasix) for the treatment of FVE. Which serum potassium level should the nurse anticipate?
1. 2.7 mEq/L
2. 3.7 mEq/L
3. 4.5 mEq/L
4. 6.2 mEq/L

16. A nurse is counseling an obese client who is considering gastric bypass surgery. When discussing the client's risk for fluid and electrolyte imbalances, which information should the nurse provide to this client?
1. An obese person has less fluid than a lean person of the same body weight and is at increased risk for imbalances.
2. An obese person has more fluid than a lean person of the same body weight and is at increased risk for imbalances.
3. An obese person has double the fluid of a lean person of the same body weight and is at increased risk for imbalances.
4. An obese person has the same amount of fluid as a lean person of the same body weight and is at the same risk for imbalances.

17. A nurse assesses a 3-day-old infant who has had difficulty latching onto its mother's breast. Worrying that her baby is not getting enough to drink, the mother has been giving the infant water from a bottle. Other than an increased intake of water, which factor should the nurse identify as predisposing this infant to fluid imbalances?
1. Decreased cardiac output
2. Decreased kidney function
3. Decreased body surface area
4. Decreased extracellular fluid

18. A nurse is assessing the lungs of a client admitted with gastrointestinal bleeding who is receiving a second unit of blood. On auscultation, the nurse hears bilateral crackles in the lower bases. Earlier, another nurse had reported clear lung sounds in this client. Which actions should the nurse take *immediately*? **Select all that apply.**
1. Stop the transfusion
2. Slow down the transfusion
3. Continue the transfusion at the current rate
4. Notify the health-care provider
5. Administer 20 mg of IV furosemide (Lasix)

19. A nurse administers digoxin and a loop diuretic to a client diagnosed with FVE related to CHF. The nurse identifies that this client is at increased risk for digoxin toxicity based on which rationale?
1. The administration of a loop diuretic decreases the effect of digoxin.
2. The sodium-depleting effect of the loop diuretic causes the client to develop FVE.
3. The magnesium-sparing effect of the loop diuretic inhibits the excretion of digoxin.
4. The potassium-depleting effect of the loop diuretic increases the effect of digoxin.

20. A nurse administers digoxin to an older adult client diagnosed with atrial fibrillation and systolic heart failure. In addition to the atrial fibrillation, for what other reason should the nurse administer digoxin to this client?
1. To increase the heart rate
2. To decrease the potassium loss
3. To increase cardiac output
4. To decrease urinary output

21. A nurse collects data from a client who is receiving digoxin. Which manifestations reported by the client should the nurse associate with the development of digoxin toxicity?
1. Increased appetite, muscle weakness, and tinnitus
2. Decreased appetite, nausea, and muscle cramps
3. Lethargy, hemoptysis, and diarrhea
4. Euphoria, headache, and productive cough

22. A nurse is reviewing a client's laboratory data. Which laboratory result should the nurse associate with the development of FVE?
1. Increased hematocrit
2. Decreased hematocrit
3. Increased hemoglobin
4. Decreased hemoglobin

23. A nurse is preparing to transfuse 2 units of packed red blood cells to a client with a history of CHF. Which infusion rate should the nurse use for a 4-hour transfusion?
1. 50 mL/hr
2. 100 mL/hr
3. 150 mL/hr
4. 200 mL/hr

24. A nurse is caring for a client with a history of multiple chronic illnesses. Which illness should the nurse identify as placing the client at greatest risk for FVE?
1. Type 2 diabetes
2. Myocardial infarction
3. Hypertension
4. End-stage renal disease

25. A nurse evaluates a client who has received diuretic therapy for FVE. Which finding should indicate to the nurse that the therapy has been effective?
1. Decrease in body weight
2. Increase in respiratory rate
3. Decrease in urine output
4. Increase in blood pressure

26. After an initial assessment, a nurse suspects that a client has FVE related to left-sided heart failure. Which assessment finding most likely caused the nurse's suspicion?
1. Peripheral edema
2. Persistent nonproductive cough
3. Jugular venous distention
4. Hepatic enlargement

27. When teaching a client who is taking long-term corticosteroid therapy, which statement by the nurse is correct?
1. "Corticosteroids may cause you to develop FVE by weakening your immune system."
2. "Corticosteroids may cause you to develop FVE through the retention of sodium."
3. "Corticosteroids may cause you to develop FVE by increasing your appetite."
4. "Corticosteroids may cause you to develop FVE by increasing your calcium excretion."

28. A nurse is planning care for a client on fluid restriction because of FVE. Which solution should the nurse plan to use when diluting the client's medications?
1. Hypertonic solution
2. Isotonic solution
3. Smallest volume possible
4. Dextrose solution

29. A nurse is preparing to infuse 0.9% normal saline solution intravenously to an infant. To prevent FVE, what is the safest way to implement this order?
1. Calculate the gravity drip rate and assess the infusion every hour.
2. Calculate the drip rate and control the infusion using an infusion pump.
3. Calculate the drip rate and control the infusion using a 150-mL calibrated buret (Soluset or Buretrol).
4. Calculate the gravity drip rate and assess the infusion every 15 minutes.

30. When evaluating a client being treated for FVE, a nurse determines that the FVE has *not* resolved based on which finding?
1. Level of consciousness improved to alert and oriented
2. Decrease in urine specific gravity and increase in urine output
3. Bilateral lower extremity edema decreased to scant
4. Crackles increased bilaterally in anterior and posterior lung fields

31. A client who is on fluid restriction because of acute renal failure reports discomfort, thirst, and an extremely dry mouth. The client asks a nurse, "Why is it necessary to limit fluids when I already feel so dry?" Which response is most appropriate?
1. "Your heart cannot adequately pump any extra fluid at this time."
2. "Your primary health-care provider has ordered the fluid restriction; perhaps you should ask him the reason."
3. "Your kidneys are unable to filter and excrete extra fluid at this time."
4. "Your fluid intake will need to be decreased permanently, so you will need to adapt to the sensation of a dry mouth."

32. A nurse evaluating the education of a client with FVE determines that the client has an adequate understanding of the teaching based on which statement?
1. "I will notify my health-care provider if I lose more than 1 lb in a day."
2. "I will notify my health-care provider if I gain more than 2 lb in a week."
3. "I will notify my health-care provider if I gain more than 2 lb in a day."
4. "I will notify my health-care provider if my daily weight remains unchanged."

33. A nurse is developing a care plan for a client with FVE and pitting edema. Based on this information, which nursing diagnosis should be included in the care plan?
1. Risk for Imbalanced Fluid Volume
2. Risk for Impaired Skin Integrity
3. Risk for Activity Intolerance
4. Decreased Cardiac Output

34. A nurse is caring for an elderly client who is experiencing a fluid imbalance. Which age-related changes should the nurse associate with fluid imbalance in an older adult? **Select all that apply.**
1. Higher percentage of total body water than younger or middle-aged adults
2. Less efficient sodium and water regulation as renal blood flow and glomerular filtration decline
3. Decreased perception of thirst, interfering with the thirst mechanism
4. Efficient temperature regulation
5. Limited access to fluids because of physical disabilities associated with age-related illnesses

35. A physician orders a 100-mg IV bolus of furosemide (Lasix) for a client diagnosed with FVE. To administer this medication safely, which action should the nurse take?
1. Administer IV push (IVP) over 1 minute.
2. Administer IVP over 2 minutes.
3. Administer IVP over 3 minutes.
4. Administer IVP over 5 minutes.

36. A nurse is educating a client regarding a prescribed loop diuretic. Which instructions should the nurse include in the client's education? **Select all that apply.**
   1. Take a double dose if one dose is missed, to avoid edema.
   2. Change positions slowly to avoid orthostatic hypotension.
   3. Notify the health-care provider of a weight gain of more than 2 lb in 1 day.
   4. Follow a low-potassium diet.
   5. Use sunscreen and protective clothing when outdoors.

37. When evaluating a client's education regarding furosemide (Lasix), which client statement demonstrates an understanding of the potential side effects of loop diuretics?
   1. "I will stop taking this medication when I have lost more than 3 lb in a week."
   2. "I will notify my health-care provider if I urinate more frequently."
   3. "I will notify my health-care provider if I hear a persistent ringing in my ears."
   4. "I will take the last daily dose of this medication at bedtime."

38. A client's IV solution of 5% dextrose in normal saline solution with 20 mEq/L potassium chloride is infusing at 150 mL/hr as ordered. After 4 hours of infusion, the client reports shortness of breath and develops a cough. Which intervention should be the nurse's *priority*?
   1. Assess the client's lung sounds
   2. Elevate the client's legs
   3. Notify the health-care provider
   4. Continue to only monitor the client

39. A client develops moist crackles and dyspnea while receiving an IV infusion at 150 mL/hr. Based on this information, which intervention should be the nurse's *first* priority?
   1. Elevate the head of the bed to 90 degrees.
   2. Encourage the client to turn, cough, and deep-breathe.
   3. Administer oxygen via nasal cannula at 2 L/min.
   4. Stop the infusion and notify the health-care provider.

40. A medical resident writes orders for a client diagnosed with hypervolemia. Which orders should a nurse *question*? **Select all that apply.**
   1. Administer oral fluids as tolerated
   2. Auscultate lung sounds every 4 hours and as needed
   3. Weigh once per week
   4. Administer hypertonic IV fluids as ordered
   5. Administer isotonic IV fluids as ordered

41. A nurse performing a client assessment suspects the client has FVE related to right-sided heart failure. Which finding, if identified in this client, should the nurse associate with the development of right-sided heart failure?
   1. Peripheral edema
   2. Bilateral crackles in both lung fields
   3. S_4 heart sound
   4. Hypotension

42. A nurse is evaluating the education of a client with FVE. Which statement by the client indicates that additional education is needed?
   1. "I do not need to worry about my diet because I am taking furosemide (Lasix)."
   2. "I plan to avoid all cold cuts."
   3. "I will notify my health-care provider if I gain weight."
   4. "I do not need to restrict the amount of fresh vegetables in my diet."

43. A nurse observes an elderly client who is developing edema because of right-sided heart failure. Without intervention, which physiological events are likely to occur? Order each event in the correct sequence (1–7).

_______ The right side of the heart weakens and is unable to pump blood efficiently into the pulmonary blood vessels.

_______ Visible edema forms.

_______ Capillary hydrostatic pressure increases above the hydrostatic pressure in the interstitial space.

_______ As blood backs up into the venous system, venous hydrostatic pressure increases.

_______ Venous hydrostatic pressure causes capillary hydrostatic pressure to increase.

_______ Excess filtration of fluid from the capillaries into the interstitial space occurs.

_______ The volume of blood in the right side of the heart increases.

44. A registered nurse (RN) is assigned to care for the following clients. Which client could the RN most appropriately delegate to a licensed practical nurse (LPN)?
   1. An elderly client admitted with dehydration who is receiving IV fluids.
   2. A client in renal failure who is receiving emergent dialysis.
   3. A client with active gastrointestinal bleeding who is receiving a blood transfusion.
   4. A new postoperative client who has uncontrolled pain.

45. A nurse assesses the edematous extremities of a 6-month-old client. The nurse should document that the client has which grade of edema?

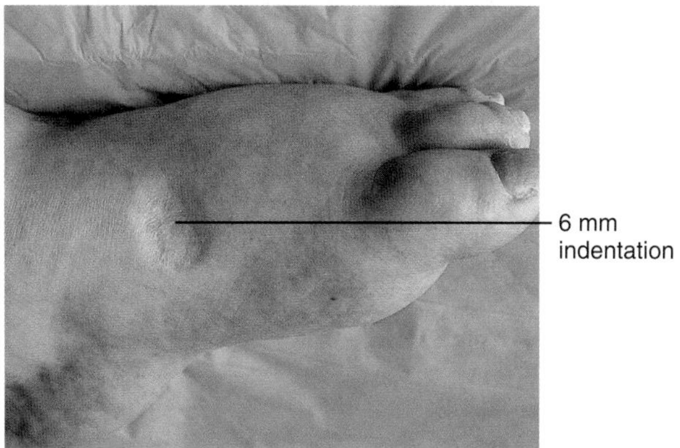

1. Grade: 1+
2. Grade: 2+
3. Grade: 3+
4. Grade: 4+

REVIEW ANSWERS

1. ANSWER: 2.

Rationale:

1. An infant has more (not less) fluid per total body weight compared with an adult.
2. An infant has more fluid per total body weight and is at greater risk for fluid and electrolyte imbalances.
3. The body of an adult is approximately 60% water, and the body of an infant is 70% to 80% water.
4. An infant has more (not the same amount of) fluid per total body weight than an adult.

TEST-TAKING TIP: Recall that clients who have a greater percentage of body fluid, such as infants and children, are at greater risk for fluid and electrolyte imbalances. Review the basics of fluid balances if you had difficulty with this question.

Content Area: Child Health
Integrated Processes: Nursing Process: Planning
Client Need: Physiological Integrity
Cognitive Level: Knowledge
Reference: *Williams, L. S., and Hopper, P. D. (2011). Understanding Medical-Surgical Nursing (4th ed.). Philadelphia, PA: F. A. Davis.*

2. ANSWER: 4.

Rationale:

1. Aldosterone decreases (not increases) fluid excretion in the kidneys.
2. Aldosterone is secreted by the adrenal cortex; it does not suppress the adrenal cortex.
3. Aldosterone acts directly on the nephron, not on either of the specific arterioles.
4. The primary function of aldosterone is the protection of sodium balance and the regulation of fluid balance by increasing sodium reabsorption from the renal tubules. Aldosterone is a hormone excreted by the adrenal cortex when the sodium level in the extracellular fluid is decreased. Aldosterone prevents water and sodium loss by triggering the nephrons of the kidney to reabsorb sodium and water from the urine back into the blood.

TEST-TAKING TIP: Review the function of aldosterone if you were unable to answer this question correctly.

Content Area: Adult Health
Integrated Processes: Nursing Process: Analysis
Client Need: Physiological Integrity
Cognitive Level: Knowledge
Reference: *Ignatavicius, D. D., and Workman, M. L. (2012). Medical-Surgical Nursing: Patient-Centered Collaborative Care (7th ed.). St. Louis, MO: Saunders.*

3. ANSWER: 1, 3, 4.

Rationale:

1. The regulators of fluid balance include sodium, protein, and albumin. Body fluids are composed of water and particles that are dissolved or suspended in the water. The processes of filtration, diffusion, and osmosis are important in controlling fluid and electrolyte balance and work together to maintain the internal environment. Solutes that help maintain fluid balance, primarily by influencing the rate of diffusion, are sodium, protein, and albumin. Sodium is the major cation in the ECF and maintains ECF osmolarity, whereas protein and albumin are larger molecules that do not readily diffuse from the ECF, also increasing osmolarity.
2. Calcium is an electrolyte that does not regulate fluid balance. Calcium plays a major role in the transmission of nerve impulses, maintenance of bone density and strength, activation of enzymes, skeletal and cardiac muscle contraction, and blood clotting.
3. The regulators of fluid balance include sodium, protein, and albumin.
4. The regulators of fluid balance include sodium, protein, and albumin.
5. Adrenaline (epinephrine) is a hormone and neurotransmitter that increases heart rate, strengthens the force of the heart's contraction, opens up airways in the lungs, and has numerous other effects. It does not regulate fluid balance.

TEST-TAKING TIP: Rule out incorrect options. Remember that calcium (option 2) and adrenaline (option 5) have no role in the regulation of fluid balance.

Content Area: Adult Health
Integrated Processes: Teaching/Learning
Client Need: Physiological Integrity
Cognitive Level: Knowledge
Reference: *Ignatavicius, D. D., and Workman, M. L. (2012). Medical-Surgical Nursing: Patient-Centered Collaborative Care (7th ed.). St. Louis, MO: Saunders.*

4. ANSWER: 2.

Rationale:

1. ACE inhibitors, such as captopril, suppress the renin-angiotensin system, which is activated in response to decreased renal blood flow; they do not *cause* a decrease in renal blood flow.
2. Captopril is an ACE inhibitor that decreases fluid overload. ACE inhibitors ultimately block aldosterone, preventing sodium and water retention, which decreases fluid overload.
3. ACE inhibitors prevent the conversion of angiotensin I to angiotensin II, resulting in arterial dilation, decreased arterial resistance, and increased stroke volume.
4. ACE inhibitors have no impact on the production of renin.

TEST-TAKING TIP: Review the pharmacodynamics of ACE inhibitors if you were unable to answer this question correctly.

Content Area: Adult Health
Integrated Processes: Nursing Process: Implementation
Client Need: Physiological Integrity
Cognitive Level: Comprehension
Reference: *Ignatavicius, D. D., and Workman, M. L. (2012). Medical-Surgical Nursing: Patient-Centered Collaborative Care (7th ed.). St. Louis, MO: Saunders.*

5. ANSWER: 3.

Rationale:

1. Bologna is a luncheon meat that is high in sodium.
2. Spaghetti with meat sauce contains sausage, which is high in sodium.
3. The meal consisting of baked chicken breast, corn on the cob, dinner roll, and milk is the only option that does not include foods either naturally or artificially high in sodium.
4. Cheese sauce is high in sodium.

TEST-TAKING TIP: Refer to Box 1.2, "Foods High in Sodium," if you were unable to answer this question correctly. It is important to become familiar with foods that are high in sodium and potassium because you will use that information frequently in practice.
Content Area: Adult Health
Integrated Processes: Nursing Process: Implementation
Client Need: Physiological Integrity
Cognitive Level: Comprehension
***Reference:** Lemone, P., and Burke, K. (2010). Medical-Surgical Nursing: Critical Thinking in Patient Care (5th ed.). Upper Saddle River, NJ: Pearson Prentice Hall.*

6. ANSWER: 2, 4.
Rationale:
1. Increased cardiac output, decreased fluid intake, and decreased sodium intake are often related to fluid volume deficit (FVD).
2. The nurse should recognize decreased fluid output and increased sodium intake as factors associated with FVE. FVE is caused by excessive fluid intake, decreased fluid output (secondary to renal failure or decreased cardiac output), and excessive sodium intake. Water follows sodium; hypernatremia (a high sodium level) causes water to be pulled into the interstitial tissues via osmosis, resulting in edema.
3. FVE may be caused by excessive fluid intake, not decreased fluid intake, in combination with a weakened cardiac muscle or renal failure.
4. The nurse should recognize decreased fluid output and increased sodium intake as factors associated with FVE, which is caused by excessive fluid intake, decreased fluid output (secondary to renal failure or decreased cardiac output), and excessive sodium intake. Water follows sodium; hypernatremia causes water to be pulled into the interstitial tissues via osmosis, resulting in edema.
5. Increased cardiac output, decreased fluid intake, and decreased sodium intake are often related to FVD, not FVE.
TEST-TAKING TIP: Use the process of elimination by ruling out options associated with FVD.
Content Area: Adult Health
Integrated Processes: Nursing Process: Implementation
Client Need: Physiological Integrity
Cognitive Level: Application
***Reference:** Wilkinson, J. M., and Van Leuven, K. (2011). Fundamentals of Nursing (2nd ed.). Philadelphia, PA: F. A. Davis.*

7. ANSWER: 3, 4, 5.
Rationale:
1. Polyuria is associated with FVD (not FVE).
2. Weak pulse is a sign of FVD, not FVE.
3. The nurse should associate weight gain with FVE. Other signs of FVE include presence of crackles in lungs on auscultation, increased respiratory rate, oliguria (not polyuria), bounding pulse (not weak pulse), increased blood pressure, and venous distention.
4. The nurse should associate crackles in lungs with FVE. Other signs of FVE include weight gain, increased respiratory rate, oliguria (not polyuria), bounding pulse (not weak pulse), increased blood pressure, and venous distention.
5. The nurse should associate increased respirations with FVE. Other signs of FVE include weight gain, presence of crackles in lungs on auscultation, oliguria (not polyuria), bounding pulse (not weak pulse), increased blood pressure, and venous distention.
TEST-TAKING TIP: Remember that "too much fluid" (FVE) usually means increased (or "too much") weight, abnormal lung sounds, and increased blood volume (bounding pulse and jugular venous distention).
Content Area: Older Adult Health
Integrated Processes: Nursing Process: Assessment
Client Need: Physiological Integrity
Cognitive Level: Application
***Reference:** Wilkinson, J. M., and Van Leuven, K. (2011). Fundamentals of Nursing (2nd ed.). Philadelphia, PA: F. A. Davis.*

8. ANSWER: 3.
Rationale:
1. Peripheral edema may be present, but for edema to become apparent, total body water must increase by at least 5%, or approximately 500 mL, for a 1-year-old child.
2. Paroxysmal nocturnal dyspnea may be a sign of fluid retention, but it is not the most reliable indicator.
3. The nurse should identify sudden weight gain as the most reliable indicator of fluid retention.
4. Increased respiratory rate is a sign of fluid retention, but it is not the most reliable indicator.
TEST-TAKING TIP: The key words are "most reliable indicator" of fluid retention.
Content Area: Child Health
Integrated Processes: Nursing Process: Assessment
Client Need: Physiological Integrity
Cognitive Level: Application
***Reference:** Ward, S. L., and Hisley, S. M. (2011). Maternal-Child Nursing Care: Optimizing Outcomes for Mothers, Children and Families. Philadelphia, PA: F. A. Davis.*

9. ANSWER: 2.
Rationale:
1. A weight gain of 2% or greater over a 48-hour period indicates FVE.
2. The nurse should classify a sudden 2% increase in total body weight as mild FVE.
3. Moderate FVE is characterized by a 5% increase in total body weight.
4. Severe FVE is characterized by an 8% increase in total body weight.
TEST-TAKING TIP: Calculate that a 2% increase in total body weight in a 100-lb client would be about 2 lb over 48 hours, suggesting mild FVE.
Content Area: Adult Health
Integrated Processes: Nursing Process: Analysis
Client Need: Physiological Integrity
Cognitive Level: Application
***Reference:** Berman, A. J., Snyder, S. J., Kozier, B., and Erb, G. (2011). Kozier and Erb's Fundamentals of Nursing: Concepts, Process, and Practice (9th ed.). Upper Saddle River, NJ: Pearson Education.*

10. **ANSWER: 1,100.**

Rationale: 600-mL oral intake + 500-mL parenteral intake = 1,100-mL total intake. The 350 mL the client voided is output, not intake.

TEST-TAKING TIP: If a client reports oral intake in ounces, recall that 1 oz equals 30 mL. Use that conversion to calculate intake and output accurately.

Content Area: Adult Health

Integrated Processes: Nursing Process: Implementation

Client Need: Physiological Integrity

Cognitive Level: Application

Reference: *Berman, A. J., Snyder, S. J., Kozier, B., and Erb, G. (2011). Kozier and Erb's Fundamentals of Nursing: Concepts, Process, and Practice (9th ed.). Upper Saddle River, NJ: Pearson Education.*

11. **ANSWER: 4.2.**

Rationale:

185 lb × 5% = 9.25 lb

9.25 lb ÷ 2.2 lb/kg = 4.2 kg

TEST-TAKING TIP: Remember that 2.2 lb = 1 kg.

Content Area: Adult Health

Integrated Processes: Nursing Process: Implementation

Client Need: Physiological Integrity

Cognitive Level: Application

Reference: *Berman, A. J., Snyder, S. J., Kozier, B., and Erb, G. (2011). Kozier and Erb's Fundamentals of Nursing: Concepts, Process, and Practice (9th ed.). Upper Saddle River, NJ: Pearson Education.*

12. **ANSWER: 31.5.**

Rationale:

46 lb ÷ 2.2 lb/kg = 21 kg

3 mg × 21 kg = 63 mg/day

63 mg ÷ 2 doses = 31.5 mg every 12 hours

TEST-TAKING TIP: Key words are "every 12 hours." Be sure to divide the total daily dosage by 2.

Content Area: Child Health

Integrated Processes: Nursing Process: Implementation

Client Need: Physiological Integrity

Cognitive Level: Application

Reference: *Deglin, J. H., Vallerand, A. H., and Sanoski, C. A.(2011). Davis's Drug Guide for Nurses (12th ed.). Philadelphia, PA: F. A. Davis.*

13. **ANSWER: 1.6.**

Rationale:

36 lb ÷ 2.2 lb/kg = 16.36 kg

2 mg × 16.36 kg = 32.73 mg/day

32.73 mg ÷ 2 doses = 16.36 mg every 12 hours

10 mg/1 mL = 16.36/X mL (cross-multiply) = (10X = 16.36) = 16.36/10 = 1.6 mL every 12 hours

TEST-TAKING TIP: If rounding is necessary, do so at the end of the calculation.

Content Area: Child Health

Integrated Processes: Nursing Process: Implementation

Client Need: Physiological Integrity

Cognitive Level: Application

Reference: *Deglin, J. H., Vallerand, A. H., and Sanoski, C. A.(2011). Davis's Drug Guide for Nurses (12th ed.). Philadelphia, PA: F. A. Davis.*

14. **ANSWER: 4.**

Rationale:

400 mg ÷ 50 mg/tablet = 8 tablets/day

8 tablets ÷ 2 doses = 4 tablets every 12 hours (twice daily)

TEST-TAKING TIP: Calculate the total number of tablets daily and divide by 2. Key words are "two divided doses" and "every 12 hours."

Content Area: Adult Health

Integrated Processes: Nursing Process: Implementation

Client Need: Physiological Integrity

Cognitive Level: Application

Reference: *Deglin, J. H., Vallerand, A. H., and Sanoski, C. A.(2011). Davis's Drug Guide for Nurses (12th ed.). Philadelphia, PA: F. A. Davis.*

15. **ANSWER: 1.**

Rationale:

1. **The nurse should anticipate a serum potassium level of 2.7 mEq/L (hypokalemia) because furosemide is a non–potassium-sparing loop diuretic.**
2. Serum potassium levels of 3.7 mEq/L and 4.5 mEq/L are within the normal reference range and would be expected only if the client were also taking a potassium supplement.
3. Serum potassium levels of 3.7 mEq/L and 4.5 mEq/L are within the normal reference range and would be expected only if the client were also taking a potassium supplement.
4. A serum potassium level of 6.2 mEq/L would not be expected in a client taking a potassium-depleting diuretic.

TEST-TAKING TIP: Recall that the normal serum potassium level in an adult client is between 3.5 and 5 mEq/L. Knowledge of normal adult serum potassium levels is tested on the NCLEX® examination.

Content Area: Adult Health

Integrated Processes: Nursing Process: Analysis

Client Need: Physiological Integrity

Cognitive Level: Application

Reference: *Van Leeuwen, A. M., Poelhuis-Leth, D. J., and Bladh, M. L.(2011). Davis's Comprehensive Handbook of Laboratory and Diagnostic Tests With Nursing Implications (4th ed.). Philadelphia, PA: F. A. Davis.*

16. **ANSWER: 1.**

Rationale:

1. **The nurse should teach the client that a person who is obese has *less* total fluid than a lean person of the same body weight because fat cells contain almost no water. This places an obese client at increased risk for fluid and electrolyte imbalances compared with a lean client. A client's age and gender also affect the amount and distribution of body fluids.**
2. An obese person has *less* fluid than a lean person of the same body weight but is at increased risk for fluid imbalances.
3. An obese person does not have double the fluid of a lean person of the same body weight but is at increased risk for fluid imbalances.
4. An obese person does not have the same amount of fluid as a lean person of the same body weight and is at increased risk for fluid imbalances.

TEST-TAKING TIP: Recall that older adults, infants, children, and obese clients are at risk for fluid and electrolyte imbalances.

Content Area: Adult Health
Integrated Processes: Teaching/Learning
Client Need: Physiological Integrity
Cognitive Level: Application
***Reference:** Ignatavicius, D. D., and Workman, M. L. (2012). Medical-Surgical Nursing: Patient-Centered Collaborative Care (7th ed.). St. Louis, MO: Saunders.*

17. ANSWER: 2.
Rationale:
1. An infant has a proportionally greater body surface area, an increased amount of extracellular fluid, and a higher cardiac output per kilogram of body weight.
2. The nurse should identify that the infant is predisposed to fluid and electrolyte imbalances because of decreased kidney function. An infant's kidneys are functionally immature at birth and excrete waste inefficiently. Immature kidneys are also unable to concentrate or dilute urine efficiently, conserve or excrete sodium, and acidify urine. An infant is less able to handle large quantities of solute-free water than an older child and is more likely to become dehydrated when given concentrated formulas or overhydrated when given excessive water or dilute formula.
3. An infant has a proportionally greater body surface area, an increased amount of extracellular fluid, and a higher cardiac output per kilogram of body weight.
4. An infant has a proportionally greater body surface area, an increased amount of extracellular fluid, and a higher cardiac output per kilogram of body weight.
TEST-TAKING TIP: Recall that young clients with immature kidneys and elderly clients with decreased kidney function are at greater risk for fluid and electrolyte imbalances.
Content Area: Child Health
Integrated Processes: Nursing Process: Assessment
Client Need: Physiological Integrity
Cognitive Level: Application
***Reference:** Ward, S. L., and Hisley, S. M. (2011). Maternal-Child Nursing Care: Optimizing Outcomes for Mothers, Children and Families. Philadelphia, PA: F. A. Davis.*

18. ANSWER: 2, 4.
Rationale:
1. The nurse should not stop the transfusion because there are no signs of a transfusion reaction.
2. The nurse should immediately slow the transfusion and notify the health-care provider because the development of bilateral lung crackles is a sign of fluid overload.
3. Continuing the transfusion would increase FVE in the client.
4. The nurse should immediately slow the transfusion and notify the health-care provider because the development of bilateral lung crackles is a sign of fluid overload.
5. The administration of furosemide requires a health-care provider's order and should not be performed without first notifying the health-care provider of the situation.
TEST-TAKING TIP: The key word is "immediately." Select the actions the nurse should take first.
Content Area: Adult Health
Integrated Processes: Nursing Process: Implementation
Client Need: Physiological Integrity
Cognitive Level: Application
***Reference:** Ignatavicius, D. D., and Workman, M. L. (2012). Medical-Surgical Nursing: Patient-Centered Collaborative Care (7th ed.). St. Louis, MO: Saunders.*

19. ANSWER: 4.
Rationale:
1. Loop diuretics increase (not decrease) the effects of digoxin.
2. Sodium levels are not significantly affected by loop diuretics and do not increase the client's risk for digoxin toxicity.
3. Magnesium levels are not significantly affected by loop diuretics and do not increase the client's risk for digoxin toxicity.
4. The nurse should determine that a client taking a loop diuretic is at increased risk for digoxin toxicity because of the potassium-depleting effects of the diuretic. Hypokalemia increases the sensitivity of cardiac muscle to digoxin and may result in digoxin toxicity even when the digoxin level is in the therapeutic range. Digoxin toxicity may cause cardiac dysrhythmias, most commonly premature ventricular contractions.
TEST-TAKING TIP: Associate the use of any loop diuretic with potential potassium imbalances, usually hypokalemia.
Content Area: Adult Health
Integrated Processes: Nursing Process: Implementation
Client Need: Physiological Integrity
Cognitive Level: Application
***Reference:** Deglin, J. H., Vallerand, A. H., and Sanoski, C. A.(2011). Davis's Drug Guide for Nurses (12th ed.). Philadelphia, PA: F. A. Davis.*

20. ANSWER: 3.
Rationale:
1. Digoxin does not increase the heart rate.
2. Digoxin does not decrease potassium loss.
3. The nurse should administer digoxin not only to treat atrial fibrillation but also to treat heart failure by increasing the cardiac output. An increase in cardiac output promotes diuresis, reducing FVE. The therapeutic effects of digoxin include increased cardiac output (positive inotropic effect) and slowing of the heart rate (negative chronotropic effect).
4. Digoxin does not decrease urinary output.
TEST-TAKING TIP: Be familiar with the actions of digoxin, a commonly prescribed medication.
Content Area: Older Adult Health
Integrated Processes: Nursing Process: Implementation
Client Need: Physiological Integrity
Cognitive Level: Application
***Reference:** Deglin, J. H., Vallerand, A. H., and Sanoski, C. A.(2011). Davis's Drug Guide for Nurses (12th ed.). Philadelphia, PA: F. A. Davis.*

21. ANSWER: 2.
Rationale:
1. Increased appetite, muscle weakness, and tinnitus are not manifestations of digoxin toxicity.
2. The nurse should recognize decreased appetite, nausea, vomiting, muscle cramps, paresthesias, and confusion as manifestations of digoxin toxicity.
3. Lethargy, hemoptysis, and diarrhea are not manifestations of digoxin toxicity.
4. Euphoria, headache, and productive cough are not manifestations of digoxin toxicity.

TEST-TAKING TIP: Key words are "digoxin toxicity." Options 1, 3, and 4 can be ruled out because they are not signs of digoxin toxicity.
Content Area: Adult Health
Integrated Processes: Nursing Process: Assessment
Client Need: Physiological Integrity
Cognitive Level: Application
Reference: *Deglin, J. H., Vallerand, A. H., and Sanoski, C. A.(2011). Davis's Drug Guide for Nurses (12th ed.). Philadelphia, PA: F. A. Davis.*

22. ANSWER: 2.
Rationale:
1. Hematocrit does not increase with the development of FVE.
2. The nurse should recognize that a decreased hematocrit is associated with the development of FVE. FVE involves excessive retention of sodium and water in the extracellular fluid. The increase in fluid volume results in hemodilution and causes BUN, hematocrit, and urine specific gravity to decrease.
3. Hemoglobin (the oxygen-carrying protein in red blood cells) is not affected by FVE.
4. Hemoglobin is not affected by FVE, although a decreased hemoglobin can worsen the client's oxygenation status if FVE occurs simultaneously.
TEST-TAKING TIP: Know the difference between hemoglobin and hematocrit, and determine which factor may be affected by hemodilution.
Content Area: Adult Health
Integrated Processes: Nursing Process: Implementation
Client Need: Physiological Integrity
Cognitive Level: Application
Reference: *Wilkinson, J. M., and Van Leuven, K. (2011). Fundamentals of Nursing (2nd ed.).Philadelphia, PA: F. A. Davis.*

23. ANSWER: 2.
Rationale:
1. An infusion rate of 50 mL/hr would not deliver the units within the 4-hour time limit.
2. The nurse should use an infusion rate of 100 mL/hr when administering packed red blood cells to a client diagnosed with CHF. Circulatory overload can occur when a blood product is infused too quickly. Older adults are at the greatest risk for this complication.
3. An infusion rate of 150 mL/hr is not recommended for this client because it is too rapid and increases the client's risk of FVE.
4. An infusion rate of 200 mL/hr is not recommended for this client because it is too rapid and increases the client's risk of FVE.
TEST-TAKING TIP: Review the administration of blood products if you were unable to answer this question correctly.
Content Area: Adult Health
Integrated Processes: Nursing Process: Planning
Client Need: Physiological Integrity
Cognitive Level: Application
Reference: *Ignatavicius, D. D., and Workman, M. L. (2012). Medical-Surgical Nursing: Patient-Centered Collaborative Care (7th ed.). St. Louis, MO: Saunders.*

24. ANSWER: 4.
Rationale:
1. Although type 2 diabetes increases the client's risk for renal failure, it does not place the client at greatest risk for FVE.
2. Although myocardial infarction may increase the client's risk for renal failure, it does not place the client at greatest risk for FVE.
3. Hypertension increases the client's risk for renal failure; however, hypertension alone does not place the client at greatest risk for FVE.
4. The nurse should identify end-stage renal disease as placing this client at greatest risk for FVE. FVE is a sign that fluid intake or retention is greater than the body's fluid needs. The conditions most commonly associated with FVE are those related to excessive intake or inadequate excretion of fluid. They include excessive fluid replacement, renal failure, heart failure, long-term corticosteroid therapy, SIADH, psychiatric disorders involving polydipsia, and water intoxication.
TEST-TAKING TIP: Select the condition that would definitely prevent the client from eliminating excess fluid.
Content Area: Adult Health
Integrated Processes: Nursing Process: Implementation
Client Need: Physiological Integrity
Cognitive Level: Application
Reference: *Ignatavicius, D. D., and Workman, M. L. (2012). Medical-Surgical Nursing: Patient-Centered Collaborative Care (7th ed.). St. Louis, MO: Saunders.*

25. ANSWER: 1.
Rationale:
1. A decrease in body weight should indicate to the nurse that therapy for FVE has been effective. A decrease in body weight corresponds to a decrease in excess fluid, which is the goal of diuretic therapy.
2. An increase in respiratory rate is a sign of FVE.
3. A decrease in urine output is a potential cause or sign of FVE.
4. An increase in blood pressure is a sign of FVE.
TEST-TAKING TIP: Use the process of elimination. Rule out options 2, 3, and 4 because these are signs of FVE.
Content Area: Adult Health
Integrated Processes: Nursing Process: Evaluation
Client Need: Physiological Integrity
Cognitive Level: Application
Reference: *Ignatavicius, D. D., and Workman, M. L. (2012). Medical-Surgical Nursing: Patient-Centered Collaborative Care (7th ed.). St. Louis, MO: Saunders.*

26. ANSWER: 2.
Rationale:
1. Peripheral edema, jugular venous distention, and hepatic enlargement are signs of right-sided (not left-sided) heart failure, which may be caused by left ventricular failure, right ventricular myocardial infarction, or pulmonary hypertension. In this type of heart failure, the right ventricle cannot empty completely, which causes increased volume and pressure in the venous system and results in jugular venous distention, hepatic enlargement, and peripheral edema.

2. The nurse should suspect FVE related to left-sided heart failure if the client develops a persistent nonproductive cough. In left-sided heart failure, as the amount of blood ejected from the left ventricle diminishes, hydrostatic pressure builds in the pulmonary venous system and results in fluid-filled alveoli and pulmonary congestion. Cough is often an early manifestation of heart failure. A client in early heart failure describes the cough as irritating, frequently nocturnal, and usually nonproductive.
3. Jugular venous distention is a manifestation of right-sided (not left-sided) heart failure.
4. Hepatic enlargement is associated with the development of right-sided (not left-sided) heart failure.
TEST-TAKING TIP: Review the signs of left-sided and right-sided heart failure if you were unable to answer this question correctly. Realize that clients may manifest all these signs if they are experiencing both right-sided and left-sided heart failure.
Content Area: Adult Health
Integrated Processes: Nursing Process: Assessment
Client Need: Physiological Integrity
Cognitive Level: Application
Reference: *Ignatavicius, D. D., and Workman, M. L. (2012). Medical-Surgical Nursing: Patient-Centered Collaborative Care (7th ed.). St. Louis, MO: Saunders.*

27. ANSWER: 2.
Rationale:
1. Weakening of the immune system is a side effect of corticosteroid therapy but does not cause FVE.
2. The nurse should ensure that the client understands that corticosteroids contribute to the development of FVE because they cause sodium retention, which results in body water retention. Where sodium goes, water follows.
3. Increased appetite is a side effect of corticosteroid therapy but does not cause FVE.
4. An increase in calcium secretion is a side effect of corticosteroid therapy but does not cause FVE.
TEST-TAKING TIP: Consider each option carefully. Select the option most likely to cause FVE.
Content Area: Adult Health
Integrated Processes: Nursing Process: Analysis
Client Need: Physiological Integrity
Cognitive Level: Application
Reference: *Deglin, J. H., Vallerand, A. H., and Sanoski, C. A.(2011). Davis's Drug Guide for Nurses (12th ed.). Philadelphia, PA: F. A. Davis.*

28. ANSWER: 3.
Rationale:
1. A hypertonic solution may exacerbate the client's FVE because it could increase vascular volume as the body attempts to dilute the solution.
2. An isotonic solution may be appropriate for dilution of the client's IV medications, but it is not the best answer.
3. When fluid restriction is required, the nurse should ensure that IV medications are diluted in the smallest volume possible and delivered using a syringe pump or manual IV push. For example, 1 gm of antibiotic could be diluted in 10 mL of normal saline solution instead of the more common 50 mL.
4. A dextrose solution, depending on its tonicity and volume, may be appropriate for dilution of the client's IV medications, but it is not the best answer.
TEST-TAKING TIP: Recall that the administration of IV fluids increases FVE. Choose the option that increases the volume administered the least.
Content Area: Adult Health
Integrated Processes: Nursing Process: Planning
Client Need: Physiological Integrity
Cognitive Level: Application
Reference: *Ignatavicius, D. D., and Workman, M. L. (2012). Medical-Surgical Nursing: Patient-Centered Collaborative Care (7th ed.). St. Louis, MO: Saunders.*

29. ANSWER: 2.
Rationale:
1. Calculating the gravity drip rate and assessing the infusion every hour is not the safest way to infuse the IV solution and could potentially cause great harm to the infant if the IV infusion is not monitored and controlled much more precisely.
2. The safest way to administer an IV solution to an infant is to calculate the drip rate and control the infusion with an infusion pump. An infusion pump should always be used for infants receiving IV therapy; it infuses fluids accurately and provides the prescribed amount of solution, minimizing the possibility of overloading the infant's circulation.
3. Calculating the drip rate and controlling the infusion using a 150-mL calibrated buret is not the safest way to infuse the IV solution.
4. Calculating the gravity drip rate and assessing the infusion every 15 minutes is not the safest way to infuse the IV solution.
TEST-TAKING TIP: Clients with a higher percentage of body fluid are at greater risk for fluid and electrolyte imbalances. Great care should always be taken when administering IV fluids to infants and children. Choose the option that provides the strictest control of the IV solution.
Content Area: Child Health
Integrated Processes: Nursing Process: Planning
Client Need: Physiological Integrity
Cognitive Level: Application
Reference: *Perry, S. E., Hockenberry, M. J., Lowdermilk, D. L., and Wilson, D. (2010). Maternal Child Nursing Care (4th ed.). St. Louis, MO: Mosby.*

30. ANSWER: 4.
Rationale:
1. Return to a normal level of consciousness reflects resolution of FVE.
2. A decrease in urine specific gravity and increase in urine output indicate resolution of FVD, *not* FVE.
3. Reduction to scant peripheral edema indicates resolution of FVE.
4. The nurse should determine that the presence of bilateral crackles indicates that FVE has not resolved. The client's lungs should be clear bilaterally after the excess fluid has been removed or excreted.

TEST-TAKING TIP: Consider each option carefully. Note that the question is asking which sign indicates that the problem is *not* resolved, so choose the option that denotes continued FVE.
Content Area: Adult Health
Integrated Processes: Nursing Process: Evaluation
Client Need: Physiological Integrity
Cognitive Level: Application
Reference: *Ignatavicius, D. D., and Workman, M. L. (2012). Medical-Surgical Nursing: Patient-Centered Collaborative Care (7th ed.). St. Louis, MO: Saunders.*

31. ANSWER: 3.
Rationale:
1. Acute renal failure does not cause the heart to pump extra circulatory volume inadequately.
2. Deferring the question to the primary health-care provider is usually not the best option because it leaves the client worried and potentially confused.
3. The statement "Your kidneys are unable to filter and excrete extra fluid at this time" is the most appropriate response because a diagnosis of acute renal failure means that the kidneys are unable to rid the body of extra fluid adequately.
4. The nurse is incorrect in stating that fluid restriction will be permanent because a client in acute renal failure may recover adequate function.
TEST-TAKING TIP: Key words are "acute renal failure." Select the option that relates to kidney function.
Content Area: Adult Health
Integrated Processes: Communication and Documentation
Client Need: Physiological Integrity
Cognitive Level: Application
Reference: *Wilkinson, J. M., and Van Leuven, K. (2011). Fundamentals of Nursing (2nd ed.).Philadelphia, PA: F. A. Davis.*

32. ANSWER: 3.
Rationale:
1. Weight loss is a desired effect and would not need to be reported to the health-care provider.
2. A weight gain of more than 2 lb in 1 week is not significant and would not need to be reported to the health-care provider.
3. The nurse determines that the client's understanding is adequate when the client states, "I will notify my health-care provider if I gain more than 2 lb in a day." Daily weight is one of the most important gauges of fluid balance. Acute weight gain or loss represents fluid gain or loss. Weight gain of 1 kg (2.2 lb) is equivalent to fluid gain of 1 L.
4. An unchanged weight is not significant and would not need to be reported to the health-care provider.
TEST-TAKING TIP: A gain of 2% of total body weight indicates mild FVE. For a 100-lb client, this would be a weight gain of 2 lb.
Content Area: Adult Health
Integrated Processes: Nursing Process: Evaluation
Client Need: Physiological Integrity
Cognitive Level: Application
Reference: *Lemone, P., and Burke, K. (2010). Medical-Surgical Nursing: Critical Thinking in Patient Care (5th ed.). Upper Saddle River, NJ: Pearson Prentice Hall.*

33. ANSWER: 2.
Rationale:
1. Because the client is already experiencing a fluid volume imbalance, a nursing diagnosis of Risk for Imbalanced Fluid Volume is inappropriate at this time.
2. The nurse should include the nursing diagnosis Risk for Impaired Skin Integrity in the client's care plan. Tissue edema decreases oxygen and nutrient delivery to the skin and subcutaneous tissue.
3. The nursing diagnosis Risk for Activity Intolerance is related to concurrent electrolyte imbalances, not to FVE and pitting edema.
4. The nursing diagnosis Decreased Cardiac Output is related to concurrent electrolyte imbalances, not to FVE and pitting edema.
TEST-TAKING TIP: Key terms are "FVE" and "pitting edema," which should lead to the nursing diagnosis of Risk for Impaired Skin Integrity.
Content Area: Adult Health
Integrated Processes: Nursing Process: Planning
Client Need: Physiological Integrity
Cognitive Level: Application
Reference: *Lemone, P., and Burke, K. (2010). Medical-Surgical Nursing: Critical Thinking in Patient Care (5th ed.). Upper Saddle River, NJ: Pearson Prentice Hall.*

34. ANSWER: 2, 3, 5.
Rationale:
1. Older adults have a lower (not higher) percentage of total body water than younger adults, increasing the risk for fluid imbalance.
2. The nurse should associate less efficient sodium and water regulation with fluid imbalance in an older adult client.
3. The nurse should associate decreased perception of thirst with fluid imbalance in an older adult client.
4. Older adults have less efficient (not more efficient) temperature regulation than younger adults, increasing the risk for fluid imbalance.
5. The nurse should associate limited access to fluids because of physical disabilities with fluid imbalance in an older adult client.
TEST-TAKING TIP: Recall that older adults experience a "slowing down" or "decrease" in functioning and have less body water than younger adults or children.
Content Area: Older Adult Health
Integrated Processes: Nursing Process: Implementation
Client Need: Physiological Integrity
Cognitive Level: Application
Reference: *Lemone, P., and Burke, K. (2010). Medical-Surgical Nursing: Critical Thinking in Patient Care (5th ed.). Upper Saddle River, NJ: Pearson Prentice Hall.*

35. ANSWER: 4.
Rationale:
1. Administering the dose over 1 minute is too rapid and increases the risk of ototoxicity.
2. Administering the dose over 2 minutes is too rapid and increases the risk of ototoxicity.
3. Administering the dose over 3 minutes is too rapid and increases the risk of ototoxicity.

4. The nurse should administer the furosemide IVP over 5 minutes, which is a safe rate. Hearing loss is most common after rapid or high-dose IV administration of furosemide in clients with decreased renal function or clients taking other ototoxic drugs. A more rapid administration does not increase the effectiveness of the drug.

TEST-TAKING TIP: Key words are "to administer this medication safely." Review guidelines for the administration of furosemide if you were unable to answer this question correctly.

Content Area: Adult Health
Integrated Processes: Nursing Process: Implementation
Client Need: Physiological Integrity
Cognitive Level: Application
***Reference:** Deglin, J. H., Vallerand, A. H., and Sanoski, C. A.(2011). Davis's Drug Guide for Nurses (12th ed.). Philadelphia, PA: F. A. Davis.*

36. ANSWER: 2, 3, 5.

Rationale:

1. The client should be instructed to take missed doses as soon as possible but never to take a double dose.
2. The nurse should instruct the client to change positions slowly to minimize orthostatic hypotension.
3. The nurse should instruct the client to notify a health-care professional of weight gain greater than 2 lb in 1 day or 3 lb in 1 week because rapid weight gain is the best indication of fluid retention and FVE.
4. The nurse should instruct the client to consult a health-care professional regarding a diet that is high (not low) in potassium, because loop diuretics can cause hypokalemia.
5. The nurse should instruct the client to use sunscreen and protective clothing to prevent photosensitivity reactions.

TEST-TAKING TIP: Review guidelines for the administration of loop diuretics. Associate loop diuretics with "less fluid" and "less potassium," and include those concepts when caring for clients prescribed this type of medication.

Content Area: Adult Health
Integrated Processes: Teaching/Learning
Client Need: Physiological Integrity
Cognitive Level: Application
***Reference:** Deglin, J. H., Vallerand, A. H., and Sanoski, C. A.(2011). Davis's Drug Guide for Nurses (12th ed.). Philadelphia, PA: F .A. Davis.*

37. ANSWER: 3.

Rationale:

1. The statement "I will stop taking this medication when I have lost more than 3 lb in a week" demonstrates an inadequate understanding of the indications for the medication's use, and this would have to be corrected.
2. The statement "I will notify my health-care provider if I urinate more frequently" is incorrect because an increase in urination is an expected effect of the diuretic.
3. The nurse should determine that the client understands the potential side effects of loop diuretics when he or she states, "I will report persistent ringing in the ears (tinnitus)." Audiometry is recommended for clients receiving prolonged high-dose IV therapy.
4. The statement "I will take the last daily dose of this medication at bedtime" is incorrect. Clients who take a diuretic more than once a day are advised to take the last dose at the evening meal to avoid nocturnal diuresis.

TEST-TAKING TIP: Review the side effects of loop diuretics if you were unable to answer this question correctly.

Content Area: Adult Health
Integrated Processes: Nursing Process: Evaluation
Client Need: Physiological Integrity
Cognitive Level: Analysis
***Reference:** Deglin, J. H., Vallerand, A. H., and Sanoski, C. A.(2011). Davis's Drug Guide for Nurses (12th ed.). Philadelphia, PA: F. A. Davis.*

38. ANSWER: 1.

Rationale:

1. The nurse's priority should be to assess the client's lung sounds. Assessment of vital signs, heart sounds, lung sounds, and volume of peripheral pulses is critical when monitoring for FVE. Gas exchange may be impaired by edema of pulmonary interstitial tissues. Acute pulmonary edema is a serious and potentially life-threatening complication of pulmonary congestion. Auscultation of the lungs to check for the presence or worsening of crackles and wheezes should be done routinely and with any change in the client's status.
2. Elevating the client's legs could worsen his or her respiratory status because vascular volume is increased by gravity.
3. The health-care provider should be notified after the assessment.
4. Continuing to only monitor the client may result in the development of major complications as the FVE increases.

TEST-TAKING TIP: Follow the nursing process: Assess *first*, then implement.

Content Area: Adult Health
Integrated Processes: Nursing Process: Implementation
Client Need: Physiological Integrity
Cognitive Level: Analysis
***Reference:** Lemone, P., and Burke, K. (2010). Medical-Surgical Nursing: Critical Thinking in Patient Care (5th ed.). Upper Saddle River, NJ: Pearson Prentice Hall.*

39. ANSWER: 4.

Rationale:

1. The client should be placed in a semi-Fowler's position to ease respiratory effort.
2. "Turn, cough, and deep-breathe" is an intervention used to prevent and treat atelectasis. That would not improve this client's respiratory status because moist crackles and dyspnea are classic signs of fluid overload, not atelectasis.
3. Although it is appropriate to administer oxygen via nasal cannula, this should not be the nurse's first priority.
4. The nurse's *first* priority in this situation is to stop the infusion and notify the health-care provider. Moist crackles and dyspnea are classic signs of fluid overload. IV fluids should be stopped to prevent further FVE, and the health-care provider should be notified.

TEST-TAKING TIP: When a client experiences a complication during an IV infusion, *the nurse's first action should be to stop the infusion.*

Content Area: Adult Health
Integrated Processes: Nursing Process: Implementation
Client Need: Physiological Integrity
Cognitive Level: Analysis
***Reference:** Ignatavicius, D. D., and Workman, M. L. (2012). Medical-Surgical Nursing: Patient-Centered Collaborative Care (7th ed.). St. Louis, MO: Saunders.*

40. ANSWER: 1, 3, 4, 5.
Rationale:
1. The nurse should question the order to administer oral fluids as tolerated. Cautious administration of oral fluids is advised while adhering to any prescribed fluid restriction.
2. Auscultation of the lungs for the presence or worsening of crackles and wheezes should be performed on an ongoing basis and is an appropriate order for a client diagnosed with hypervolemia.
3. The nurse should question the order to weigh the client once per week. Recording daily (not weekly) weights is recommended because this is one of the most important gauges of fluid balance.
4. The nurse should question the order to administer hypertonic IV fluids. IV fluids would not normally be administered to a client with hypervolemia.
5. The nurse should question the order to administer isotonic IV fluids. IV fluids would not normally be administered to a client with hypervolemia.
TEST-TAKING TIP: Recall that the administration of oral or IV fluids increases FVE.
Content Area: Adult Health
Integrated Processes: Nursing Process: Analysis
Client Need: Physiological Integrity
Cognitive Level: Analysis
Reference: *Lemone, P., and Burke, K. (2010). Medical-Surgical Nursing: Critical Thinking in Patient Care (5th ed.). Upper Saddle River, NJ: Pearson Prentice Hall.*

41. ANSWER: 1.
Rationale:
1. The nurse should associate peripheral edema with the development of right-sided heart failure. Edema develops with changes in normal hydrostatic pressure that occur in right-sided heart failure. Right-sided heart failure may be caused by left ventricular failure, right ventricular myocardial infarction, or pulmonary hypertension. In this type of heart failure, the right ventricle cannot empty completely, which causes increased volume and pressure in the venous system and results in jugular venous distention, hepatic enlargement, and peripheral edema.
2. Bilateral crackles in both lung fields are a sign of left-sided heart failure.
3. An S_4 heart sound is a sign of left-sided heart failure.
4. Hypotension is more often a sign of FVD, not of right-sided or left-sided heart failure. Heart failure is associated with the development of FVE, not FVD.
TEST-TAKING TIP: Review the signs of left-sided and right-sided heart failure if you were unable to answer this question correctly.
Content Area: Adult Health
Integrated Processes: Nursing Process: Assessment
Client Need: Physiological Integrity
Cognitive Level: Analysis
Reference: *Ignatavicius, D. D., and Workman, M. L. (2012). Medical-Surgical Nursing: Patient-Centered Collaborative Care (7th ed.). St. Louis, MO: Saunders.*

42. ANSWER: 1.
Rationale:
1. The statement "I do not need to worry about my diet because I am taking furosemide (Lasix)" should indicate to the nurse that the client needs additional education. Teaching clients about diuretic therapy is essential to prevent electrolyte imbalances. If a non–potassium-sparing diuretic is prescribed, teach the client which foods are high in potassium. A client must closely monitor electrolyte levels, especially potassium, when taking a loop diuretic such as furosemide.
2. The statement "I plan to avoid all cold cuts" is correct. The client with FVE must also demonstrate an ability to incorporate a low-sodium diet into his or her lifestyle.
3. The statement "I will notify my health-care provider if I gain weight" is correct. The client with FVE must also demonstrate an understanding of the signs and symptoms of fluid excess that should be reported to the health-care provider.
4. The statement "I do not need to restrict the amount of fresh vegetables in my diet" is correct.
TEST-TAKING TIP: Look for the incorrect statement.
Content Area: Adult Health
Integrated Processes: Teaching/Learning
Client Need: Physiological Integrity
Cognitive Level: Analysis
Reference: *Williams, L. S., and Hopper, P. D. (2011). Understanding Medical-Surgical Nursing (4th ed.). Philadelphia, PA: F. A. Davis.*

43. ANSWER: 1, 7, 4, 5, 3, 6, 2.
Rationale: A client diagnosed with right-sided heart failure develops edema because the right side of the heart is weakened and is unable to pump blood efficiently into the pulmonary blood vessels. This increases the volume of blood in the right side of the heart. As blood backs up into the venous system, venous hydrostatic pressure increases and causes capillary hydrostatic pressure to increase. Capillary hydrostatic pressure increases above the hydrostatic pressure in the interstitial space; this causes excess filtration of fluid from the capillaries into the interstitial space, resulting in visible edema.
TEST-TAKING TIP: Envision the physiological process of edema formation. Use logic to determine the order of events.
Content Area: Older Adult Health
Integrated Processes: Nursing Process: Analysis
Client Need: Physiological Integrity
Cognitive Level: Analysis
Reference: *Ignatavicius, D. D., and Workman, M. L. (2012). Medical-Surgical Nursing: Patient-Centered Collaborative Care (7th ed.). St. Louis, MO: Saunders.*

44. ANSWER: 1.
Rationale:
1. It is most appropriate for the RN to delegate the care of the older adult client with dehydration to the LPN. This client is the most stable; all the others require frequent assessment by the RN.
2. A client in renal failure who is receiving emergent dialysis requires frequent assessment by the RN.

3. A client with active gastrointestinal bleeding who is receiving a blood transfusion requires frequent assessment by the RN.
4. A new postoperative client with uncontrolled pain requires frequent assessment by the RN.
TEST-TAKING TIP: The RN should delegate the care of the client who does not require ongoing assessment.
Content Area: *Adult Health*
Integrated Processes: *Nursing Process: Planning*
Client Need: *Safe and Effective Care Environment*
Cognitive Level: *Analysis*
Reference: *Ignatavicius, D. D., and Workman, M. L. (2012). Medical-Surgical Nursing: Patient-Centered Collaborative Care (7th ed.). St. Louis, MO: Saunders.*

45. ANSWER: 3.
Rationale:
1. A 2-mm indentation = 1+ pitting edema.
2. A 4-mm indentation = 2+ pitting edema.
3. The nurse should document that the client has grade 3+ edema, indicated by a 6-mm indentation. Edema is the presence of excess interstitial fluid, and pitting refers to the degree to which the skin remains indented or pitted after pressure, usually by a finger.
4. An 8-mm indentation = 4+ pitting edema.
TEST-TAKING TIP: Review Figure 1.3 if you were unable to answer this question correctly.
Content Area: *Child Health*
Integrated Processes: *Nursing Process: Assessment*
Client Need: *Physiological Integrity*
Cognitive Level: *Analysis*
Reference: *Berman, A. J., Snyder, S. J., Kozier, B., and Erb, G. (2011). Kozier and Erb's Fundamentals of Nursing: Concepts, Process, and Practice (9th ed.). Upper Saddle River, NJ: Pearson Education.*

Chapter 2

Fluid Volume Deficit

KEY TERMS

Cellular dehydration—Intracellular fluid deficit that leaves the cells without adequate water to carry on normal function

Colloid solution—Intravenous solution containing large proteins and molecules; these solutions usually stay within the vascular space

Crystalloid solution—Intravenous solution containing varying concentrations of electrolytes; these solutions closely resemble body fluids in composition

Dehydration—Deficit of water in the extracellular fluid

Fluid volume deficit—Clinical sign of a disorder in which fluid intake or retention is less than the body's fluid needs; not a disease

Hypertonic dehydration—Fluid deficit caused primarily by the loss of water; water loss exceeds sodium loss, making the blood hypertonic to normal body fluids

Hypertonic solution—A solution that has more solutes than body fluids (is more concentrated); causes fluid to shift out of the cells and into the intravascular space

Hypotonic dehydration—Fluid deficit caused by the loss of water and sodium; more sodium than water is lost, making the blood hypotonic to normal body fluids

Hypotonic solution—A solution that has fewer solutes than body fluids (is less concentrated); causes fluid to shift into cells and out of the intravascular space

Hypovolemia—Abnormal decrease in the volume of water in the bloodstream (intravascular space)

Insensible fluid loss—Fluid loss that occurs without the person's awareness, such as through perspiration, respiration, and solid feces

Isotonic dehydration—Fluid deficit caused by a decrease in plasma volume while the serum osmolality of the blood remains unchanged; the most common type of fluid volume deficit

Isotonic solution—A solution that has the same concentration of solutes as body fluids (the same tonicity); does not cause fluid to shift into or out of the cells

Relative dehydration—Dehydration that occurs without an actual loss of total body water; occurs when fluid shifts out of the bloodstream (intravascular space) and into the interstitial space

Sensible fluid loss—Fluid loss that is measurable and apparent to the individual, such as through urination and vomitus

I. Description

Fluid volume deficit (FVD) occurs when there is not enough fluid to meet the body's needs. Fluid, consisting primarily of water and sodium, is lost from the body and is not adequately replaced, resulting in a decrease in body weight. This may be caused by excess water loss, inadequate intake of water, excess sodium loss, or inadequate intake of sodium. FVD can also occur without an *actual* loss of total body water, such as when water shifts from the bloodstream (intravascular space) into the interstitial space, causing **relative dehydration.** An extracellular fluid (ECF) deficit may eventually cause an intracellular fluid (ICF) deficit, resulting in **cellular dehydration,** which leaves the cells without adequate water to carry on their normal functions.

DID YOU KNOW?

Fluid volume deficit is a clinical sign of an underlying disorder in which there is not enough water to meet the body's fluid needs. It is not a disease.

A. Daily fluid requirements
   1. Adequate fluid intake is crucial in maintaining hydration status.
   2. Water, juice, or any other fluid that does not contain caffeine or alcohol can be used to maintain hydration.
   3. To prevent FVD, an adult client weighing 40 kg (88 lb) or more requires at least 30 mL/kg/day of free liquid intake. Figure 2.1 shows normal fluid balance.

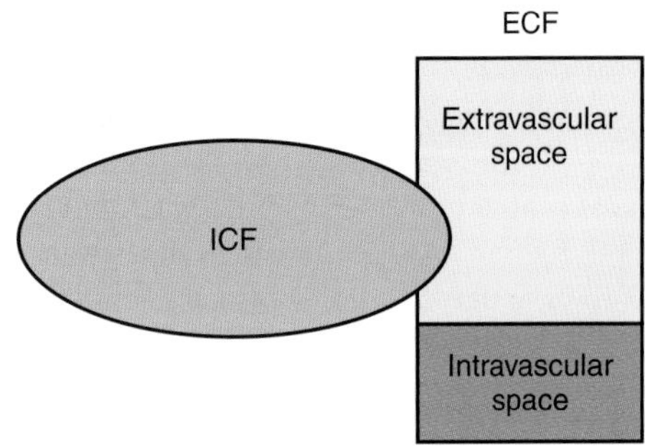

Fig 2.1

4. Fluid requirements for infants and children can be calculated based on body weight according to the Holliday-Segar method (Table 2.1).
5. Fluid requirements are better estimated by weight than age because a child may be underweight or overweight for his or her age (see Table 2.1).
6. It is important to note that daily fluid requirements are higher when increased fluid losses occur, such as with fever, diarrhea, vomiting, or excessive sweating.
7. When calculating fluid requirements, remember that pounds must be converted into kilograms before performing the calculation. See Box 2.1 for help with this conversion.

II. Types of Fluid Volume Deficit

There are three main types of fluid volume deficit: isotonic dehydration, hypotonic dehydration, and hypertonic dehydration. Each type of dehydration causes water to move into or out of the cells in a different way. It is important to understand how each type of FVD affects the fluid balance in the body.

A. Isotonic dehydration
1. A loss of both water and sodium (Fig. 2.2).
2. The most common type of FVD, accounting for about 80% of cases.
3. There is little or no change in the concentration of water and sodium in the bloodstream.
4. Water is neither pulled from the cells into the circulation nor pulled from the circulation into the cells.

Table 2.1 Holliday-Segar Method for Calculating Fluid Requirements

Body Weight	Free Liquid Intake	Urine Output
Infants and Children		
0–10 kg (0–22 lb)	*100 mL/kg*	
5 kg (11 lb)	500 mL (16.67 oz)	Infant: More than 2–3 mL/kg/hr or wet diaper every 3 hours
6 kg (13.2 lb)	600 mL (20 oz)	
7 kg (15.4 lb)	700 mL (23.33 oz)	
8 kg (17.6 lb)	800 mL (26.67 oz)	
9 kg (19.8 lb)	900 mL (30 oz)	
10 kg (22 lb)	1,000 mL (33.33 oz)	
11–20 kg (24.2–44 lb)	*1,000 mL + 50 mL/kg for each kg over 10*	
11 kg (24.2 lb)	1,050 mL (35 oz)	Child: More than 1–2 mL/kg/hr
12 kg (26.4 lb)	1,100 mL (36.67 oz)	
13 kg (28.6 lb)	1,150 mL (38.33 oz)	
14 kg (30.8 lb)	1,200 mL (40 oz)	
15 kg (33 lb)	1,250 mL (41.67 oz)	
16 kg (35.2 lb)	1,300 mL (43.33 oz)	
17 kg (37.4 lb)	1,350 mL (45 oz)	
18 kg (39.6 lb)	1,400 mL (46.67 oz)	
19 kg (41.8 lb)	1,450 mL (48.33 oz)	
20 kg (44 lb)	1,500 mL (50 oz)	
More than 20 kg (44 lb)	*1,500 mL + 20 mL/kg for each kg over 20*	
25 kg (55 lb)	1,600 mL (53.33 oz)	Teen: More than 0.5–1 mL/kg/hr
30 kg (66 lb)	1,700 mL (56.67 oz)	
35 kg (77 lb)	1,800 mL (60 oz)	
40 kg (88 lb)	1,900 mL (63.33 oz)	
Adult		
More than 40 kg (88 lb)	30 mL/kg/day	More than 0.5 mL/kg/hr or 30 mL/hr

Box 2.1 Useful Conversions for Fluid Requirements

1 kilogram (kg) = 2.2 pounds (lb)
1 cup = 240 milliliters (mL)
1 ounce (oz) = 30 milliliters (mL)
1 liter (L) = 1 kilogram (kg)

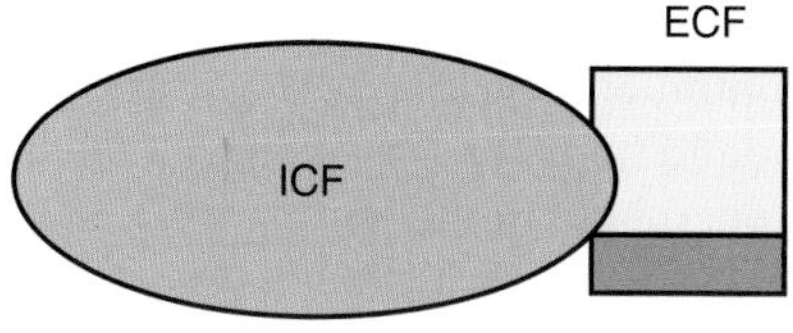

Isotonic dehydration

Equal loss of water and electrolytes; ICF volume remains normal.

Fig 2.2

5. Fluid is lost only from the vascular and interstitial spaces (ECF); the ICF volume remains normal.
6. The serum osmolarity of the blood remains relatively normal: 275 to 295 mOsm/kg.

B. Hypotonic dehydration
1. A loss of more sodium than water, resulting in sodium deficiency in the ECF (Fig. 2.3).
2. Water is pulled *out of* the ECF and *into* the cells (where the sodium concentration is greater) to prevent cellular dehydration.
3. The serum osmolarity of the blood decreases to less than 250 mOsm/kg, causing electrolyte imbalances.

C. Hypertonic dehydration
1. A loss of more water than sodium, usually caused by excessive sodium intake without proportional water intake (Fig. 2.4).
2. Excess sodium in the ECF pulls water *out of* the cells and *into* the ECF, causing cellular dehydration.
3. The serum osmolarity of the blood increases to greater than 295 mOsm/L, causing electrolyte imbalances.

III. Causes of Fluid Volume Deficit

Fluid volume deficit can be caused by inadequate intake or loss of water, inadequate intake or loss of sodium, excessive intake of sodium, water-sodium imbalance, or the shifting of fluid into and out of the cells. There are many conditions, disease processes, medications, and therapies that can result in FVD. To develop a clear understanding of these causes, it is helpful to categorize the most common causes of FVD by type: isotonic, hypotonic, or hypertonic. Table 2.2 provides a snapshot of the causes of FVD.

A. Causes of isotonic dehydration
1. Excessive loss of isotonic fluids through hemorrhage, diarrhea, vomiting, suctioning, profuse sweating, drainage, and diuretic therapy may cause isotonic dehydration.
   a. Hemorrhage (blood loss) is a proportional loss of fluid, electrolytes, protein, and blood cells that, if not quickly controlled, may result in hypovolemia, shock, and eventual death.
   b. Illness-related diarrhea, or the passage of three or more loose or liquid stools per day, results in the loss of both water and sodium in relatively equal proportions.
   c. *Diarrhea is the most common cause of isotonic dehydration*; severe diarrhea should be

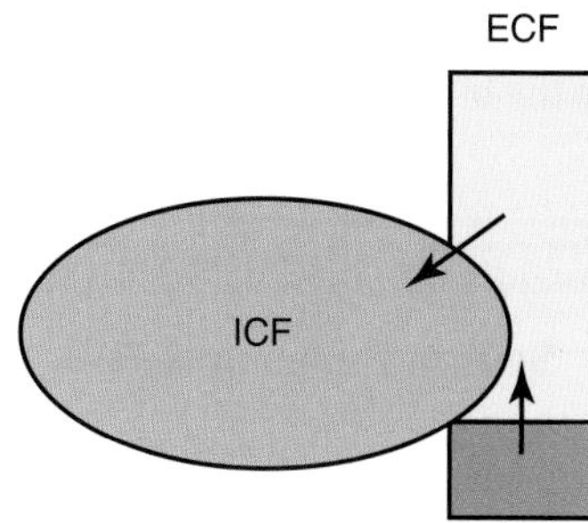

Hypotonic dehydration

More sodium than water is lost making the serum sodium level low. Water moves out of the ECF and into the cell to prevent cellular dehydration.

Fig 2.3 Hypotonic dehydration: more sodium than water is lost, resulting in a low serum sodium level. Water moves out of the ECF and into the cells to prevent cellular dehydration.

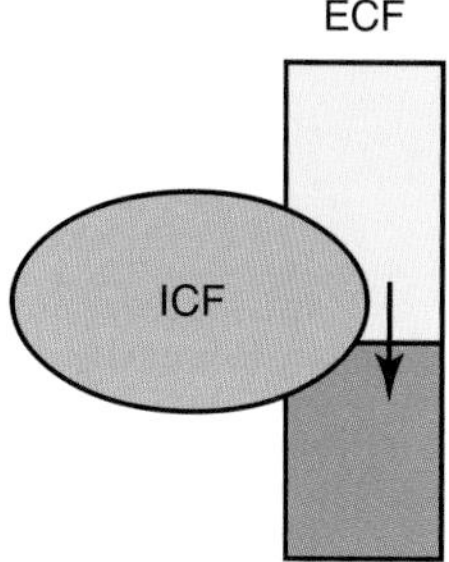

Hypertonic dehydration

More water than sodium is lost, making the serum sodium level high. Water moves out of the cell into the ECF. Then water shifts into the intravascular space minimizing intravascular volume depletion.

Fig 2.4 Hypertonic dehydration: more water than sodium is lost, resulting in a high serum sodium level. Water moves out of the cells and into the intravascular space to prevent intravascular volume depletion.

treated promptly by a health-care provider (Box 2.2).

DID YOU KNOW?

According to the World Health Organization (WHO), dehydration secondary to diarrhea is the second leading cause of death worldwide in children younger than 5 years.

c. Vomiting (emesis) can result in dehydration, especially if it occurs frequently or is prolonged. FVD may result because it is difficult to replace fluids orally if someone has nausea and is unable to tolerate liquids.

Table 2.2 Causes of Fluid Volume Deficit

Type	Causes
Isotonic dehydration *(hypovolemia)*	Excessive loss of isotonic fluids • Hemorrhage • Illness-related diarrhea • Vomiting Removal or loss of other body fluids • Continuous nasogastric suctioning • Wound suction or drainage • Drainage from tubes, fistulas, or ostomies • Profuse sweating • Heatstroke • Severe burns • Diuretic therapy • Carbon monoxide poisoning
Hypotonic dehydration	Inadequate sodium intake during rehydration • After diarrhea and/or vomiting • Excessive perspiration Excessive sodium loss • Salt-wasting renal conditions • Adrenal insufficiency • Adrenal failure • Adrenalectomy • Long-term use or overuse of thiazide diuretics
Hypertonic dehydration	Inadequate water intake • Clients who cannot obtain water independently • Anorexia • Nausea • Dysphagia Severe isotonic fluid loss Increased sodium ingestion • Concentrated parenteral and enteral feedings • Concentrated infant formula Diabetic ketoacidosis (DKA) • Hyperglycemia Excessive loss of water with sodium retention • Hyperventilation • Diabetes insipidus (DI)

Box 2.2 Definition of Severe Diarrhea

Any age—Stools hourly for more than 5 hours
Age older than 2 years—More than 19 stools in 24 hours
Age 1–2 years—More than 14 stools in 24 hours
Age younger than 1 year—More than 9 stools in 24 hours

d. Removal or loss of other body fluids through continuous nasogastric (NG) suctioning; wound suctioning or drainage; and drainage from tubes, fistulas (permanent, abnormal passageways between two organs in the body or between an organ and the exterior of the body through which body fluids are lost), and ostomies results in fluid and electrolyte losses in relatively proportional amounts.

e. Diuretic therapy increases the amount of urine produced by the kidneys, resulting in the loss of water and sodium. Diuretics are first-line treatment for hypertension and congestive heart failure; they cause the intravascular volume to decrease, thus reducing the pressure in the cardiovascular system.

2. Profuse sweating caused by fever, medically induced diaphoresis, or environmental heat results in the loss of both water and sodium.
   a. Heatstroke occurs when the rate of heat production in the body exceeds the rate of heat dissipation, even in the presence of profuse sweating; it may be caused by a malfunction in the body's temperature-regulating system or failure of the cardiovascular system during exercise in a hot environment.

(!) Heatstroke is a medical emergency. A delay in treatment can be fatal.

3. Severe burns can cause FVD, beginning at the onset of the burn and lasting for 48 to 72 hours.

MAKING THE CONNECTION

Severe Burns and FVD

During the first 48 to 72 hours after a severe burn, fluid shifts out of the blood vessels and into the interstitial spaces, decreasing blood volume (relative dehydration). Damaged capillaries become more permeable, allowing fluid and electrolytes to "leak" into the body tissue, causing edema. Because the integrity of the skin is damaged, massive **insensible fluid loss** occurs as the exposed body fluids evaporate. Additional insensible loss occurs during respiration, which may be increased in rate. After the first 48 to 72 hours, edema fluid in the tissue shifts back into the blood vessels, and blood volume increases, resulting in the opposite problem—fluid *overload.*

4. Carbon monoxide (CO) poisoning may result in FVD. (See Making the Connection). CO is produced by incomplete combustion in motor vehicles, gasoline-powered tools, gas heaters, and gas-powered cooking equipment.

B. Causes of hypotonic dehydration
   1. Inadequate sodium intake during rehydration results in sodium deficiency in the ECF; hypotonic ECF causes water to move into the cells (where the concentration of sodium is higher) to balance the sodium concentration on both sides of the cell membrane and to prevent cellular dehydration.
      a. After experiencing diarrhea or vomiting, sodium-containing beverages and foods should be consumed to replace water and sodium lost during illness.
      b. Excessive perspiration, caused by extreme heat or physical activity, can result in hypotonic dehydration when water is consumed but sodium-containing foods are not.
   2. Excessive sodium loss is a common cause of hypotonic dehydration; sodium can be lost secondary to diarrhea, kidney disease, adrenal gland disorders, draining of body fluids, and long-term diuretic therapy.
      a. Salt-wasting renal conditions, such as chronic kidney disease, impair the kidneys' ability to reabsorb sodium and water, causing abnormal urinary sodium loss in persons ingesting normal amounts of sodium chloride; it is characterized by vomiting, dehydration, and vascular collapse.
      b. Adrenal insufficiency, adrenal failure, and adrenalectomy result in a significant decrease or complete loss of the hormone aldosterone, produced by the adrenal glands; impaired aldosterone production inhibits the kidneys' ability to reabsorb sodium and water, resulting in dehydration, hypotension, and, if left untreated, shock. Aldosterone is part of the renin-angiotensin-aldosterone mechanism.
      c. Long-term use or overuse of thiazide diuretics, such as hydrochlorothiazide (HCTZ), can cause excessive sodium loss. These drugs work by increasing sodium reabsorption and excretion by the kidneys; because water follows sodium, water is also absorbed and excreted by the kidneys, decreasing the amount of circulating fluid in the bloodstream and thus lowering blood pressure.

C. Causes of hypertonic dehydration
   1. Inadequate water intake results in an increased concentration of solutes in the ECF, which causes water to be pulled *out of* the cells and into the ECF, resulting in cellular dehydration.
      a. Clients who cannot obtain water independently, such as infants, the elderly, and bedridden or disabled clients, develop hypertonic dehydration as water is lost from the body and ever-increasing concentrations of solutes are left behind.
      b. Clients with anorexia, nausea, or dysphagia may be unable to swallow or to tolerate fluid intake.
      c. Prolonged NPO (nothing by mouth) status without IV fluid replacement also results in inadequate water intake that may lead to hypertonic dehydration.
   2. Severe isotonic fluid loss occurs following hyperemesis or prolonged watery diarrhea.
      a. This extreme fluid loss may deplete the body of so much water that the kidneys no longer have water to conserve.
      b. The ECF eventually becomes hypertonic and begins to pull water out of the cells, causing cellular dehydration.
   3. Increased solute intake without proportional water intake results in hypertonic dehydration.
      a. Sodium ingestion through the consumption of salt tablets or high-sodium beverages and foods (also seawater) without adequate water intake can cause hypertonic dehydration.
      b. Concentrated parenteral (IV) and enteral (tube) feedings that are not properly diluted can cause hypertonic dehydration when solutes such as amino acids, proteins, glucose, minerals, and electrolytes (including sodium) are administered without adequate amounts of water.
      c. Concentrated infant formula that is not properly diluted can also cause this type of dehydration.

MAKING THE CONNECTION

Carbon Monoxide Poisoning and FVD

Carbon monoxide gas is difficult to detect, and when it is inhaled even in relatively small amounts, it binds to hemoglobin, the principal oxygen-carrying compound in blood. Carbon monoxide binds much more easily to hemoglobin than oxygen does, forming a compound called "carboxyhemoglobin" that deprives the tissues of oxygen (hypoxia). If left untreated, anaerobic respiration occurs, resulting in acid production (respiratory acidosis), which causes profound vasodilation. When the blood vessels dilate, the vascular space expands, resulting in FVD (relative dehydration) even though no *actual* fluid loss has occurred. This fluid shift may result in severe hypotension, shock, or death. A classic postmortem sign of CO poisoning is the presence of bright pink cheeks.

4. Hyperglycemia and diabetic ketoacidosis (DKA), caused by insulin deficiency, can result in hypertonic dehydration.
   a. Hyperglycemia results in glucose overloading in the kidneys.
   b. When the kidneys can no longer absorb glucose, the excess spills over into the urine.
   c. Osmotic diuresis occurs, resulting in dehydration, which exacerbates the acidosis.
5. Excessive loss of water with sodium retention causes hypertonic dehydration.
   a. Hyperventilation results in the insensible loss of water with each respiration, leaving sodium and other electrolytes behind.
   b. Diabetes insipidus (DI) is a condition in which the kidneys are unable to conserve water due to a deficiency of antidiuretic hormone (ADH) (central DI) or due to the kidneys' insensitivity to ADH (nephrogenic DI). DI is characterized by intense, uncontrollable thirst and the excretion of massive amounts of extremely diluted urine, even when fluid intake is restricted.

DID YOU KNOW?

When hypertonic dehydration occurs, fluid is pulled out of the cells and into the vascular space, increasing blood volume, so hypovolemia (a classic sign of dehydration) is not present.

MAKING THE CONNECTION

Diabetes Mellitus and Osmotic Diuresis

You have learned that polydipsia and polyuria are classic signs of diabetes mellitus (DM), but what causes a client with DM to experience extreme thirst and excessive urination? The answer is osmotic diuresis. Osmotic diuresis is excessive urination caused by the presence of certain substances, such as glucose, that cannot be reabsorbed in the small tubules of the kidneys. These substances cause an increase in the osmotic pressure in the kidney tubule, resulting in water retention in the lumen of the kidney and a subsequent increase in urine output (diuresis). Compounding the problem, the solutes in the blood become more concentrated as water is excreted by the kidneys, increasing the osmolarity of the blood. Once the blood has a higher osmolarity than the body fluids, water is pulled *into* the bloodstream from the interstitial space, providing even more water for the kidneys to excrete as urine. Thus osmotic diuresis results in dehydration from polyuria, which causes polydipsia, the classic signs of DM.

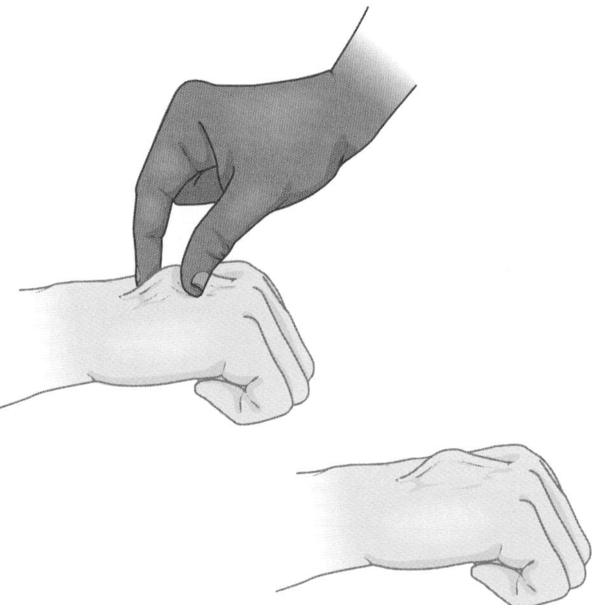

Fig 2.5 Assessing skin turgor in an adult (nonelderly): 1. Gently pinch the skin on the posterior surface of the forearm or over the sternum between your thumb and forefinger and then release it. 2. Assess how quickly the skin returns to its normal position. Hydrated skin should return to normal within 3 seconds. If the skin remains tented or returns more gradually to its original position, the turgor is described as decreased, poor, nonelastic, or nonresilient, or it can be described by the amount of time it takes for the skin to return to normal. Assess turgor in an older adult client over the sternum, clavicle, or forehead. Because of the loss of elasticity related to aging, skin on the hands and arms may remain tented even if the client is well hydrated.

IV. Nursing Assessment for Fluid Volume Deficit

The nurse should conduct a focused nursing assessment for FVD, beginning with a thorough nursing history. Interview the client and family members to reveal any risk factors or preexisting conditions that would contribute to FVD, such as age; vomiting or diarrhea; drainage through operative wounds, burns, or fistulas; diaphoresis; DM; or inflammatory diseases of the skin that are associated with fluid loss. The nurse should also assess the client's ability to drink and tolerate oral fluids and obtain a current dietary history, inquiring about recent changes in appetite. The nursing history should also cover lifestyle factors and current medication use. A thorough physical assessment is necessary because FVD affects many body systems. Assess the client's skin turgor for signs of dehydration (Figs. 2.5 and 2.6). Measure and record the client's vital signs. Assess each body system, observing for signs and symptoms of FVD, and review the client's laboratory data to assess for the presence of FVD and any associated electrolyte imbalances (Table 2.3).

V. Nursing Interventions for a Client with Fluid Volume Deficit

A. Identify high-risk clients
  1. Infants and young children
    a. Require more water for size than adults.
    b. Lose water more easily than adults.
    c. Have immature kidneys (until age 2 years) that cannot efficiently compensate for fluid loss.
    d. Have a larger body surface area and a higher metabolism, causing them to lose more water; fevers also tend to be higher and last longer than in adults.
  2. Adults older than 60 years
    a. Have more body fat than younger adults.
    b. Reduced kidney function makes older adults less glucose tolerant, increasing their risk for hyperglycemia.
    c. Diminished thirst mechanism places older adult clients at risk for FVD.
    d. Small water losses have a greater impact on older adults because of these factors.
  3. Women and obese clients
    a. Have a higher percentage of fat that holds less water, reducing the amount of total body water and increasing the risk for dehydration.
  4. Clients with acute or chronic illnesses
    a. Surgery, draining wounds, and wound suctioning can result in the loss of blood and body fluids.

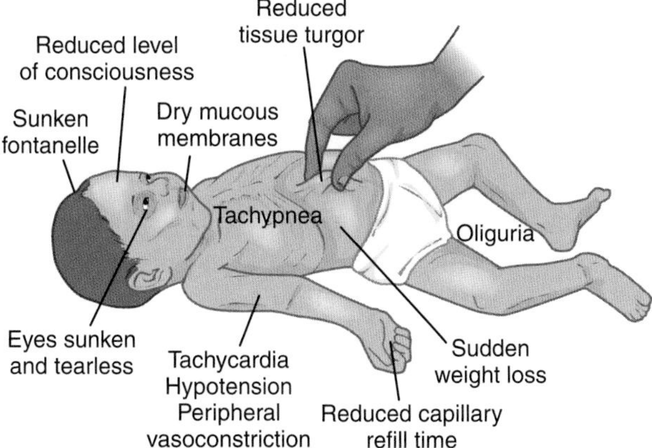

Fig 2.6 Assessing skin turgor in an infant: 1. Gently pinch the loose skin of the abdomen between your thumb and forefinger and then release it. 2. Assess how quickly the skin returns to its normal position. Hydrated skin should return to normal within 3 seconds. If the skin remains tented or returns more gradually to its original position, the turgor is described as decreased, poor, nonelastic, or nonresilient, or it can be described by the amount of time it takes for the skin to return to normal.

Table 2.3 Signs and Symptoms of Fluid Volume Deficit

Vital Signs	
Blood pressure	Decreased, orthostatic hypotension
Heart rate	Increased, weak pulse volume
Pulse pressure	Decreased
Respiratory rate	Increased
Temperature	Within normal limits or elevated
Weight	Sudden weight loss • Mild FVD: loss of 2%–5% body weight • Moderate FVD: loss of 6%–9% body weight • Severe FVD: loss of greater than 10% body weight • Death: loss of 15% body weight is usually fatal
Signs and Symptoms by Body System	
Cardiovascular	• Weak, rapid pulse • Diminished peripheral veins • Heart palpitations
Gastrointestinal	• Dry mouth • Nausea and vomiting
Integumentary	• Pale, cool, dry skin • Decreased skin turgor • Sunken eyeballs • Sunken fontanelles in infants • Dry mucous membranes • No tears when crying • Sweating may stop
Musculoskeletal	• Muscle weakness • Fatigue
Neurological	• Thirst • Lightheadedness • Orthostatic hypotension • Confusion • Altered mental status • Decreased level of consciousness
Renal	• Amber or dark-colored urine • Decreased urine output
Respiratory	• Increased respiratory rate
Laboratory Values	
Blood urea nitrogen (BUN)	Increased
Increased, serum hyperosmolality	Hematocrit
Serum osmolality	Depends on type of FVD
Urine specific gravity	High

    b. Gastrointestinal illnesses that cause nausea, vomiting, or diarrhea result in fluid and electrolyte losses; difficulty chewing or swallowing can lead to decreased consumption of liquids and fluid-rich foods.

c. Liver disease results in the decreased production of albumin, which is needed to maintain adequate vascular volume.
d. Renal disease adversely affects the kidneys' ability to regulate water and sodium.
e. Cancer can cause fluid shifts in the body; radiation and chemotherapy can cause nausea, vomiting, and extreme fatigue, resulting in the reduced intake of fluids and foods.
f. Psychological disorders, such as anorexia nervosa, bulimia, and other eating disorders, can result in FVD; addictive disorders, such as alcoholism and illicit drug use, can result in liver damage and malnutrition-related FVD.

B. Weigh the client daily
1. Evaluate the client's weight gain over 1 to 3 days.
   a. Weigh the client at the same time each day, preferably before breakfast, with the same amount of clothing on and using the same scale.

DID YOU KNOW?
Weight is the most reliable indicator of fluid loss or gain.

C. Monitor the client
1. Obtain the client's vital signs as prescribed and compare to baseline.
   a. Observe for changes in heart rate, blood pressure, and respiratory rate.
   b. Pulse oximetry values below 95% are considered "low" for clients with healthy lungs; normal baseline may be decreased in smokers and in clients with preexisting heart or lung disorders.
2. Monitor the client's respiratory status.
   a. Observe for signs of overhydration during IV fluid replacement: shortness of breath, coughing, labored breathing, rapid breathing (tachypnea), difficulty breathing when lying down (orthopnea), pale skin (pallor), blue skin color (cyanosis), or anxiety.
   b. Auscultate for abnormal heart sounds and moist crackles (rales) in the lungs; rales usually begin in the bases and then move into the upper lung fields.
   c. Normal respiratory rate for an adult is 12 to 20 breaths per minute.
3. Obtain and evaluate laboratory values.
   a. Monitor for changes in hematocrit, blood urea nitrogen (BUN), serum sodium, serum potassium, and other electrolyte levels; FVD may accompany electrolyte imbalances (depending on etiology).
   b. Observe for changes in mental status.
   c. Be alert for signs of overcorrection (fluid volume excess) (see Chapter 1, p 7).

D. Measure intake and output
1. Measure intake.
   a. At least every 8 hours, record the type and amount of all fluids received and describe the route as oral, parenteral, rectal, or by enteric tube.
   b. Record ice chips as fluid at approximately one-half their volume.
   c. Compare the client's intake with the intake of an average adult.
2. Measure output.
   a. Record the type and amount of all fluids the client has lost, and indicate the route; describe output as urine, liquid stool, vomitus, tube drainage (including from chest, closed wound drainage, and nasogastric tubes), and any fluid aspirated from a body cavity.
   b. Measure the amount of irrigation fluid instilled; subtract it from the total output when irrigating a nasogastric or other tube or the bladder.
   c. Measure drainage in a calibrated container. Observe it at eye level, and record the reading at the bottom of the meniscus.
   d. Compare the client's output with that of an average adult; intake and output should be relatively equivalent.

E. Administer oral fluids
1. Administer oral rehydration therapy as prescribed by the health-care provider.
   a. Provide an adult client with at least 30 mL/kg/day of fluids; mild FVD generally responds well to oral fluid replacement.
   b. Determine whether the client has any special fluid needs (e.g., thickened fluids, fluid restriction).
   c. Plan the type and timing of fluid intake with the client and caregivers. Encourage the client to indicate preferences.
   d. Encourage fluid intake of 60 to 120 mL every hour for a client with FVD or at high risk for FVD; provide a straw, change water routinely, and accommodate client preferences.
   e. Offer fluids regularly (every hour) to a confused or bedridden client.
   f. Offer small amounts of fluid every hour to older adult or bedridden clients who may be unable to drink independently.
   g. Avoid carbonated beverages, fruit juices, gelatin desserts, and instant fruit drink mixes if the client is experiencing nausea, vomiting, or diarrhea.
   h. Offer solutions containing glucose and electrolytes that are easily absorbed even in the presence of vomiting and diarrhea.
   i. Pedialyte, Equalyte, Oralyte, and Rehydralyte are readily available.

F. Provide comfort measures
 1. Provide oral hygiene and mouth care to the client, including the application of lip moisturizer.
 2. Apply moisturizers to the client's skin.

G. Administer IV fluids
 1. Administer IV fluids as ordered.
  a. Use an IV administration route for moderate to severe FVD or if the client is unable to ingest fluids.
  b. The type of IV solution prescribed depends on the type of fluid and electrolyte replacement needed (Table 2.4).
  c. Anticipate a rapid effect when IV fluids are administered.
 2. Know the drop factor.
  a. Determine the manufacturer's drop factor for each IV administration set used; the larger the bore of the tubing, the faster the fluid flows.
  b. Drop factors range from 10 gtt/mL (largest diameter) to 60 gtt/mL (smallest diameter). Other drop factors are 12, 15, and 20 gtt/mL.
  c. When the drop factor is between 10 and 20, it is called "macrodrip tubing," whereas a drop factor of 60 gtt/mL is called "microdrip tubing."

Table 2.4 Types of Solutions

Crystalloid Solutions

Isotonic Solutions	*Action/Use*	*Nursing Considerations*
Isotonic saline solution • 0.9% sodium chloride solution (normal saline [NS], NaCl)	• Contains sodium chloride as the solute, dissolved in sterile water • Increases vascular and ECF volumes • Replaces sodium • Causes no fluid shift	• May cause hyperglycemia, osmotic diuresis, or both • May cause fluid overload and generalized edema • Dilutes hemoglobin and lowers hematocrit levels • May cause other electrolyte imbalances • Inflammatory in high doses
Balanced electrolyte solutions • Ringer's solution • Lactated Ringer's solution (LR)	• Ringer's solution contains sodium chloride, potassium chloride, and calcium chloride dissolved in sterile water • Lactated Ringer's solution contains sodium chloride, sodium lactate, potassium chloride, and calcium chloride dissolved in sterile water • Lactate is metabolized by the liver to form bicarbonate, which is useful in treating metabolic acidosis	• May cause fluid overload and generalized edema • Dilutes hemoglobin and lowers hematocrit levels • May cause other electrolyte imbalances • Use with caution in clients with renal insufficiency, congestive heart failure, and conditions in which potassium retention is present • May be contraindicated in clients with hyperkalemia and hypernatremia • Excessive administration of lactated Ringer's solution may result in metabolic alkalosis
Hypotonic Solutions	*Action/Use*	*Nursing Considerations*
Dextrose solutions • Dextrose 5% in water (D_5W) • Dextrose 5% in 0.225% saline solution (D_5 ¼ NS) • Dextrose 5% in 0.45% saline solution (D_5 ½ NS)	• Carbohydrate solution, using glucose as the solute • Provides calories and free water • Provides glucose for metabolism, sparing muscle mass; hydrates cells • Treats hyperkalemia via dilutional effect • Promotes sodium diuresis • Shifts fluid from the intravascular space into the intracellular and interstitial spaces	• May cause fluid overload, water intoxication, or both • D_5W is isotonic when infused and quickly becomes hypotonic in the body, as dextrose is metabolized rapidly • D_5W is often used as a mixing solution (diluent) for IV medications • Check compatibility before adding medications to dextrose solution • May irritate veins • May worsen hypotension • May increase edema • May cause hyponatremia
Hypotonic saline solutions • 0.225% saline solution (¼ NS) • 0.45% saline solution (½ NS)	• Hydrates cells • Replaces fluids when sodium intake must be restricted • Shifts fluid out of the intravascular space into the intracellular and interstitial spaces, causing cells to swell	• May cause fluid overload • May worsen hypotension because water moves out of the vascular space • May increase edema because water moves into the cells and interstitial spaces • May cause dilutional hyponatremia (see Chapter 3) because the sodium content is less than that of plasma

Continued

Table 2.4 Types of Solutions—cont'd

Crystalloid Solutions

Hypertonic Solutions	*Action/Use*	*Nursing Considerations*
Dextrose solutions • Dextrose 5% in 0.9% sodium chloride solution (D_5NS) • Dextrose 5% in lactated Ringer's solution (D_5LR)	• Supplies fluid and calories to the body • Decreases edema • Replaces electrolytes • Shifts fluid from the intracellular compartment into the intravascular space, expanding vascular volume	• May cause fluid overload • D_5NS may cause hypernatremia related to sodium content • Hypertonic solutions may be irritating to veins • Check compatibility before adding medications to dextrose solution
Hypertonic saline solutions • 3% sodium chloride solution (3% saline) • 5% sodium chloride solution (5% saline)	• Supplies sodium to the body; treats hyponatremia • Decreases inflammation and increases capillary permeability • Shifts fluid from the intracellular compartment into the intravascular space	• May cause fluid overload • May cause cells to shrink (cellular dehydration) as fluid is drawn out of the cells • Hypertonic solutions may be irritating to veins • May cause hypernatremia • Use with extreme caution
Total parenteral nutrition (TPN) or partial parenteral nutrition (PPN) • Concentrated dextrose in water (20%, 40%, 50%, 60%, or 70%): added to amino acid solutions	• May contain all electrolytes, carbohydrates, proteins, lipids, vitamins, insulin, and trace elements • Provides nutrition when client is unable to tolerate or absorb nutrients via the gastrointestinal system • Customized based on client's nutrient and electrolyte needs • TPN provides all the daily nutritional requirements but not the caloric requirements • Best for short-term use	• May cause fluid volume overload and electrolyte imbalances • TPN is administered via central venous catheter • PPN is administered via peripheral IV catheter • Medication should never be added to a TPN or PPN solution • Catheter-related bacterial infection is the most common complication of TPN • TPN or PPN should be administered using an infusion pump • Usually administered to critically ill clients

Colloid Solutions

Types	*Action/Use*	*Nursing Considerations*
Albumin (human plasma protein) • 5% and 25% concentrations	• Natural plasma protein prepared from donor plasma • Maintains vascular volume by keeping fluid in the intravascular space • Replaces protein and treats shock and burns • 25% concentration is used to treat hypoproteinemia • Encourages movement of fluid from the interstitial space to the intravascular space • Decreases third spacing	• May cause fluid overload • May cause pulmonary edema • 5% albumin is equivalent to plasma protein; isotonic • 25% albumin solution is equivalent to 500 mL of plasma or 2 units of whole blood • 25% albumin solution must not be used in dehydrated clients without supplemental fluids May cause anaphylaxis (observe for hives, fever, chills, and headache)
Dextran (polysaccharide) • Low molecular weight dextran (dextran 40) • High molecular weight dextran (dextran 70)	• Synthetic colloid made of glucose polysaccharides • Expands volume • Mobilizes interstitial edema • Prolongs hemodynamic response when given with hetastarch • Shifts fluid from the cells and interstitial spaces into the intravascular space	• May cause hypersensitivity and fluid overload • Increases risk of bleeding • Contraindicated in clients with bleeding disorders, congestive heart failure, and renal failure
Hetastarch • 6% and 10% concentrations	• Synthetic colloid made from corn, diluted in normal saline solution • Expands volume • Shifts fluid from the cells and interstitial spaces into the intravascular space	• May cause hypersensitivity • May cause fluid overload • Increases risk of bleeding • Contraindicated in clients with bleeding disorders, congestive heart failure, and renal failure
Plasma protein fraction • 5% concentration	• Human plasma protein in normal saline solution • Expands volume • Similar to albumin • Increases osmotic pressure • Shifts fluid from the cells and interstitial spaces into the intravascular space	• May cause fluid overload • May cause hypertension • Used interchangeably with albumin • Lacks clotting factors and should not be considered a plasma substitute

Table 2.4 Types of Solutions—cont'd

Blood and Blood Products

Types	*Action/Use*	*Nursing Considerations*
Whole blood	• Rarely used • May be given emergently to an exsanguinating client • Contains all blood components	No medications or IV fluids should be added to or mixed with blood products, except for normal saline solution • All blood and blood products should be administered using an in-line filter primed with normal saline solution When administering any blood product, observe for: • Acute hemolytic reaction: fever, chills, flushing, low back pain, tachycardia, hypotension, vascular collapse, cardiac arrest • Allergic reaction: hives, urticaria, flushing, fever • Anaphylaxis: urticaria, restlessness, wheezing, shock, cardiac arrest • Bacteremia: fever, chills, vomiting, diarrhea, hypotension, septic shock • Circulatory overload: pulmonary congestion, restlessness, cough, shortness of breath, hypertension, distended neck veins • Febrile, nonhemolytic reaction: fever, chills, flushing, headache, muscle aches, respiratory distress, cardiac dysrhythmias
Packed red blood cells (PRBCs)	• Used to treat acute anemia, chronic anemia, and blood loss • Contains red blood cells in approximately 20% plasma • Contains no clotting factors or platelets	
Platelets	• Used to increase low platelet counts or to treat coagulopathies • Usually given in pools of 6–10 units • One unit generally increases the platelet count by 6,000 units	
Fresh frozen plasma (FFP)	• Used to replace clotting factors • Contains plasma and clotting factors • Not usually administered until more than 6 units of PRBCs have been infused • Reverses effects of warfarin (Coumadin)	
Cryoprecipitate	• Used to treat hemophilia, fibrinogen deficiency, and disseminated intravascular coagulation • Contains clotting factors	

You must know the drop factor of the tubing being used to calculate the drip rate.

3. Calculate the hourly rate if it is not specified in the order.Divide the volume to be infused by the number of hours it is to be infused.

   Example: 1,000 mL ÷ 8 hours = 125 mL/hr

4. Calculate the drip rate.
   a. Multiply the volume to be infused by the drop factor (number of drops per milliliter).
   b. Divide the result by the time in minutes to obtain the drip rate.

   Example: 500 mL × 10 (drop factor) ÷ 60 minutes = 83.3 gtt/min

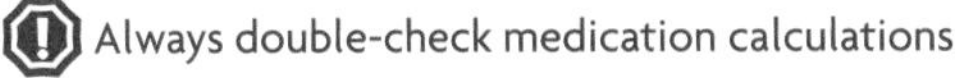
Always double-check medication calculations.

5. Begin the infusion, and monitor hourly.
   a. Follow the manufacturer's instructions for priming the tubing.
   b. Attach the tubing to the client's IV access site per institution policy.
   c. Regulate the speed of flow using the roller clamp; use a watch with a second hand, and count the number of drops entering the chamber in 1 minute.
   d. Ensure that the flow rate has not inadvertently changed.

H. Use intravenous infusion pumps
1. Control the flow rate of fluids or blood products administered through an IV catheter by using an IV pump.
2. Use microdrip tubing with a drop factor of 60 gtt/mL when using an IV pump.
   a. Simplify the calculations based on an infusion time of 60 minutes (1 hour) because pumps are routinely programmed in milliliters per hour rather than drops per minute.
   b. Follow the manufacturer's instructions for priming the tubing and loading the administration set into the pump.
3. Program the pump with the infusion rate and the volume to be infused.
   a. Enter the total volume of the IV bag minus 25 to 50 mL so the infusion does not "run dry."
   b. Attach the tubing to the client's IV access site per institution policy.
4. Start the infusion.
   a. Ensure that all alarms are turned on and in working order.
5. Monitor hourly.
   a. Ensure that the flow rate has not inadvertently changed.

The use of IV pumps DOES NOT relieve the nurse of responsibility for calculating and monitoring the flow rate.

6. Perform a fluid challenge if ordered.
   a. Rapidly administer a designated amount of IV fluid when ordered.
   b. A fluid challenge is used to evaluate fluid volume status when cardiac or renal function is questionable, usually when blood pressure or urine output is decreased.

I. Administer medications as ordered
   1. Antidiarrheal medications: administered to decrease or eliminate diarrhea by thickening the stool or slowing intestinal spasms.
      a. bismuth subsalicylate (Pepto-Bismol)
      b. diphenoxylate/atropine (Lomotil) and loperamide (Imodium) to slow intestinal motility and propulsion
      c. kaolin/pectin (Kaopectate)
      d. octreotide (Sandostatin) in certain types of cancer
      e. polycarbophil (FiberCon) in certain circumstances
   2. Antiemetics: administered to reduce or eliminate nausea and prevent vomiting.
      a. diphenhydramine (Benadryl)
      b. dolasetron (Anzemet)
      c. granisetronHCl (Kytril)
      d. meclizine (Antivert, Antrizine, Bonine, Meni-D) to prevent nausea and vomiting related to motion sickness
      e. metoclopramide (Reglan)
      f. ondansetron (Zofran) to manage nausea and vomiting related to surgery, anesthesia, antineoplastic therapy, and radiation therapy
      g. palonosetron (Aloxi) and aprepitant (Emend) to manage nausea and vomiting during the administration of emetogenic chemotherapy
   3. Antimicrobials: administered to kill or inhibit the growth of microorganisms, such as bacteria, fungi, or protozoa.
      a. Specific to the underlying infection.
   4. Antipyretics: administered to decrease body temperature and reduce fluid loss.
      a. acetaminophen (Tylenol)
      b. ibuprofen (Advil, Medipren, Motrin, Nuprin)

J. Educate the client
   1. Teach the client or caregiver the causes of FVD.
   2. Provide specific information regarding the client's medical diagnosis and related interventions and treatments.
   3. Teach the client how to prevent FVD.
      a. Encourage a client with vomiting and diarrhea to modify his or her diet and to use medications to control symptoms and minimize water loss.
      b. Advise the client to use acetaminophen or ibuprofen to control fever.
      c. Instruct the client to replace fluids by frequently drinking small amounts of clear fluids.
   4. Teach the client how to identify signs and symptoms of FVD.
      a. Instruct the client and family to notify the primary health-care provider if the client becomes confused or lethargic; if there is persistent, uncontrolled fever, vomiting, or diarrhea; or if they have any other specific concerns.
   5. Ensure that the client or caregiver understands the specifics, rationale, potential side effects, and desired effects of the treatment regimen.
      a. Include medication administration, nutrition, hydration, and dietary restrictions (foods high in sodium) in client teaching.

(!) Call 911 or obtain emergency medical services for any individual with altered mental status—confusion, lethargy, or coma.

K. Evaluate and document
   1. Document all interventions and the client's response to them, per institution policy.
   2. Evaluate and document the client's response to interventions and education.
      a. Vital signs and weight should return to baseline.
      b. Laboratory values should return to the normal reference range.
      c. Urinary output should be at least 30 mL/hr for an adult client.
      d. Level of consciousness should return to baseline.
      e. Underlying cause of FVD should be resolved.

VI. Types of Intravenous Solutions

IV solutions can be divided into three basic categories: (1) crystalloid solutions, (2) colloid solutions, and (3) whole blood and blood products.

A. **Crystalloid solutions** contain water and dextrose or electrolytes (or both) and are commonly used to treat various fluid and electrolyte imbalances. These solutions are the primary fluids used for IV therapy. Crystalloid solutions affect the movement of fluid in the body, depending on the tonicity (concentration of electrolytes)of the solution. They are classified into three types: isotonic, hypotonic, and hypertonic.
   1. **Isotonic solutions** have the same amount of electrolytes as plasma (Fig. 2.7).
   2. **Hypotonic solutions** have fewer electrolytes than plasma (Fig. 2.8).
   3. **Hypertonic solutions** have more electrolytes than plasma (Fig. 2.9).

B. **Colloid solutions**, such as albumin and dextran, contain proteins and molecules that are so large they cannot pass through the capillary walls into the cells. These solutions remain in the intravascular space for a longer time than crystalloid solutions and are used

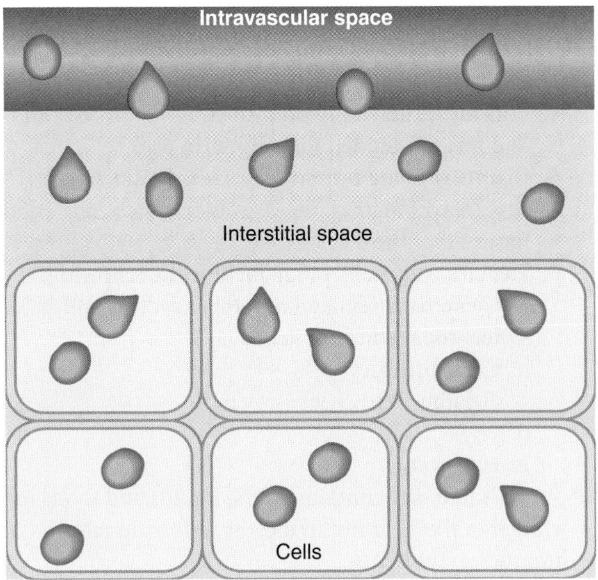

Fig 2.7 Isotonic IV solutions increase intravascular volume without causing fluid to move into or out of the cells.

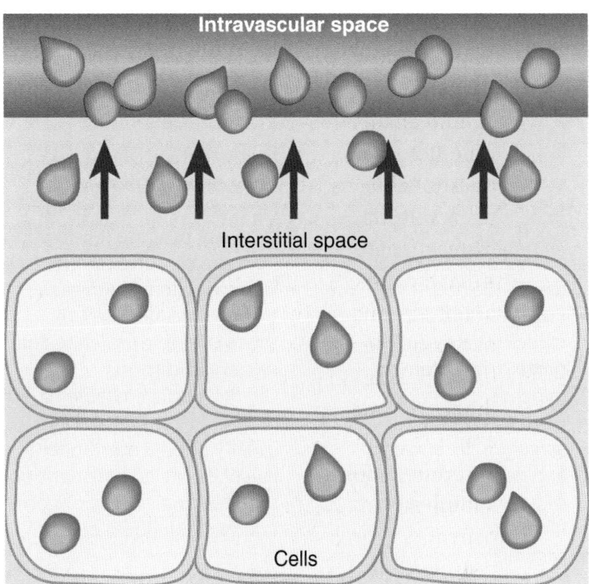

Fig 2.9 Hypertonic IV solutions cause fluid to move out of the cells and into the intravascular space, restoring intravascular volume and reducing edema.

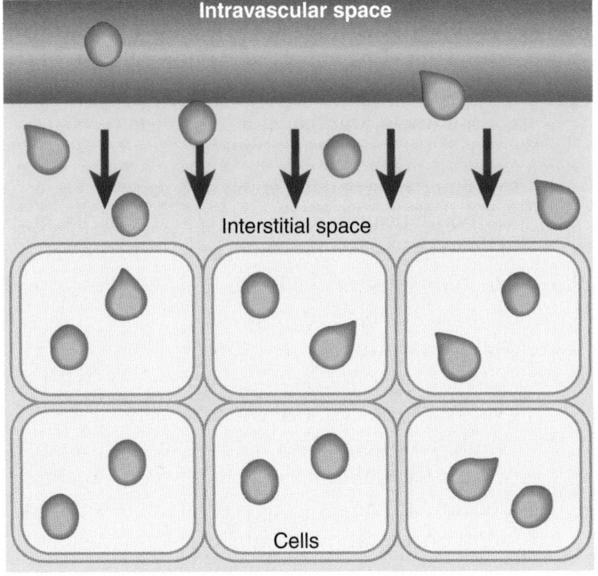

Fig 2.8 Hypotonic IV solutions cause fluid to move out of the intravascular space and into the cells, preventing or correcting cellular dehydration.

as volume expanders. Colloid solutions can cause cells to lose too much water and become dehydrated.

C. **Whole blood and blood products**, such as packed red blood cells (PRBCs), platelets, fresh frozen plasma (FFP), and cryoprecipitate, are preferred for the replacement of blood and blood components. One advantage of whole blood and PRBCs over crystalloid and colloid solutions is the ability of the hemoglobin to transport oxygen to the cells.

DID YOU KNOW?

The type of IV solution prescribed for each client is based on the etiology of fluid loss and the client's need for electrolyte replacement.

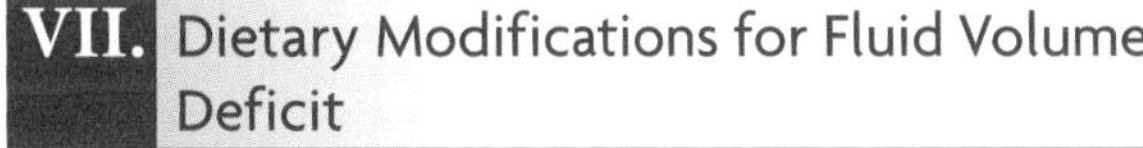

VII. Dietary Modifications for Fluid Volume Deficit

In the presence of a gastrointestinal disturbance, it may be necessary to limit the client's intake—starting with a clear liquid diet, then progressing to a full liquid diet and finally to solid food as tolerated. Current recommendations are for the client to continue eating a normal diet during vomiting or diarrhea, if possible. The BRAT diet (bananas, rice, applesauce, and toast) has fallen out of favor. The nurse should instruct the client to avoid foods that are high in fats and simple sugars, which may increase vomiting and diarrhea. Yogurt is often recommended and may be helpful in reestablishing gastric flora.

A. A clear liquid diet consists of clear drinks and foods that are liquid or become liquid at body temperature (Table 2.5).
   1. Foods or drinks with color are considered "clear" as long as one can see through them.
   2. The clear liquid diet provides fluid and carbohydrates but no protein, fat, vitamins, or minerals.

Table 2.5 Clear Liquid and Full Liquid Diets

Clear Liquid Diet	Full Liquid Diet
• Consists of drinks and liquid foods that are clear; they may have color as long as you can see through them • Intended for short-term use (24–36 hours) • Provides fluid and carbohydrates but no protein, fat, vitamins, minerals, or calories • Used to prepare for surgery, after surgery, and during acute stages of gastrointestinal illnesses • Minimizes stimulation of the gastrointestinal tract while providing hydration and relieving thirst	• Contains only liquids or foods that become liquid at body temperature • Not recommended for long-term use because it is low in iron, protein, and calories • Used for clients with gastrointestinal illnesses or those unable to tolerate solid or semisolid foods • Clients who are unable to progress to solid food are usually given a nutritionally balanced oral supplement or tube feeding instead of continuing a full liquid diet
Foods Permitted	**Foods Permitted**
Clear decaffeinated beverages (coffee, tea, clear sodas, strained lemonade or limeade) Clear broth (bouillon) Clear fruit juice (apple, cranberry, or grape) Gelatin Popsicles Ice chips Hard candy Jelly without seeds Honey	Every option on clear liquid diet Cream, milk, milkshakes Fruit juices, vegetable juices Ice cream, sherbet, Italian ice Yogurt Puddings, custards Refined or strained cereals (e.g., oatmeal) Strained soups Smooth peanut butter
Foods to Be Omitted	**Foods to Be Omitted**
Citrus juices Milk products Any solid	Breads Cheeses Fruits Meats Vegetables

3. This diet minimizes stimulation of the gastrointestinal tract while providing hydration and relieving thirst.
4. This diet is generally prescribed for 24 to 36 hours and is not intended for long-term use.
5. Clients who are prescribed a clear liquid diet should avoid citrus juices, milk products, and solid foods.
6. The clear liquid diet may include the following:
   a. Clear, decaffeinated beverages such as coffee, tea, soda, and fruit juices
   b. Clear broth
   c. Gelatin
   d. Popsicles
   e. Hard candy

B. A full liquid diet contains all the liquids and foods included in the clear liquid diet, as well as nonclear items (see Table 2.5).

1. The full liquid diet provides fluid, carbohydrates, and small amounts of iron and protein.
2. This diet is used for clients with gastrointestinal illnesses or those who cannot tolerate solid or semisolid foods; it is not recommended for long-term use.
3. Clients who are prescribed a full liquid diet should avoid bread, cheese, fruits, vegetables, and meats.
4. The full liquid diet may include the following:
   a. Milk, ice cream, and milkshakes
   b. Fruit juices, sherbet, and Italian ice
   c. Yogurt, pudding, and custard
   d. Refined or strained cereals and soups
   e. Smooth peanut butter

CASE STUDY: Putting It All Together

Subjective Data

A 68-year-old woman presents to the emergency department with fatigue, nausea, malaise, and dizziness when standing. Her family reports that she has been intermittently confused since she awoke that morning. The client reports a 3-day history of nausea, vomiting, and diarrhea; denies discomfort; and states that she has lost 6 lb (2.7 kg) in the past 3 days. She was recently diagnosed with congestive heart failure and fluid volume excess (FVE), necessitating acute treatment with IV furosemide (Lasix) and maintenance therapy consisting of a low-sodium diet, daily weighing, furosemide and potassium by mouth (PO), and an increase in her metoprolol dosage. She has no known allergies, and her current medications are:

- metoprolol (Toprol-XL) 100 mg PO daily
- aspirin 81 mg PO daily
- potassium chloride (K-Lor) 20 mEq PO daily
- furosemide (Lasix) 40 mg PO daily

Objective Data

Nursing Assessment

1. Reports intermittent confusion but is currently oriented to person, place, and time
2. Heart sounds S_1 and S_2 are soft and regular; no murmur
3. Respirations are shallow and slightly rapid
4. Lung sounds clear in all fields
5. Presence of dry oral mucous membranes
6. Orthostatic hypotension
7. Skin pale and cool
8. Poor skin turgor; skin at sternum remains tented longer than 3 seconds
9. Pedal and radial pulses regular, 1+, and weak bilaterally

Vital Signs	
Current weight:	135 lb (61 kg)
Temperature:	99.8°F (37.7°C) orally
Blood pressure (sitting):	90/60 mm Hg
Heart rate:	124 bpm, regular
Respiratory rate:	24 per minute
O_2 saturation:	94%

Laboratory Results	
Serum K^+:	5.5 mEq/L
Serum Ca^{++}:	4.8 mg/dL
Serum CO_2:	23 mEq/L
Serum chloride:	110 mEq/L
Blood glucose:	72 mg/dL
Serum BUN:	46 mg/dL
Serum creatinine:	1.5 mg/dL
Urinalysis:	negative

Health-Care Provider Orders

1. Administer O_2 at 2 L/min via nasal cannula.
2. Keep client nothing by mouth (NPO).
3. Begin rehydration with IV normal saline 200 mL over 1 hour, then decrease to 100 mL/hr.
4. Repeat basic metabolic panel and call with results.
5. Vital signs every 15 minutes × 1 hour and then every 30 minutes × 1 hour.
6. Administer 12.5 mg promethazine (Phenergan) intravenously now.
7. Hold furosemide (Lasix), K-Lor, and Toprol-XL.

Case Study Questions

A. What *subjective* assessment findings indicate that the client is experiencing a health alteration?

1. ______
2. ______
3. ______
4. ______
5. ______
6. ______
7. ______
8. ______

Continued

CASE STUDY: Putting It All Together *cont'd*

Case Study Questions

B. What *objective* assessment findings indicate that the client is experiencing a health alteration?

1. ______
2. ______
3. ______
4. ______
5. ______
6. ______
7. ______
8. ______
9. ______
10. ______

C. After analyzing the data collected, what **primary** nursing diagnosis should the nurse assign to this client?

______

D. What interventions should the nurse plan and/or implement to meet this client's needs?

1. ______
2. ______
3. ______
4. ______
5. ______
6. ______
7. ______
8. ______
9. ______
10. ______

E. What client outcomes should the nurse plan to evaluate the effectiveness of the nursing interventions?

1. ______
2. ______
3. ______
4. ______
5. ______
6. ______

REVIEW QUESTIONS

1. When assessing the fluid status of a client, how should a nurse expect normal fluid intake to compare with output?
   1. Less than the urine output
   2. More than the sensible and insensible output
   3. The same amount as the sensible and insensible output
   4. Equal to the urine output

2. A client who is receiving a hypertonic IV solution may experience excess fluid in the intravascular compartment secondary to fluid shifts caused by which type of pressure?
   1. Hydrostatic pressure
   2. Intraocular pressure
   3. Hyperbaric pressure
   4. Osmotic pressure

3. A nurse is caring for a child diagnosed with FVD. The nurse recognizes that increased production of aldosterone and ADH caused by FVD would elicit a decrease in which physiological parameter?
   1. Urine output
   2. Blood pressure
   3. Serum sodium
   4. Body temperature

4. A full-term infant is placed under phototherapy lights to treat hyperbilirubinemia. A nurse should recognize that this intervention increases the infant's risk for FVD related to which side effect of treatment?
   1. Decreased urinary output
   2. Increased absorption of bilirubin
   3. Decreased sodium absorption
   4. Increased insensible water loss

5. A health-care provider writes orders for a client diagnosed with FVD secondary to influenza. Which medication should a nurse plan to administer if the client experiences nausea?
   1. acetaminophen (Tylenol)
   2. oseltamivir (Tamiflu)
   3. promethazine (Phenergan)
   4. loperamide (Imodium)

6. A nurse assesses a client who reports vomiting and diarrhea. Which information is *most important* for the nurse to obtain?
   1. When the client ate or drank last
   2. What medications the client is taking
   3. Who has been caring for the client at home
   4. How long the client has had these symptoms

7. An older adult client has had nausea, vomiting, and diarrhea for 3 days. Assessment by a nurse reveals dry oral mucosa, amber urine, and decreased skin turgor. Which measurement should the nurse obtain to best determine the client's current fluid status?
   1. Respiratory rate
   2. Temperature
   3. Blood pressure
   4. Pulse oximetry

8. A client is admitted with FVD caused by severe blood loss. What should a nurse identify as the most likely rationale for oliguria in this client?
   1. An increase in serum osmolarity causes conservation of fluid.
   2. A decrease in antidiuretic hormone (ADH) level causes conservation of fluid.
   3. Activation of atrial natriuretic factor causes conservation of fluid.
   4. The renin-angiotensin-aldosterone mechanism causes conservation of fluid.

9. Which client should a nurse classify as being at greatest risk for FVD?
   1. A toddler learning to drink from a cup
   2. An adolescent playing outside with moderate exertion in warm weather
   3. An adult with moderate diarrhea
   4. An older adult with hypertension

10. Which urine output value in an adult client should a nurse associate with the development of FVD?
    1. 20 mL/hr
    2. 40 mL/hr
    3. 60 mL/hr
    4. 80 mL/hr

11. A nurse takes the vital signs of a client who collapsed while working outdoors. Which parameter in the client's blood pressure measurement should the nurse associate with FVD?
    1. Increasing diastolic blood pressure
    2. Decreasing systolic blood pressure
    3. Prominent Korotkoff sounds
    4. Widening pulse pressure

12. A nurse is admitting a client with vomiting and diarrhea. Which action should the nurse perform **first**?
    1. Weigh the client.
    2. Begin an IV infusion.
    3. Administer an oral electrolyte solution.
    4. Administer an antidiarrheal.

13. A nurse reviews a care plan for a client and notes an order for a clear liquid diet. Which choice should the nurse offer this client?
   1. Vanilla ice cream
   2. Ginger ale
   3. Cream soup
   4. Carnation Instant Breakfast

14. A nurse is teaching a client to evaluate fluid status by weight. Which is the appropriate instruction to provide this client?
   1. Weigh yourself twice a day wearing the same amount of clothing.
   2. Weigh yourself 1 hour before meals and before urinating.
   3. Weigh yourself at the same time every morning and after urinating.
   4. Weigh yourself after breakfast using the same scale.

15. Which intervention should a nurse include when planning care for a confused client with FVD?
   1. Explain to the client the rationale for increasing the fluid intake.
   2. Ensure that the certified nursing assistant maintains fresh ice water at the client's bedside at all times.
   3. Provide fluids at the client's bedside, at the desired temperature, at all times.
   4. Assist the client in drinking fluids every hour.

16. How should a nurse who is calculating a client's intake and output include the irrigating fluid of the client's continuous bladder irrigation?
   1. Add the amount to the total intake.
   2. Deduct the amount from the urine output.
   3. Subtract the amount from the IV intake.
   4. Record the amount in the urine output.

17. How should a nurse include a client's wound drainage when calculating intake and output?
   1. Add the total amount to the client's intake.
   2. Subtract the amount from the total output.
   3. Add the amount to the total output.
   4. Subtract the amount from the oral intake.

18. When teaching a client who is breastfeeding a newborn, which instruction should a nurse provide to the new mother to reduce the newborn's risk of developing FVD?
   1. Maintain an adequate fluid intake.
   2. Limit breastfeedings to every 4 hours.
   3. Decrease caloric intake to promote weight loss.
   4. Feed from both breasts during each feeding.

19. A neonate weighing 2,500 gm is to receive a transfusion of 10 mL/kg packed red blood cells (PRBCs) to treat FVD resulting from abruptio placentae at delivery. How many milliliters of PRBCs should a nurse administer to this client? Record your answer as a whole number.

____

20. A pediatrician writes an order for an infant to receive a minimum of 140 mL of formula every 12 hours. To achieve this, how many milliliters of formula should a nurse administer to the infant every 4 hours? Record your answer using one decimal place.

____

21. An infant weighing 11 lb has voided 180 mL at the end of a 12-hour shift. How many mL/kg/hr of urine has this infant voided? Record your answer as a whole number.

____

22. A client is admitted to the emergency department with a closed head injury and multiple fractures. Which IV solution should a nurse plan to administer?
   1. 0.9% saline solution
   2. 0.25% saline solution
   3. 0.5% saline solution
   4. Dextrose 5% in water

23. A client presents to an urgent care center after a reported 3-day history of nausea, vomiting, and diarrhea. A nurse suspects this client is severely dehydrated. Which information is *most important* for the nurse to obtain when assessing this client?
   1. Vital signs
   2. Skin turgor
   3. Thirst level
   4. BUN and creatinine

24. Which client information should a nurse associate with a nursing diagnosis of Deficient Fluid Volume Secondary to Dehydration?
   1. Decreased pulse rate
   2. Decreased hemoglobin level and hematocrit
   3. Jugular venous distention
   4. Blood pressure 96/54 mm Hg

25. An older adult client presents at a health-care provider's office and reports dizziness and "heart racing" while gardening outdoors. Which question should the nurse include in the initial assessment of this client?
1. "Are you wearing sunscreen when you garden?"
2. "Have you noticed an increase in thirst when you garden?"
3. "What time of day do you garden, and for how long?"
4. "Do you have a plan in place if you pass out while gardening?"

26. A client diagnosed with liver failure presents to an acute care facility with moderate ascites and reports shortness of breath. Vital signs are as follows: blood pressure, 90/50 mm Hg; heart rate, 104 bpm and weak; and respiratory rate, 26 and shallow. The client's skin and mucous membranes are dry. Based on this information, which nursing diagnosis should be the priority?
1. Excess Fluid Volume Related to Third Spacing Fluid Shifts Secondary to Liver Failure
2. Deficient Fluid Volume Related to Third Spacing Fluid Shifts Secondary to Liver Failure
3. Risk for Decreased Cardiac Output Related to Decreased Plasma Volume and Electrolyte Deficits Secondary to Liver Failure
4. Risk for Shock Related to Decreased Plasma Volume Secondary to Liver Failure

27. Which intervention should a nurse include in the plan of care for a client diagnosed with FVD?
1. Offer fluids with meals.
2. Monitor for an increase in temperature.
3. Administer diuretics as ordered.
4. Monitor for crackles and orthopnea.

28. A nurse who is planning care for a client with severe FVD and hyponatremia should anticipate an order for the infusion of which IV solution?
1. 0.45% saline solution
2. 0.25% saline solution
3. 0.9% saline solution
4. 3% saline solution

29. A nurse receives a phone call from the parent of an infant who is listless and has had vomiting and diarrhea for 2 days. Which is the **most** appropriate instruction for the nurse to give the parent?
1. Give the infant 2 to 4 oz of oral electrolyte replacement solution every 1 to 2 hours.
2. Monitor the infant's urine output for 24 hours.
3. Bring the infant to the pediatrician or emergency department.
4. Withhold all oral intake until vomiting has resolved.

30. A client has had nausea, vomiting, and diarrhea for 3 days. A nurse suspects the client has FVD and plans to assess the client for orthostatic hypotension. Which method should the nurse use in this assessment? Place each action in the correct sequence (1–5).

_____ Check the client's blood pressure and pulse rate in the standing position.

_____ Compare the client's blood pressures and pulse rates.

_____ Check the client's blood pressure and pulse rate in the supine position.

_____ Document the results of the assessments.

_____ Check the client's blood pressure and pulse rate in the sitting position.

31. Which urine output value in an adult client should a nurse associate with the development of FVD?
1. 500 mL/day or 20 mL/hr
2. 700 mL/day or 29 mL/hr
3. 1,680 mL/day or 70 mL/hr
4. 2,400 mL/day or 100 mL/hr

32. A nurse is planning care for a confused but otherwise healthy 70-kg adult client at risk for FVD. What is the *minimum* number of milliliters of fluid per day the nurse should plan for the client to ingest? Record your answer using a whole number.

____

33. A pregnant client with hyperemesis gravidarum has had continuous nausea and vomiting for 3 days. IV fluid replacement is planned. A nurse should anticipate orders from the client's obstetrician for which type of IV solution?
1. Hypertonic
2. Isotonic
3. Hypotonic
4. Atonic

34. A nurse is caring for a client diagnosed with FVD secondary to DKA who is experiencing nausea, vomiting, and abdominal pain. A health-care provider orders NPO status for the client to decrease nausea and vomiting and then starts to write orders for IV fluid replacement therapy. Which IV solutions should the nurse identify as appropriate for this client? **Select all that apply.**
1. Normal saline solution
2. Dextrose 5% in water
3. Dextrose 5% in normal saline solution
4. 0.45% saline solution
5. 3% sodium chloride solution
6. Lactated Ringer's solution

35. A nurse caring for a client who is hypovolemic anticipates orders from a health-care provider for IV fluid replacement therapy. Which IV solutions should the nurse identify as appropriate for this client? **Select all that apply.**
1. Normal saline solution
2. Dextrose 5% in water
3. Dextrose 5% in normal saline solution
4. 0.45% saline solution
5. 3% sodium chloride solution
6. Lactated Ringer's solution

36. A nurse planning oral rehydration for a client with FVD should include which choices in a clear liquid diet? **Select all that apply.**
1. Orange juice
2. Diet ginger ale
3. Chicken bouillon
4. Chicken noodle soup
5. Grape juice

37. A nurse who is calculating intake and output from 0700 to 1900 for a client with FVD notes that the client has ingested two 120-mL portions of juice, 240 mL of water, and 240 mL of milk and has been receiving IV 0.9% saline solution at 100 mL/hr via electronic pump. The client has voided 275 mL, 300 mL, and 200 mL of urine and has vomited twice with an estimated volume of 100 mL at each occurrence. The client has also had one liquid stool measuring 300 mL. What should the nurse enter on the intake and output record for this time period? Record your answers as whole numbers.
Intake ________ Output ________

38. A nurse is evaluating IV fluid administration orders for a client with FVD secondary to vomiting. Which IV solutions should the nurse identify as appropriate for this client? **Select all that apply.**
1. 0.45% saline solution
2. 0.9% saline solution
3. Lactated Ringer's solution
4. Dextrose 5% in normal saline solution
5. Dextrose 5% in lactated Ringer's solution
6. Albumin

39. A nurse plans to assess the skin turgor of a young adult client. In which location should the nurse assess the skin turgor of this client?

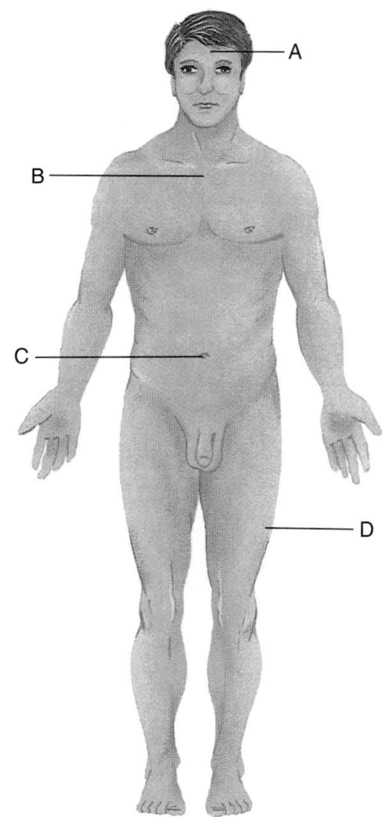

1. A
2. B
3. C
4. D

40. For which potential complication should a nurse monitor in a client receiving IV hypotonic saline solution?
1. Decreased ECF
2. Hypernatremia
3. Increased urine output
4. Mental status changes

41. Which vital sign readings should a nurse associate with the development of FVD?
   1. Blood pressure (BP) 140/70 mm Hg, pulse (P) 96 bpm, respiratory rate (RR) 24
   2. BP 110/80 mm Hg, P 84 bpm, RR 24
   3. BP 100/70 mm Hg, P 60 bpm, RR 20
   4. BP 80/60 mm Hg, P 110 bpm, RR 24

42. Which clinical manifestation should a nurse associate with effective IV fluid replacement therapy for a client diagnosed with FVD?
   1. Jugular venous distention
   2. Urine output of 50 mL/hr
   3. Blood pressure of 90/60 mm Hg
   4. Temperature of 99.9°F (37.7°C)

43. Which order given for a client with a closed head injury, multiple fractures, and blood loss should a nurse question?
   1. Neurological checks every hour
   2. Vital signs every 4 hours
   3. IV normal saline at 150 mL/hr
   4. Strict intake and output measurement

44. A nurse who is assessing intake and output for a client with severe burns notes that the client's intake is 2,000 mL greater than output. Which rationales should the nurse associate with this discrepancy? **Select all that apply.**
   1. The client is experiencing vasoconstriction.
   2. The client is experiencing increased insensible output.
   3. The client has been incontinent of urine and stool.
   4. The client has been dangerously overhydrated.
   5. The client is experiencing third spacing.

45. Which manifestations should a nurse associate with the development of FVD in a client receiving diuretic therapy? **Select all that apply.**
   1. Dry oral mucosa
   2. Hypertension
   3. Hypotension
   4. Jugular venous distention
   5. Tachycardia with peripheral pulses 3+ bilaterally

REVIEW ANSWERS

1. ANSWER: 3.

Rationale:

1. If the client's fluid intake is less than or equal to the urine output, the client will develop FVD. Urine output is one measure of sensible fluid loss and does not include insensible losses or other routes of sensible output.
2. If the client's intake is greater than the total fluid output, the client will develop FVE.
3. **A client's fluid intake should be approximately the same as fluid output, which includes sensible and insensible fluid losses.**
4. Fluid output includes sensible and insensible fluid losses. Urine output is one measure of sensible loss and does not include insensible losses or other routes of sensible output.

TEST-TAKING TIP: Recall that urine output is only one source of fluid loss.

Content Area: Adult Health
Integrated Processes: Nursing Process: Assessment
Client Need: Physiological Integrity
Cognitive Level: Knowledge
Reference: Williams, L., and Hopper, P. (2011). Understanding Medical-Surgical Nursing (4th ed.). Philadelphia, PA: F. A. Davis.

2. ANSWER: 4.

Rationale:

1. Hydrostatic pressure is the pressure water molecules exert on the walls of the space in which they are confined. The amount of water in any body fluid compartment determines the hydrostatic pressure of that space. Compared with osmotic pressure, hydrostatic pressure is less dependent on the amount of solute.
2. Intraocular pressure is the fluid pressure within the eye.
3. Hyperbaric pressure refers to gas pressure greater than atmospheric pressure and is associated with hyperbaric oxygen therapy. This therapy, which delivers oxygen at an increased concentration and pressure, is most commonly used to treat decompression sickness.
4. **Hypertonic or hyperosmotic fluids (fluids with osmolarities greater than 300 mOsm/L) have a greater osmotic pressure than isotonic fluids. If a hypertonic IV solution were infused into a client with normal ECF osmolarity, the infused fluid would make the client's intravascular compartment hyperosmotic (or hypertonic). In an attempt to achieve balance, the client's interstitial fluid would be pulled into the intravascular compartment to dilute the blood osmolarity back to normal, resulting in expansion of the plasma volume and shrinkage of the interstitial volume. Osmotic pressure is also called "oncotic pressure."**

TEST-TAKING TIP: Read each option carefully and use the process of elimination to rule out incorrect answers.

Content Area: Adult Health
Integrated Processes: Nursing Process: Planning
Client Need: Physiological Integrity
Cognitive Level: Knowledge
Reference: Ignatavicius, D., and Workman, M. (2012). Medical-Surgical Nursing: Patient-Centered Collaborative Care (7th ed.). St. Louis, MO: Saunders.

3. ANSWER: 1.

Rationale:

1. **An increase in the production of aldosterone and ADH would cause a decrease in the child's urine output. Both aldosterone and ADH promote the conservation of water and sodium and cause a decrease in urine output as the kidneys increase their reabsorption of water and sodium.**
2. Following an increase in the production of aldosterone and ADH, the client's blood pressure should increase as vascular volume is restored.
3. Because sodium reabsorption is also increased by an increase in the production of aldosterone and ADH, the serum sodium does not decrease.
4. Aldosterone and ADH have no effect on body temperature.

TEST-TAKING TIP: Recall that signs of FVD include a decrease in blood pressure, an increase in heart rate and respiratory rate, and a decrease in urine output.

Content Area: Child Health
Integrated Processes: Nursing Process: Analysis
Client Need: Physiological Integrity
Cognitive Level: Comprehension
Reference: Wilkinson, J., and Treas, L. (2011). Fundamentals of Nursing: Theory, Concepts & Applications(2nd ed.). Philadelphia, PA: F. A. Davis.

4. ANSWER: 4.

Rationale:

1. A decrease in urinary output may be a sign that FVD has developed in the infant placed under phototherapy lights. Decreased urinary output is not a cause of FVD.
2. Increased absorption of bilirubin does not place the client at risk for FVD.
3. Although phototherapy may cause decreased sodium absorption, this is not the cause of FVD in this client.
4. **The nurse should recognize that an infant placed under phototherapy lights is at risk for FVD related to insensible water loss. Infants exposed to phototherapy, particularly low-birth-weight infants and those placed under a radiant warmer, have a significant increase in insensible water losses. These infants also have increased water losses in stool.**

TEST-TAKING TIP: Recall that phototherapy increases insensible fluid loss secondary to heat.

Content Area: Child Health
Integrated Processes: Nursing Process: Implementation
Client Need: Physiological Integrity
Cognitive Level: Comprehension
Reference: Perry, S., Hockenberry, M., Lowdermilk, D., and Wilson, D. (2010). Maternal Child Nursing Care (4th ed.). St. Louis, MO: Mosby.

5. ANSWER: 3.

Rationale:

1. Acetaminophen (Tylenol) is an analgesic-antipyretic medication used to control flu symptoms but is not indicated for nausea.
2. Oseltamivir (Tamiflu) is a neuraminidase inhibitor that stops the spread of the flu virus in the body. Oseltamivir helps shorten the duration of flu symptoms, such as a stuffy or runny nose, sore throat, cough, muscle or joint aches, tiredness, headache, fever, and chills. It is not indicated for nausea.

3. **If the client begins to experience nausea, the nurse should plan to administer promethazine (Phenergan), an antiemetic used to control nausea. Control of nausea is an important nursing intervention for a client admitted with dehydration secondary to flu symptoms.**
4. Loperamide (Imodium) is an antidiarrheal medication used to control flu symptoms but is not indicated for nausea.
TEST-TAKING TIP: Consider the expected effect of each medication. Select the medication that is classified as an antiemetic.
Content Area: Adult Health
Integrated Processes: Nursing Process: Planning
Client Need: Physiological Integrity
Cognitive Level: Comprehension
Reference: *Deglin, J. H., Vallerand, A. H., and Sanoski, C. A. (2013). Davis's Drug Guide for Nurses (13th ed.). Philadelphia, PA: F. A. Davis.*

6. ANSWER: 4.
Rationale:
1. When the client last ate or drank would be important information to obtain in a preoperative client. It is not a priority for a client who reports vomiting and diarrhea.
2. What medications the client is taking is important, but not as important as how long the client has had vomiting and diarrhea.
3. Who has been caring for the client is not important at this time.
4. **It is most important for the nurse to determine how long the client has been experiencing vomiting and diarrhea to assess the severity of the potential FVD. A client who has experienced these symptoms for several days is more likely to be moderately to severely dehydrated than someone who has been experiencing these symptoms for just a few hours.**
TEST-TAKING TIP: Think about why the nurse would need to know each piece of information. Use the process of elimination to determine which information is *most* important.
Content Area: Adult Health
Integrated Processes: Nursing Process: Assessment
Client Need: Physiological Integrity
Cognitive Level: Application
Reference: *Williams, L., and Hopper, P. (2011). Understanding Medical-Surgical Nursing (4th ed.). Philadelphia, PA: F. A. Davis.*

7. ANSWER: 3.
Rationale:
1. Although the respiratory rate may be affected by FVD, it would not reveal the client's fluid status as precisely as decreased blood pressure.
2. Although temperature may be affected by FVD, it would not reveal the client's fluid status as precisely as decreased blood pressure.
3. **To best determine the client's fluid status, the nurse should assess the blood pressure. The client has signs and symptoms of FVD (nausea, vomiting, and diarrhea for 3 days; dry oral mucosa; amber urine; and decreased skin turgor). A decrease in blood pressure is the best indicator of FVD related to a lack of circulating vascular volume.**
4. Pulse oximetry should not be affected by the client's fluid status.
TEST-TAKING TIP: Key words are "to best determine the client's current fluid status." Consider each option, and select the most sensitive indicator of fluid status.
Content Area: Older Adult Health
Integrated Processes: Nursing Process: Assessment
Client Need: Physiological Integrity
Cognitive Level: Application
Reference: *Williams, L., and Hopper, P. (2011). Understanding Medical-Surgical Nursing (4th ed.). Philadelphia, PA: F. A. Davis.*

8. ANSWER: 4.
Rationale:
1. An increase in serum osmolarity would trigger the client's thirst sensation and may be a result of hemorrhage, but it would not affect urine output.
2. A decrease in the client's ADH level would prompt an increase in urine output, not a decrease.
3. Activation of atrial natriuretic factor would prompt an increase in urine output, not a decrease.
4. **The nurse should identify that the most likely reason for oliguria in a client admitted with FVD caused by severe blood loss is activation of the renin-angiotensin-aldosterone mechanism due to a decrease in the client's blood pressure.**
TEST-TAKING TIP: Review the pathophysiology related to FVD if you had difficulty answering this question.
Content Area: Adult Health
Integrated Processes: Nursing Process: Analysis
Client Need: Physiological Integrity
Cognitive Level: Application
Reference: *Williams, L., and Hopper, P. (2011). Understanding Medical-Surgical Nursing (4th ed.). Philadelphia, PA: F. A. Davis.*

9. ANSWER: 3.
Rationale:
1. Although the toddler is at increased risk for FVD, this client is not at greatest risk for FVD.
2. The adolescent playing outside in warm weather would lose fluid but should be able to compensate with adequate intake and is not at greatest risk for FVD.
3. **The nurse should identify the client with moderate diarrhea as being at greatest risk for FVD because he or she is losing fluid and electrolytes with each stool.**
4. Although the older adult with hypertension is at increased risk for FVD, this individual is not at greatest risk for FVD.
TEST-TAKING TIP: Key words are "greatest risk for FVD." Recall the conditions that place a client at risk for FVD and compare them with the conditions that actually cause FVD.
Content Area: Adult Health
Integrated Processes: Nursing Process: Analysis
Client Need: Physiological Integrity
Cognitive Level: Application
Reference: *Williams, L., and Hopper, P. (2011). Understanding Medical-Surgical Nursing (4th ed.). Philadelphia, PA: F. A. Davis.*

10. ANSWER: 1.
Rationale:
1. **The nurse should identify a urine output of 20 mL/hr as indicative of FVD. The minimal urine output for an adult client is 30 mL/hr, and the average urine output is 35 to 40 mL/hr. Dehydration should be considered in any adult with a urine output of less than 30 mL/hr.**

2. For an adult client, 40 mL/hr is within the range of average hourly urine output and is not associated with the development of FVD.
3. For an adult client, 60 mL/hr is a greater than average hourly urine output and is not associated with the development of FVD.
4. For an adult client, 80 mL/hr is a greater than average hourly urine output and is not associated with the development of FVD.
TEST-TAKING TIP: Recall that the signs of FVD include a decrease in blood pressure, an increase in heart rate and respiratory rate, and a decrease in urine output.
Content Area: Adult Health
Integrated Processes: Nursing Process: Assessment
Client Need: Physiological Integrity
Cognitive Level: Application
Reference: *Williams, L., and Hopper, P. (2011). Understanding Medical-Surgical Nursing (4th ed.). Philadelphia, PA: F. A. Davis.*

11. ANSWER: 2.
Rationale:
1. The diastolic blood pressure would also decrease, not increase, in FVD, although not as noticeably as the systolic blood pressure.
2. The nurse should associate a decrease in systolic blood pressure with the development of FVD. The systolic blood pressure decreases as a direct result of FVD.
3. Korotkoff sounds (the sounds heard through a stethoscope when taking a client's blood pressure) would become less prominent or remain unchanged in FVD, depending on the severity of the deficit.
4. Pulse pressure, the difference in the systolic and diastolic blood pressures, narrows in FVD.
TEST-TAKING TIP: Select the option that is a sign of FVD. Rule out the other options, which are signs of FVE.
Content Area: Adult Health
Integrated Processes: Nursing Process: Analysis
Client Need: Physiological Integrity
Cognitive Level: Application
Reference: *Ignatavicius, D., and Workman, M. (2012). Medical-Surgical Nursing: Patient-Centered Collaborative Care (7th ed.). St. Louis, MO: Saunders.*

12. ANSWER: 1.
Rationale:
1. The nurse's first action should be to weigh the client. Weight is the best indicator of fluid balance in the body.
2. An IV infusion may be needed, depending on the degree of FVD, but the priority intervention is to assess for FVD and determine whether IV or oral rehydration is indicated.
3. Administration of an oral electrolyte solution is inappropriate at this time because the client is vomiting. The cause of vomiting must be addressed before oral fluids can be tolerated.
4. Administration of an antidiarrheal may be indicated, but the priority intervention is the assessment component.
TEST-TAKING TIP: Remember to use the nursing process, which involves assessing the client before performing interventions. Weighing the client is part of the nursing assessment.
Content Area: Adult Health
Integrated Processes: Nursing Process: Implementation
Client Need: Physiological Integrity
Cognitive Level: Application
Reference: *Williams, L., and Hopper, P. (2011). Understanding Medical-Surgical Nursing (4th ed.). Philadelphia, PA: F. A. Davis.*

13. ANSWER: 2.
Rationale:
1. Vanilla ice cream is not included in a clear liquid diet. It may be included in a full liquid diet.
2. The nurse should offer the client ginger ale as part of a clear liquid diet. A clear liquid diet includes water, tea, coffee, clear broths, strained or clear juices (usually apple, grape, or cranberry juice), popsicles, ginger ale or other carbonated beverages, and plain gelatin. "Clear" does not mean "colorless."
3. Cream soup is not included in a clear liquid diet. It may be included in a full liquid diet.
4. Carnation Instant Breakfast is not included in a clear liquid diet. It may be included in a full liquid diet.
TEST-TAKING TIP: Consider each option, and rule out foods and beverages that are not clear (i.e., items you cannot see through).
Content Area: Adult Health
Integrated Processes: Nursing Process: Implementation
Client Need: Physiological Integrity
Cognitive Level: Application
Reference: *Berman, A., Snyder, S., Kozier, B., and Erb, G. (2012). Kozier & Erb's Fundamentals of Nursing: Concepts, Process, and Practice (9th ed.). Upper Saddle River, NJ: Pearson.*

14. ANSWER: 3.
Rationale:
1. Weighing twice a day is not advised because weight fluctuates throughout the day.
2. Weighing 1 hour before meals is not advised because mealtimes may vary from day to day, and the results may be unreliable.
3. The nurse should instruct clients to weigh themselves using the same scale, at the same time each day (usually in the morning), after urinating (to disregard the amount of fluid in the bladder and colon, because this weight does not reflect fluid status), and wearing the same amount of clothing.
4. Weighing after breakfast is not advised because mealtimes may vary from day to day, and the results may be unreliable.
TEST-TAKING TIP: Read each option carefully and select the one that best reduces the variables that might affect the client's weight.
Content Area: Adult Health
Integrated Processes: Teaching/Learning
Client Need: Health Promotion and Maintenance
Cognitive Level: Application
Reference: *Williams, L., and Hopper, P. (2011). Understanding Medical-Surgical Nursing (4th ed.). Philadelphia, PA: F. A. Davis.*

15. ANSWER: 4.
Rationale:
1. Explaining the rationale for increasing the fluid intake would not ensure that a confused client receives the appropriate amount of fluid to meet needs.
2. Ensuring that the certified nursing assistant maintains fresh ice water at the client's bedside at all times is

important but does not guarantee that a confused client will ingest the desired amount.
3. Providing fluids at the client's bedside, at the desired temperature, and at all times is important but does not guarantee that a confused client will ingest the desired amount.
4. The nurse should plan to assist the confused client in drinking fluids every hour to ensure that he or she gets the daily recommended fluid intake. Assistance includes reminders to drink and helping the client in the process of drinking.
TEST-TAKING TIP: Key words are "confused client," indicating the need for additional help.
Content Area: Adult Health
Integrated Processes: Nursing Process: Planning
Client Need: Physiological Integrity
Cognitive Level: Application
***Reference:** Williams, L., and Hopper, P. (2011). Understanding Medical-Surgical Nursing (4th ed.). Philadelphia, PA: F. A. Davis.*

16. ANSWER: 1.
Rationale:
1. To measure fluid intake, the nurse should record each fluid item taken in by the client, including oral fluids, ice chips, foods that are liquid or tend to become a liquid at room temperature, tube feedings, parenteral fluids, IV medications, and catheter or tube irrigation fluids.
2. Bladder irrigating fluid should be recorded as intake, not deducted from the client's urine output.
3. Bladder irrigating fluid should be recorded as intake, not subtracted from the IV intake.
4. Bladder irrigating fluid should be recorded as intake, not output. To measure fluid output, measure and record urine output; vomitus and liquid feces; and drainage, such as gastric or intestinal tube drainage, wound drainage, and draining fistulas.
TEST-TAKING TIP: Read each option carefully and use the process of elimination to rule out incorrect answers.
Content Area: Adult Health
Integrated Processes: Nursing Process: Implementation
Client Need: Physiological Integrity
Cognitive Level: Application
***Reference:** Berman, A., Snyder, S., Kozier, B., and Erb, G. (2012). Kozier & Erb's Fundamentals of Nursing: Concepts, Process, and Practice (9th ed.). Upper Saddle River, NJ: Pearson.*

17. ANSWER: 3.
Rationale:
1. Wound drainage should be added to the client's total output, not intake. To measure fluid intake, the nurse should record each fluid item consumed by the client on the intake and output form; this includes oral fluids, ice chips, foods that are liquid or tend to become a liquid at room temperature, tube feedings, parenteral fluids, IV medications, and catheter or tube irrigation fluids.
2. Wound drainage should be added to, not subtracted from, total output.
3. To measure fluid output, the nurse should measure and record urine output; vomitus and liquid feces; and drainage, such as gastric or intestinal tube drainage, wound drainage, and draining fistulas.
4. Wound drainage should be added to total output, not subtracted from oral intake.
TEST-TAKING TIP: Recall that wound drainage is included in the client's output, eliminating options 1 and 4.
Content Area: Adult Health
Integrated Processes: Nursing Process: Implementation
Client Need: Physiological Integrity
Cognitive Level: Application
***Reference:** Berman, A., Snyder, S., Kozier, B., and Erb, G. (2012). Kozier & Erb's Fundamentals of Nursing: Concepts, Process, and Practice (9th ed.). Upper Saddle River, NJ: Pearson.*

18. ANSWER: 1.
Rationale:
1. The nurse should instruct the new mother to maintain an adequate fluid intake to reduce the risk of FVD developing in her breastfeeding infant. The mother's fluid intake must be adequate to maintain milk production. Her level of thirst is the best indicator of fluid consumption.
2. Newborns typically nurse every 2 to 3 hours, which helps maintain the supply of breast milk. Limiting breastfeeding to every 4 hours could increase the newborn's risk of FVD.
3. Maternal caloric intake should not be decreased; 1,800 kcal/day is required during lactation.
4. Feeding from one or both breasts should not affect the newborn's hydration.
TEST-TAKING TIP: Read each option carefully and use the process of elimination to rule out incorrect responses.
Content Area: Maternal Health
Integrated Processes: Teaching/Learning
Client Need: Health Promotion and Maintenance
Cognitive Level: Application
***Reference:** Lowdermilk, D. L., Perry, S. E., Cashion, K., and Alden, K. R. (2010). Maternity and Women's Health Care (10thed.). St. Louis, MO: Mosby.*

19. ANSWER: 25.
Rationale:

2,500 gm = 2.5 kg

2.5 kg (given weight) × 10 mL (volume ordered) =
25 mL PRBCs to be infused

TEST-TAKING TIP: Recall that there are 1,000 kg in 1 gm.
Content Area: Child Health
Integrated Processes: Nursing Process: Implementation
Client Need: Physiological Integrity
Cognitive Level: Application
***Reference:** Beaman, N. (2008). Pharmacology Clear and Simple: A Drug Classifications and Dosage Calculations Approach. Philadelphia, PA: F. A. Davis.*

20. ANSWER: 48.5.
Rationale: If the infant eats every 4 hours, there will be three feedings in a 12-hour period.

140 mL (minimum amount) ÷ 3 (number of feedings) =
48.5 mL every 4 hours

TEST-TAKING TIP: Read the question carefully. There are three 4-hour periods in 12 hours.
Content Area: Child Health
Integrated Processes: Nursing Process: Implementation
Client Need: Physiological Integrity
Cognitive Level: Application

Reference: *Beaman, N. (2008). Pharmacology Clear and Simple: A Drug Classifications and Dosage Calculations Approach. Philadelphia, PA: F. A. Davis.*

21. ANSWER: 3 mL/kg.

Rationale:

$$11 \text{ lb} \div 2.2 \text{ lb/kg} = 5 \text{ kg}$$

$$[180 \text{ mL (volume excreted)} \div 5 \text{ kg (current weight)}] \div 12 \text{ hr} = 3 \text{ mL/kg/hr}$$

TEST-TAKING TIP: Be sure to convert an infant's weight to kilograms before performing medication calculations.
Content Area: Child Health
Integrated Processes: Nursing Process: Implementation
Client Need: Physiological Integrity
Cognitive Level: Application
Reference: *Beaman, N. (2008). Pharmacology Clear and Simple: A Drug Classifications and Dosage Calculations Approach. Philadelphia, PA: F. A. Davis.*

22. ANSWER: 1.

Rationale:

1. **The nurse should plan to administer an isotonic IV solution because hypotonic IV solutions (e.g., 0.25% sodium chloride, 0.5% sodium chloride, dextrose 5% in water) are contraindicated in clients with acute brain injuries. Cerebral cells are more sensitive to swelling than the cells of other tissues, and hypotonic solutions shift fluid out of the intravascular space and into the intracellular space, causing cerebral cell edema.**
2. In clients with acute brain injuries, 0.25% saline solution is contraindicated because it is a hypotonic solution.
3. In clients with acute brain injuries, 0.5% saline solution is contraindicated because it is a hypotonic solution.
4. In clients with acute brain injuries, dextrose 5% in water is contraindicated because it is a hypotonic solution.

TEST-TAKING TIP: Know which IV solutions are hypotonic, isotonic, and hypertonic and the indications for the administration of each.
Content Area: Adult Health
Integrated Processes: Nursing Process: Planning
Client Need: Physiological Integrity
Cognitive Level: Application
Reference: *Ignatavicius, D., and Workman, M. (2012). Medical-Surgical Nursing: Patient-Centered Collaborative Care (7th ed.). St. Louis, MO: Saunders.*

23. ANSWER: 1.

Rationale:

1. **When assessing a client for FVD, it is most important for the nurse to obtain the client's vital signs. Although skin turgor, thirst level, and renal function are important when assessing a client with FVD, vital signs are most important to direct the course of therapy and assess for cardiovascular and respiratory manifestations of dehydration.**
2. Although skin turgor is an important assessment for a client with FVD, vital sign assessment is the most important.
3. Although thirst level is an important assessment for a client with FVD, vital sign assessment is the most important.
4. Although BUN and creatinine are important assessments for a client with FVD, vital sign assessment is the most important.

TEST-TAKING TIP: Recall that the most accurate method of assessing fluid volume status is to monitor the client's vital signs and body weight.
Content Area: Adult Health
Integrated Processes: Nursing Process: Assessment
Client Need: Physiological Integrity
Cognitive Level: Application
Reference: *Ignatavicius, D., and Workman, M. (2012). Medical-Surgical Nursing: Patient-Centered Collaborative Care (7th ed.). St. Louis, MO: Saunders.*

24. ANSWER: 4.

Rationale:

1. An increased, not a decreased, pulse rate is associated with FVD.
2. Clients with isotonic and hypotonic dehydration with plasma volume deficits show hemoconcentration, or an increased hemoglobin level and hematocrit; decreased hemoglobin and hematocrit values may be indicative of hemorrhage or FVE.
3. Jugular venous distention would be present with FVE, not FVD.
4. **The nurse should associate a blood pressure of 96/54 mm Hg with a nursing diagnosis of Deficient Fluid Volume Secondary to Dehydration. Common manifestations of dehydration include increased pulse rate, thready pulse, and decreased blood pressure.**

TEST-TAKING TIP: Select the option that is most indicative of FVD.
Content Area: Adult Health
Integrated Processes: Nursing Process: Assessment
Client Need: Physiological Integrity
Cognitive Level: Application
Reference: *Ignatavicius, D., and Workman, M. (2012). Medical-Surgical Nursing: Patient-Centered Collaborative Care (7th ed.). St. Louis, MO: Saunders.*

25. ANSWER: 3.

Rationale:

1. Asking the client about sunscreen does not help assess the cause of the client's symptoms.
2. Assessing thirst in an older adult client is unreliable because the thirst mechanism may be compromised in older adult clients.
3. **Asking the client about the time of day and the length of time spent gardening is correct because it is important to ask specific questions about activities and environmental conditions that may contribute to dehydration.**
4. It would be important to create a plan to address the possibility of the client experiencing syncope after the client is stabilized, but not at the time of the initial assessment.

TEST-TAKING TIP: Recall that older adult clients are at increased risk for FVD because they have less total body water than younger adults.
Content Area: Older Adult Health
Integrated Processes: Nursing Process: Analysis
Client Need: Physiological Integrity
Cognitive Level: Application
Reference: *Ignatavicius, D., and Workman, M. (2012). Medical-Surgical Nursing: Patient-Centered Collaborative Care (7th ed.). St. Louis, MO: Saunders.*

26. ANSWER: 2
Rationale:
1. Although a client with third spacing may eventually exhibit weight gain and FVE as a result of third spacing, the primary problem is the FVD that results from a decrease in the ECF volume.
2. When caring for a client with liver failure, dry skin, and dry mucous membranes, the priority nursing diagnosis should be Deficient Fluid Volume Related to Third Spacing Fluid Shifts Secondary to Liver Failure. Although a client with third spacing may eventually exhibit weight gain and FVE as a result of third spacing, the primary problem is the FVD that results from a decrease in the ECF volume.
3. Risk for decreased cardiac output is a potential problem, not an actual problem, and should not be the priority.
4. Risk for shock is a potential problem, not an actual problem, and should not be the priority.
TEST-TAKING TIP: Rule out "Risk for ..." diagnoses when prioritizing nursing diagnoses. Actual problems always take priority over potential problems.
Content Area: Adult Health
Integrated Processes: Nursing Process: Analysis
Client Need: Physiological Integrity
Cognitive Level: Application
Reference: *Ignatavicius, D., and Workman, M. (2012). Medical-Surgical Nursing: Patient-Centered Collaborative Care (7th ed.). St. Louis, MO: Saunders.*

27. ANSWER: 2.
Rationale:
1. A client with FVD should receive fluids hourly, not just with meals.
2. The nurse should include monitoring for an increase in body temperature when caring for a client with FVD because an increase in temperature can exacerbate FVD. Fever greater than 100.5°F (38°C) should be treated to decrease insensible fluid loss.
3. Diuretics are usually withheld in a client with FVD.
4. Crackles and orthopnea are signs of FVE, not FVD.
TEST-TAKING TIP: Rule out options contraindicated in FVD or associated with FVE.
Content Area: Adult Health
Integrated Processes: Nursing Process: Planning
Client Need: Physiological Integrity
Cognitive Level: Application
Reference: *Williams, L., and Hopper, P. (2011). Understanding Medical-Surgical Nursing (4th ed.). Philadelphia, PA: F. A. Davis.*

28. ANSWER: 4.
Rationale:
1. The hypotonic 0.45% saline solution is not appropriate in this situation.
2. The hypotonic 0.25% saline solution is not appropriate in this situation.
3. The isotonic 0.9% saline solution is not appropriate in this situation.
4. The nurse should anticipate an order for 3% saline solution. Clients experiencing both FVD and hyponatremia require the replacement of both fluid and electrolytes, specifically sodium. This replacement is achieved with an IV infusion of a hypertonic solution. The only hypertonic solution among the options is 3% saline.
TEST-TAKING TIP: Recall that human plasma has approximately the same tonicity as 0.9% normal saline solution. To correct hyponatremia, a health-care provider would need to order an IV solution containing more sodium than normal saline, or a hypertonic solution.
Content Area: Adult Health
Integrated Processes: Nursing Process: Planning
Client Need: Physiological Integrity
Cognitive Level: Application
Reference: *Wilkinson, J., and Treas, L. (2010). Fundamentals of Nursing: Theory, Concepts & Applications (2nd ed.). Philadelphia, PA: F. A. Davis.*

29. ANSWER: 3.
Rationale:
1. Oral replacement therapy is not the appropriate treatment for severe FVD.
2. Monitoring the infant's output is not the appropriate treatment for severe FVD.
3. The nurse should instruct the parent to bring the infant to the pediatrician or emergency department because this infant is exhibiting signs of significant FVD. Infants and toddlers are at higher risk than adults for FVD. Water and electrolyte disturbances in children occur more frequently and more quickly and take longer to treat. Parents should be taught the importance of reporting early signs and symptoms of dehydration to a physician or other health-care provider.
4. It is unnecessary to withhold all oral intake until vomiting has resolved because the infant may be able to absorb some portion of the oral fluid.
TEST-TAKING TIP: Recall that infants are at increased risk for FVD because of their higher percentage of total body water.
Content Area: Child Health
Integrated Processes: Nursing Process: Implementation
Client Need: Physiological Integrity
Cognitive Level: Application
Reference: *Williams, L., and Hopper, P. (2011). Understanding Medical-Surgical Nursing (4th ed.). Philadelphia, PA: F. A. Davis.*

30. ANSWER: 3, 4, 1, 5, 2.
Rationale: Orthostatic, or postural, hypotension is determined by measuring the blood pressure and pulse rate first in the supine position, then in the sitting position, and finally in the standing position. A significant change in both blood pressure and pulse rate signifies hypovolemia or dehydration. A positive result occurs if the client becomes dizzy or loses consciousness or if the pulse rate increases by 20 bpm or more and the systolic blood pressure decreases by 20 mm Hg within 3 minutes of changing from supine to sitting or from sitting to standing.
TEST-TAKING TIP: Review the procedure for assessing orthostatic hypotension.
Content Area: Adult Health
Integrated Processes: Nursing Process: Implementation
Client Need: Physiological Integrity
Cognitive Level: Application
Reference: *Wilkinson, J., and Treas, L. (2010). Fundamentals of Nursing: Theory, Concepts & Applications (2nd ed.). Philadelphia, PA: F. A. Davis.*

31. ANSWER: 2.

Rationale:

1. A urine output of 500 mL/day or 20 mL/hr indicates that FVD has already occurred in this client; it is not in the process of developing.

2. The nurse should associate a urine output of 700 mL/day or 29 mL/hr with the development of FVD. The minimal urine output for an adult client is 30 mL/hr; the average urine output is 35 to 40 mL/hr, which equals 840 to 960 mL/day.

3. A urine output of 1,680 mL/day or 70 mL/hr is within normal limits for an adult client.

4. A urine output of 2,400 mL/day or 100 mL/hr is within normal limits for an adult client.

TEST-TAKING TIP: Read the question carefully. Recall that the minimum urine output for an adult client is 30 mL/hr.

Content Area: Adult Health

Integrated Processes: Nursing Process: Analysis

Client Need: Physiological Integrity

Cognitive Level: Application

Reference: Williams, L., and Hopper, P. (2011). Understanding Medical-Surgical Nursing (4th ed.). Philadelphia, PA: F. A. Davis.

32. ANSWER: 2,100.

Rationale: Adults need a minimum of 30 mL/kg/day of fluid.

70 kg × 30 mL= 2,100 mL/day (24-hour period) to meet the minimum requirement.

TEST-TAKING TIP: Recall that the minimum fluid intake for an adult client is 30 mL/kg/day.

Content Area: Adult Health; Category of Health Alteration: Fluid Volume Deficit

Integrated Processes: Nursing Process: Planning

Client Need: Physiological Integrity: Basic Care and Comfort: Nutrition and Oral Hydration

Cognitive Level: Application

Reference: Williams, L., and Hopper, P. (2011). Understanding Medical-Surgical Nursing (4th ed.). Philadelphia, PA: F. A. Davis.

33. ANSWER: 2.

Rationale:

1. Hypertonic fluids should be avoided in a client who needs to replace both fluids and electrolytes because they can cause cellular dehydration as fluid shifts from cells.

2. The nurse should anticipate orders for an isotonic IV solution. A client with hyperemesis gravidarum needs to replace both fluid and electrolytes. Isotonic fluids are typically administered in this case.

3. Hypotonic fluids should be avoided in a client who needs to replace both fluids and electrolytes because they will not adequately replace losses.

4. "Atonic" is not a type of IV fluid; it is a term that refers to the loss or lack of normal muscle tone or strength, as in atonic uterus.

TEST-TAKING TIP: Consider each type of IV fluid and visualize how each solution affects the movement of fluids and electrolytes into and out of the cells.

Content Area: Maternal Health

Integrated Processes: Nursing Process: Planning

Client Need: Physiological Integrity

Cognitive Level: Application

Reference: Venes, D., et al (Eds.). (2013). Taber's Cyclopedic Medical Dictionary (22nd ed.). Philadelphia, PA: F. A. Davis.

34. ANSWER: 2, 3, 4, 6.

Rationale:

1. Normal saline is an isotonic solution used to increase intravascular volume, but it does not cause fluid to shift back into the cells, where it is needed in this client diagnosed with FVD secondary to DKA.

2. The nurse should identify dextrose 5% in water as an appropriate IV solution for this client. Clients with DKA are hyperglycemic (blood glucose greater than 300 mg/dL). The elevated serum glucose pulls fluid out of the cells and into the vascular and interstitial compartments, causing cellular dehydration. *Hypotonic* solutions, such as dextrose 5% in water, dextrose 5% in normal saline, and 0.45% saline, pull fluid from the intravascular and interstitial compartments into the cells, correcting the imbalance. Hypotonic fluids must be administered slowly, however, to prevent a sudden fluid shift from the intravascular space into the cells. Dextrose solutions are often avoided in clients with DKA because the blood sugar is already elevated, but they may be used when the client is NPO and receiving a high insulin dose.

3. The hypotonic solution dextrose 5% in normal saline is an appropriate IV solution for this client.

4. The hypotonic solution 0.45% saline is an appropriate IV solution for this client.

5. The hypertonic solution 3% sodium chloride pulls fluid out of the cells and into the intravascular and interstitial spaces, which would worsen cellular dehydration in a client with DKA.

6. Lactated Ringer's solution (which produces bicarbonate when metabolized in the liver) may be used to counteract the client's acidotic state and to replace needed electrolytes.

TEST-TAKING TIP: Consider each type of IV fluid, identify the type of solution, and visualize how each solution affects the movement of fluids and electrolytes into and out of the cells.

Content Area: Adult Health

Integrated Processes: Nursing Process: Planning

Client Need: Physiological Integrity

Cognitive Level: Application

Reference: Wilkinson, J., and Treas, L. (2010). Fundamentals of Nursing:T heory, Concepts & Applications(2nd ed.). Philadelphia, PA: F. A. Davis.

35. ANSWER: 1, 6.

Rationale:

1. The nurse should identify normal saline solution and lactated Ringer's solution as appropriate for this client. Clients who are hypovolemic require fluid replacement with isotonic solutions such as normal saline solution and lactated Ringer's solution, which are similar in osmolarity to blood serum and remain in the intravascular space, increasing intravascular volume.

2. The hypotonic solution dextrose 5% in water is not an appropriate choice for a client with hypovolemia because it

would promote the movement of fluid from the intravascular and interstitial compartments into the cells; this could create an excess of cellular fluid and would not correct the hypovolemia.
3. The hypertonic solution dextrose 5% in normal saline is not an appropriate choice for a client with hypovolemia because it would pull fluid from the cells into the intravascular and interstitial compartments, worsening the client's fluid imbalance.
4. The hypotonic solution 0.45% saline is not an appropriate choice for a client with hypovolemia because it would promote the movement of fluid from the intravascular and interstitial compartments into the cells; this could create an excess of cellular fluid and would not correct the hypovolemia.
5. The hypertonic solution 3% sodium chloride is not an appropriate choice for a client with hypovolemia because it would pull fluid from the cells into the intravascular and interstitial compartments, worsening the client's fluid imbalance on the cellular level.
6. The nurse should identify normal saline solution and lactated Ringer's solution as appropriate for this client. Clients who are hypovolemic require fluid replacement with isotonic solutions such as normal saline solution and lactated Ringer's solution, which are similar in osmolarity to blood serum and remain in the intravascular space, increasing intravascular volume.
TEST-TAKING TIP: Recall that hypovolemia simply means that there is decreased volume in the intravascular compartment.
Content Area: Adult Health
Integrated Processes: Nursing Process: Planning
Client Need: Physiological Integrity
Cognitive Level: Application
Reference: *Wilkinson, J., and Treas, L. (2010). Fundamentals of Nursing: Theory, Concepts & Applications(2nd ed.). Philadelphia, PA: F. A. Davis.*

36. ANSWER: 2, 3, 5.
Rationale:
1. Orange juice is appropriate for a full liquid diet, not a clear liquid diet.
2. The nurse should include diet ginger ale as part of the client's clear liquid diet. A clear liquid diet includes water, tea, coffee, clear broths, strained or clear juices (usually apple, grape, or cranberry juice), popsicles, ginger ale or other carbonated beverages, and plain gelatin. "Clear" does not mean "colorless."
3. The nurse should include chicken bouillon as part of the client's clear liquid diet.
4. Chicken noodle soup, although primarily liquid, also contains solid food (noodles and possibly chicken), making it inappropriate for a liquid diet.
5. The nurse should include grape juice as part of the client's clear liquid diet.
TEST-TAKING TIP: Recall that clear liquids are transparent but not necessarily colorless.
Content Area: Adult Health
Integrated Processes: Nursing Process: Planning
Client Need: Physiological Integrity
Cognitive Level: Application
Reference: *Berman, A., Snyder, S., Kozier, B., and Erb, G. (2012). Kozier & Erb's Fundamentals of Nursing: Concepts, Process, and Practice (9th ed.). Upper Saddle River, NJ: Pearson*

37. ANSWER: Intake: 1,920 mL; Output: 1,275 mL.
Rationale: To calculate intake and output, add oral and IV intake, remembering that 0700 to 1900 includes 12 hours of IV fluid infusion; then total all measurable output, remembering that the client has experienced two episodes of emesis for a total of 200 mL, plus stool and urine.
TEST-TAKING TIP: Remember to include stool and emesis when calculating output.
Content Area: Adult Health
Integrated Processes: Nursing Process: Analysis
Client Need: Physiological Integrity
Cognitive Level: Application
Reference: *Beaman, N. (2008). Pharmacology Clear and Simple: A Drug Classifications and Dosage Calculations Approach. Philadelphia, PA: F. A. Davis.*

38. ANSWER: 2, 3.
Rationale:
1. Because this client needs replacement of both fluid and electrolytes, an isotonic fluid would be administered; 0.45% saline is a hypotonic solution.
2. The nurse should identify 0.9% saline (normal saline) solution as appropriate for this client, who needs replacement of both fluid and electrolytes. Isotonic fluids are typically administered in this situation.
3. The nurse should identify lactated Ringer's solution as appropriate for this client, who needs replacement of both fluid and electrolytes. Isotonic fluids are typically administered in this situation.
4. Dextrose 5% in normal saline is a hypertonic solution. Although hypertonic solutions contain a large amount of electrolytes, they are not the first choice for routine fluid replacement in a client with losses secondary to vomiting.
5. Dextrose 5% in lactated Ringer's solution is a hypertonic solution. Although hypertonic solutions contain a large amount of electrolytes, they are not the first choice for routine fluid replacement in a client with losses secondary to vomiting.
6. Albumin is a hypertonic solution. Although hypertonic solutions contain a large amount of electrolytes, they are not the first choice for routine fluid replacement in a client with losses secondary to vomiting.
TEST-TAKING TIP: Memorize which IV solutions are isotonic, hypotonic, and hypertonic to determine which solutions are appropriate or inappropriate for clients.
Content Area: Adult Health
Integrated Processes: Nursing Process: Analysis
Client Need: Physiological Integrity
Cognitive Level: Application
Reference: *Williams, L., and Hopper, P. (2011). Understanding Medical-Surgical Nursing (4th ed.). Philadelphia, PA: F. A. Davis.*

39. ANSWER: 2.
Rationale:
1. Because older adults have decreased skin elasticity, especially in the hands and arms, skin turgor is usually assessed over the sternum or clavicle in these clients; the forehead is also a reliable location to assess skin turgor.

2. For a young adult client, the nurse should plan to assess skin turgor over the client's sternum, clavicle, or dorsal aspect of the hand and lower forearm. To assess skin turgor, the nurse gently pinches up the skin in an unexposed area, noting how quickly it returns to the original position when released.
3. In infants, skin turgor is assessed over the abdomen.
4. The thigh is not routinely used to assess skin turgor in clients of any age.
TEST-TAKING TIP: When selecting a site to assess skin turgor, consider the age and physical characteristics of the client.
Content Area: Adult Health
Integrated Processes: Nursing Process: Assessment
Client Need: Physiological Integrity
Cognitive Level: Application
Reference: *Wilkinson, J., and Treas, L. (2010). Fundamentals of Nursing: Theory, Concepts & Applications(2nd ed.). Philadelphia, PA: F. A. Davis.*

40. ANSWER: 4.
Rationale:
1. The vascular space is part of the ECF and would be expected to increase with the IV infusion, not decrease.
2. The infusion of a hypotonic solution would result in hyponatremia, not hypernatremia, as a result of the dilutional effect of the increased fluids.
3. Increased urine output would be an expected side effect.
4. In a client receiving a hypotonic IV solution, the nurse should plan to monitor for mental status changes. Cerebral cells are especially sensitive to fluid gains from hypotonic IV solutions. If the solution is infused too rapidly, the cerebral cells will be the first to swell, resulting in neurological changes.
TEST-TAKING TIP: Review the effects of hypotonic IV solutions.
Content Area: Adult Health
Integrated Processes: Nursing Process: Analysis
Client Need: Physiological Integrity
Cognitive Level: Application
Reference: *Ignatavicius, D., and Workman, M. (2012). Medical-Surgical Nursing: Patient-Centered Collaborative Care (7th ed.). St. Louis, MO: Saunders.*

41. ANSWER: 4.
Rationale:
1. An increase in blood pressure (140/70 mm Hg) and respiratory rate (24) with a high-normal pulse rate (96 bpm) would be indicative of FVE, not FVD.
2. A normal blood pressure (110/80 mm Hg), normal pulse rate (84 bpm), and increased respiratory rate (24) are not indicative of a fluid imbalance. The increased respiratory rate would need to be evaluated further to determine its cause.
3. A low-normal blood pressure (100/70 mm Hg), low-normal pulse rate (60 bpm), and normal respiratory rate (20) are not indicative of a fluid imbalance.
4. The nurse should recognize a decrease in blood pressure (80/60 mm Hg) and an increase in pulse rate (110 bpm) as indicative of FVD. In adults, the normal accepted range for systolic blood pressure is 100 to 120 mm Hg; for diastolic blood pressure it is 60 to 80 mm Hg. The normal resting heart rate in adults ranges from 60 to 100 bpm. The normal respiratory rate in adults ranges from 12 to 20 breaths per minute.
TEST-TAKING TIP: Recall that signs of FVD include a decrease in blood pressure, an increase in heart rate and respiratory rate, and a decrease in urine output.
Content Area: Adult Health
Integrated Processes: Nursing Process: Assessment
Client Need: Physiological Integrity
Cognitive Level: Analysis
Reference: *Wilkinson, J., and Treas, L. (2011). Fundamentals of Nursing:Theory, Concepts &Applications(2nd ed.). Philadelphia, PA: F. A. Davis.*

42. ANSWER: 2.
Rationale:
1. Jugular venous distention indicates that fluid resuscitation has been too aggressive and the client is now experiencing FVE, an undesired effect of IV therapy.
2. The nurse should associate a urine output of 50 mL/hr with effective IV fluid replacement therapy. Urine output in a client without kidney disease should equal at least 30 mL/hr; 50 mL/hr reflects adequate hydration.
3. A blood pressure of 90/60 mm Hg indicates that the client's circulating volume is still decreased, given that average blood pressure in a healthy adult is 120/80 mm Hg.
4. A low-grade fever would be associated with ongoing FVD.
TEST-TAKING TIP: Select the option that describes a "normal" assessment finding.
Content Area: Adult Health
Integrated Processes: Nursing Process: Evaluation
Client Need: Physiological Integrity
Cognitive Level: Analysis
Reference: *Williams, L., and Hopper, P. (2011). Understanding Medical-Surgical Nursing (4th ed.). Philadelphia, PA: F. A. Davis.*

43. ANSWER: 2.
Rationale:
1. Conducting neurological checks at least every hour is an appropriate order for a client with a closed head injury, multiple fractures, and blood loss. More frequent monitoring may be necessary in the acute phase of the injuries.
2. The nurse should question the order to obtain vital signs every 4 hours. Monitoring vital signs is an important intervention when caring for clients with fluid loss. Clients in the acute phase of FVD require continuous or hourly monitoring of vital signs.
3. IV normal saline at 150 mL/hr is an appropriate order for a client with a closed head injury, multiple fractures, and blood loss. Normal saline is an isotonic solution that replaces vascular volume. Blood products may also be used, depending on the severity of the blood loss.
4. Strict intake and output measurement is an appropriate order for a client with a closed head injury, multiple fractures, and blood loss. Monitoring intake and output provides crucial information about the client's fluid balance and kidney function.
TEST-TAKING TIP: Recognize that a client who has experienced blood loss is at risk for FVD and should be monitored closely.
Content Area: Adult Health
Integrated Processes: Nursing Process: Analysis

Client Need: Physiological Integrity
Cognitive Level: Analysis
Reference: *Ignatavicius, D., and Workman, M. (2012). Medical-Surgical Nursing: Patient-Centered Collaborative Care (7th ed.). St. Louis, MO: Saunders.*

44. ANSWER: 1, 2, 5.
Rationale:
1. When caring for a client with severe burns, the nurse should reason that intake would exceed output because this client would have vasoconstriction, increased insensible output, and third spacing. Vasoconstriction causes decreased renal perfusion and a decrease in urinary output. Third spacing occurs after initial vasoconstriction when blood vessels near the burn dilate and leak fluid into the interstitial space, increasing insensible loss. The amount of fluid shifted depends on the extent and severity of the injury.
2. When caring for a client with severe burns, the nurse should reason that intake would exceed output because this client would have vasoconstriction, increased insensible output, and third spacing. Vasoconstriction causes decreased renal perfusion and a decrease in urinary output. Third spacing occurs after initial vasoconstriction when blood vessels near the burn dilate and leak fluid into the interstitial space, increasing insensible loss. The amount of fluid shifted depends on the extent and severity of the injury.
3. A client with severe burns would be on strict intake and output measurement, including an indwelling urinary catheter and fecal containment system to reduce the risk of miscalculation owing to incorrect information or incontinence.
4. The management of severe burns may require massive amounts of fluid infusions, necessitating that the client be monitored for fluid overload throughout the healing phase. The question contains inadequate data to infer that the client has been dangerously overhydrated.
5. When caring for a client with severe burns, the nurse should reason that intake would exceed output because this client would have vasoconstriction, increased insensible output, and third spacing. Vasoconstriction causes decreased renal perfusion and a decrease in urinary output. Third spacing occurs after initial vasoconstriction when blood vessels near the burn dilate and leak fluid into the interstitial space, increasing insensible loss. The amount of fluid shifted depends on the extent and severity of the injury.
TEST-TAKING TIP: Recall that clients with severe burns are at risk for FVD related to vasoconstriction, third spacing, and increased insensible fluid loss.
Content Area: Adult Health
Integrated Processes: Nursing Process: Assessment
Client Need: Physiological Integrity
Cognitive Level: Analysis
Reference: *Ignatavicius, D., and Workman, M. (2012). Medical-Surgical Nursing: Patient-Centered Collaborative Care (7th ed.). St. Louis, MO: Saunders.*

45. ANSWER: 1, 3.
Rationale:
1. The nurse should associate dry oral mucosa with the development of FVD.
2. Hypertension is a sign of FVE, not FVD.
3. The nurse should associate hypotension with the development of FVD.
4. Jugular venous distention is a sign of FVE, not FVD.
5. Tachycardia is found in both FVD and FVE, but pulse strength is decreased in FVD and increased in FVE; 3+ represents increased pulse strength.
TEST-TAKING TIP: Differentiate manifestations of FVD from manifestations of FVE. Select only the options related to FVD.
Content Area: Adult Health
Integrated Processes: Nursing Process: Assessment
Client Need: Physiological Integrity
Cognitive Level: Analysis
Reference: *Wilkinson, J., and Treas, L. (2011). Fundamentals of Nursing: Theory, Concepts & Applications(2nd ed.). Philadelphia, PA: F. A. Davis.*

UNIT II

Electrolyte Imbalances

Chapter 3

Sodium and Chloride Imbalances

KEY TERMS

Chloride—Major anion in the extracellular fluid (ECF) that balances the concentration of fluid and solutes between the intracellular fluid (ICF) and the ECF; helps maintain proper blood volume, blood pressure, and pH of body fluids

Diaphoresis—Excessive sweating

Diuresis—Excessive urination

Euvolemic hypernatremia—Decreased total body water with near-normal total body sodium

Euvolemic hyponatremia—Increased total body water while sodium content remains the same; the ECF volume is increased minimally to moderately, but without the presence of edema

Hyperchloremia—Serum chloride (Cl^-) greater than 108 mEq/L; chloride excess

Hypernatremia—Serum sodium (Na^+) greater than 145 mEq/L; sodium excess

Hypervolemic hypernatremia—Increased sodium with normal or increased total body water

Hypervolemic hyponatremia—Increased total body sodium, with total body water increased to a greater extent; the ECF is increased markedly, with the presence of edema.

Hypochloremia—Serum chloride (Cl^-) less than 95 mEq/L; chloride deficit

Hyponatremia—Serum sodium (Na^+) less than 135 mEq/L; sodium deficit

Hypovolemic hypernatremia—Decreased total body water and sodium, with a relatively greater decrease in total body water

Hypovolemic hyponatremia—Decreased total body water, with total body sodium decreased to a greater extent; the ECF volume is decreased

I. Description

Sodium (Na^+) is the major **cation** in the extracellular fluid (ECF) and plays a significant role in fluid balance and the regulation of fluid volume. Sodium balance is regulated primarily by aldosterone and antidiuretic hormone (ADH), and sodium moves into and out of the cells via active transport across the cellular membrane. Sodium is obtained through the diet, is absorbed continuously by the intestines, and is excreted by the kidneys via the urine. When combined with chloride, the resulting substance is table salt. Sodium is found in most body secretions and performs the following functions:

1. Maintains blood volume and blood pressure
2. Is essential in the electrical transmission of nerve impulses
3. Helps maintain the acid-base balance of the blood
4. Is a vital component of the sodium-potassium pump, which keeps sodium outside the cells and potassium inside the cells

DID YOU KNOW?

The recommended daily intake of sodium is no more than 2.3 gm/day, the amount contained in slightly more than 1 teaspoon of table salt. Most Americans consume 4 to 6 gm of salt per day, which contributes to the development of hypertension and heart disease. Sodium is often "hidden" in processed foods, canned foods, seasonings, and medications such as antacids, cough syrups, and cold remedies.

Normal Lab Value The normal serum sodium level is 135 to 145 mEq/L (mmol/L).

II. Sodium Imbalance

Sodium imbalance occurs when there is a decrease or increase in the sodium content of the blood in relation to the amount of water in the body.

A. **Hyponatremia**, or sodium deficit, is a serum sodium level less than 135 mEq/L.
   1. Hyponatremia is the most common electrolyte imbalance in the United States.
   2. Onset may be sudden (acute) or gradual, but a sudden onset is more dangerous for clients. Signs and symptoms are usually not apparent until serum sodium levels decrease to less than 120 mEq/L.
      a. A rapid decline of serum sodium that occurs over less than 48 hours may cause symptoms at levels greater than 120 mEq/L.
      b. With a gradual decline of serum sodium that occurs over several days to weeks, levels may fall to 110 mEq/L with few symptoms.
   3. A decrease in serum sodium causes water to move *out of* the ECF and *into* the intracellular fluid (ICF), resulting in cellular edema, which reduces cell function and the transmission of impulses. Box 3.1 lists conditions that place clients at risk for hyponatremia.

B. **Hypernatremia**, or sodium excess, is a serum sodium level greater than 145 mEq/L.
   1. Hypernatremia is most common in older adults, who may have a decreased thirst sensation or may be unable to access fluids independently.
   2. Onset may be sudden or gradual, but a sudden onset is more dangerous for clients.
   3. An increase in serum sodium causes water to move *out of* the ICF and *into* the ECF, resulting in cellular dehydration and the stimulation or overstimulation of excitable cells.

Box 3.1 Conditions That Place Clients at Risk for Hyponatremia

- Nothing by mouth (NPO)
- Excessive diaphoresis (sweating)
- Diuretics
- Gastrointestinal suctioning
- Syndrome of inappropriate antidiuretic hormone secretion (SIADH)
- Excessive ingestion of hypotonic fluids
- Freshwater near-drowning
- Decreased aldosterone

(!) A critical serum sodium level—less than 120 mEq/L or greater than 160 mEq/L—is a medical emergency and can lead to seizures, respiratory arrest, coma, and death.

MAKING THE CONNECTION

Sodium and Plasma Osmolality

Sodium has a profound effect on fluid balance in the body because, as a general rule, wherever sodium goes, water follows. Thus, the shifting of water into and out of the cells (ICF) depends primarily on the sodium concentration of the blood (plasma osmolality) and other extracellular fluids. Under normal circumstances, the osmolalities of the ECF and the ICF are about equal (isotonic), even though these fluids are composed of different solutes. However, a higher-than-normal (hypertonic) concentration of sodium in the ECF causes water to move *out of* the cells via osmosis to equalize the sodium concentration between the ECF and the ICF. Conversely, a lower-than-normal (hypotonic) concentration of sodium in the ECF causes water to shift *into* the cells to reestablish the sodium balance between the ICF and the ECF. The plasma osmolality of blood (normally 275 to 295 mOsm/kg) can be roughly estimated by doubling the serum sodium laboratory value (normally 135 to 145 mEq/L). If the plasma osmolality is elevated, this means that the solutes (mainly sodium) in the blood are concentrated and that water is moving out of the cells, placing the client at risk for cellular dehydration and other electrolyte imbalances.

III. Types of Sodium Imbalance

There are three types of both hyponatremia and hypernatremia: euvolemic, hypovolemic, and hypervolemic. These terms describe the relationship between a client's fluid status and serum sodium level. The specific sodium imbalance depends on how much the sodium content decreases or increases in proportion to total body water (Table 3.1).

A. Euvolemic sodium imbalance occurs when the amount of water in the body is normal or near normal.
   1. **Euvolemic hyponatremia** is a decrease in serum sodium that occurs when the amount of water in the body is normal or near normal.
   2. **Euvolemic hypernatremia** is an increase in serum sodium that occurs when the amount of water in the body is normal or near normal.

B. Hypovolemic sodium imbalance occurs when the amount of water in the body is decreased—fluid volume deficit (FVD).
   1. **Hypovolemic hyponatremia** occurs when there is not enough water (FVD) and not enough sodium in the bloodstream.

Table 3.1 Types of Sodium Imbalance

Imbalance	Description	
Hyponatremia		
Euvolemic	Sodium content remains near normal while total body water increases • Client becomes hyponatremic because sodium ions are diluted by the increase in body water • This may occur with severe pain or nausea, trauma, or the syndrome of inappropriate antidiuretic hormone secretion (SIADH)	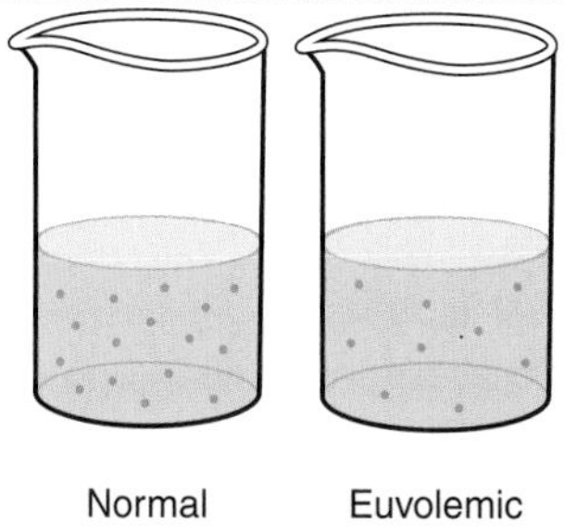 Normal Euvolemic
Hypervolemic	Sodium content and total body water increase • Client becomes hyponatremic because total body water increases more than sodium content increases • This may occur with liver cirrhosis, congestive heart failure, nephrotic syndrome, and excessive edema	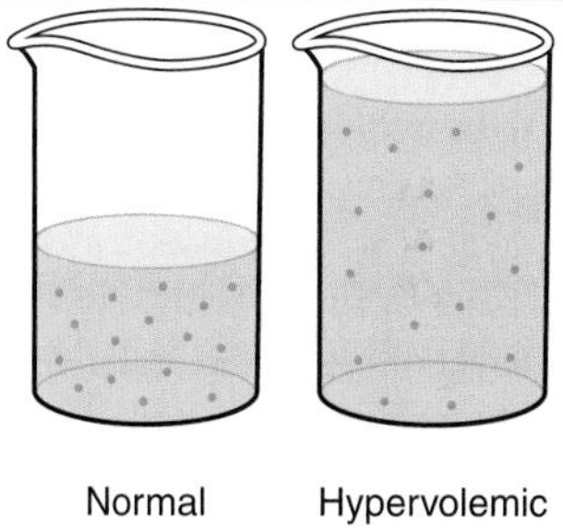 Normal Hypervolemic
Hypovolemic	Sodium content and total body water decrease • Client becomes hyponatremic because sodium content decreases more than total body water decreases • This may occur with prolonged vomiting, decreased oral intake, severe diarrhea, low-salt diet, and certain medications	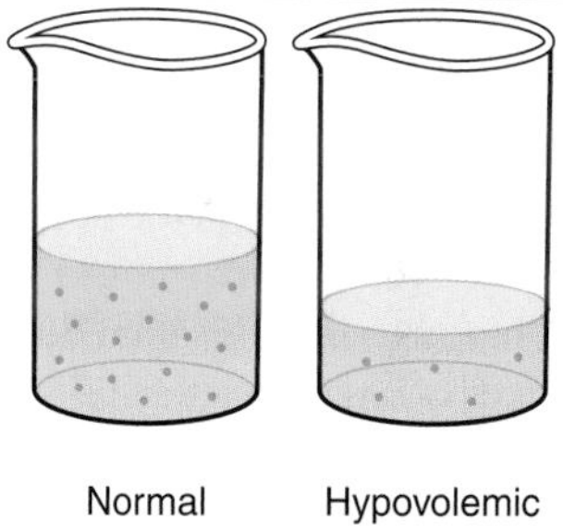 Normal Hypovolemic
Hypernatremia		
Euvolemic	Sodium content remains near normal while total body water decreases • Client becomes hypernatremic because total body water decreases and sodium ions become more concentrated • This may occur with diabetes insipidus, pituitary gland disease, or chronic kidney disease	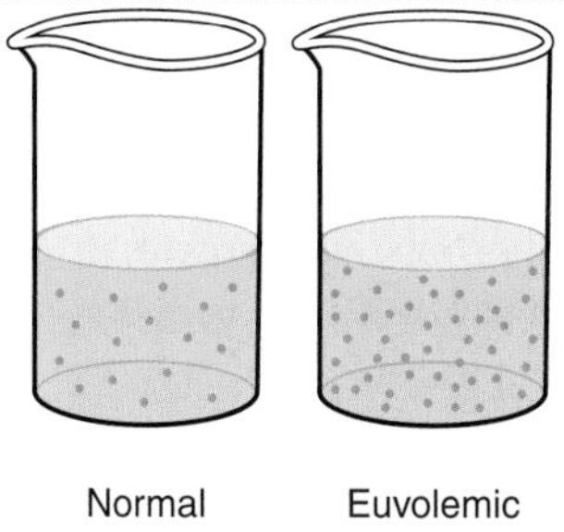 Normal Euvolemic
Hypervolemic	Sodium content increases while total body water remains the same *or* increases • Client becomes hypernatremic because sodium content increases more than total body water increases • This occurs with excessive administration of hypertonic fluids, ingestion of seawater, or steroid use	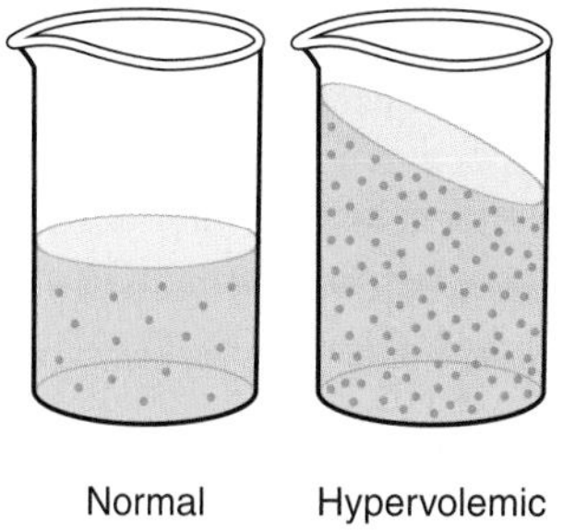 Normal Hypervolemic

Continued

Table 3.1 Types of Sodium Imbalance—cont'd

Imbalance	Description
Hypovolemic	Sodium content and total body water decrease • Client becomes hypernatremic because total body water decreases more than sodium content decreases • This occurs with inadequate intake of water, excess loss of water, or severe watery diarrhea

Normal Hypovolemic

2. **Hypovolemic hypernatremia** occurs when there is not enough water in the bloodstream (FVD); the lack of water concentrates the normal sodium content in the body, increasing the serum sodium level of the blood (relative sodium increase). There may be an actual sodium excess as well.

C. Hypervolemic sodium imbalance occurs when the amount of water in the body is increased—fluid volume excess (FVE).
   1. **Hypervolemic hyponatremia** occurs when there is too much water in the bloodstream (FVE); the excess water dilutes the normal sodium content in the body, lowering the serum sodium level of the blood (relative sodium decrease). There may be an actual sodium deficit as well.
   2. **Hypervolemic hypernatremia** occurs when there is too much water and too much sodium in the bloodstream.

IV. Causes of Sodium Imbalance

Changes in water and sodium balance may result in actual or relative increases or decreases in sodium content (Table 3.2). An *actual* increase or decrease in sodium occurs as a direct result of sodium gain or loss. A *relative* increase or decrease in sodium occurs as a result of water gain or loss; this is also referred to as a "dilutional" sodium imbalance.

A. Actual hyponatremia may be caused by sodium loss or inadequate sodium intake, resulting in an *actual* decrease in sodium content in the body.
   1. Actual loss of sodium from the body.
      a. Gastrointestinal (GI) system: loss of sodium through vomiting, diarrhea, nasogastric (NG) suctioning, tap water enemas, and GI surgery.
      b. Integumentary system: loss of sodium through **diaphoresis** (excessive sweating), severe burns, and wound drainage or suctioning.
      c. Renal system: loss of sodium through **diuresis** (excessive urination).
      d. Endocrine system: loss of sodium caused by decreased aldosterone secretion by the adrenal glands.
      e. Medications: diuretics, angiotensin-converting enzyme (ACE) inhibitors, and angiotensin II inhibitors act directly on the kidneys to increase urine production, promoting sodium loss.
   2. Inadequate sodium intake.
      a. Intake of salt-free solutions, such as water, without adequate dietary sodium intake.
      b. Lack of salt in the diet may result in chronic hyponatremia.
      c. Anorexia and other eating disorders may lead to sodium deficiency.

B. Relative hyponatremia may be caused by water gain or third spacing, resulting in a *relative* (dilutional) decrease in sodium content in the body.
   1. Excessive intake of hypotonic fluids.
      a. Excessive intake of salt-free solutions, such as water (water intoxication).
      b. Psychogenic polydipsia (excessive water drinking in the absence of a physiologic stimulus to drink).
      c. Administration of hypotonic IV solutions, such as 0.225% saline solution (¼ NS) or 0.45% saline solution (½ NS).
   2. Adrenal insufficiency or adrenal failure.
      a. Decreased aldosterone secretion by the adrenal glands causes an increase in water retention by the kidneys, resulting in greater dilution of sodium in the blood.
   3. Hyperglycemia increases the osmolality of the ECF, causing water to be pulled out of the cells and into the ECF, resulting in increased ECF volume, dilution of serum electrolytes, and cellular dehydration.
   4. Syndrome of inappropriate antidiuretic hormone secretion (SIADH) causes ADH to be secreted in excessive amounts, resulting in water retention and dilutional hyponatremia.

Table 3.2 Causes of Sodium Imbalance

Hyponatremia	
Actual decrease in sodium	Relative decrease in sodium (dilutional)

Sodium loss
• Vomiting
• Nasogastric suctioning
• Diarrhea
• Excessive diaphoresis
• Burns
• Wound drainage
• Consumption of large quantities of beer
• Use of the recreational illicit substance "ecstasy"
• Kidney disease
• Medications that act directly on the kidney to produce hyponatremia:
  • ACE inhibitors
  • Angiotensin II receptor blockers
  • Carbonic anhydrase inhibitors
  • Diuretics
Inadequate sodium intake
• Nothing by mouth (NPO) status
• Low-salt diet
	Water gain
	• Adrenal insufficiency
	• Excessive intake of hypotonic fluids (water, IV D_5W, tube feeding)
	  • Psychogenic polydipsia
	  • Tap water enemas
	  • Infants fed tap water for 1–2 days
	  • Postoperative administration of hypotonic fluids
	  • Drinking excessive water during exercise
	  • Freshwater near-drowning
	• Nephrotic syndrome
	• Wound irrigation with hypotonic fluids
	• Heart failure or congestive heart failure
	• Hyperglycemia
	• Syndrome of inappropriate antidiuretic hormone secretion (SIADH)
	Third spacing
	• Edema
	• Ascites (liver failure, liver cirrhosis)

Hypernatremia	
Actual increase in sodium	Relative increase in sodium (dilutional)
Sodium gain • Excessive oral sodium intake • Administration of hypertonic tube feedings without adequate water • Administration of hypertonic IV solutions (hypertonic saline solution, sodium bicarbonate, total parenteral nutrition) Sodium retention • Hyperaldosteronism • Cushing's syndrome • Corticosteroids • Acute renal failure	Water loss • Kidney disease • Osmotic diuresis (glucose, urea) • Vomiting • Diarrhea • Excessive diaphoresis • Burns • Diabetes insipidus • Mineralocorticoid excess • Increased insensible loss Inadequate water intake • Inability to ingest water • Decreased fluid intake

5. Third spacing, the accumulation of fluid in the body where fluid does not normally collect, results in a relative (dilutional) loss of sodium and may be caused by any condition associated with edema or ascites, such as congestive heart failure (CHF) or liver failure.

C. Actual hypernatremia may be caused by sodium gain or sodium retention, resulting in an *actual* increase in sodium content in the body.
   1. Sodium gain may be caused by the excessive intake of sodium via oral and IV routes.

MAKING THE CONNECTION

SIADH

The syndrome of inappropriate antidiuretic hormone secretion (SIADH) is a condition in which antidiuretic hormone (ADH) is secreted by the hypothalamus in excessive amounts or at the wrong time. Too much ADH causes the body to retain water, diluting the concentration of sodium, which results in relative hyponatremia. SIADH tends to occur in clients diagnosed with congestive heart failure or in individuals with a diseased hypothalamus—the part of the brain that works directly with the pituitary gland to produce hormones. SIADH is most often caused by central nervous system disorders, malignancies, or pulmonary diseases. The condition may also be drug induced or occur postoperatively because of the stress of surgery. SIADH is usually treated by restricting fluid intake, restoring sodium balance, and administering demeclocycline, a potent inhibitor of ADH, or other medications.

      a. Excessive oral sodium intake can occur through the diet or by near drowning in saltwater.
      b. Concentrated parenteral (IV) and enteral (tube) feedings that are not properly diluted can cause hypernatremia, dehydration, and other electrolyte imbalances.
      c. Concentrated infant formula that is not properly diluted may also result in hypernatremia and dehydration.
      d. Administration of IV hypertonic solutions, such as 3% sodium chloride (3% saline) or 5% sodium chloride (5% saline) solutions, can cause hypernatremia.
   2. Sodium retention.
      a. Hyperaldosteronism is a condition in which too much aldosterone is produced by the adrenal glands; it causes water and sodium retention.
      b. Corticosteroid use can have side effects such as hypertension, hypokalemia (low potassium levels in the blood), and hypernatremia (high sodium levels in the blood); corticosteroids may also cause immunosuppression and impaired wound healing.
      c. Acute kidney injury adversely affects the kidneys' ability to filter and remove water and sodium.

D. Relative hypernatremia may be caused by excessive water loss or inadequate water intake, resulting in a relative increase in sodium content in the body.
   1. Excessive water loss.
      a. Water may be lost through vomiting, watery diarrhea, diuretic therapy, burns,

MAKING THE CONNECTION

Diabetes Insipidus and Hypernatremia

Diabetes insipidus (DI) is a disorder characterized by intense thirst and the excretion of large amounts of dilute urine (polyuria). The kidneys are unable to conserve water, usually because of a decrease in the secretion of ADH. Water is lost through the urine, but sodium is retained, resulting in relative hypernatremia. If DI is caused by a decrease in the secretion of ADH, it is called *central DI*. Central DI can be caused by damage to the hypothalamus or pituitary gland as a result of head injury, infection, malignancy, or surgery. If ADH is present but the kidneys are unable to respond to the hormone, it is called *nephrogenic DI*. This type of DI is caused by genetic defects; certain drugs, such as lithium, amphotericin B, and demeclocycline; high levels of calcium in the body (hypercalcemia); and kidney disease. Diabetes mellitus (DM) and DI are different disorders and are not related.

perspiration, fever, or other forms of insensible water loss.
   b. Osmotic diuresis is excessive urination that causes solutes in the blood, especially sodium, to become more concentrated as water is excreted by the kidneys, increasing the blood's osmolarity.
2. Inadequate water intake.
   a. Inability to ingest water or decreased fluid intake.
   b. Infants, young children, and older clients are at greatest risk.

V. Nursing Assessment for Sodium Imbalance

The nurse should conduct a focused nursing assessment for sodium imbalance, beginning with a thorough nursing history. Interview the client and family members to reveal any risk factors or preexisting conditions that would contribute to sodium imbalance, such as vomiting, nasogastric suctioning, diarrhea, acute kidney injury, or other conditions associated with sodium loss or gain. The nurse should assess the client's ability to drink and tolerate oral fluids and obtain a current dietary history, inquiring about dietary sodium intake. The nursing history should also include lifestyle factors, such as the consumption of beer, the use of certain illicit substances, and current medication use. A thorough physical assessment is necessary because sodium imbalance can affect many body systems. Assess each body system, observing for signs and symptoms of sodium imbalance as well as any associated fluid imbalance. Measure and record the client's vital signs, and review the client's laboratory data to assess for the presence of hypo- or hypernatremia (Table 3.3).

DID YOU KNOW?

Seizure activity is associated with both hypo- and hypernatremia.

VI. Nursing Interventions for Clients With Sodium Imbalance

A. Identify high-risk clients.
   1. Infants and young children are at greater risk for FVD and related sodium imbalances.
   2. Older adults, aged 60 and older, have a decreased thirst mechanism and decreased renal function, placing them at greater risk for fluid and sodium imbalances.
   3. Clients taking certain medications.
      a. Loop diuretics, corticosteroid medications, certain antibiotics, and IV saline solutions increase the client's risk for hypernatremia.
      b. Over-the-counter (OTC) medications such as Alka-Seltzer, aspirin, cough syrups, and cold preparations often contain sodium.
   4. Clients with high-salt diets.
      a. Fast food, soda pop, and processed foods are often very high in sodium.
      b. Many food seasonings are a source of hidden sodium.
B. Implement the health-care provider's orders to treat the underlying cause of the imbalance.
   1. The health-care provider may order oral or IV fluid administration, oral or IV sodium administration, fluid restriction, and medication administration.
C. Monitor the client and the client's serum sodium and other levels.
   1. Monitor the client's serum sodium level as ordered by the health-care provider.
      a. Normal reference range for serum sodium is 135 to 145 mEq/L.
   2. Monitor other laboratory values associated with sodium imbalance.
      a. Serum chloride: normal reference range is 95 to 108 mEq/L.
      b. Serum potassium: normal reference range is 3.5 to 5.0 mEq//L.
      c. Serum osmolality: less than 275 mOsm/L indicates hyponatremia; greater than 295 mOsm/L indicates hypernatremia.
   3. Monitor for cerebral changes.
      a. Establish the client's usual cognitive and behavioral patterns.
      b. Observe the client's behavior, level of consciousness, and mental status.
      c. Monitor for seizure activity.

Table 3.3 Signs and Symptoms of Sodium Imbalance

Vital Signs		
	Hyponatremia	*Hypernatremia*
Blood pressure	Decreased, orthostatic hypotension, or normal to elevated	Decreased, orthostatic hypotension, or normal to elevated
Heart rate	Increased	Increased
Respiratory rate	Decreased	Severely decreased; may produce respiratory arrest
Temperature	Within normal limits	Elevated (related to fluid volume deficit)
Signs and Symptoms by Body System		
	Hyponatremia	*Hypernatremia*
Cardiovascular	• Hyponatremia with hypovolemia • Tachycardia • Weak, thready pulse • Decreased blood pressure progressing to severe orthostatic hypotension • Hyponatremia with hypervolemia • Bounding pulse • Normal or elevated blood pressure	• Tachycardia • Orthostatic hypotension, if hypovolemic • Hypertension, if hypervolemic
Cerebral	• Lethargy, fatigue • Headache • Irritability • Confusion • Restlessness • Decreased level of consciousness • Hallucinations • Seizures • Coma, signs of brainstem herniation	(!) Thirst is usually the first symptom to appear • Agitation • Confusion • Restlessness • Loss of short-term memory • Seizures • Coma possible
Gastrointestinal	• Anorexia • Nausea, vomiting • Abdominal cramping • Hyperactive bowel sounds • Frequent, watery bowel movements	None
Neuromuscular	• Weakness (generalized) • Decreased deep tendon reflexes (DTRs) • Muscle spasm or cramps; twitching	• Muscle spasm, cramps, or twitching; progressing to severe weakness • Decreased to absent DTRs with severe hypernatremia
Renal	• Urinary retention	• Hypernatremia with hypovolemia • Small amounts of dark, yellow urine • Hypernatremia with kidney dysfunction • Large amounts of clear, water-like urine
Respiratory	• Hypoventilation • Bradypnea	• Severely decreased • Respiratory arrest possible
Laboratory Values		
	Hyponatremia	*Hypernatremia*
Serum sodium	Less than 135 mEq/L (mmol/L)	Greater than 145 mEq/L (mmol/L)
Serum osmolality	May be decreased or normal, depending on etiology of hyponatremia • Normal plasma osmolality is 275–299 mOsm/kg	May be increased or normal, depending on etiology of hypernatremia • Normal plasma osmolality is 275–299 mOsm/kg

DID YOU KNOW?

Cerebral cells are highly sensitive to changes in sodium level and fluid volume. Brain cells swell (cerebral edema) in the presence of hyponatremia and shrink in the presence of hypernatremia, which, when severe, may lead to seizure activity, coma, or death.

4. Monitor for cardiovascular changes.
   a. Auscultate the apical pulse rate.
   b. Observe for jugular venous distention.
   c. Palpate peripheral pulses.
   d. Check orthostatic blood pressure.
   e. Observe for peripheral edema.

5. Monitor for neuromuscular changes.
   a. Establish a baseline for the client's deep tendon reflexes, muscle strength, and tone.
   b. Monitor the client for muscle weakness, muscle twitching, or irregular muscle contractions during each nursing shift.

(!) If muscle weakness is present, immediately assess the client's respiratory status: ventilation depends on adequate strength of the respiratory muscles.

6. Monitor for gastrointestinal changes.
   a. Auscultate bowel sounds in all four quadrants.
   b. Observe frequency and consistency of bowel movements.

D. Weigh the client daily.
1. Evaluate the client's weight gain or loss over 1 to 3 days.
2. Weigh the client at the same time each day, preferably before breakfast, with the same amount of clothing on and using the same scale.
3. An increase or decrease in body weight may indicate fluid gain or loss influenced by or causing a sodium imbalance.

E. Measure intake and output.
1. Measure intake.
   a. At least every 8 hours, record the type and amount of all fluids received and describe the route as oral, parenteral, rectal, or by enteric tube.
   b. Record ice chips as fluid at approximately one-half their volume.
   c. Compare the client's intake with that of an average adult.
2. Measure output.
   a. Record the type and amount of all fluids the client has lost, and indicate the route; describe output as urine, liquid stool, vomitus, tube drainage (including from chest, closed wound drainage, and nasogastric tubes), and any fluid aspirated from a body cavity.
   b. Measure the amount of irrigation fluid instilled; subtract it from the total output when irrigating a nasogastric or other tube or the bladder.
   c. Measure drainage in a calibrated container. Observe it at eye level, and record the reading at the bottom of the meniscus.
   d. Compare the client's output with that of an average adult; intake and output should be relatively equivalent.

F. Ensure client safety.
1. Reduce environmental stimuli.
   a. Provide a quiet room.
   b. Limit the client's visitors.
   c. Darken the client's room.
   d. Speak in soft tones.
2. Implement seizure precautions related to neuromuscular irritability.
   a. Pad side rails.
   b. Have oxygen and suction equipment available.
   c. Ensure the patency of IV access devices.
   d. Administer emergency medications as ordered.
   e. Prepare for possible endotracheal intubation.
   f. Prepare for cardiac defibrillation if necessary.
3. Implement fall precautions related to muscle weakness caused by hyponatremia and severe hypernatremia (Box 3.2).

VII. Nursing Interventions Specific to Hyponatremia and Hypernatremia

A. Control sodium and water intake
1. Hyponatremia
   a. Increase oral sodium intake.
   b. Restrict free water.
   c. For acute or chronic hyponatremia with severe symptoms:
      1) Administer small volumes of IV hypertonic (2% to 3%) saline solution as ordered—only enough to increase the serum sodium level by 4 to 6 mEq/L over the first 1 to 2 hours.
      2) Monitor the cardiac rhythm of clients receiving hypertonic IV saline solutions.
      3) Delay achieving a normal sodium level or hypernatremia for the first 48 hours.
      4) Treat hypovolemic hyponatremia with IV normal saline solution (0.9%) as ordered to restore both sodium and fluid volume.

(!) Avoid increasing the serum sodium level too quickly because this may cause central nervous system irritation, pulmonary edema, or both.

Box 3.2 Implementing Fall Precautions

- Perform a fall risk assessment.
- Maintain the bed in a low position with locked wheels.
- Remove all obstacles from pathways, especially to the toilet.
- Monitor the environment for safety hazards (e.g., torn carpet, liquid spills on floors).
- Place assistive devices (walkers, canes) within the client's reach.
- Use nightlights.
- Instruct the client to request assistance to ambulate.
- Ensure the availability of the call light.
- Assess footwear, and provide appropriate footwear if necessary; clients must use antiskid soles.
- Keep items (e.g., telephone, fluids) close to the client.
- Request that family members remain with the client if necessary.
- Position the client to allow close observation by staff members.
- Communicate the client's fall risk during the shift report and as necessary.

2. Hypernatremia
   a. Decrease oral sodium intake.
   b. Ensure adequate water intake.
   c. Administer hypotonic IV solutions (usually 0.225% or 45% NaCl) as ordered if fluid loss is the cause of hypernatremia.
   d. Administer isotonic IV normal saline solution (0.9%) as ordered if both fluid and sodium losses have occurred.

B. Administer medications as ordered

1. Hyponatremia
   a. Analgesics to decrease pain related to headache: acetaminophen (Tylenol) or other NSAIDs.
   b. Antiemetics to treat nausea and vomiting: promethazine (Phenergan).
   c. Antiepileptics to treat seizures: phenytoin (Dilantin).
   d. Arginine vasopressin receptor antagonists to increase free water excretion without sodium excretion—used only in euvolemic or hypervolemic hyponatremia: approved by the Food and Drug Administration—conivaptan (Vaprisol), tolvaptan (Samsca)
   e. Corticosteroids to decrease cerebral edema: methylprednisolone (Solu-Medrol).
2. Hypernatremia
   a. Loop diuretics or thiazide diuretics to promote sodium loss by increasing urine excretion.
      1) Loop diuretic: furosemide (Lasix)
      2) Thiazide diuretic: hydrochlorothiazide (Diuril)

C. Educate the client

1. Hyponatremia
   a. Teach the client or caregiver the causes of sodium deficit.
   b. Provide specific information regarding the client's medical diagnosis and related interventions and treatments.
   c. Teach the client how to prevent sodium deficiency by drinking water in moderation and ingesting drinks that contain electrolytes to replace fluids lost during exercise, strenuous activities, and hot weather.
   d. Teach the client how to identify the signs and symptoms of sodium deficiency, and instruct the client and family to notify the primary health-care provider if the client exhibits signs or symptoms of hyponatremia or if they have any other specific concerns.
   e. Ensure that the client or caregiver understands the specifics, rationale, potential side effects, and desired effects of the treatment regimen.
   f. Include medication administration, nutrition, hydration, dietary restrictions, and foods high in sodium in client teaching; clients with fluid volume excess related to chronic conditions may be on long-term fluid and sodium restrictions.
2. Hypernatremia
   a. Teach the client or caregiver the causes of sodium excess.
   b. Provide specific information regarding the client's medical diagnosis and related interventions and treatments.
   c. Teach the client how to prevent sodium excess.
      1) Teach the client to avoid high-sodium foods (see Box 1.2, page 12, for a list of high-sodium foods).
      2) Instruct the client that recommendations for a low-sodium diet range from 400 to 2,000 mg/day.
      3) Teach the client the specific definitions of reduced-sodium food products.
         a) Low sodium: Less than 140 mg per serving
         b) Very low sodium: Less than 35 mg per serving
         c) Salt free or sodium free: Less than 5 mg sodium per serving
      4) Recommend the use of salt substitutes, if allowed by the primary health-care provider.
      5) Teach the client and family how to read food labels that list the amount of sodium contained in each serving and list other sodium-containing compounds such as monosodium glutamate (MSG), baking soda, disodium phosphate, sodium alginate, and sodium nitrate or nitrite (Fig. 3.1).
      6) Recommend the seasoning of foods with spices, herbs, lemon juice, or pepper.
      7) Instruct the client to avoid medications that contain sodium (Alka-Seltzer, Bromo-Seltzer).
      8) Advise the client to avoid using salt-softened water for drinking and cooking because it contains significant amounts of added salt.
   d. Teach the client how to identify the signs and symptoms of sodium excess, and instruct the client and family to notify the primary health-care provider if the client exhibits signs or symptoms of hypernatremia or if they have any other specific concerns.
   e. Ensure that the client or caregiver understands the specifics, rationale, potential side effects, and desired effects of treatment regimen.
   f. Include medication administration, nutrition, hydration, dietary restrictions, and foods high in sodium in client teaching.

Nutrition Facts
Serving Size 0 cup (000 g)
Servings Per Container 0

Amount Per Serving	
Calories 000	Calories from Fat 000
	% Daily Value*
Total Fat 00g	00%
Saturated Fat 0g	00%
Cholesterol 00mg	00%
Sodium 000mg	00%
Total Carbohydrate 00g	00%
Dietary Fiber 0g	0%
Sugars 00g	
Protein 00g	
Vitamin A 0% •	Vitamin C 0%
Calcium 00% •	Iron 0%

Percent Daily Values are based on a 2,000 calorie diet. Your daily values may be higher or lower depending on your calorie needs.

	Calories	2,000	2,500
Total Fat	Less than	65g	80g
*Sat. Fat	Less than	20g	25g
Cholesterol	Less than	300mg	300mg
Sodium	Less than	2,400mg	2,400mg
Total Carbohydrate		300g	375g
Dietary Fiber		25g	30g

Calories per gram
Fat 9 • Carbohydrate 4 • Protein 4

Fig 3.1 Assist the client in locating the sodium content in milligrams on every product label. Instruct the client that the total daily sodium intake should not exceed 2,400 mg/day for individuals who are not on restricted-sodium diets.

D. Evaluate and document
1. Document all assessment findings and interventions per institution policy.
2. Evaluate and document the client's response to interventions and education.
   a. Serum sodium level should return to the normal reference range of 135 to 145 mEq/L.
   b. Other laboratory values should return to the normal reference range.
   c. Vital signs should return to baseline.
   d. Underlying cause of sodium imbalance should be resolved.
   e. Level of consciousness should return to baseline.

VIII. Chloride Imbalance

Chloride (Cl^-) is the major **anion** in the ECF and functions primarily with sodium and water to maintain a balance between intracellular and extracellular fluids. When sodium is retained, chloride is also retained; thus, decreases in sodium are accompanied by decreases in chloride. There is no recommended daily allowance for chloride, and most diets contain enough sodium chloride (salt) to meet the normal needs of the body. Chloride is absorbed continuously by the intestines along with sodium. The kidneys are responsible for the reabsorption and excretion of chloride (along with sodium), which are regulated by aldosterone and ADH. Within the body, chloride performs the following functions:

1. Maintains a balance between intracellular and extracellular fluids
2. Combines with hydrogen in the stomach to produce hydrochloric acid
3. Activates certain enzymes
4. Is essential in maintaining acid-base balance
5. Works with magnesium and calcium to maintain nerve transmission and normal muscle contraction and relaxation

Normal Lab Value The normal serum chloride level is 95 to 108 mEq/L (mmol/L).

DID YOU KNOW?
Wherever sodium goes, chloride follows.

IX. Types of Chloride Imbalance

Hypochloremia, or chloride deficit, is a serum chloride level less than 95 mEq/L. A decrease in serum chloride is usually accompanied by a decrease in serum sodium, potassium, or both. **Hyperchloremia**, or chloride excess, is a serum chloride level greater than 108 mEq/L. An increase in serum chloride is usually accompanied by an increase in serum sodium, potassium, or both.

(!) Critical serum chloride levels are less than 80 mEq/L or greater than 115 mEq/L.

X. Causes of Chloride Imbalance

Changes in water and sodium balance affect chloride balance because sodium and chloride are attracted by a chemical bond and move through the body together. Chloride imbalance may also occur as a result of chloride loss or gain and abnormal retention or excretion, resulting in an *actual* increase or decrease in chloride. The shifting of chloride between intracellular and extracellular compartments, or water gain or loss, results in a *relative* decrease in chloride content (Table 3.4).

A. Hypochloremia may be caused by excess chloride loss, inadequate chloride intake or absorption, or chloride shifts between intracellular and extracellular compartments.
1. Excess chloride loss.
   a. Vomiting results in the loss of hydrochloric acid from the stomach.
   b. Gastric suctioning decreases serum chloride by removing hydrogen chloride (HCl) from the stomach.
   c. Diarrhea results in water, sodium, and chloride loss.

Table 3.4 Causes of Chloride Imbalance

Hypochloremia	
Actual decrease in chloride	Relative decrease in chloride (dilutional)
Chloride loss • Renal disease • Excessive vomiting • Prolonged diarrhea • Prolonged gastric suctioning • Excessive diaphoresis • Burns • SIADH • Addison's disease • Diuretics (loop and thiazide) and other medications Inadequate chloride intake or absorption • Prolonged or excessive administration of 5% dextrose IV therapy • Inadequate dietary intake • Acute renal failure (nephrotic syndrome) • Anorexia	Shifts between intracellular and extracellular compartments • Metabolic alkalosis • Diabetic ketoacidosis • Increase in serum bicarbonate (ingestion of excessive antacids) • Hypervolemic congestive heart failure • Burns
Hyperchloremia	
Actual increase in chloride	Relative increase in chloride (dilutional)
Chloride gain • Hyperparathyroidism • Hypernatremia • Oral or nasogastric intake • Administration of IV NaCl (normal saline solution) • Saline enemas • Administration of medications *-acetazolamide (Diamox)* *-ammonium chloride* *-boric acid* *-bromide (excessive intake)* *-triamterene (Dyrenium)* Decreased excretion of chloride • Renal insufficiency • Acute renal failure • Severe dehydration • Loss of pancreatic secretions	Shifts between intracellular and extracellular compartments • Hypernatremia • Metabolic acidosis • Respiratory alkalosis

   d. Diaphoresis (excessive sweating) may cause chloride loss because chloride is found in perspiration.
   e. Some medications act directly on the kidneys to increase urine production or decrease serum sodium levels.
2. Inadequate chloride intake or absorption.
   a. Excessive administration of 5% dextrose IV solution, which does not contain sodium or chloride.
   b. Inadequate dietary intake.
   c. Nephrotic syndrome.
   d. Anorexia or malnutrition.
3. Shifts between intracellular and extracellular compartments.
   a. Metabolic alkalosis (a metabolic condition in which the pH of tissue increases above the normal range of 7.35 to 7.45).
   b. Excessive ingestion of antacid.
   c. Diabetic ketoacidosis (a potentially life-threatening complication of diabetes mellitus in which the pH of tissue decreases below 7.35).
   d. Burn injuries.

B. Hyperchloremia may be caused by excess chloride intake, decreased excretion or retention of chloride by the kidneys, or chloride shifts between intracellular and extracellular compartments.
1. Excess chloride intake.
   a. Oral or nasogastric chloride intake.
   b. Administration of IV sodium chloride solution.
   c. In the presence of hypernatremia.
2. Decreased excretion or retention of chloride.
   a. Renal insufficiency.
   b. Severe dehydration.
3. Chloride shifts between intracellular and extracellular compartments.
   a. In the presence of hypernatremia.

DID YOU KNOW?

Chloride imbalances almost never occur alone; check for imbalances in sodium, bicarbonate, and potassium as well.

XI. Nursing Assessment for Chloride Imbalance

The nurse should conduct a focused nursing assessment for chloride imbalance, beginning with a thorough nursing history. Interview the client and family members to reveal any risk factors or preexisting conditions that would contribute to sodium or chloride imbalances. Include a current dietary history, inquiring about the intake of dietary sodium chloride (table salt) or potassium chloride–based salt substitutes. The nursing history should also include lifestyle factors and current medication use. A thorough physical assessment is necessary because chloride imbalance affects many body systems. Assess each body system, observing for signs and symptoms of chloride imbalance as well as any associated electrolyte imbalances. Measure and record the client's vital signs, and review the client's laboratory data to assess for the presence of hypo- or hyperchloremia (Table 3.5).

XII. Nursing Interventions for Clients With Chloride Imbalance

A. Implement the health-care provider's orders to treat the underlying cause of the imbalance. These orders may include oral or IV fluid administration, oral or

Table 3.5 Signs and Symptoms of Chloride Imbalance

Vital Signs		
	Hypochloremia	*Hyperchloremia*
Blood pressure	Decreased, orthostatic hypotension, or normal to elevated	Decreased, orthostatic hypotension, or normal to elevated
Heart rate	Increased	Increased
Respiratory rate	Decreased	Decreased or increased
Temperature	Within normal limits or elevated	Elevated (related to fluid volume deficit)
Signs and Symptoms by Body System		
	Hypochloremia	*Hyperchloremia*
Cardiovascular	• Hypotension (with severe hypochloremia and ECF loss)	• Hypertension • Pitting edema
Cerebral	• Disorientation • Confusion	• Agitation • Headache • Confusion • Stupor • Unconsciousness to coma
Gastrointestinal	None	• Nausea
Neuromuscular	• Paralysis • Muscle spasm or cramps; twitching	• Weakness • Lethargy
Respiratory	• Hypoventilation • Bradypnea • Shallow respirations	• Kussmaul respirations (deep, gasping respirations associated with acidosis; the body's attempt to eliminate carbon dioxide and acid) • Tachypnea • Dyspnea
Laboratory Values		
	Hypochloremia	*Hyperchloremia*
Serum chloride	Less than 95 mEq/L	Greater than 108 mEq/L
Serum sodium	Usually less than 135 mEq/L	Usually greater than 145 mEq/L
Serum potassium	Usually less than 3.5 mEq/L	Usually greater than 5.0 mEq/L

IV sodium administration, fluid restrictions, and medication administration.

B. Monitor the client and the client's serum chloride levels.
1. Monitor the client's serum chloride level as ordered by the health-care provider.
   a. Normal reference range for serum chloride is 95 to 108 mEq/L.
2. Monitor other laboratory values associated with chloride imbalance.
   a. Serum sodium: normal reference range is 135 to 145 mEq/L.
   b. Serum potassium: normal reference range is 3.5 to 5.0 mEq/L.
   c. Bicarbonate: normal reference range is 22 to 30 mEq/L.
3. Measure intake and output.
4. Assess vital signs, especially blood pressure.
5. Document observations, and notify the health-care provider as ordered.

C. Control chloride intake
1. Hypochloremia
   a. Increase oral chloride and sodium intake.
      1) Salt tablets
      2) Salty broth or other oral fluids
   b. Restrict free water.
2. Hyperchloremia
   a. Decrease oral chloride and sodium intake.
   b. Ensure adequate water intake.
   c. Discontinue medications that contain chloride.

D. Administer IV medications
1. Hypochloremia
   a. Administer medications as ordered. Electrolyte replenishers to increase the serum chloride level include IV ammonium chloride, IV potassium chloride (in metabolic acidosis), and IV NaCl solution if the client is unable to tolerate replacement or if levels are critically low.

2. Hyperchloremia
   a. Administer medications as ordered. Alkalinizing agents to increase the serum bicarbonate levels and to encourage the renal excretion of chloride include IV lactated Ringer's solution (to convert bicarbonate in the liver and correct acidosis) and IV sodium bicarbonate for severe hyperchloremic acidosis.

E. Educate the client
1. Hypochloremia
   a. Teach the client or caregiver the causes of chloride deficit.
   b. Instruct the client that because most dietary chloride comes from table salt, he or she should increase the amount of salt used, as ordered by the health-care provider.
   c. Teach the client how to prevent chloride deficiency.
   d. Teach the client that the following are good sources of chloride: fresh fruits and vegetables (dates, bananas, spinach, celery, olives); canned vegetables and soups; rye; meat, fish, and poultry; eggs; milk and cheese; processed foods.
   e. Ensure that the client or caregiver understands the specifics, rationale, potential side effects, and desired effects of the treatment regimen.
   f. Include medication administration, nutrition, hydration, dietary restrictions, and foods high in chloride in client teaching.
2. Hyperchloremia
   a. Teach the client or caregiver the causes of chloride excess.
   b. Provide specific information regarding the client's medical diagnosis and related interventions and treatments.
   c. Teach the client how to prevent chloride excess.
   d. Instruct the client to avoid high-chloride foods (see specific foods listed under hypochloremia).
   e. Ensure that the client or caregiver understands the specifics, rationale, potential side effects, and desired effects of the treatment regimen.

F. Evaluate and document
1. Document all assessment findings and interventions per institution policy.
2. Evaluate and document the client's response to interventions and education.
   a. Serum chloride level should return to the normal reference range of 95 to 108 mEq/L.
   b. Other laboratory values should return to the normal reference range.
   c. Vital signs should return to baseline.
   d. Underlying cause of chloride imbalance should be resolved.
   e. Level of consciousness should return to baseline.

CASE STUDY: Putting It All Together

Subjective Data

A 6-year-old client is scheduled for an outpatient tonsillectomy and adenoidectomy. The client has a history of frequent tonsillitis and strep throat, necessitating antibiotic therapy at least three times a year; the client has no known allergies and is receiving no medications at this time. The procedure is performed uneventfully under general anesthesia, with minimal blood loss. The client receives 500 mL of D_5W IV intraoperatively and returns to a postoperative outpatient recovery room. The client reports a "sore throat" and nausea.

Objective Data

Nursing Assessment

1. Lethargic with confusion since admission to the postoperative unit
2. Vomiting frequent small amounts of clear, blood-tinged fluid
3. Tachycardia with a weak, thready pulse
4. Decreased blood pressure
5. Heart sounds S_1 and S_2 soft and regular; no murmur
6. Respirations shallow, slow
7. Lung sounds clear in all fields
8. Skin pale, cool
9. Pedal and radial pulses regular, 1+, and weak bilaterally

Vital Signs	
Temperature:	100°F (37.8°C) axillary
Blood pressure:	90/48 mm Hg
Heart rate:	154 bpm, regular
Respiratory rate:	10
O_2 saturation:	94%

Laboratory Results	
Serum Na^+:	125 mEq/L
Serum Cl^-:	90 mEq/L
Blood glucose:	76 mg/dL
Serum BUN:	12 mg/dL
Serum creatinine:	0.6 mg/dL

Health-Care Provider Orders

1. Administer O_2 at 2 L/min via nasal cannula.
2. Measure vital signs every 15 minutes × 2 hours, then every 30 minutes.
3. Discontinue D_5W now.
4. Administer IV normal saline solution: 100 mL over 1 hour, then 50 mL/hr × 1 L; correct serum sodium over 24 hours, no faster than 1 to 2 mEq/hr.
5. Administer IV ondansetron (Zofran) 0.15 mg/kg every 6 hours as necessary for nausea.
6. Repeat basic metabolic panel every 4 hours × 2 after normal saline IV fluid started; notify health-care provider of results.
7. Monitor intake and output.
8. Assess neurological status every hour × 8.
9. Implement seizure precautions.
10. Provide clear liquid diet when awake; avoid free water; use electrolyte supplemental fluids (Pedialyte, Gatorade) as tolerated.
11. Admit to facility as inpatient.

Case Study Questions

A. What *subjective* assessment findings indicate that the client is experiencing a health alteration?

1. ______
2. ______
3. ______
4. ______

CASE STUDY: Putting It All Together *cont'd*

Case Study Questions

B. What *objective* assessment findings indicate that the client is experiencing a health alteration?

1. ______
2. ______
3. ______
4. ______
5. ______
6. ______
7. ______
8. ______
9. ______

C. After analyzing the data collected, what **primary** nursing diagnosis should the nurse assign to this client other than Acute Pain?

______

D. What interventions should the nurse plan or implement to meet this client's needs?

1. ______
2. ______
3. ______
4. ______
5. ______
6. ______
7. ______
8. ______
9. ______
10. ______

E. What client outcomes should the nurse plan to evaluate the effectiveness of the nursing interventions?

1. ______
2. ______
3. ______
4. ______
5. ______
6. ______

REVIEW QUESTIONS

1. A nursing instructor is educating students about sodium imbalance. Which statement by the nursing instructor is correct?
   1. Sodium is the most abundant cation in the ECF.
   2. Sodium is the least abundant cation in the ECF.
   3. Sodium is the most abundant anion in the ECF.
   4. Sodium is the least abundant anion in the ECF.

2. A nurse assesses the laboratory values of an adult client. Which imbalance should a nurse associate with a serum sodium level of 150 mEq/L?
   1. Hyponatremia
   2. Hypernatremia
   3. Hypokalemia
   4. Hyperkalemia

3. A nurse assessing a client who experienced a seizure during a water-drinking contest should associate the client's seizure with which electrolyte imbalance?
   1. Hyponatremia related to actual decrease in sodium
   2. Hyponatremia related to relative decrease in sodium
   3. Hypernatremia related to actual increase in sodium
   4. Hypernatremia related to relative increase in sodium

4. A nurse assesses a newly admitted client with a serum sodium level of 120 mEq/L. The nurse should observe the client for which clinical manifestations? **Select all that apply.**
   1. Disorientation
   2. Constipation
   3. Generalized weakness
   4. Tachypnea
   5. Headache

5. A nurse is providing discharge instructions to a client diagnosed with end-stage renal disease. The nurse explains that the client is at risk for developing hypernatremia. Which manifestation should the nurse instruct the client to report immediately to a health-care provider?
   1. Euphoria
   2. Weight gain of 3 lb in 1 day
   3. Nausea for 1 day
   4. Single episode of diarrhea

6. A nurse instructing a client on a low-sodium diet should advise the client that it is appropriate to consume which condiment?
   1. Mayonnaise
   2. Barbecue sauce
   3. Catsup
   4. Chili sauce

7. A nurse instructing a client on a low-sodium diet should advise the client to *avoid* which beverage?
   1. Lemonade
   2. Iced tea
   3. Root beer
   4. Kool-Aid

8. A nurse is evaluating the laboratory data of clients on a medical-surgical unit. Which laboratory result should a nurse report to a health-care provider?

Result A	Result C
Serum sodium: 130 mEq/L Serum potassium: 3.6 mEq/L *Serum osmolality: 285 mOsm/kg*	Serum sodium: 140 mEq/L Serum potassium: 3.6 mEq/L Serum osmolality: 288 mOsm/kg
Result B	**Result D**
Serum sodium: 137 mEq/L Serum potassium: 3.7 mEq/L *Serum osmolality: 287 mOsm/kg*	Serum sodium: 145 mEq/L Serum potassium: 3.6 mEq/L Serum osmolality: 290 mOsm/kg

   1. Result A
   2. Result B
   3. Result C
   4. Result D

9. Which factor in a client's history should a nurse associate with the development of hypochloremia?
   1. Anorexia nervosa
   2. Bulimia nervosa
   3. Binge eating
   4. Pica

10. A nurse is teaching an older adult client diagnosed with hyponatremia. Which substance should the nurse instruct the client to *avoid*?
    1. Potassium
    2. Chloride
    3. Sodium
    4. Water

11. A home health nurse is educating a client diagnosed with SIADH. What should the nurse advise the client to do regarding the intake of fluids? **Select all that apply.**
    1. Limit fluid intake.
    2. Increase fluid intake.
    3. Measure fluid intake.
    4. Record fluid intake.
    5. Discontinue fluid intake.

12. A nurse is instructing a client on a high-sodium diet. Which foods should the nurse recommend as part of a high-sodium diet?
    1. Fish and plain baked potato
    2. Baked chicken and buttered egg noodles
    3. Salad with balsamic vinaigrette dressing
    4. Ham and cheese sandwich

13. A nurse is caring for a client diagnosed with hypovolemic hyponatremia. Which IV solution order should the nurse anticipate?
    1. Dextrose 5% in half-normal saline solution
    2. Dextrose 5% in water
    3. 0.9% saline solution
    4. 3% saline solution

14. A nurse is planning care for a client diagnosed with severe hyponatremia. Which action should the nurse take when implementing seizure precautions for this client?
    1. Pad the side rails and headboard.
    2. Elevate the head of the client's bed at a 30-degree angle.
    3. Place a bite block in the client's mouth.
    4. Remove all pillows from the area.

15. Which serum chloride level should a nurse anticipate when evaluating the laboratory data of a client diagnosed with hypernatremia?
    1. 90 mEq/L
    2. 100 mEq/L
    3. 108 mEq/L
    4. 118 mEq/L

16. Which manifestations should a nurse identify as the most serious complications associated with hyponatremia?
    1. Anorexia, nausea, and vomiting
    2. Generalized weakness, muscle cramps, and twitching
    3. Lethargy, acute confusion, and decreased level of consciousness
    4. Tachycardia, weak, thready pulses, and decreased blood pressure

17. A nurse is instructing a client on how to reduce the amount of sodium in the diet. Which meal choices, if made by the client, should indicate to the nurse that the client understands the dietary instructions?
    1. Canned tomato soup with a grilled cheese sandwich
    2. Italian sub with a small bag of baked potato chips
    3. Grilled chicken with a broccoli and carrot medley
    4. Smoked salmon with a seasoned baked potato

18. A nurse admitting a client with a serum sodium level of 128 mEq/L and a serum chloride level of 88 mEq/L obtains a list of the client's current medications. Which medication should the nurse identify as having the potential to decrease serum sodium and chloride levels?
    1. Acetaminophen with phenylephrine and dextromethorphan (Tylenol Cold)
    2. Metoprolol and hydrochlorothiazide (Lopressor HCT)
    3. Simvastatin (Zocor)
    4. Esomeprazole (Nexium)

19. Which measure, if included in the care plan for a client diagnosed with diabetes insipidus, should a nurse identify as *most* effective in restoring sodium balance?
    1. Administer IV 3% saline solution.
    2. Administer thiazide diuretics as ordered.
    3. Provide the client with a list of foods that are high in sodium.
    4. Assess the central nervous system for neurological changes.

20. Which statement, if made by a client on a sodium-restricted diet, should indicate to a nurse that the client needs further instruction?
    1. "I will limit the amount of table salt I put on my food."
    2. "I will use natural herbs as seasoning when I cook."
    3. "I will choose canned items that are low in sodium content."
    4. "I will read the product label of my diet soft drinks to assess sodium content."

21. Which foods should a nurse instruct a client to *avoid* to reduce dietary sodium intake? **Select all that apply.**
    1. Luncheon meats
    2. Fresh fruit
    3. Green leafy vegetables
    4. Canned soup
    5. Dry cereal

22. A nurse reviews the laboratory data of a dehydrated older adult client and notes that the client has a serum sodium level of 150 mEq/L. Which manifestations, if identified during assessment, should a nurse associate with this result? **Select all that apply.**
    1. Increased thirst
    2. Orthostatic hypotension
    3. Bradycardia
    4. Decreased temperature
    5. Bounding pulses

23. Which factors, if noted in a client's history, should a nurse associate with the development of hyponatremia? **Select all that apply.**
1. Hyperaldosteronism
2. NPO for 12 hours preoperatively
3. SIADH
4. Gastrointestinal suctioning
5. Excessive diaphoresis

24. A nurse is teaching a client diagnosed with hypertension how to read food labels to assist in choosing foods that are lower in sodium. When discussing the following exhibit with the client, which statement by the nurse is correct?

Nutrition Facts
Per 2 slices (64 g)

Amount	
Calories 160	
	% Daily Value*
Fat 5g	2%
Saturated Fat 0.3g + Trans 0.5g	4%
Cholesterol 0mg	0%
Sodium 290mg	12%
Total Carbohydrate 26g	9%
Dietary Fiber 3g	12%
Sugars 2g	
Protein 5g	
Vitamin A 0% •	Vitamin C 0%
Calcium 4% •	Iron 10%

1. "This food contains too much sodium and should be avoided."
2. "This food is low in sodium and can be part of a low-sodium diet."
3. "You should eat only one slice of this food to maintain a low-sodium diet."
4. "You can eat this food as long as you do not exceed 1,500 mg of sodium per day."

25. Which client should a nurse identify as being at highest risk for hypernatremia?
1. A young child on NPO status before surgery
2. An older adult client admitted with vomiting and diarrhea
3. A client admitted with congestive heart failure
4. An older adult client who has hypertension

26. Which gastrointestinal manifestation, if identified in a client admitted with heart failure, should a nurse associate with the development of hyponatremia?
1. Constipation
2. Diarrhea
3. Gastrointestinal ulcer
4. Hypoactive bowel sounds

27. When hypernatremia is caused by rapid fluid loss, which IV solution should a nurse anticipate being ordered to restore the client's fluid and electrolyte balance?
1. 0.45% NaCl (half-normal saline)
2. 0.9% NaCl (normal saline)
3. 3% NaCl
4. Sterile water

28. Which factor in a client admission assessment should a nurse identify as a cause of hypernatremia?
1. History of heart failure
2. Watery diarrhea present
3. Large amount of dilute urine
4. Excessive diaphoresis

29. Which statement by a student nurse best demonstrates an understanding of the body's attempt to restore sodium balance in a client who is hyponatremic?
1. "ADH and aldosterone are released by the body."
2. "ADH is released and aldosterone is inhibited."
3. "ADH and aldosterone release are both inhibited."
4. "ADH is inhibited and aldosterone is released."

30. A nurse identifies Risk for Falls Related to Skeletal Muscle Weakness as a diagnosis for a client admitted with hypernatremia secondary to chronic renal failure. Which nursing interventions would assist in maintaining this client's safety? **Select all that apply.**
1. Health-care providers will perform hourly checks.
2. The client will call for assistance when getting out of the bed.
3. The nurse will assess the client's neuromuscular status once every shift.
4. A nursing assistant will weigh the client daily at the same time and using the same scale.

31. Which laboratory result should a nurse anticipate when assessing an infant who has persistent projectile vomiting secondary to hypertrophic pyloric stenosis?
1. Serum chloride 118 mEq/L
2. Serum chloride 108 mEq/L
3. Serum chloride 100 mEq/L
4. Serum chloride 90 mEq/L

32. A 6-year-old client is brought to the emergency department after a near-drowning experience in the Pacific Ocean. For which electrolyte imbalance should the nurse assess?
1. Hyponatremia related to actual decrease in sodium
2. Hyponatremia related to relative decrease in sodium
3. Hypernatremia related to actual increase in sodium
4. Hypernatremia related to relative increase in sodium

33. A nurse is preparing to administer IV 3% NaCl solution to a child weighing 60 lb who has been diagnosed with acute hyponatremia. A physician orders 0.5 mEq/kg/hr of 3% saline; 3% NaCl solution contains 50 mEq of sodium per 100 mL. How many milliliters of this IV solution should the nurse administer hourly? Record your answer using a whole number.

____

34. An older adult client in an extended care facility has been vomiting for 2 days. A nurse understands that this client is at increased risk for developing fluid volume deficit and hyponatremia and prepares to infuse 750 mL IV 0.9% saline solution at 125 mL/hr, as ordered by a physician. The nurse selects IV tubing that has a drop factor of 15 gtt/mL. How many drops per minute should the nurse infuse to administer the prescribed 125 mL/hr? Record your answer using a whole number.

____

35. A nurse determines that a client's laboratory test reveals severe hypochloremia. Which nursing diagnosis should be the nurse's priority for this client?
1. Ineffective Breathing Pattern
2. Risk for Injury
3. Risk for Falls
4. Impaired Memory

36. Which manifestations, if identified during the assessment of a client, should a nurse associate with the development of hypernatremia? **Select all that apply.**
1. Confusion
2. Restlessness
3. Hypertension
4. Polyuria
5. Increased thirst

37. A nurse assesses a client diagnosed with hyperchloremia. Which findings would require immediate investigation by the nurse? **Select all that apply.**
1. Respiratory rate: 20
2. Blood pressure: 132/82 mm Hg
3. Increased lethargy
4. Kussmaul respirations
5. Decreased urinary output

38. A nurse is assessing a client with a possible fluid and electrolyte imbalance. Which manifestation, if identified in this client, should the nurse associate with the development of *either* hyponatremia *or* hypernatremia?
1. Hypertension
2. Bradycardia
3. Confusion
4. Diarrhea

39. A nurse is planning care for a client with severe hypernatremia. Which safety intervention should be the nurse's priority?
1. Fall precautions
2. Aspiration precautions
3. Seizure precautions
4. Isolation precautions

40. A nurse is caring for a client who has been diagnosed with H1N1 virus. After 3 days of severe vomiting and diarrhea, the client is now lethargic and hypotensive. A health-care provider writes orders for the client. Which orders should the nurse question? **Select all that apply.**
1. Restrict fluid intake.
2. Monitor and record intake and output.
3. Administer IV 3% sodium chloride solution at 150 mL/hr.
4. Administer IV 0.9% saline solution at 150 mL/hr.
5. Administer furosemide (Lasix) 40 mg daily by mouth.
6. Weigh the client daily.

41. A nurse assists a client who is experiencing a seizure secondary to hyponatremia. When prioritizing care for this client, which actions should the nurse take? Place each intervention in the correct order (1–6).

_______ Document the details of the episode.
_______ Turn the client on his or her side.
_______ Assess respiratory status and apply oxygen if needed.
_______ Suction if needed.
_______ Loosen restrictive clothing.
_______ Remain with the client.

42. A nurse identifies that a client with hyponatremia is confused and restless and has a bounding pulse, a blood pressure of 145/96 mm Hg, and decreased serum osmolarity. Based on these findings, which cause of sodium imbalance should the nurse suspect?
1. Diuretic overdose
2. Excessive diaphoresis
3. Prolonged NPO status
4. Heart failure

43. For a client admitted with severe hyponatremia, which should be the *priority* intervention for a nurse who plans to achieve the goal "Client will remain free from injury"?
1. Adhere to sodium restrictions as ordered.
2. Maintain accurate intake and output records.
3. Monitor neurological status and initiate seizure precautions.
4. Weigh the client daily at the same time and using the same equipment.

44. Which laboratory result should a nurse anticipate in a client diagnosed with SIADH? **Select all that apply.**
    1. Increased serum sodium
    2. Increased urine sodium
    3. Decreased urine osmolality
    4. Decreased plasma osmolality

45. A nurse is planning care for a client diagnosed with hyperchloremia. On which intervention should the nurse place the highest priority?
    1. Place the client on seizure precautions.
    2. Administer IV 0.45% saline solution.
    3. Monitor the client for hypertension.
    4. Evaluate the client's serum sodium level.

REVIEW ANSWERS

1. ANSWER: 1.

Rationale:

1. **Sodium is the most abundant cation in the ECF. The normal serum sodium level is 135 to 145 mEq/L. Cations are positively charged ions, whereas anions are negatively charged. Cations in the body include sodium, potassium, calcium, and magnesium.**
2. The least abundant cation in the ECF is potassium, with a normal serum level of 3.5 to 5.0 mEq/L.
3. Sodium is a cation, not an anion. Anions in the body include bicarbonate, chloride, phosphorus, sulfate, certain organic acids, and certain protein compounds.
4. Sodium is a cation, not an anion.

TEST-TAKING TIP: Review the physiology related to sodium if you had difficulty answering this question. Memorize the normal reference range for sodium because this information is tested on the NCLEX examination.

Content Area: Adult Health

Integrated Processes: Nursing Process: Implementation

Client Need: Physiological Integrity

Cognitive Level: Knowledge

Reference: *Ignatavicius, D., and Workman, M. (2012). Medical-Surgical Nursing: Patient-Centered Collaborative Care (7th ed.). St. Louis, MO: Saunders.*

2. ANSWER: 2.

Rationale:

1. Hyponatremia is defined as a serum sodium level less than 135 mEq/L.
2. **The nurse should associate a serum sodium level of 150 mEq/L with hypernatremia. Hypernatremia is defined as a serum sodium level greater than 145 mEq/L.**
3. Hypokalemia is defined as a serum potassium level less than 3.5 mEq/L.
4. Hyperkalemia is defined as a serum potassium level greater than 5.0 mEq/L.

TEST-TAKING TIP: Be familiar with key terms. Differentiate between hyponatremia and hypernatremia and hypokalemia and hyperkalemia. Memorize the normal reference ranges for sodium and potassium because this information is tested on the NCLEX examination.

Content Area: Adult Health

Integrated Processes: Nursing Process: Assessment

Client Need: Physiological Integrity

Cognitive Level: Comprehension

Reference: *Williams, L., and Hopper, P. (2011). Understanding Medical-Surgical Nursing (4th ed.). Philadelphia, PA: F. A. Davis.*

3. ANSWER: 2.

Rationale:

1. A client who experienced a seizure during a water-drinking contest is most likely experiencing hyponatremia, but not related to an actual decrease in sodium. Based on the history of recent ingestion of excessive amounts of water, the client is experiencing a relative decrease in sodium secondary to the increase in plasma volume, causing a dilution of serum sodium.
2. **The nurse should associate the client's seizure with hyponatremia related to a relative decrease in sodium. Based on the history of recent ingestion of excessive amounts of water, the client is experiencing a relative decrease in sodium secondary to the increase in plasma volume, causing a dilution of serum sodium.**
3. A client who experienced a seizure during a water-drinking contest is most likely experiencing hyponatremia, not hypernatremia.
4. A client who experienced a seizure during a water-drinking contest is most likely experiencing hyponatremia, not hypernatremia.

TEST-TAKING TIP: Differentiate between actual and relative decreases or increases in electrolytes. Relative decreases and increases are always due to alterations in fluid volume.

Content Area: Adult Health

Integrated Processes: Nursing Process: Assessment

Client Need: Physiological Integrity

Cognitive Level: Application

Reference: *Williams, L., and Hopper, P. (2011). Understanding Medical-Surgical Nursing (4th ed.). Philadelphia, PA: F. A. Davis.*

4. ANSWER: 1, 3, 5.

Rationale:

1. **The nurse should observe the client with hyponatremia (serum sodium level less than 135 mEq/L) for changes in mental status, including disorientation, confusion, and personality changes, which are caused by cerebral edema.**
2. Constipation is not associated with sodium imbalance. Diarrhea may occur in a client with hyponatremia (serum sodium level less than 135 mEq/L).
3. **Weakness, nausea, vomiting, and diarrhea may also occur in a client with hyponatremia (serum sodium level less than 135 mEq/L).**
4. Tachypnea is not associated with sodium imbalance.
5. **Cerebral edema is directly responsible for headache, which may be an indication of the development of hyponatremia; observe a client with hyponatremia (serum sodium level less than 135 mEq/L) for signs of headache.**

TEST-TAKING TIP: Recall the signs and symptoms of hyponatremia. Use the process of elimination to rule out incorrect options when there may be multiple correct answers.

Content Area: Adult Health

Integrated Processes: Nursing Process: Assessment

Client Need: Physiological Integrity

Cognitive Level: Application

Reference: *Williams, L., and Hopper, P. (2011). Understanding Medical-Surgical Nursing (4th ed.). Philadelphia, PA: F. A. Davis.*

5. ANSWER: 2.

Rationale:

1. The client with end-stage renal disease is at risk for hypernatremia and fluid retention. Sodium imbalances are associated with agitation and confusion, not euphoria.
2. **The nurse should instruct the client diagnosed with end-stage renal disease to report a weight gain of 3 lb in 1 day immediately to a health-care provider. A client with end-stage renal disease is at risk for hypernatremia and fluid retention (remember, where sodium goes, water follows). A weight gain of 3 lb in 1 day reflects fluid retention of approximately 1,500 mL, a potentially dangerous amount of fluid.**
3. The client with end-stage renal disease is at risk for hypernatremia and fluid retention. Nausea is associated

with hyponatremia. It should be monitored and potentially reported to the health-care provider if it does not resolve.
4. Although diarrhea can potentially lead to sodium imbalance, one episode indicates only the need for monitoring.
TEST-TAKING TIP: Recall that each 1 lb of weight gained is equivalent to about 0.5 L of water retained.
Content Area: Adult Health
Integrated Processes: Teaching/Learning
Client Need: Physiological Integrity
Cognitive Level: Application
Reference: *Williams, L., and Hopper, P. (2011). Understanding Medical-Surgical Nursing (4th ed.). Philadelphia, PA: F. A. Davis.*

6. ANSWER: 1.
Rationale:
1. The nurse should advise the client that it is appropriate to consume mayonnaise as part of a low-sodium diet. Although it is high in fat, 1 tablespoon of mayonnaise contains approximately 80 mg of sodium—a lower sodium content than any of the other options.
2. Barbecue sauce is considered a high-sodium food additive and should be avoided on a low-sodium diet.
3. Catsup is considered a high-sodium food additive and should be avoided on a low-sodium diet.
4. Chili sauce is considered a high-sodium food additive and should be avoided on a low-sodium diet.
TEST-TAKING TIP: Consider each option and eliminate food items known to be high in sodium.
Content Area: Adult Health
Integrated Processes: Teaching/Learning
Client Need: Physiological Integrity
Cognitive Level: Application
Reference: *Lemone, P., and Burke, K. (2010). Medical-Surgical Nursing: Critical Thinking in Client Care (5th ed.). Upper Saddle River, NJ: Pearson Prentice Hall.*

7. ANSWER: 3.
Rationale:
1. Lemonade (8 fl oz) contains 5 to 19 mg of sodium, depending on the type of lemonade (powdered mix has a higher amount than frozen concentrate or fresh). It could be recommended on a low-sodium diet.
2. Tea (6 to 8 fl oz) contains 7 to 24 mg of sodium, depending on the type of tea (instant, lemon-flavored tea sweetened with *sodium saccharide* has the highest amount of sodium). It could be recommended on a low-sodium diet.
3. The nurse should instruct the client to avoid drinking root beer because it contains 48 mg of sodium per 12 fl oz, making it the option with the greatest amount of sodium.
4. Kool-Aid contains no sodium and could be recommended on a low-sodium diet.
TEST-TAKING TIP: Choose the option with the most sodium per serving as the appropriate beverage to avoid on a low-sodium diet.
Content Area: Adult Health
Integrated Processes: Teaching/Learning
Client Need: Physiological Integrity
Cognitive Level: Application
Reference: *U.S. Department of Agriculture, Agricultural Research Service. (2009). USDA National Nutrient Database for Standard Reference. Release 22. Nutrient Data Laboratory Home Page. http://www.ars.usda.gov/ba/bhnrc/ndl.*

8. ANSWER: 1.
Rationale:
1. The nurse should report Result A (serum sodium 130 mEq/L, serum potassium 3.6 mEq/L, serum osmolality 285 mOsm/kg) to the health-care provider because this reflects hyponatremia (low serum sodium level). The normal reference range for serum sodium is 135 to 145 mEq/L. A serum sodium level less than 135 mEq/L is considered hyponatremia. A serum sodium level greater than 145 mEq/L is considered hypernatremia.
2. Result B (serum sodium 137 mEq/L, serum potassium 3.7 mEq/L, serum osmolality 287 mOsm/kg) is within normal limits.
3. Result C (serum sodium 140 mEq/L, serum potassium 3.6 mEq/L, serum osmolality 288 mOsm/kg) is within normal limits.
4. Result D (serum sodium 145 mEq/L, serum potassium 3.6 mEq/L, serum osmolality 290 mOsm/kg) is within normal limits.
TEST-TAKING TIP: Memorize the normal reference range for serum sodium because this information is tested on the NCLEX examination.
Content Area: Adult Health
Integrated Processes: Nursing Process: Evaluation
Client Need: Physiological Integrity
Cognitive Level: Application
Reference: *Williams, L., and Hopper, P. (2011). Understanding Medical-Surgical Nursing (4th ed.). Philadelphia, PA: F. A. Davis.*

9. ANSWER: 2.
Rationale:
1. Anorexia nervosa is self-induced starvation and would result in multiple electrolyte imbalances and nutritional deficiencies, not just hypochloremia.
2. The nurse should associate a history of bulimia nervosa with the development of hypochloremia. Bulimia nervosa is an eating disorder characterized by binge eating followed by purging through self-induced vomiting, the excessive use of laxatives and diuretics, or both. Although chloride imbalances usually occur as a result of other electrolyte imbalances, chloride loss from excessive vomiting is an exception because the client loses chloride in the form of hydrochloric acid in the gastric secretions.
3. Binge eating alone should not produce electrolyte abnormalities.
4. Pica, the desire to consume nonfood substances such as ice, clay, and laundry starch, does not cause any specific electrolyte disturbances and usually does not cause significant nutritional deficiencies.
TEST-TAKING TIP: Consider each option carefully and select the one associated with the direct loss of hydrochloric acid (gastric secretions).
Content Area: Adult Health
Integrated Processes: Nursing Process: Analysis
Client Need: Physiological Integrity
Cognitive Level: Application
Reference: *Ignatavicius, D., and Workman, M. (2012). Medical-Surgical Nursing: Patient-Centered Collaborative Care (7th ed.). St. Louis, MO: Saunders.*

10. ANSWER: 4.
Rationale:
1. Restriction of potassium would not influence the client's sodium levels.
2. Restriction of chloride would not influence the client's sodium levels.
3. An increase in dietary sodium, not a decrease, would be appropriate for the client diagnosed with hyponatremia.
4. The nurse should instruct the client diagnosed with hyponatremia to avoid water. Restriction of free water is necessary to help the body hemoconcentrate sodium and correct dilutional hyponatremia.
TEST-TAKING TIP: Clients experiencing hyponatremia should always restrict their free water intake.
Content Area: Older Adult Health
Integrated Processes: Teaching/Learning
Client Need: Physiological Integrity
Cognitive Level: Application
Reference: *Williams, L., and Hopper, P. (2011). Understanding Medical-Surgical Nursing (4th ed.). Philadelphia, PA: F. A. Davis.*

11. ANSWER: 1, 3, 4.
Rationale:
1. The nurse should advise the client diagnosed with SIADH to limit fluid intake. In SIADH, excessive amounts of water are reabsorbed by the kidneys, creating potentially disastrous dilutional hyponatremia. Water must be restricted to prevent water intoxication.
2. Increasing fluid intake would worsen the water reabsorption and relative sodium deficit.
3. The nurse should also advise the client diagnosed with SIADH to measure all fluid intake to maintain an accurate record and detect a potential fluid imbalance.
4. The nurse should also advise the client diagnosed with SIADH to record all fluid intake to maintain an accurate record and detect a potential fluid imbalance.
5. It is not appropriate to instruct any client to discontinue fluid intake completely. It is necessary to ingest some fluids to maintain homeostasis.
TEST-TAKING TIP: Review each option carefully, and eliminate those that recommend increasing or discontinuing fluid intake.
Content Area: Adult Health
Integrated Processes: Teaching/Learning
Client Need: Physiological Integrity
Cognitive Level: Application
Reference: *Williams, L., and Hopper, P. (2011). Understanding Medical-Surgical Nursing (4th ed.). Philadelphia, PA: F. A. Davis.*

12. ANSWER: 4.
Rationale:
1. Fish and plain baked potato would be appropriate for a low-sodium, not a high-sodium, diet.
2. Baked chicken and buttered egg noodles would be appropriate for a low-sodium, not a high-sodium, diet.
3. Salad with balsamic vinaigrette dressing would be appropriate for a low-sodium, not a high-sodium, diet.
4. The nurse should recommend a ham and cheese sandwich as part of a high-sodium diet. Sandwich meat and processed cheese are the choices with the highest sodium content.
TEST-TAKING TIP: Key words are "high-sodium." Select the option that contains the *most* sodium.
Content Area: Adult Health
Integrated Processes: Teaching/Learning
Client Need: Physiological Integrity
Cognitive Level: Application
Reference: *U.S. Department of Agriculture, Agricultural Research Service. (2009). USDA National Nutrient Database for Standard Reference. Release 22. Nutrient Data Laboratory Home Page. http://www.ars.usda.gov/ba/bhnrc/ndl.*

13. ANSWER: 3.
Rationale:
1. The client with hypovolemic hyponatremia requires replacement of both sodium and fluid. Dextrose 5% in half-normal (0.45%) saline solution replaces minimal sodium and increases the client's risk for exacerbation of hyponatremia.
2. The client with hypovolemic hyponatremia requires replacement of both sodium and fluid. D_5W replaces no sodium at all and increases the client's risk for exacerbation of hyponatremia.
3. A nurse caring for a client diagnosed with hypovolemic hyponatremia should anticipate orders for 0.9% saline solution (normal saline). The client with hypovolemic hyponatremia requires replacement of both sodium and fluid, and 0.9% saline solution is the best choice because it replaces both.
4. The client with hypovolemic hyponatremia requires replacement of both sodium and fluid; 3% saline solution replaces only sodium, leaving the client at risk for hypernatremia because a fluid deficit still exists.
TEST-TAKING TIP: Select an isotonic IV solution when replacing both fluid volume and sodium.
Content Area: Adult Health
Integrated Processes: Nursing Process: Implementation
Client Need: Physiological Integrity
Cognitive Level: Application
Reference: *Williams, L., and Hopper, P. (2011). Understanding Medical-Surgical Nursing (4th ed.). Philadelphia, PA: F. A. Davis.*

14. ANSWER: 1.
Rationale:
1. To protect the client diagnosed with severe hyponatremia, the nurse should pad the side rails and headboard of the bed to prevent injury should a seizure occur. Severe hyponatremia increases this client's risk for seizure activity.
2. Elevating the head of the bed 30 degrees is unnecessary and is not included in seizure precautions.
3. Current guidelines state that one should never force open the client's airway or place anything in the client's mouth during a seizure, making the placement of a bite block in the client's mouth an inappropriate intervention.
4. Removing all pillows from the area is unnecessary and is not included in seizure precautions.
TEST-TAKING TIP: Recall that seizure precautions include padding side rails, keeping the client's call light in reach, assisting the client when ambulating, and keeping suction at the bedside.
Content Area: Adult Health
Integrated Processes: Nursing Process: Implementation

Client Need: Safe and Effective Care Environment
Cognitive Level: Application
Reference: Williams, L., and Hopper, P. (2011). Understanding Medical-Surgical Nursing (4th ed.). Philadelphia, PA: F. A. Davis.

15. ANSWER: 4.
Rationale:
1. The nurse should expect the client with hypernatremia to exhibit hyperchloremia because chloride imbalances are usually the result of other electrolyte imbalances, most frequently sodium. The serum chloride level of 90 mEq/L is below normal limits (hypochloremia), not above normal limits.
2. The nurse should expect the client with hypernatremia to exhibit hyperchloremia because chloride imbalances are usually the result of other electrolyte imbalances, most frequently sodium. The serum chloride level of 100 mEq/L is within normal limits.
3. The nurse should expect the client with hypernatremia to exhibit hyperchloremia because chloride imbalances are usually the result of other electrolyte imbalances, most frequently sodium. The serum chloride level of 108 mEq/L is within normal limits.
4. The nurse should expect the client with hypernatremia to exhibit hyperchloremia because chloride imbalances are usually the result of other electrolyte imbalances, most frequently sodium. The serum chloride level of 118 mEq/L is higher than normal and should be interpreted as hyperchloremia. Serum chloride levels of 100 and 108 mEq/L are within normal limits, and 90 mEq/L is below normal limits.
TEST-TAKING TIP: Remember that chloride follows sodium. Review the normal ranges for sodium and chloride if you had difficulty with this question.
Content Area: Adult Health
Integrated Processes: Nursing Process: Analysis
Client Need: Physiological Integrity
Cognitive Level: Application
Reference: Ignatavicius, D., and Workman, M. (2012). Medical-Surgical Nursing: Patient-Centered Collaborative Care (7th ed.). St. Louis, MO: Saunders.

16. ANSWER: 3.
Rationale:
1. Anorexia, nausea, and vomiting are not the most serious complications associated with hyponatremia.
2. Generalized weakness, muscle cramps, and twitching are not the most serious complications associated with hyponatremia.
3. The nurse should identify lethargy, acute confusion, and decreased level of consciousness as the most serious changes associated with hyponatremia. These signs may indicate the development of cerebral edema. Cerebral edema is usually associated with serum sodium levels less than 110 mEq/L and can lead to respiratory arrest and death. The other manifestations are not as serious as neurological changes.
4. Tachycardia; weak, thready pulses; and decreased blood pressure are not the most serious complications associated with hyponatremia.
TEST-TAKING TIP: Key words are "most serious." Recall that cerebral edema results in increased intracranial pressure, hypoxia, irreversible brain damage, and death.
Content Area: Adult Health
Integrated Processes: Nursing Process: Assessment
Client Need: Physiological Integrity
Cognitive Level: Application
Reference: Ignatavicius, D., and Workman, M. (2012). Medical-Surgical Nursing: Patient-Centered Collaborative Care (7th ed.). St. Louis, MO: Saunders.

17. ANSWER: 3.
Rationale:
1. Canned soups and cheese are high in sodium content and would not be included in a lower-sodium diet.
2. Luncheon meats and potato chips are high in sodium content and would not be included in a lower-sodium diet.
3. If the client chooses grilled chicken with broccoli and carrots, the nurse should recognize that the client understands the dietary instructions to decrease sodium. Canned soups, cheese, luncheon meats, smoked fish, and potato chips are all high in sodium content and would not be included in a lower-sodium diet.
4. Smoked fish is high in sodium content and would not be included in a lower-sodium diet.
TEST-TAKING TIP: Read the question carefully, and select the option that indicates client understanding.
Content Area: Adult Health
Integrated Processes: Nursing Process: Evaluation
Client Need: Physiological Integrity
Cognitive Level: Application
Reference: Ignatavicius, D., and Workman, M. (2012). Medical-Surgical Nursing: Patient-Centered Collaborative Care (7th ed.). St. Louis, MO: Saunders.

18. ANSWER: 2.
Rationale:
1. Cold remedies have the potential to increase, not decrease, sodium and chloride levels.
2. The nurse should identify Lopressor HCT as the medication most likely to decrease the client's serum sodium and chloride levels. Lopressor HCT contains the diuretic hydrochlorothiazide, which can deplete serum sodium, chloride, and potassium levels.
3. Zocor does not affect sodium or chloride levels.
4. Nexium does not affect sodium or chloride levels.
TEST-TAKING TIP: Consider the potential side effects of each medication before selecting your answer.
Content Area: Adult Health
Integrated Processes: Nursing Process: Analysis
Client Need: Physiological Integrity
Cognitive Level: Application
Reference: Ignatavicius, D., and Workman, M. (2012). Medical-Surgical Nursing: Patient-Centered Collaborative Care (7th ed.). St. Louis, MO: Saunders.

19. ANSWER: 2.
Rationale:
1. Administering 3% saline solution would be contraindicated because the client diagnosed with diabetes insipidus is likely hypernatremic, and this intervention would exacerbate the sodium imbalance.
2. The nurse should identify the administration of thiazide diuretics as most effective in restoring sodium balance in the client diagnosed with diabetes insipidus. Diabetes insipidus is a water metabolism disorder caused

by a deficiency of ADH, which results in the excretion of large volumes of dilute urine and the retention of sodium (hypovolemic hypernatremia). Thiazide diuretics are administered to promote sodium excretion.
3. Simply providing the client diagnosed with diabetes insipidus with a list of high-sodium foods, without appropriately teaching the client to avoid these foods, would not assist in restoring sodium balance and would not be more effective than administering a thiazide diuretic.
4. Assessing for central nervous system changes in the client diagnosed with diabetes insipidus is important to identify potential problems associated with the diagnosis but does not assist in restoring sodium balance.
TEST-TAKING TIP: Recall that diabetes insipidus leads to fluid loss and sodium retention.
Content Area: *Adult Health*
Integrated Processes: *Nursing Process: Analysis*
Client Need: *Physiological Integrity*
Cognitive Level: *Application*
Reference: *Ignatavicius, D., and Workman, M. (2012). Medical-Surgical Nursing: Patient-Centered Collaborative Care (7th ed.). St. Louis, MO: Saunders.*

20. ANSWER: 1.
Rationale:
1. The statement "I will limit the amount of table salt I put on my food" should indicate to the nurse that the client needs further instruction. Clients on sodium-restricted diets should *completely avoid* the use of table salt. They should use natural herbs to season foods when cooking, choose canned items low in sodium content, and read the product labels of drinks to assess sodium content.
2. Clients on sodium-restricted diets should use natural herbs to season foods when cooking. This statement indicates that the client does not need further instruction on a sodium-restricted diet.
3. Clients on sodium-restricted diets should choose canned items low in sodium content. This statement indicates that the client does not need further instruction on a sodium-restricted diet.
4. Clients on sodium-restricted diets should read the product labels of drinks to assess the sodium content. This statement indicates that the client does not need further instruction on a sodium-restricted diet.
TEST-TAKING TIP: Read the question carefully and choose the statement that indicates the client has provided an incorrect response and needs more instruction.
Content Area: *Adult Health*
Integrated Processes: *Nursing Process: Evaluation*
Client Need: *Physiological Integrity*
Cognitive Level: *Application*
Reference: *Ignatavicius, D., and Workman, M. (2012). Medical-Surgical Nursing: Patient-Centered Collaborative Care (7th ed.). St. Louis, MO: Saunders.*

21. ANSWER: 1, 4.
Rationale:
1. To reduce dietary sodium intake, the nurse should instruct the client to avoid luncheon meats and canned soups, which are high in sodium content.
2. Clients should be advised to include fresh fruits and vegetables in a low-sodium diet.
3. Clients should be advised to include fresh fruits and vegetables in a low-sodium diet.
4. To reduce dietary sodium intake, the nurse should instruct the client to avoid luncheon meats and canned soups, which are high in sodium content.
5. Dry cereal does not contain significant amounts of sodium and would be appropriate for a low-sodium diet.
TEST-TAKING TIP: Review the nutritional content of common foods if you had difficulty with this question.
Content Area: *Adult Health*
Integrated Processes: *Teaching/Learning*
Client Need: *Physiological Integrity*
Cognitive Level: *Application*
Reference: *Williams, L., and Hopper, P. (2011). Understanding Medical-Surgical Nursing (4th ed.). Philadelphia, PA: F. A. Davis.*

22. ANSWER: 1, 2.
Rationale:
1. The nurse should associate increased thirst with hypovolemic hypernatremia because the fluid volume is decreased (hypovolemia) and the serum sodium level is increased (hypernatremia) in this client (dehydrated, older adult, with a serum sodium level of 150 mEq/L). Tachycardia, not bradycardia, would be noted. This client may also experience an elevation in temperature and weak, thready pulses.
2. The nurse should associate orthostatic hypotension with hypovolemic hypernatremia because the fluid volume is decreased (hypovolemia) and the serum sodium level is increased (hypernatremia) in this client (dehydrated, older adult, with a serum sodium level of 150 mEq/L).
3. Tachycardia, not bradycardia, would be noted in a dehydrated older adult client with a serum sodium level of 150 mEq/L.
4. A dehydrated older adult client with a serum sodium level of 150 mEq/L may experience an elevation in temperature, not a decrease in temperature.
5. A dehydrated older adult client with a serum sodium level of 150 mEq/L would manifest weak, thready pulses, not bounding pulses.
TEST-TAKING TIP: Be familiar with the various types of fluid imbalances associated with hypernatremia and the signs and symptoms associated with these imbalances.
Content Area: *Adult Health*
Integrated Processes: *Nursing Process: Evaluation*
Client Need: *Physiological Integrity*
Cognitive Level: *Application*
Reference: *Ignatavicius, D., and Workman, M. (2012). Medical-Surgical Nursing: Patient-Centered Collaborative Care (7th ed.). St. Louis, MO: Saunders.*

23. ANSWER: 3, 4, 5.
Rationale:
1. Hyperaldosteronism is a common cause of hypernatremia, not hyponatremia (aldosterone protects sodium balance by preventing sodium loss).
2. Although a low-sodium diet and prolonged NPO status may cause hyponatremia, being NPO for only 12 hours would not.
3. The nurse should associate a history of SIADH with the development of hyponatremia because this factor contributes to excess sodium losses.

4. The nurse should associate gastrointestinal suctioning with the development of hyponatremia because this factor contributes to excess sodium losses.
5. The nurse should associate excessive diaphoresis with the development of hyponatremia because this factor contributes to excess sodium losses.
TEST-TAKING TIP: Determine how each option would affect a client's serum sodium level. Eliminate options that would contribute to hypernatremia.
Content Area: Adult Health
Integrated Processes: Nursing Process: Analysis
Client Need: Physiological Integrity
Cognitive Level: Application
Reference: *Ignatavicius, D., and Workman, M. (2012). Medical-Surgical Nursing: Patient-Centered Collaborative Care (7th ed.). St. Louis, MO: Saunders.*

24. ANSWER: 4.
Rationale:
1. Although this is not a low-sodium food, it may be consumed if it is factored into the client's total recommended daily sodium allowance. Other foods may need to be restricted to accommodate the low-sodium instructions.
2. This is not a low-sodium food because it contains more than 140 mg of sodium per serving and constitutes 12% of an adult's recommended daily allowance.
3. One slice of this food contains 145 mg of sodium, so it is not considered a low-sodium food because it has more than 140 mg of sodium per serving and constitutes 12% of an adult's recommended daily allowance. Although eating only one slice is better than eating two, it is still not a low-sodium food.
4. The nurse should inform the client that this food can be eaten as long as the client's daily sodium intake does not exceed 1,500 mg. One slice of this food contains 145 mg of sodium, so it is not considered a low-sodium food because it has more than 140 mg of sodium per serving and constitutes 12% of an adult's recommended daily allowance. The American Heart Association recommends that adults consume no more than 1,500 mg of sodium per day to lower blood pressure and reduce the risk of developing cardiovascular disease. Americans on average consume 3,436 mg of sodium a day.
TEST-TAKING TIP: Recall that 1 teaspoon of salt contains 2,300 mg of sodium.
Content Area: Adult Health
Integrated Processes: Teaching/Learning
Client Need: Physiological Integrity
Cognitive Level: Application
Reference: *American Heart Association. (2010). Sodium (salt or sodium chloride): Reducing sodium in your diet. http://www.americanheart.org/presenter.jhtml?identifier=4708.*

25. ANSWER: 2.
Rationale:
1. NPO status before surgery is usually not long enough to develop hypernatremia, even for a young child.
2. The nurse should identify the older adult client with vomiting and diarrhea as being at high risk for relative hypernatremia secondary to dehydration. Because of the fluid loss, the client retains sodium in an effort to reabsorb water.
3. The client with congestive heart failure is at risk for hyponatremia, not hypernatremia.
4. Hypertension alone would not increase the client's risk for hypernatremia. There are many underlying causes of increased blood pressure in older adult clients.
TEST-TAKING TIP: Recall that children and older adult clients are generally, but not always, at greatest risk for electrolyte imbalances.
Content Area: Adult Health
Integrated Processes: Nursing Process: Assessment
Client Need: Physiological Integrity
Cognitive Level: Application
Reference: *Ignatavicius, D., and Workman, M. (2012). Medical-Surgical Nursing: Patient-Centered Collaborative Care (7th ed.). St. Louis, MO: Saunders.*

26. ANSWER: 2.
Rationale:
1. Constipation is not associated with hyponatremia.
2. The nurse should associate diarrhea with the development of hyponatremia. The gastrointestinal system responds to decreased serum sodium with increased motility, causing nausea and diarrhea.
3. Gastrointestinal ulcers are not associated with hyponatremia.
4. The nurse should associate hyperactive, not hypoactive, bowel sounds and frequent watery bowel movements with a diagnosis of hyponatremia.
TEST-TAKING TIP: Review the signs and symptoms of hyponatremia if you had difficulty answering this question.
Content Area: Adult Health
Integrated Processes: Nursing Process: Assessment
Client Need: Physiological Integrity
Cognitive Level: Application
Reference: *Ignatavicius, D., and Workman, M. (2012). Medical-Surgical Nursing: Patient-Centered Collaborative Care (7th ed.). St. Louis, MO: Saunders.*

27. ANSWER: 1.
Rationale:
1. The nurse should anticipate that the health-care provider will order a hypotonic IV solution for the client diagnosed with hypernatremia caused by rapid fluid loss. Hypotonic solutions, such as half-normal saline, help restore fluid balance without exacerbating the client's hypernatremia.
2. The nurse should anticipate that the health-care provider will order a hypotonic IV solution for the client diagnosed with hypernatremia caused by rapid fluid loss; normal saline solution is isotonic, not hypotonic.
3. The nurse should anticipate that the health-care provider will order a hypotonic IV solution for the client diagnosed with hypernatremia caused by rapid fluid loss; 3% NaCl solution is hypertonic, not hypotonic.
4. Sterile H_2O is never used for IV administration because severe cell hemolysis and cell death may result.
TEST-TAKING TIP: Recall that hypotonic solutions shift fluids *out* of the vessels and *into* the cells, rehydrating the cells without increasing serum sodium levels.
Content Area: Adult Health
Integrated Processes: Nursing Process: Planning

Client Need: Physiological Integrity
Cognitive Level: Application
***Reference:** Ignatavicius, D., and Workman, M. (2012). Medical-Surgical Nursing: Patient-Centered Collaborative Care (7th ed.). St. Louis, MO: Saunders.*

28. ANSWER: 2.
Rationale:
1. A history of heart failure would most likely cause hyponatremia, not hypernatremia.
2. The nurse should identify watery diarrhea, leading to increased water loss, as a cause of hypernatremia (hypovolemic hypernatremia).
3. Diuresis (large amounts of dilute urine) would most likely cause hyponatremia, not hypernatremia.
4. Diaphoresis would most likely cause hyponatremia, not hypernatremia.
TEST-TAKING TIP: Become familiar with the types and causes of hypernatremia.
Content Area: Adult Health
Integrated Processes: Nursing Process: Analysis
Client Need: Physiological Integrity
Cognitive Level: Application
***Reference:** Ignatavicius, D., and Workman, M. (2012). Medical-Surgical Nursing: Patient-Centered Collaborative Care (7th ed.). St. Louis, MO: Saunders.*

29. ANSWER: 4.
Rationale:
1. In a client who is hyponatremic, ADH is inhibited, not released, and aldosterone is released in an attempt to restore sodium balance.
2. In a client who is hyponatremic, ADH is inhibited, not released, and aldosterone is released, not inhibited, in an attempt to restore sodium balance.
3. In a client who is hyponatremic, ADH is inhibited and aldosterone is released, not inhibited, in an attempt to restore sodium balance.
4. The statement by the student nurse that best demonstrates an understanding of the body's attempt to restore sodium balance is "ADH is inhibited and aldosterone is released." Decreased serum sodium levels inhibit the secretion of ADH and trigger aldosterone secretion. When ADH is inhibited, less water is reabsorbed and more is lost from the body in urine. Aldosterone acts on the distal tubules of the kidney nephrons, triggering them to reabsorb sodium from the urine and deposit it back into the blood. Both these mechanisms help restore sodium balance.
TEST-TAKING TIP: Review the effects of ADH and aldosterone on the body if you had difficulty answering this question.
Content Area: Adult Health
Integrated Processes: Nursing Process: Evaluation
Client Need: Physiological Integrity
Cognitive Level: Application
***Reference:** Ignatavicius, D., and Workman, M. (2012). Medical-Surgical Nursing: Patient-Centered Collaborative Care (7th ed.). St. Louis, MO: Saunders.*

30. ANSWER: 1, 2.
Rationale:
1. Performing hourly checks is an important intervention to maintain client safety.
2. Assisting the client when getting out of bed is an important intervention to maintain client safety.
3. Neuromuscular checks should be performed more frequently than every shift.
4. Weighing the client is an important intervention to determine fluid volume status but is not applicable to injury prevention.
TEST-TAKING TIP: Key words are "Risk for Falls." Eliminate options that do not pertain to client safety.
Content Area: Adult Health
Integrated Processes: Nursing Process: Planning
Client Need: Safe and Effective Care Environment
Cognitive Level: Application
***Reference:** Ignatavicius, D., and Workman, M. (2012). Medical-Surgical Nursing: Patient-Centered Collaborative Care (7th ed.). St. Louis, MO: Saunders.*

31. ANSWER: 4.
Rationale:
1. The nurse should expect the infant with pyloric stenosis to exhibit hypochloremia. A chloride level of 118 mEq/L is higher than the normal range (hyperchloremia), not lower.
2. The nurse should expect the infant with pyloric stenosis to exhibit hypochloremia. A serum chloride level of 108 mEq/L is within normal limits.
3. The nurse should expect the infant with pyloric stenosis to exhibit hypochloremia. A serum chloride level of 100 mEq/L is within normal limits.
4. The nurse should expect the infant with pyloric stenosis to exhibit hypochloremia. Hypertrophic pyloric stenosis usually develops in the first few weeks of life, causing projectile vomiting, dehydration, metabolic alkalosis, and failure to thrive. The nurse should note decreased serum levels of sodium and potassium, but of greater diagnostic value is a decrease in serum chloride levels. Excessive vomiting causes the client to lose chloride in the form of hydrochloric acid. A serum chloride level of 90 mEq/L reflects hypochloremia.
TEST-TAKING TIP: Recall specific risk factors for chloride imbalance and apply them to the client's situation. The normal reference range for serum chloride is 95 to 108 mEq/L (although it varies by laboratory).
Content Area: Child Health
Integrated Processes: Nursing Process: Analysis
Client Need: Physiological Integrity
Cognitive Level: Application
***Reference:** Perry, S., Hockenberry, M., Lowdermilk, D., and Wilson, D. (2010). Maternal Child Nursing Care (4th ed.). St. Louis, MO: Mosby.*

32. ANSWER: 3.
Rationale:
1. A near-drowning experience in any ocean would lead to hypernatremia, not hyponatremia, because of excessive ingestion of sodium in salt water.
2. A near-drowning experience in any ocean would lead to hypernatremia, not hyponatremia, because of excessive ingestion of sodium in salt water.
3. The nurse should assess the child for signs of hypernatremia related to an actual increase in sodium. A near-drowning experience in any ocean would lead to hypernatremia because of excessive ingestion (actual increase) of sodium in salt water.

4. The nurse should assess the child for signs of hypernatremia related to an actual, not a relative, increase in sodium. A near-drowning experience in any ocean would lead to hypernatremia because of excessive ingestion (actual increase) of sodium in salt water.
TEST-TAKING TIP: Key words are "near-drowning experience in the Pacific Ocean." Consider the impact that ingesting large amounts of saltwater would have on sodium balance.
Content Area: Child Health
Integrated Processes: Nursing Process: Assessment
Client Need: Physiological Integrity
Cognitive Level: Application
Reference: *Ignatavicius, D., and Workman, M. (2012). Medical-Surgical Nursing: Patient-Centered Collaborative Care (7th ed.). St. Louis, MO: Saunders.*

33. ANSWER: 27.
Rationale:

60 lb ÷ 2.2 lb/kg = 27.27 kg
27.27 kg × 0.5 mEq/kg = 13.64 mEq
50 mEq/100 mL = 0.5 mEq/mL
13.64 mEq ÷ 0.5 mEq/mL = 27.28 mL = 27 mL/hr

TEST-TAKING TIP: Always double-check calculations before administering a medication. Accidental administration of hypertonic NaCl solution has resulted in life-threatening electrolyte imbalances.
Content Area: Child Health
Integrated Processes: Nursing Process: Analysis
Client Need: Physiological Integrity
Cognitive Level: Application
Reference: *Deglin, J. H., Vallerand, A. H., and Sanoski, C. A.(2013). Davis's Drug Guide for Nurses (13th ed.). Philadelphia, PA: F. A. Davis.*

34. ANSWER: 31.
Rationale:

Volume × Drop factor/Time = Rate
125 mL/hr × 15 gtt/mL/60 min= 31.25 = 31 gtt/min

TEST-TAKING TIP: Read the question carefully. It is asking you to calculate a manual drip rate to infuse a solution at 125 mL/hr, using tubing with a drop factor of 15 gtt/min. When performing this particular calculation, the total amount of solution to be infused is irrelevant.
Content Area: Older Adult Health
Integrated Processes: Nursing Process: Analysis
Client Need: Physiological Integrity
Cognitive Level: Application
Reference: *Deglin, J. H., Vallerand, A. H., and Sanoski, C. A.(2013). Davis's Drug Guide for Nurses (13th ed.). Philadelphia, PA: F. A. Davis.*

35. ANSWER: 1.
Rationale:
1. The nurse should assign priority to the diagnosis of Ineffective Breathing Pattern for a client with severe hypochloremia. This client is at increased risk for hypoventilation and respiratory distress or failure secondary to hypochloremia. Risk for Injury, Risk for Falls, and Impaired Memory are all applicable, but they are not the priority for this client.
2. Risk for Injury is applicable but is not the priority for a client with severe hypochloremia.
3. Risk for Falls is applicable but is not the priority for a client with severe hypochloremia.
4. Impaired Memory is applicable but is not the priority for a client with severe hypochloremia.
TEST-TAKING TIP: Remember the "ABCs." Protection of the client's airway and breathing should always be the first priority.
Content Area: Adult Health
Integrated Processes: Nursing Process: Planning
Client Need: Safe and Effective Care Environment
Cognitive Level: Analysis
Reference: *Ignatavicius, D., and Workman, M. (2012). Medical-Surgical Nursing: Patient-Centered Collaborative Care (7th ed.). St. Louis, MO: Saunders.*

36. ANSWER: 1, 2, 3, 5.
Rationale:
1. The nurse should associate confusion with the development of hypernatremia. Signs and symptoms related to alterations in mental status, including agitation, restlessness, and confusion, are all potentially associated with hypernatremia.
2. The nurse should associate restlessness with the development of hypernatremia. Signs and symptoms related to alterations in mental status, including agitation, restlessness, and confusion, are all potentially associated with hypernatremia.
3. The nurse should associate hypertension with the development of hypernatremia. Hypertension may be seen when hypernatremia is accompanied by fluid volume excess.
4. Polyuria, or increased urinary output, would not be seen in hypernatremia because the body would try to dilute the elevated serum sodium by conserving, rather than excreting, water.
5. The nurse should associate increased thirst with the development of hypernatremia. Thirst is usually one of the first symptoms to appear in clients with hypernatremia.
TEST-TAKING TIP: Recall the signs and symptoms of hypernatremia. Use the process of elimination to rule out incorrect options when there may be multiple correct answers.
Content Area: Adult Health
Integrated Processes: Nursing Process: Assessment
Client Need: Physiological Integrity
Cognitive Level: Analysis
Reference: *Williams, L., and Hopper, P. (2011). Understanding Medical-Surgical Nursing (4th ed.). Philadelphia, PA: F. A. Davis.*

37. ANSWER: 3, 4.
Rationale:
1. A respiratory rate of 20 breaths per minute is within normal limits and would not require immediate investigation by the nurse.
2. A blood pressure of 132/82 mm Hg is within normal limits and would not require immediate investigation by the nurse.
3. A nurse caring for a client with hyperchloremia should intervene immediately if the client displays increased lethargy, indicating a deterioration in neurological status.
4. A nurse caring for a client with hyperchloremia should intervene immediately if the client displays Kussmaul respirations, an ineffective breathing pattern.

5. Decreased urinary output is an expected finding in hyperchloremia that would not necessitate intervention by the nurse.

TEST-TAKING TIP: Review the signs and symptoms of hyperchloremia. Rule out options that are within normal limits.

Content Area: Adult Health

Integrated Processes: Nursing Process: Analysis

Client Need: Physiological Integrity

Cognitive Level: Analysis

Reference: *Ignatavicius, D., and Workman, M. (2012). Medical-Surgical Nursing: Patient-Centered Collaborative Care (7th ed.). St. Louis, MO: Saunders.*

38. ANSWER: 3.

Rationale:

1. Hypertension is more likely to indicate hypernatremia with fluid volume excess. It is not associated with hyponatremia.

2. Bradycardia usually does not result from sodium imbalances and would not be associated with either hypernatremia or hyponatremia.

3. The nurse should associate confusion with the development of either hyponatremia or hypernatremia. Neurological changes, such as confusion, are common in hyponatremia and hypernatremia.

4. Diarrhea is found with hyponatremia but not hypernatremia.

TEST-TAKING TIP: Review the signs and symptoms of sodium imbalances, and select the manifestation that is common to both conditions.

Content Area: Adult Health

Integrated Processes: Nursing Process: Assessment

Client Need: Physiological Integrity

Cognitive Level: Analysis

Reference: *Williams, L., and Hopper, P. (2011). Understanding Medical-Surgical Nursing (4th ed.). Philadelphia, PA: F. A. Davis.*

39. ANSWER: 3.

Rationale:

1. Fall precautions would be important for a client with hypernatremia but are not the priority for this client.

2. Aspiration precautions may be indicated for a client with hypernatremia but are not the priority for this client.

3. The nurse should place priority on seizure precautions when planning care for a client with severe hypernatremia. This imbalance places the client at high risk for seizures, which can lead to traumatic injury, asphyxiation, and death, making seizure precautions the priority intervention. Specific seizure precautions vary, depending on health-care agency policy. The nurse should focus on observing the seizure and responding appropriately to the type of seizure.

4. Isolation precautions are unnecessary for a client with hypernatremia; they should be used for clients with specific infectious processes.

TEST-TAKING TIP: When prioritizing care, select the intervention for the most life-threatening event. Recall that hypernatremia causes neuromuscular irritability.

Content Area: Adult Health

Integrated Processes: Nursing Process: Planning

Client Need: Safe and Effective Care Environment

Cognitive Level: Analysis

Reference: *Ignatavicius, D., and Workman, M. (2012). Medical-Surgical Nursing: Patient-Centered Collaborative Care (7th ed.). St. Louis, MO: Saunders.*

40. ANSWER: 1, 3, 5.

Rationale:

1. The client is displaying signs of fluid volume deficit and is at risk for an actual decrease in sodium. The nurse should question the health-care provider's order to restrict fluid intake, which would worsen the client's fluid volume deficit.

2. The client is displaying signs of fluid volume deficit and is at risk for an actual decrease in sodium. Monitoring and recording intake and output are necessary to evaluate the client's fluid volume status. It would not be appropriate to question this order.

3. The client is displaying signs of fluid volume deficit and is at risk for an actual decrease in sodium. The nurse should question the health-care provider's order to administer IV 3% NaCl solution (a hypertonic solution), which would worsen the client's fluid volume deficit and potentially correct hyponatremia too rapidly.

4. The client is displaying signs of fluid volume deficit and is at risk for an actual decrease in sodium. Normal saline solution (0.9% saline) is an appropriate intervention because it would correct the client's fluid volume deficit and hyponatremia. It would not be appropriate to question this order.

5. The client is displaying signs of fluid volume deficit and is at risk for an actual decrease in sodium. The nurse should question the health-care provider's order to administer furosemide (Lasix). Furosemide administration is contraindicated in any client with fluid volume deficit because, as a diuretic, it would increase the client's fluid loss and worsen the client's FVD.

6.The client is displaying signs of fluid volume deficit and is at risk for an actual decrease in sodium. Weighing the client daily is necessary to evaluate the client's fluid volume status. It would not be appropriate to question this order.

TEST-TAKING TIP: Key words are "Which orders should the nurse question?" Select the options that would be incorrect orders in this situation.

Content Area: Adult Health

Integrated Processes: Nursing Process: Analysis

Client Need: Physiological Integrity

Cognitive Level: Analysis

Reference: *Williams, L., and Hopper, P. (2011). Understanding Medical-Surgical Nursing (4th ed.). Philadelphia, PA: F. A. Davis.*

41. ANSWER: 6, 3, 4, 5, 2, 1.

Rationale: The primary objective when caring for a client who is experiencing a seizure is to prevent injury to the client. To protect the client, the nurse should (1) remain with the client, (2) loosen restrictive clothing, (3) turn the client on his or her side to prevent airway occlusion or aspiration, (4) assess respiratory status and apply oxygen if needed, (5) suction the client's airway if necessary, and (6) document the details of the episode.

TEST-TAKING TIP: Visualize the correct nursing actions in your mind, and think about the logical sequence of implementing those actions.

Content Area: *Adult Health*
Integrated Processes: *Nursing Process: Implementation*
Client Need: *Safe and Effective Care Environment*
Cognitive Level: *Analysis*
Reference: *Williams, L., and Hopper, P. (2011). Understanding Medical-Surgical Nursing (4th ed.). Philadelphia, PA: F. A. Davis.*

42. ANSWER: 4.
Rationale:
1. Diuretic overdose would lead to hyponatremia with fluid volume deficit, which would manifest as a decreased blood pressure and a weak, thready pulse, not a bounding pulse, a blood pressure of 145/96 mm Hg, and decreased serum osmolarity.
2. Excessive diaphoresis would lead to hyponatremia with fluid volume deficit, which would manifest as a decreased blood pressure and a weak, thready pulse, not a bounding pulse, a blood pressure of 145/96 mm Hg, and decreased serum osmolarity.
3. Prolonged NPO status would lead to hyponatremia with fluid volume deficit, which would manifest as a decreased blood pressure and a weak, thready pulse, not a bounding pulse, a blood pressure of 145/96 mm Hg, and decreased serum osmolarity.
4. The nurse should suspect that the client is experiencing heart failure because a bounding pulse, elevated blood pressure, and decreased serum osmolarity indicate hyponatremia with fluid volume excess.
TEST-TAKING TIP: Review the signs, symptoms, and causes of fluid volume excess if you had difficulty answering this question. Recall that relative hyponatremia is caused by fluid volume excess.
Content Area: *Adult Health*
Integrated Processes: *Nursing Process: Analysis*
Client Need: *Physiological Integrity*
Cognitive Level: *Analysis*
Reference: *Ignatavicius, D., and Workman, M. (2012). Medical-Surgical Nursing: Patient-Centered Collaborative Care (7th ed.). St. Louis, MO: Saunders.*

43. ANSWER: 3.
Rationale:
1. Adhering to sodium restrictions is an important intervention in the treatment of a client with hyponatremia, but it is not the priority intervention to maintain client safety.
2. Maintaining accurate intake and output records is an important intervention in the treatment of a client with hyponatremia, but it is not the priority intervention to maintain client safety.
3. Monitoring neurological status and initiating seizure precautions should be the nurse's priority to achieve the goal "Client will remain free from injury." These interventions address the mental status changes that occur with severe hyponatremia and are the appropriate safety precautions for this client.
4. Weighing the client daily at the same time and using the same equipment is an important intervention in the treatment of a client with hyponatremia, but it is not the priority intervention to maintain client safety.
TEST-TAKING TIP: Key words are "Client will remain free from injury." Select the option that addresses client safety.
Content Area: *Adult Health*
Integrated Processes: *Nursing Process: Analysis*
Client Need: *Safe and Effective Care Environment*
Cognitive Level: *Analysis*
Reference: *Ignatavicius, D., and Workman, M. (2012). Medical-Surgical Nursing: Patient-Centered Collaborative Care (7th ed.). St. Louis, MO: Saunders.*

44. ANSWER: 2, 4.
Rationale:
1. The nurse should anticipate that a client diagnosed with SIADH will have decreased, not increased, serum sodium. In SIADH, the body retains water, causing dilutional hyponatremia (decreased serum sodium).
2. The nurse should anticipate that a client diagnosed with SIADH will have an increase in urine sodium and a decrease in plasma osmolality. SIADH is a disorder of the posterior pituitary gland in which vasopressin (ADH) is secreted even when plasma osmolarity is normal or low. As a result, the body retains water, causing dilutional hyponatremia (decreased serum sodium). The retained water increases the plasma volume (lowering plasma osmolality), which causes an increase in the glomerular filtration rate and concentrates the urine. This effect increases sodium loss in the urine.
3. The nurse should anticipate that a client diagnosed with SIADH will have increased, not decreased, urine osmolality. In SIADH, the body retains water, causing dilutional hyponatremia (decreased serum sodium). The retained water increases the plasma volume (lowering plasma osmolality), which causes an increase in the glomerular filtration rate, concentrates the urine, and results in increased urine osmolality.
4. The nurse should anticipate that a client diagnosed with SIADH will have a decrease in plasma osmolality and an increase in urine sodium. SIADH is a disorder of the posterior pituitary gland in which vasopressin (ADH) is secreted even when plasma osmolarity is normal or low. As a result, the body retains water, causing dilutional hyponatremia (decreased serum sodium). The retained water increases the plasma volume (lowering plasma osmolality), which causes an increase in the glomerular filtration rate and concentrates the urine. This effect increases sodium loss in the urine.
TEST-TAKING TIP: Recall that SIADH leads to sodium loss andfluid retention.
Content Area: *Adult Health*
Integrated Processes: *Nursing Process: Analysis*
Client Need: *Physiological Integrity*
Cognitive Level: *Analysis*
Reference: *Ignatavicius, D., and Workman, M. (2012). Medical-Surgical Nursing: Patient-Centered Collaborative Care (7th ed.). St. Louis, MO: Saunders.*

45. ANSWER: 1.
Rationale:
1. The nurse's highest priority should be to place the client on seizure precautions. Chloride imbalances are usually the result of other electrolyte imbalances, such as hypernatremia. The nurse should infer that the client's serum sodium level is also elevated, putting this client at risk for seizures.

2. Administering IV 0.45% saline solution is an appropriate intervention for a client diagnosed with hyperchloremia, but it should not be the nurse's priority.
3. Monitoring for hypertension is an appropriate intervention for a client diagnosed with hyperchloremia, but it should not be the nurse's priority.
4. Evaluating the serum sodium level is an appropriate intervention for a client diagnosed with hyperchloremia, but it should not be the nurse's priority.

TEST-TAKING TIP: Ensuring client safety should always be the nurse's first priority.
Content Area: *Adult Health*
Integrated Processes: *Nursing Process: Planning*
Client Need: *Physiological Integrity*
Cognitive Level: *Analysis*
Reference: *Ignatavicius, D., and Workman, M. (2012). Medical-Surgical Nursing: Patient-Centered Collaborative Care (7th ed.). St. Louis, MO: Saunders.*

Chapter 4

Potassium Imbalances

KEY TERMS

Actual hyperkalemia—Elevated serum potassium level with an increased number of potassium ions in the extracellular fluid (ECF).

Actual hypokalemia—Reduced serum potassium level with a decreased number of potassium ions in the ECF.

Adenosine triphosphate—A substance present in all living cells that contains a large amount of chemical energy; when adenosine triphosphate breaks down, it releases that energy, which is used for many metabolic processes; considered as the "universal energy currency for metabolism."

Bradycardia—An apical heart rate less than 60 bpm (in an adult client).

Dysrhythmia—Abnormal or irregular cardiac rhythm caused by a disturbance in the electrical conduction of the heart.

Hyperkalemia—Serum potassium (K^+) greater than 5 mEq/L.

Hypokalemia—Serum potassium (K^+) less than 3.5 mEq/L.

Relative hyperkalemia—Elevated serum potassium level without an actual increase in the number of potassium ions; caused by the movement of potassium out of the cells into the ECF.

Relative hypokalemia—Reduced serum potassium level without an actual decrease in the number of potassium ions; caused by the movement of potassium out of the ECF into the cells.

Sodium-potassium pump—Mechanism within the cell membrane of every cell in the body that actively transports potassium back into the cell and sodium back into the ECF to maintain electrolyte balance in the ECF.

Tachycardia—An apical heart rate greater than 100 bpm (in an adult client).

Ventricular fibrillation—A medical emergency in which the ventricles of the heart quiver rather than contract properly.

I. Description

Potassium (K^+) is the most common cation in the intracellular fluid (ICF). The ICF contains approximately 98% of the body's potassium, while approximately 2% remains in the extracellular fluid (ECF). Potassium plays a significant role in neuromuscular activity and helps maintain acid-base balance. Dietary intake is usually sufficient to meet daily requirements. Guidelines suggest that most adults should consume at least 4,700 mg of potassium daily, but surveys show that Americans consume less than half that amount because the typical Western diet is low in fruits and vegetables. Potassium is absorbed in the intestines and excreted by the kidneys. To maintain homeostasis in the body, serum potassium levels must be tightly controlled. Minimal changes in potassium concentration can cause major alterations in the body. Potassium performs the following functions:

1. Facilitates nerve impulse conduction
2. Is essential for the normal electrical activity of the heart
3. Plays a key role in skeletal and smooth muscle contraction, making it important for normal digestive and muscular functioning
4. Assists in making protein using amino acids
5. Aids in the regulation of acid-base balance

Normal Lab Value The normal serum potassium level is 3.5 to 5.0 mEq/L.

MAKING THE CONNECTION

Potassium Balance and the Sodium-Potassium Pump

The **sodium-potassium pump,** which is found in the cell membrane of every cell in the body, regulates the amount of potassium in the ECF. Because the concentration of potassium is much higher in the ICF than in the ECF, potassium easily moves out of the cells down the concentration gradient via diffusion. The sodium-potassium pump then transports sodium and potassium ions across cell membranes *against* their concentration gradients. This process requires the expenditure of energy, which is provided by adenosine triphosphate. Potassium is moved *out of* the ECF, where its concentration is low, and *into* the cells, where the concentration is much higher, to control the amount of potassium in the blood and other extracellular fluids. Sodium is moved in the opposite direction. The sodium-potassium pump removes three sodium ions from each cell for every two potassium ions returned to each cell (Fig. 4.1). If an underlying disorder prevents the sodium-potassium pump from working properly, potential life-threatening electrolyte imbalances can occur.

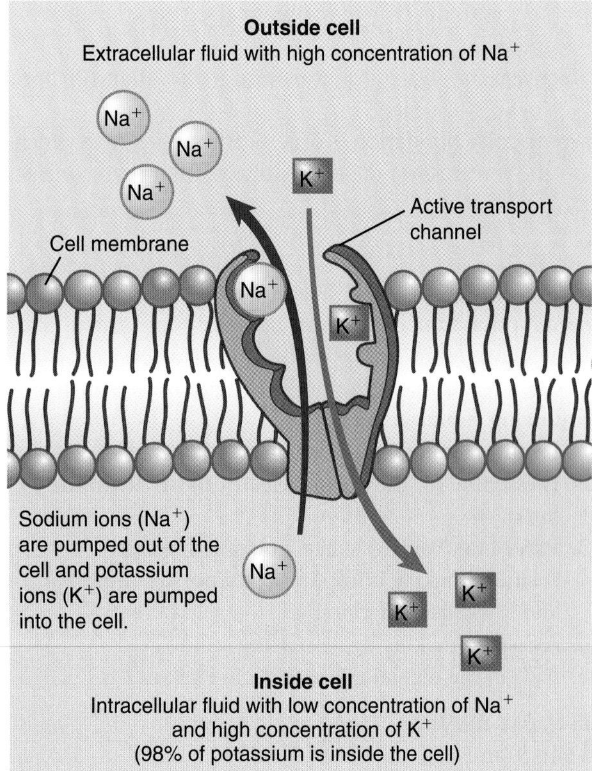

Fig 4.1 The intracellular potassium concentration is higher than the extracelluar concentration. To equalize the concentrations, potassium automatically flows out of the cell through channels in the cell membrane; however, it is also continuously pumped in via active transport by means of the sodium-potassium pump.

II. Potassium Imbalance

Potassium imbalances occur when there is a decrease or increase in the potassium content of the ECF. To remember how potassium affects the body, associate *low* potassium levels (hypokalemia) with general *hypo*activity in the body (deep tendon hyporeflexia, flattened T waves on the electrocardiogram [ECG], and hypoactive bowel sounds or constipation) because reduced potassium levels slow down nerve impulses. Associate *high* potassium levels (hyperkalemia) with general *hyper*activity in the body (irritability; tall, tented T waves on the ECG; and hyperactive bowel sounds or diarrhea) because increased potassium levels speed up nerve impulses. The greatest danger related to either type of potassium imbalance is cardiac dysrhythmia because the heart muscle (myocardium) is highly excitable and most sensitive to changes in potassium levels.

III. Types of Potassium Imbalance

A. **Hypokalemia,** or potassium deficit, is a serum potassium level less than 3.5 mEq/L.
   1. If potassium loss is gradual, the body can compensate for the change, and signs and symptoms of hypokalemia may not appear until potassium loss is extreme.
   2. Consequences of hypokalemia are worsened by alkalosis, digoxin therapy, and hypocalcemia.
   3. Hypokalemia can be life threatening because it disrupts the electrical activity in cardiac, skeletal, and smooth muscles, resulting in cardiac dysrhythmias and profound muscle weakness.
   4. Respiratory insufficiency and cardiac dysrhythmias are the most dangerous potential problems associated with hypokalemia.

DID YOU KNOW?

Chronic, moderate potassium deficiency is associated with increased blood pressure, increased sensitivity to salt, increased risk of kidney stones, and increased rate of bone remodeling.

B. **Hyperkalemia,** or potassium excess, is a serum potassium level greater than 5.0 mEq/L.
   1. Hyperkalemia is dangerous because there are often no signs or symptoms.
   2. Mild hyperkalemia is usually well tolerated.
   3. Moderate hyperkalemia can produce ECG changes.
   4. Sudden increases in serum potassium can cause severe problems at levels between 6.0 and 7.0 mEq/L, whereas gradual increases may not affect the client until the level reaches 8.0 mEq/L or greater.
   5. Severe hyperkalemia suppresses the electrical activity of the heart, causing cardiac dysrhythmias or cardiac arrest.

DID YOU KNOW?

Cardiac dysrhythmia is the most common cause of death in clients with hyperkalemia.

(!) A serum potassium level less than 2.5 mEq/L or greater than 6.5 mEq/L is a medical emergency and can lead to respiratory arrest and lethal dysrhythmias.

IV. Causes of Potassium Imbalance

Changes in fluid and potassium balance may result in *actual* or *relative* increases or decreases in potassium content. An *actual* increase or decrease in potassium occurs as a direct result of potassium gain or loss. A *relative* increase or decrease in potassium is most often caused by shifts in potassium between the ICF and ECF compartments (Table 4.1).

A. **Actual hypokalemia** may be caused by potassium loss or inadequate potassium intake or absorption, resulting in an *actual* decrease in potassium in the body.
   1. Potassium loss
      a. Vomiting and chronic diarrhea result in the loss of water, sodium, and potassium.
      b. Prolonged gastric suctioning removes fluid and hydrochloric acid, causing the pH of the blood to increase (alkalosis) (see Chapter 8, Acidosis and Alkalosis).
      c. Diaphoresis (excessive sweating) caused by heat leads to the loss of water, sodium, and potassium as the body attempts to reduce its core temperature.
      d. Renal disease adversely affects the kidneys' ability to reabsorb potassium.
      e. Hemodialysis and peritoneal dialysis lead to direct potassium loss.

Table 4.1 Causes of Potassium Imbalance

Hypokalemia	
Actual decrease in potassium	Relative decrease in potassium (dilutional)

Potassium loss
• Vomiting
• Prolonged gastric suctioning
• Chronic diarrhea
• Major surgical procedures
• Hemorrhage
• Medications (those that act on the kidneys to increase potassium excretion)
  • Corticosteroids
  • Insulins
  • Loop diuretics
  • Non–potassium-sparing diuretics
  • Thiazide diuretics
Inadequate potassium intake or absorption
• Eating disorders
  • Anorexia
  • Bulimia
  • Ingestion of clay (bentonite)
• Prolonged nothing-by-mouth status
• Hyperalimentation or total parenteral nutrition
• IV therapy with solutions that do not contain potassium
	Shifts between intracellular and extracellular compartments
	• Familial periodic paralysis
	Water gain
	• Adrenal insufficiency
	• Excessive intake of hypotonic fluids (water, IV D_5W, tube feeding)
	• Nephrotic syndrome
	• Wound irrigation with hypotonic fluids
	• Heart failure or congestive heart failure
	• Hyperglycemia
	Third spacing
	• Edema
	• Ascites (liver failure, liver cirrhosis)

Hyperkalemia	
Actual increase in potassium	Relative increase in potassium

Potassium retention
• Acute kidney injury
• Chronic kidney disease
• Glomerulonephritis
• Rejection of kidney transplant
• Addison's disease
• Medications (those that interfere with the urinary excretion of potassium)
  • ACE inhibitors
  • Angiotensin II receptor blockers
  • NSAIDs
  • Potassium-sparing diuretics
Excessive potassium intake
• Excessive intake of oral or parenteral potassium replacements
• Overuse of potassium-based salt substitutes
	Shifts between intracellular and extracellular compartments
	• Metabolic acidosis
	• Tissue trauma
	  • Burns
	  • Surgical procedures
	  • Trauma
	  • Tumor invasion
	Water loss
	• Kidney disease
	• Vomiting
	• Diarrhea
	• Burns

f. Elevated serum glucose levels lead to diuresis, causing potassium to be lost in the urine.
g. Medications, such as non–potassium-sparing diuretics, digitalis preparations, and corticosteroids, act on the kidneys to increase potassium excretion.

2. Inadequate potassium intake or absorption
   a. Malnutrition or starvation
   b. Eating disorders, such as anorexia or bulimia
   c. Prolonged nothing-by-mouth (NPO) status without IV replacement therapy
   d. Alcoholism and pica
      1) Alcoholism causes a decrease in the absorption of potassium.
      2) Pica is the chronic ingestion of nonfood materials, such as animal feces, dirt, paper, laundry starch, or ice. If clay (bentonite) is ingested, it binds with potassium and decreases potassium absorption.

DID YOU KNOW?

Hypokalemia is one of the most common electrolyte imbalances associated with chronic alcoholism. Clients who abuse alcohol may experience potassium deficiency even if they consume an adequate daily amount, owing to a lack of absorption in the small intestine.

B. **Relative hypokalemia** results when potassium shifts *out of* the ECF and *into* the cells, resulting in a relative decrease in potassium content in the body.

1. Water gain
   a. Excessive water intake dilutes the serum potassium content of the blood (dilutional hypokalemia).
2. Shifts between intracellular and extracellular compartments
   a. Alkalosis (increased blood pH) causes potassium to move into the cells; hydrogen ions then move out of the cells to compensate for the pH imbalance.
   b. Stimulation of the sympathetic nervous system, particularly with beta-2-agonists such as albuterol or terbutaline, may increase cellular potassium uptake.
   c. Familial periodic paralysis is a genetic disorder that causes a sudden intracellular shift of potassium, resulting in transient episodes of profound hypokalemia.
   d. Insulin administration for hyperglycemia causes potassium to move into the skeletal muscles and hepatic cells; intracellular shifts of potassium are often episodic and self-limited.
3. Third spacing
   a. Fluid, sodium, potassium, and other electrolytes often become "trapped" in areas that are inaccessible to the circulation.

DID YOU KNOW?

In clients taking digoxin (Lanoxin), hypokalemia increases the cardiac muscle's sensitivity to the drug, possibly resulting in digoxin toxicity.

C. **Actual hyperkalemia** is caused by excessive potassium intake or potassium retention, resulting in an actual increase of potassium in the body (see Table 4.1).

1. Excessive intake of potassium
   a. Overconsumption of potassium-rich foods (rare when the kidneys are functioning normally)
   b. Overuse of salt substitutes that contain potassium
   c. Excessive or rapid infusion of IV solutions that contain potassium

DID YOU KNOW?

In the United States, a lethal dose of potassium chloride is the last of the three drugs administered during execution by lethal injection. Potassium chloride actually causes death by stopping the heart.

2. Potassium retention
   a. Acute kidney injury and chronic kidney disease result in decreased potassium excretion by the kidneys.
   b. Medications, such as potassium-sparing diuretics and angiotensin-converting enzyme (ACE) inhibitors, inhibit the excretion of potassium by the kidneys.
   c. Addison's disease occurs when the adrenal glands do not produce enough aldosterone (adrenal insufficiency).
   d. Hyperkalemia may also be caused by fluid volume deficit or when potassium shifts out of the cells, resulting in a relative increase in potassium in the body.

D. **Relative hyperkalemia** results when potassium is concentrated by excessive water loss or when potassium shifts *out of* the ICF and *into* the ECF, resulting in a relative increase in potassium content in the body or (see Table 4.1).

1. Water loss
   a. Vomiting and diarrhea result in water loss in the ECF, which causes potassium and other electrolytes to become concentrated.
   b. Severe burns cause tissue damage and an increase in capillary permeability, resulting in profound dehydration; this water loss causes potassium to become concentrated, resulting in an elevation in the serum potassium level without an actual potassium gain.
2. Shifts between intracellular and extracellular compartments
   a. Surgical procedures, tissue trauma, and crush injuries cause damaged cells to release

potassium into the bloodstream; breakdown of muscle tissue (rhabdomyolysis) also releases the protein myoglobin into the bloodstream, causing kidney damage and the retention of potassium.

b. Metabolic acidosis, or blood pH below 7.35, causes potassium to shift out of the cells in exchange for excess hydrogen ions (acid) as the body attempts to increase the blood pH.
c. Tumor invasion destroys healthy cells, causing them to release their potassium stores into the ECF and resulting in an increase in the serum potassium level without an actual gain in potassium (relative hyperkalemia).
d. In clients with severe burns, potassium shifts out of the cells of the burned tissue and into the ECF, resulting in relative hyperkalemia.

MAKING THE CONNECTION

Addison's Disease and Hyperkalemia

Addison's disease occurs when damaged or diseased adrenal glands do not produce enough glucocorticoid hormones (such as cortisol), sex hormones (such as androgens [male] and estrogens [female]), and mineralocorticoid hormones (such as aldosterone). Aldosterone causes the kidneys to conserve sodium and secrete potassium. The lack of aldosterone leads to the excretion of sodium and the retention of potassium, resulting in increased serum potassium levels (hyperkalemia).

V. Nursing Assessment for Potassium Imbalances

The nurse should conduct a focused nursing assessment for potassium imbalance, beginning with a thorough nursing history. Interview the client and family members to identify any risk factors or preexisting conditions that would contribute to potassium imbalance, such as vomiting, nasogastric suctioning, diarrhea, acute kidney injury, or other conditions associated with potassium loss or gain. The nurse should also assess the client's ability to drink and tolerate oral fluids. Obtain a current dietary history, inquiring about the intake of potassium chloride–based salt substitutes. The nursing history should also include current medications, focusing on the use of diuretics and digoxin. Diuretic use increases the risk for potassium imbalance, and hypokalemia increases the risk of digoxin toxicity. A thorough physical assessment is necessary because potassium imbalances affect many body systems. Assess each body system, observing for signs and symptoms of potassium imbalance. Measure and record the client's vital signs, and review the client's laboratory data to assess for the presence of hypo- or hyperkalemia (Table 4.2).

VI. Electrocardiogram Changes in Potassium Imbalance

A. A hallmark finding of potassium imbalance is a change in the ECG. Potassium is needed to bring the cell membranes to a resting state after the heart contracts. Low potassium levels in the extracellular space cause the strength of the electrical current across the cell

Table 4.2 Signs and Symptoms of Potassium Imbalance

Vital Signs		
	Hypokalemia	*Hyperkalemia*
Blood pressure	Decreased, orthostatic hypotension	Decreased, orthostatic hypotension, or normal to elevated
Heart rate	Normal to decreased; may be irregular	Normal to decreased; may be irregular
Respiratory rate	May decrease in severe hypokalemia	May decrease in severe hyperkalemia
Temperature	Within normal limits	Within normal limits
Signs and Symptoms by Body System		
	Hypokalemia	*Hyperkalemia*
Cardiovascular	• Weak, thready pulse; may be irregular • Bradycardia or tachycardia, depending on etiology • Decreased blood pressure that progresses to severe orthostatic hypotension  Causes life-threatening cardiac dysrhythmias • Premature ventricular contractions (PVCs) • Ventricular tachycardia (VT) • Ventricular fibrillation • Asystole	• Irregular heartbeat, "palpitations" • Bradycardia • Slow, weak, or absent pulse • Hypotension Causes life-threatening cardiac dysrhythmias • PVCs • VT • Ventricular fibrillation • Complete heart block • Asystole

Continued

Table 4.2 Signs and Symptoms of Potassium Imbalance—cont'd

Signs and Symptoms by Body System

	Hypokalemia	*Hyperkalemia*
Cerebral	• Fatigue • Irritability • Anxiety • Decreased level of consciousness	• Frequently asymptomatic • Fatigue
Electrocardiogram (ECG) changes	• U waves increase in size; may become as prominent as T waves (prominent U wave) or fuse with T waves (see Figs 4.2 and 4.3) • QRS complexes widen • ST segments may become depressed • T waves may flatten or invert (see Fig. 4.3)	• Heart block (first degree or second degree); may become complete heart block • Bradycardia • Peaked, tented T waves • Ventricular fibrillation (see Fig. 4.4)
Gastrointestinal	• Nausea, vomiting • Abdominal distention • Hypoactive bowel sounds • Constipation	• Nausea • Hyperactive bowel sounds • Diarrhea (may be frequent)
Neuromuscular	• Weakness (generalized) • Muscle aches, cramps, twitching • Decreased deep tendon reflexes • Paralysis	• Muscle weakness • Muscle cramps and tingling, followed by circumoral and peripheral numbness as potassium level increases
Respiratory	• Shallow, ineffective respirations	• May produce respiratory arrest because of muscle weakness

Laboratory Values

	Hypokalemia	*Hyperkalemia*
Serum potassium	Less than 3.5 mEq/L	Greater than 5.0 mEq/L

membranes to increase, preventing the cell membranes of the heart from achieving a resting state. This leads to impaired cardiac conduction, which can result in premature ventricular contractions (PVCs), ventricular tachycardia, ventricular fibrillation, or asystole.

1. Hypokalemia can be identified in an ECG rhythm strip by looking for the triad of (1) ST segment depression, (2) low-amplitude T waves, and (3) prominent U waves (Fig. 4.2).

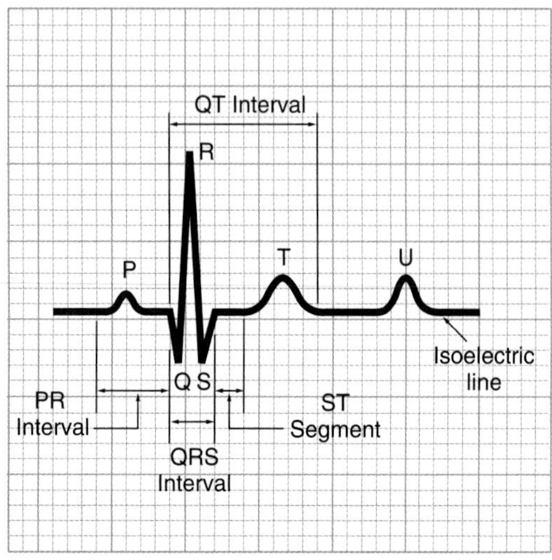

Fig 4.2 A prominent U wave in a QRS complex is associated with hypokalemia.

2. As hypokalemia worsens, U waves increase in size, QRS complexes widen, ST segments become depressed, and T waves flatten or invert (Fig. 4.3)

B. High potassium levels in the extracellular space cause the electrical current across the cell membranes to become "sluggish," prolonging the resting state of the cell membranes of the heart. This leads to impaired cardiac conduction, which can result in ventricular fibrillation or asystole.
   1. Hyperkalemia is characterized by bradycardia; peaked, tented T waves; and ventricular fibrillation (Fig. 4.4).

VII. Nursing Interventions for Clients With Potassium Imbalance (Table 4.3)

A. Identify high-risk clients.

B. Implement the health-care provider's orders to treat the underlying cause of the imbalance.
   1. The health-care provider's orders may include oral or IV fluid administration, oral or IV potassium administration, and medication administration.

C. Monitor the client and the client's serum potassium level.
   1. Monitor the client's serum potassium level as ordered by the health-care provider.
      a. Normal reference range for serum potassium is 3.5 to 5.0 mEq/L.

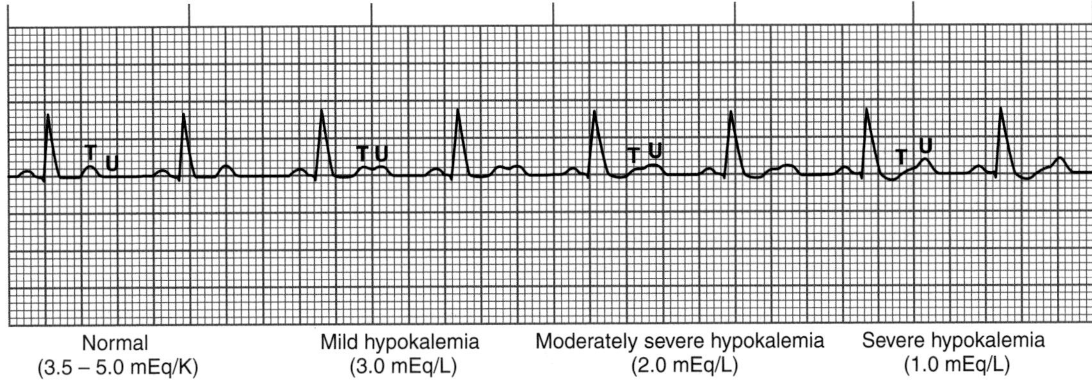

Fig 4.3 As hypokalemia worsens, U waves increase in size, QRS complexes widen, ST segments become depressed, and T waves flatten or invert.

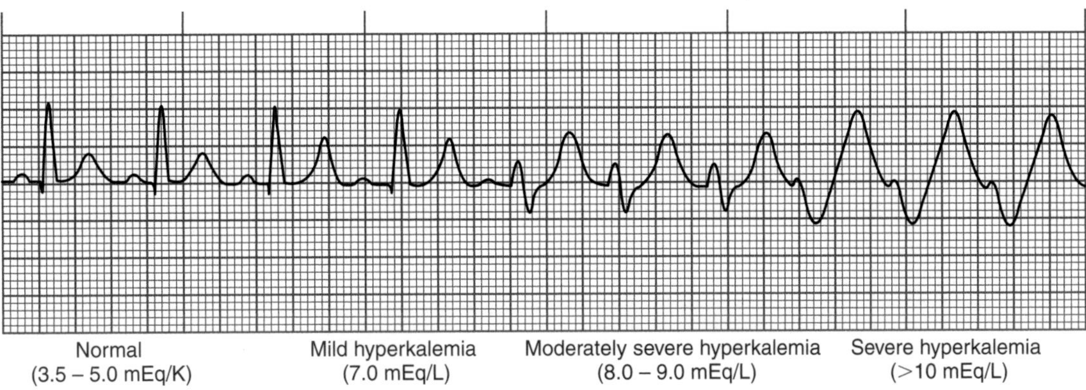

Fig 4.4 Hyperkalemia is characterized by peaked, tented T waves and ventricular fibrillation.

2. Monitor other laboratory values associated with hypokalemia. Normal reference ranges are as follows:
   a. Blood glucose: 65 to 99 mg/dL (adult, fasting)
   b. Serum calcium: 8.2 to 10.2 mg/dL (adults)
   c. Serum chloride: 95 to 108 mEq/L
   d. Urine osmolality: 250 to 900 mOsm/kg (children and adults)
3. Monitor for signs of metabolic acidosis (see Chapter 8).
4. Monitor for cardiovascular changes.
   a. Observe for ECG changes (see Figs. 4.2, 4.3, and 4.4).
   b. Palpate peripheral pulses.
   c. Check orthostatic blood pressures.

Activate the rapid response team if the client's heart rate falls below 60 bpm or if the client's T waves become spiked.

5. Monitor for neuromuscular changes.
   a. Establish a baseline for the client's deep tendon reflexes, muscle strength, and tone.
   b. Monitor the client for muscle weakness, muscle twitching, or irregular muscle contractions during each nursing shift.
6. Monitor for gastrointestinal changes.
   a. Auscultate bowel sounds in all four quadrants.
   b. Observe the frequency and consistency of bowel movements.

D. Ensure client safety
1. Implement fall precautions related to muscle weakness caused by potassium imbalances.

E. Educate the client
1. Hypokalemia
   a. Teach the client or caregiver the causes of potassium deficit.
   b. Provide specific information regarding the client's medical diagnosis and related interventions and treatments.
   c. Teach the client or caregiver how to identify the signs and symptoms of potassium deficiency.
   d. Instruct the client and family to notify the primary health-care provider if the client exhibits any of the signs or symptoms of hypokalemia or if they have any other specific concerns.
   e. Teach the client how to prevent potassium deficiency.
   f. Teach the client about foods that contain potassium; because a lack of potassium is rare, there is no recommended daily allowance for this mineral.

Table 4.3 Nursing Interventions Specific to Hypokalemia and Hyperkalemia

Hypokalemia

Increase potassium level

Mild to moderate hypokalemia

- Administer oral supplements, as ordered, to clients with serum potassium levels less than 3.5 mEq/L but greater than 3.0 mEq/L
- Dilute powders and liquids in juice or other desired liquid to improve palatability and prevent gastrointestinal irritation
- Advise the client that potassium has an extremely unpleasant taste
- Follow the manufacturer's instructions for the amount of fluid to be used as a diluent for the preparation; the most common dilution is 20 mEq potassium per 120 mL (4 oz)
  - Mix solutions thoroughly before administering them to the client
  - Administer liquid, capsule, or tablet potassium with food or meals to minimize gastrointestinal irritation
  - Do not crush tablets; do not open capsules

Severe hypokalemia

- Administer IV potassium, as ordered, to clients with serum potassium levels less than 3.0 mEq/L

IV potassium is a high-alert drug; DO NOT administer via IV push!

- Infuse IV potassium slowly at 5–10 mEq/hr; never exceed 20 mEq/hr under any circumstances

Rapid administration or high concentrations of potassium may cause cardiac arrest

- Monitor cardiac function when infusing large amounts of potassium
- Do not administer potassium intramuscularly or subcutaneously because potassium is a severe tissue irritant
- Dilute potassium before IV infusion; a dilution of no more than 1 mEq/10 mL of solution is recommended
- Monitor the client's IV site closely; infiltration of potassium is painful and may cause tissue damage, followed by necrosis and sloughing
- Potassium may cause severe irritation to veins
- Stop the infusion and notify the health-care provider if the client reports pain, even if the IV line is not infiltrated

Hyperkalemia

Decrease potassium level

Mild to moderate hyperkalemia

- Limit dietary potassium, including potassium-based salt substitutes
- Discontinue or decrease potassium supplements
- Discontinue or decrease medications that potentially cause hyperkalemia
- Hospitalize the client if ordered; usually treated without hospitalization

Severe hyperkalemia

- Treat in an acute care facility with cardiac monitoring capabilities
- Decrease the serum potassium level by direct removal (especially if renal failure is a cause)
  - Hemodialysis
  - Continuous venovenous hemofiltration
  - Continuous renal replacement therapy
- Administer IV calcium, as ordered, to treat cardiac and skeletal muscle effects of hyperkalemia
- Administer IV glucose and insulin, as ordered, to decrease serum potassium levels temporarily by increasing movement back into the cells
- Administer IV sodium bicarbonate, as ordered, to reverse hyperkalemia caused by acidosis; promotes the movement of potassium from the ECF back into the ICF
- Administer medications as ordered
  - Adrenergics to stimulate beta-2-adrenergic receptors to drive potassium back into cells

    -albuterol (Ventolin)

    -epinephrine (Ana-Guard)
  - Cationic exchange resins to reduce serum potassium levels by exchanging sodium ions for potassium ions in the intestine and removing them via the gastrointestinal tract

    -sodium polystyrene sulfonate (Kayexalate) orally or via retention enema
  - Loop diuretics to decrease total serum potassium by increasing excretion by the kidneys

    -bumetanide (Bumex)

    -ethacrynic acid (Edecrin)

    -furosemide (Lasix)

    -torsemide (Demadex)
  - Thiazide diuretics to decrease total serum potassium by increasing excretion by the kidneys

    -chlorothiazide (Diuril)

    -hydrochlorothiazide

    -metolazone (Zaroxolyn)

g. Teach the client how to prepare and take oral potassium supplements.
   1) Dilute powders and liquids in juice or another desired liquid.
   2) Follow the manufacturer's instructions for the amount of fluid to be used as a diluent for the preparation: commonly, 20 mEq potassium per 120 mL (4 oz).
   3) Mix solutions thoroughly before drinking.
   4) Administer liquid, capsule, or tablet potassium with food or meals to minimize gastrointestinal irritation.
   5) Do not crush tablets; do not open capsules.
   6) Do not take potassium supplements while taking a potassium-sparing diuretic.
   7) Do not use salt substitutes containing potassium unless prescribed by the primary health-care provider.

8) Report adverse effects, such as nausea, vomiting, diarrhea, and abdominal cramping, to the primary health-care provider.

h. Encourage the client to keep appointments for laboratory studies to evaluate serum potassium levels, because values can change dramatically; even small variations in serum potassium can have major effects on the body.

i. Ensure that client or caregiver understands the specifics, rationale, potential side effects, and desired effects of the treatment regimen.

j. Include medication administration, nutrition, hydration, dietary restrictions, and foods high in potassium in client teaching.

2. Hyperkalemia

a. Teach the client or caregiver the causes of potassium excess.

b. Provide specific information regarding the client's medical diagnosis and related interventions and treatments.

c. Teach the client or caregiver how to identify the signs and symptoms of potassium excess.

d. Instruct the client and family to notify the primary health-care provider if the client exhibits any of the signs or symptoms of hyperkalemia or if they have any other specific concerns.

e. Teach the client how to prevent potassium excess.

1) Avoid salt substitutes that contain potassium.

2) Avoid foods high in potassium (Table 4.4)

3) Choose low-potassium foods, such as eggs, apples, apricots, cherries, grapefruit (but note that grapefruit interferes with many medications), peaches, cranberries, cabbage, cauliflower, celery, eggplant, lettuce, green beans, onions, peas, and peppers.

4) Eat less red meat and more lean meats and cold-water fish.

5) Read food labels to determine the amount of potassium in each serving.

6) Drink more fluids; dehydration worsens hyperkalemia.

f. Ensure that the client or caregiver understands the specifics, rationale, potential side effects, and desired effects of the treatment regimen.

g. Include medication administration, nutrition, hydration, dietary restrictions, and foods high in potassium in client teaching.

Table 4.4 Foods High in Potassium

Food (Standard Amount)	Potassium (mg)	Calories
Sweet potato, baked, 1 potato (146 gm)	694	131
Tomato paste, ¼ cup	664	54
Beet greens, cooked, ½ cup	655	19
Potato, baked, with flesh, 1 potato (156 gm)	610	145
White beans, canned, ½ cup	595	153
Yogurt, plain, nonfat, 8-oz container	579	127
Clams, canned, 3 oz	534	126
Prune juice, ¾ cup	530	136
Carrot juice, ¾ cup	517	71
Blackstrap molasses, 1 tbsp	498	47
Soybeans, green, cooked, ½ cup	485	127
Banana, 1 medium	422	105
Spinach, cooked, ½ cup	419	21
Peaches, dried, uncooked, ¼ cup	398	96
Milk, nonfat, 1 cup	398	133
Prunes, stewed, ½ cup	382	83
Apricots, dried, uncooked, ¼ cup	378	78
Cantaloupe, ¼ medium	368	47
Honeydew melon, ⅛ medium	365	58
Orange juice, ¾ cup	355	85

F. Evaluate and document

1. Document all assessment findings and interventions per institution policy.

2. Evaluate and document the client's response to interventions and education.

a. Serum potassium level should return to the normal reference range of 3.5 to 5.0 mEq/L.

b. Other laboratory values should return to the normal reference range.

c. Vital signs should return to baseline.

d. Cardiac rate and rhythm should return to baseline.

e. Underlying cause of potassium imbalance should be resolved.

CASE STUDY: Putting It All Together

Subjective Data

A 69-year-old client presents to the emergency department reporting fatigue, muscle aches, weakness, and severe cramping for 2 days. He reports being ill recently, with nausea, vomiting, and diarrhea that lasted 3 days. The client has a history of rheumatic fever, congestive heart failure (CHF), and hypertension. The client states that he follows a low-sodium diet, weighs himself daily, and has continued this regimen throughout the current illness.

The client has no known allergies, and his current medications are:

- metoprolol (Toprol-XL) 100 mg by mouth (PO) daily
- lisinopril (Zestril) 5 mg PO daily
- digoxin (Lanoxin) 0.25 mg PO daily
- aspirin 81 mg PO daily
- potassium chloride (K-Lor) 20 mEq PO daily
- furosemide (Lasix) 40 mg PO daily

Objective Data

Nursing Assessment

1. Alert, oriented to person, place, and time
2. Heart sounds S_1 and S_2 present but irregular; no murmur
3. Orthostatic hypotension
4. Pedal and radial pulses irregular, 1+, and weak bilaterally
5. Deep tendon reflexes 1+ (hypoactive) bilaterally
6. Bowel sounds hypoactive in all four quadrants
7. Chest x-ray: cardiomegaly; no evidence of CHF
8. ECG: sinus tachycardia with intraventricular conduction defect (left anterior fascicular block), occasional to frequent PVCs, prominent U wave

Vital Signs	
Temperature:	97.8°F (36.6°C) orally
Blood pressure:	115/65 mm Hg supine, 106/58 mm Hg sitting, 92/54 mm Hg standing
Heart rate:	112 bpm, irregular
Respiratory rate:	20
O_2 saturation:	96%

Laboratory Results	
Serum Na^+:	140 mEq/L
Serum K^+:	2.7 mEq/L
Blood glucose:	80 mg/dL
Serum BUN:	30 mg/dL
Serum creatinine:	1.3 mg/dL
Digoxin level:	2.3 ng/mL (normal 0.5 to 2 ng/mL)

Health-Care Provider Orders

1. Place on telemetry
2. Fall precautions
3. Vital signs every 15 minutes × 1 hour and every 30 minutes × 1 hour, then every 4 hours if stable
4. Monitor intake and output
5. Administer IV solution now: 40 mEq of potassium diluted in 500 mL of normal saline solution at 10 mEq/hr
6. Hold digoxin, metoprolol, and lisinopril
7. Administer IV ondansetron (Zofran) 4 mg every 6 hours as needed for nausea
8. Clear liquid diet
9. Repeat ECG, serum potassium, glucose, and electrolytes in 4 to 6 hours, and notify health-care provider of results
10. Refer to primary health-care provider to restart digoxin and adjust potassium chloride, furosemide, metoprolol, and lisinopril dosages

Case Study Questions

A. What *subjective* assessment findings indicate that the client is experiencing a health alteration?

1. ____________________
2. ____________________
3. ____________________
4. ____________________
5. ____________________
6. ____________________

CASE STUDY: Putting It All Together *cont'd*

Case Study Questions

7. ______________________
8. ______________________

B. What *objective* assessment findings indicate that the client is experiencing a health alteration?

1. ______________________
2. ______________________
3. ______________________
4. ______________________
5. ______________________
6. ______________________
7. ______________________
8. ______________________

C. After analyzing the data collected, what **primary** nursing diagnosis should the nurse assign to this client?

____

D. What interventions should the nurse plan and/or implement to meet this client's needs?

1. ______________________
2. ______________________
3. ______________________
4. ______________________
5. ______________________
6. ______________________
7. ______________________
8. ______________________
9. ______________________
10. ______________________

E. What client outcomes should the nurse plan to evaluate the effectiveness of the nursing interventions?

1. ______________________
2. ______________________
3. ______________________
4. ______________________
5. ______________________
6. ______________________
7. ______________________
8. ______________________

REVIEW QUESTIONS

1. A nurse in the emergency department admits an elderly client who is diagnosed with moderate hyperkalemia secondary to a decline in renal function. The nurse anticipates administering a medication that works by exchanging sodium ions for potassium ions in the gastrointestinal tract to help reduce the client's potassium level. Which medication is being described by the nurse?
   1. Sodium bicarbonate
   2. Calcium gluconate
   3. Sodium polystyrene sulfonate
   4. Regular insulin and dextrose

2. When caring for a newborn, which condition should a nurse associate with inadequate serum potassium?
   1. Diarrhea
   2. Hyperactive bowel sounds
   3. Muscle weakness
   4. Anemia

3. Which clinical manifestation should a nurse associate with the development of hypokalemia if it is observed in a newly admitted client?
   1. Skeletal muscle weakness
   2. Widened QRS complex
   3. Diarrhea
   4. Tall T waves

4. Which outcome would be most appropriate for a nurse to establish when caring for a client who has a nursing diagnosis of Risk for Falls Related to Skeletal Muscle Weakness Secondary to Electrolyte Imbalance?
   1. The client's serum electrolyte levels will return to the normal reference range.
   2. The nurse will promote oral fluid intake as appropriate.
   3. The dietitian will teach the client how to increase dietary potassium intake.
   4. The client will remain free from injury throughout the hospital stay.

5. A nurse is caring for an elderly client who is at risk for falls secondary to muscle weakness associated with hypokalemia. Which actions should the nurse take when implementing fall precautions for this client? **Select all that apply.**
   1. Perform a fall risk assessment.
   2. Maintain the bed in the Trendelenburg position.
   3. Place assistive devices (walkers, canes) at the end of the client's bed.
   4. Instruct the client to request assistance to ambulate.
   5. Request that family members remain with the client if necessary.

6. Which assessment should a nurse perform to identify whether a client is developing a potentially dangerous side effect of the medication lisinopril (Zestril)?
   1. Assessment for deep tendon hyporeflexia
   2. Assessment for irregular heartbeat
   3. Assessment for increased urine output
   4. Assessment of the client's nutritional status

7. A nurse is reviewing the ECG strip of a client who has been diagnosed with a fluid and electrolyte imbalance. Based on the exhibit provided, which imbalance should the nurse suspect?

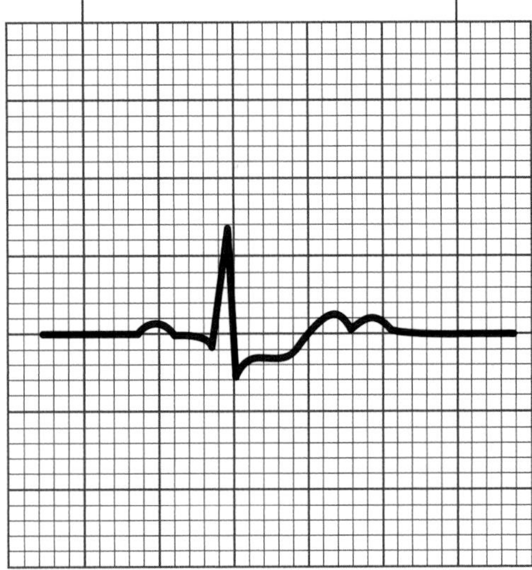

   1. Hyponatremia
   2. Hypernatremia
   3. Hypokalemia
   4. Hyperkalemia

8. An elderly client is prescribed furosemide (Lasix) 40 mg by mouth daily for the treatment of CHF. A nurse teaches the client to observe for signs of potassium imbalance while taking this medication. Which signs should the nurse include in client teaching?
   1. Muscle twitches, diarrhea, increased gastrointestinal motility
   2. Confusion, agitation, muscle twitching
   3. General muscle weakness; constipation; weak, thready pulse
   4. Increased blood pressure and heart rate, constipation

9. A nurse is caring for an adult client with a serum potassium level of 2.0 mEq/L. Which order for potassium chloride should the nurse identify as being *most appropriate* for this client?
   1. Administer potassium chloride 40 mEq/L intramuscularly now.
   2. Administer potassium chloride 40 mEq/L by mouth twice daily.
   3. Administer potassium chloride 40 mEq/L by IV push now.
   4. Administer potassium chloride 40 mEq/L by IV infusion over 4 hours.

10. A nurse evaluates the laboratory data for a hospitalized pregnant client who is diagnosed with hyperemesis gravidarum. The client has a serum potassium level of 2.8 mEq/L and is to receive IV potassium therapy. When preparing to administer IV potassium to this client, which actions should the nurse plan to take to ensure client safety? **Select all that apply.**
    1. Infuse the potassium at a rate of 30 mEq/hr, as ordered by the health-care provider.
    2. Check the concentration of the potassium solution with another registered nurse.
    3. Use a controlled infusion device to administer the potassium solution.
    4. Assess the client's IV site every 2 hours for phlebitis or infiltration.
    5. Administer IV bumetanide (Bumex) 1 mg, as ordered by health-care provider.

11. Understanding that potassium is a nutrient most likely to be lacking in the diets of childbearing women, which is the most appropriate nursing intervention to include when teaching a pregnant adolescent client?
    1. Encourage the adolescent to eat foods she likes and is accustomed to eating.
    2. Recommend the ingestion of low-calorie foods to restrict weight gain.
    3. Identify the adolescent's sources of peer pressure and dietary habits.
    4. Improve the adolescent's nutritional knowledge, meal planning, and food preparation skills.

12. A nurse is preparing to administer 40 mEq of IV potassium. To ensure that the medication is diluted properly, how many milliliters of solution would be required to obtain a concentration of 1 mEq/10 mL? Record your answer as a whole number.

    ____

13. A nurse is preparing to administer 60 mEq of potassium by mouth in three divided doses. The dosage on hand is a 20 mEq/tablet. How many tablets should the nurse plan to administer at each dose? Record your answer as a whole number.

    ____

14. A nurse is preparing to administer 10 mEq of IV potassium diluted in 100 mL of normal (0.9%) saline solution. The nurse plans to infuse the solution via peripheral IV access over 2 hours, using microdrip tubing with a drop factor of 60 gtt/mL. How many mL/hr should the nurse program the IV pump to deliver? Record your answer as a whole number.

    ____

15. A nurse notes nonsustained ventricular tachycardia (VT) on the cardiac monitor of a client with a fluid or electrolyte imbalance. Which fluid or electrolyte imbalances should the nurse associate with this finding? **Select all that apply.**
    1. Hyponatremia
    2. Hypernatremia
    3. Hypokalemia
    4. Hyperkalemia
    5. Fluid volume deficit
    6. Fluid volume excess

16. Which information obtained from a client's history should a nurse associate with the development of hyperkalemia?
    1. History of corticosteroid use
    2. History of diuretic use
    3. History of urinary incontinence
    4. History of uncontrolled diabetes mellitus

17. A nurse admits a client who is diagnosed with uncontrolled diabetes mellitus and who has a serum potassium level of 6.6 mEq/L, with no ECG changes. Which possible interventions should a nurse anticipate a health-care provider ordering to decrease this client's serum potassium level? **Select all that apply.**
    1. Administer sodium polystyrene sulfonate (Kayexalate) 15 gm in sorbitol PO four times daily.
    2. Administer IV regular insulin 7 units simultaneously with 50 mL 50% glucose at 250 mL/hr.
    3. Administer IV 10% calcium gluconate 15 mL over 5 to 10 minutes.
    4. Administer albuterol (Proventil) (5 mg/mL concentration) 20 mg inhaled over 10 minutes.

18. A nurse is caring for a client whose serum potassium is 2.5 mEq/L. Based on this information, which physician orders should the nurse question? **Select all that apply.**
    1. Implement fall precautions.
    2. Implement seizure precautions.
    3. Administer IV potassium chloride 40 mEq.
    4. Monitor telemetry continuously.
    5. Administer chlorothiazide (Diuril) 125 mg daily by mouth.

19. Which manifestation should a nurse investigate *first* when assessing an elderly client who is admitted with a 2-day history of vomiting and diarrhea?
   1. Blood pressure 100/45 mm Hg
   2. Weakness and lightheadedness
   3. Pulse 100 bpm
   4. Shallow respirations with tachypnea

20. A nurse assesses a client who has CHF and is taking the following medications: digoxin (Lanoxin), furosemide (Lasix), and benazepril (Lotensin). Which assessment finding should the nurse act on *immediately*?
   1. Mental confusion
   2. Dysrhythmias
   3. Abdominal distention
   4. Hypotension

21. Which nursing diagnoses should a nurse assign to a client who has a serum potassium level of 3.1 mEq/L? **Select all that apply.**
   1. Diarrhea Related to Spastic Colonic Activity
   2. Constipation Related to Smooth Muscle Atony
   3. Decreased Cardiac Output Related to Dysrhythmia
   4. Impaired Physical Mobility Related to Skeletal Muscle Weakness
   5. Potential for Respiratory Insufficiency Related to Muscle Weakness

22. A nurse assesses that a client with a nasogastric tube in place to allow suctioning has a potassium level of 2.8 mEq/L. Which nursing diagnosis should receive priority in this client?
   1. Impaired Physical Mobility Related to Skeletal Muscles Weakness
   2. Decreased Cardiac Output Related to Dysrhythmias
   3. Risk for Falls Related to Skeletal Muscle Weakness
   4. Constipation Related to Smooth Muscle Atony

23. An elderly client diagnosed with CHF is receiving furosemide (Lasix) 40 mg by mouth daily, increasing the client's risk for hypokalemia. Which ECG finding should a nurse identify as indicative of hypokalemia?

1.

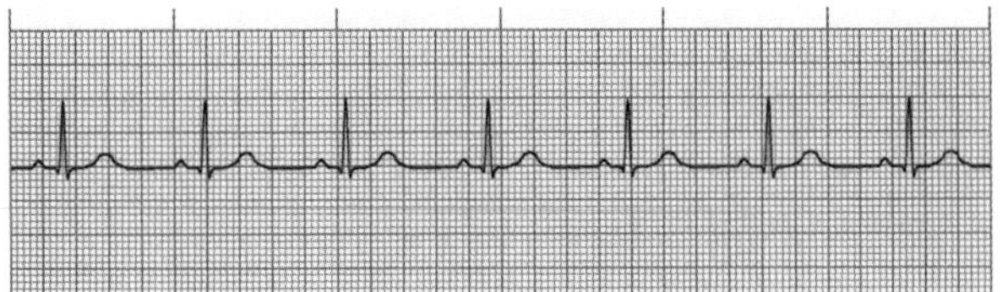

2.

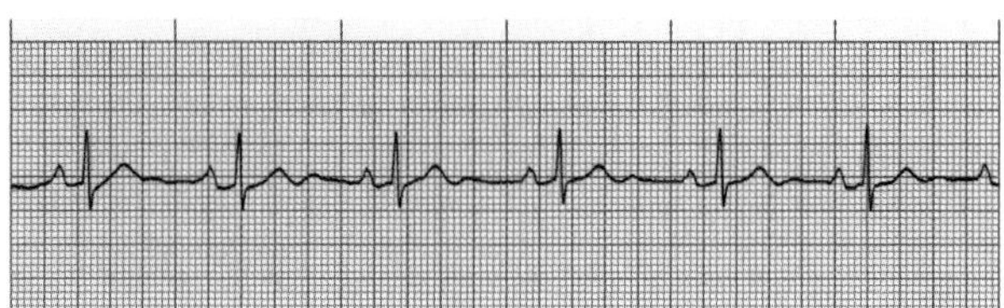

3.

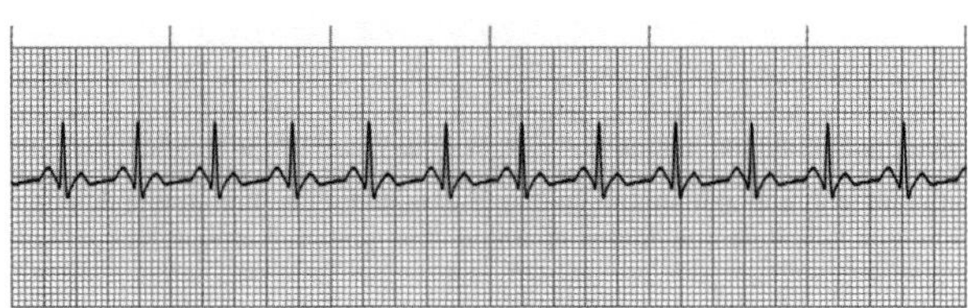

4.

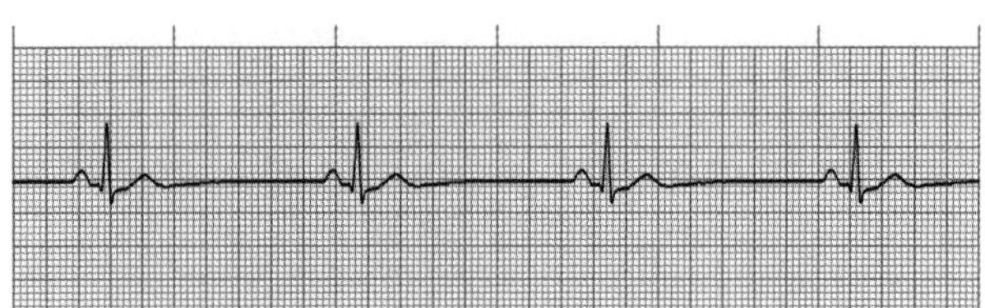

24. A client diagnosed with chronic kidney disease presents to the emergency department reporting shortness of breath, nausea, and muscle weakness. The client did not have dialysis, as scheduled yesterday and is experiencing hyperkalemia. Which ECG finding should a nurse identify as indicative of hyperkalemia?

1.

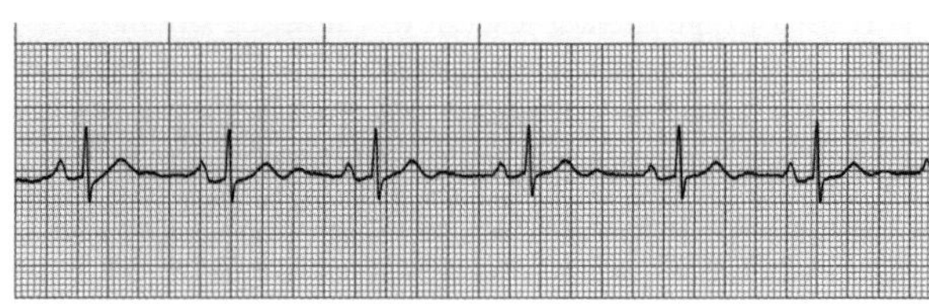

2.

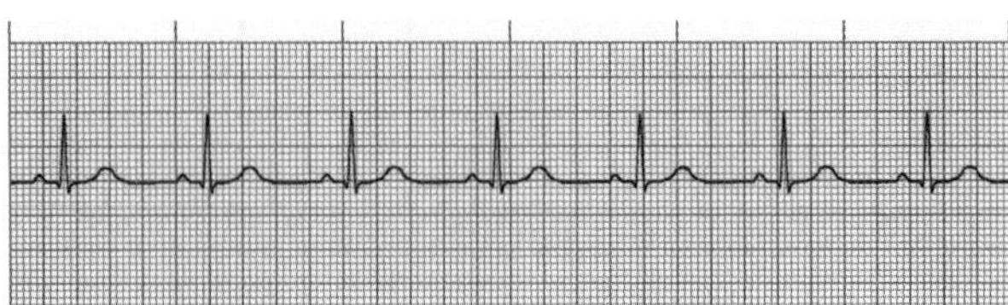

3.

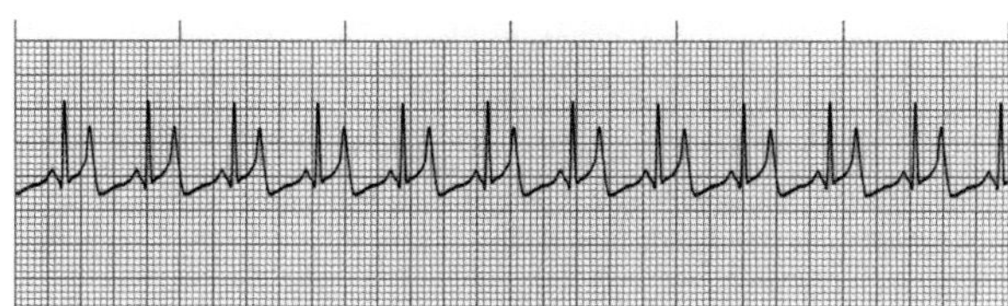

4.

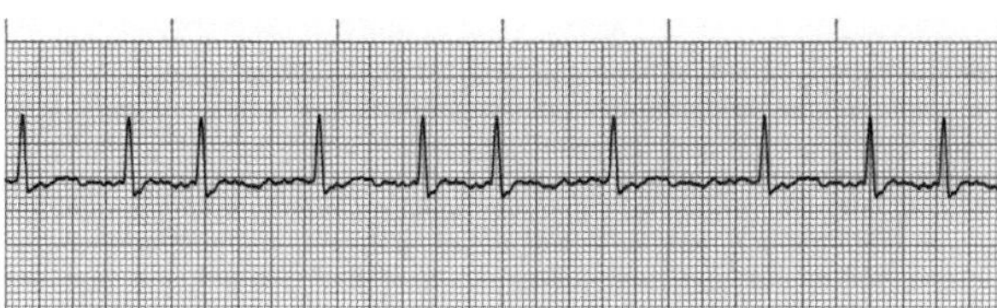

25. A nurse is caring for a client with fluid volume excess and a serum potassium level of 3.0 mEq/L. Which medication should the nurse identify as being most appropriate for this client?

1. chlorothiazide (Diuril)
2. bumetanide (Bumex)
3. spironolactone (Aldactone)
4. furosemide (Lasix)

REVIEW ANSWERS

1. ANSWER: 3.

Rationale:

1. Sodium bicarbonate works by shifting potassium from the ECF to the ICF and is used to decrease serum potassium levels quickly in the presence of severe hyperkalemia (greater than 7.0 mEq/L).
2. Calcium gluconate decreases the myocardial irritability associated with hyperkalemia but does not promote potassium loss.
3. **The nurse is describing sodium polystyrene sulfonate (Kayexalate), which is a cationic exchange resin that reduces serum potassium levels by exchanging sodium ions for potassium ions in the intestine and removes potassium via the gastrointestinal tract.**
4. Regular insulin and dextrose work by shifting potassium from the ECF to the ICF and are used to decrease serum potassium levels quickly in the presence of severe hyperkalemia (greater than 7.0 mEq/L).

TEST-TAKING TIP: Remember that sodium polystyrene sulfonate is the generic name for Kayexalate, an agent that is commonly used to treat hyperkalemia and is administered by mouth or rectally as a retention enema. In the intestine, 1 gm of Kayexalate is exchanged for 1 mEq of potassium.

Content Area: Adult Health
Integrated Processes: Nursing Process: Planning
Client Need: Physiological Integrity
Cognitive Level: Knowledge
Reference: Deglin, J. H., Vallerand, A. H., and Sanoski, C. A. (2013). Davis's Drug Guide for Nurses (13th ed.). Philadelphia, PA: F. A. Davis.

2. ANSWER: 3.

Rationale:

1. Diarrhea is associated with hyperkalemia, not hypokalemia.
2. Hyperactive bowel sounds are associated with hyperkalemia, not hypokalemia.
3. **The nurse should suspect a low serum potassium level if the infant has muscle weakness. Infants require 2 to 3 mEq/kg/day of potassium to maintain growth, acid-base balance, cellular energy, and electrical charge balance. A potassium deficiency may result in myocardial damage, dysrhythmia, hypotension, and muscle weakness.**
4. Anemia is associated with inadequate iron levels, not with potassium imbalances.

TEST-TAKING TIP: The signs of hypokalemia are similar in infants and adults. Review the signs and symptoms of hypokalemia if you had difficulty answering this question.

Content Area: Child Health
Integrated Processes: Nursing Process: Assessment
Client Need: Physiological Integrity
Cognitive Level: Application
Reference: Ward, S. L., and Hisley, S. M. (2011). Maternal-Child Nursing Care: Optimizing Outcomes for Mothers, Children and Families. Philadelphia, PA: F. A. Davis.

3. ANSWER: 1.

Rationale:

1. **The nurse should associate skeletal muscle weakness with the development of hypokalemia. Neuromuscular manifestations of hypokalemia include anxiety, lethargy, skeletal muscle weakness, and deep tendon hyporeflexia.**
2. A widened QRS complex may indicate hyperkalemia, not hypokalemia.
3. Diarrhea may indicate hyperkalemia, not hypokalemia.
4. Tall T waves may indicate hyperkalemia, not hypokalemia.

TEST-TAKING TIP: Recall that adequate serum potassium is necessary for proper muscle function.

Content Area: Adult Health
Integrated Processes: Nursing Process: Assessment
Client Need: Physiological Integrity
Cognitive Level: Application
Reference: Ignatavicius, D., and Workman, M. (2012). Medical-Surgical Nursing: Patient-Centered Collaborative Care (7th ed.). St. Louis, MO: Saunders.

4. ANSWER: 4.

Rationale:

1. The statement regarding the client's serum electrolyte level is not an appropriate outcome for a nursing diagnosis of Risk for Falls Related to Skeletal Muscle Weakness Secondary to Electrolyte Imbalance.
2. Promoting oral fluid intake is an intervention and does not pertain to client safety.
3. Teaching the client is an intervention and does not pertain to client safety.
4. **The most appropriate outcome for a client with a nursing diagnosis of Risk for Falls Related to Skeletal Muscle Weakness Secondary to Electrolyte Imbalance is to remain free from injury throughout the hospital stay.**

TEST-TAKING TIP: Rule out options that are not client outcomes.

Content Area: Adult Health
Integrated Processes: Nursing Process: Planning
Client Need: Safe and Effective Care Environment
Cognitive Level: Application
Reference: Ignatavicius, D., and Workman, M. (2012). Medical-Surgical Nursing: Patient-Centered Collaborative Care (7th ed.). St. Louis, MO: Saunders.

5. ANSWER: 1, 4, 5.

Rationale:

1. **When implementing fall precautions, the nurse should perform a fall risk assessment.**
2. The client's bed should be maintained in the lowest position with the wheels locked. In the Trendelenburg position, the client lies flat on the back (supine) with the feet higher than the head. This was previously the standard position for treating shock, but it has fallen out of favor.
3. Assistive devices should be placed beside the client's bed, not at the end of it, so they are within the client's reach.
4. **When implementing fall precautions, the nurse should instruct the client to request assistance when ambulating.**
5. **When implementing fall precautions, the nurse should request family members to remain with the client if necessary.**

TEST-TAKING TIP: Consider each option, and determine which ones would prevent a client from falling.

Content Area: Older Adult Health
Integrated Processes: Nursing Process: Implementation
Client Need: Safe and Effective Care Environment
Cognitive Level: Application
Reference: Ignatavicius, D., and Workman, M. (2012). Medical-Surgical Nursing: Patient-Centered Collaborative Care (7th ed.). St. Louis, MO: Saunders.

6. ANSWER: 2.

Rationale:

1. A potentially dangerous side effect of the medication lisinopril (Zestril) is hyperkalemia. Deep tendon hyporeflexia is seen in hypokalemia, not hyperkalemia.

2. When a client is taking lisinopril, an angiotensin-converting enzyme (ACE) inhibitor, the nurse should assess for an irregular heartbeat. ACE inhibitors may cause hyperkalemia, which may cause cardiac dysrhythmias. Cardiovascular changes are the most severe problems associated with hyperkalemia.

3. Increased urine output would be associated with the use of diuretics, not ACE inhibitors.

4. The nutritional status of the client would not be affected by the medication lisinopril (Zestril).

TEST-TAKING TIP: Recall that lisinopril (Zestril) is an ACE inhibitor that adversely affects kidney function, which may lead to hyperkalemia.

Content Area: Adult Health

Integrated Processes: Nursing Process: Assessment

Client Need: Physiological Integrity

Cognitive Level: Application

Reference: Deglin, J. H., Vallerand, A. H., and Sanoski, C. A. (2013). Davis's Drug Guide for Nurses (13th ed.). Philadelphia, PA: F. A. Davis.

7. ANSWER: 3.

Rationale:

1. Although hyponatremia does result in cardiovascular changes, it is not associated with ECG changes.

2. Although hypernatremia does result in cardiovascular changes, it is not associated with ECG changes.

3. The nurse should suspect that this client is experiencing hypokalemia. Hypokalemia causes ST segment depression, flat or inverted T waves, and increased U waves.

4. Hyperkalemia results in prolonged P-R intervals; flat or absent P waves; wide QRS complexes; and tall, peaked T waves.

TEST-TAKING TIP: Recall that in hypokalemia, electrical activity in the body slows down, resulting in depressed ST segments, flat T waves, and increased U waves visible on an ECG. Conversely, in hyperkalemia, excitable tissues are more sensitive to stimuli, resulting in prolonged P-R intervals; flat or absent P waves; wide QRS complexes; and tall, peaked T waves visible on an ECG.

Content Area: Adult Health

Integrated Processes: Nursing Process: Evaluation

Client Need: Physiological Integrity

Cognitive Level: Application

Reference: Ignatavicius, D., and Workman, M. (2012). Medical-Surgical Nursing: Patient-Centered Collaborative Care (7th ed.). St. Louis, MO: Saunders.

8. ANSWER: 3.

Rationale:

1. The administration of non–potassium-sparing diuretics, such as furosemide, places the client at risk for hypokalemia. Muscle twitches, diarrhea, and increased gastrointestinal motility are signs of hyperkalemia, not hypokalemia.

2. The administration of non–potassium-sparing diuretics, such as furosemide, places the client at risk for hypokalemia. Confusion, agitation, and muscle twitching are signs of hypernatremia, not hypokalemia.

3. The administration of non–potassium-sparing diuretics, such as furosemide, places the client at risk for hypokalemia. The nurse should teach the client to observe for general muscle weakness, constipation, and a weak, thready pulse, which may indicate that the client's serum potassium level is too low.

4. The administration of non–potassium-sparing diuretics, such as furosemide, places the client at risk for hypokalemia. Increased blood pressure, increased heart rate, and constipation are early manifestations of hypercalcemia, not hypokalemia.

TEST-TAKING TIP: Recall that furosemide is a non–potassium-sparing diuretic that may cause a decrease in serum potassium (hypokalemia). Select the option that describes the signs of hypokalemia.

Content Area: Adult Health

Integrated Processes: Teaching/Learning

Client Need: Physiological Integrity

Cognitive Level: Application

Reference: Ignatavicius, D., and Workman, M. (2012). Medical-Surgical Nursing: Patient-Centered Collaborative Care (7th ed.). St. Louis, MO: Saunders.

9. ANSWER: 4.

Rationale:

1. Potassium should not be administered intramuscularly because it is a severe tissue irritant.

2. A serum potassium level of 2.0 mEq/L is considered a severe deficit and requires an IV infusion of potassium for replacement.

3. Potassium should *never* be given by IV push or bolus because the rapid infusion of potassium chloride can result in death.

4. The nurse should identify potassium chloride 40 mEq/L by IV infusion over 4 hours as the most appropriate order to treat hypokalemia in this adult client with a serum potassium level of 2.0 mEq/L. A serum potassium level of 2.0 mEq/L is considered a severe deficit and requires an IV infusion of potassium for replacement.

TEST-TAKING TIP: Potassium is a high-alert medication. Be familiar with its administration: IV infusions of potassium should not exceed a rate of 10 mEq/hr for adults.

Content Area: Adult Health

Integrated Processes: Nursing Process: Planning

Client Need: Physiological Integrity

Cognitive Level: Application

Reference: Deglin, J. H., Vallerand, A. H., and Sanoski, C. A. (2013). Davis's Drug Guide for Nurses (13th ed.). Philadelphia, PA: F. A. Davis.

10. ANSWER: 2, 3, 4.

Rationale:

1. To ensure the safety of a client receiving IV potassium therapy, the nurse should infuse the medication slowly, at a rate of no more than 10 mEq/hr via peripheral line or 20 mEq/hr via central line, with continuous cardiac monitoring. Potassium should never be infused at a rate of 30 mEq/hr.

2. To ensure the safety of a client receiving IV potassium therapy, the nurse should plan to check the concentration of the potassium solution with another registered nurse to confirm that the medication has been properly diluted.

3. To ensure the safety of a client receiving IV potassium therapy, the nurse should plan to use a controlled infusion

device to administer the potassium solution to ensure that the medication is infused slowly, at no more than 10 mEq/hr via peripheral line or 20 mEq/hr via central line, with continuous cardiac monitoring.
4. To ensure the safety of a client receiving IV potassium therapy, the nurse should assess the client's IV site every 2 hours to monitor for signs of phlebitis or infiltration because IV potassium is extremely irritating to the veins.
5. The nurse should not administer bumetanide because it is a non–potassium-sparing diuretic, which would worsen the client's fluid volume deficit and hypokalemia.
TEST-TAKING TIP: Read each option carefully. Rule out the options that would cause harm to the client.
Content Area: Maternal Health
Integrated Processes: Nursing Process: Planning
Client Need: Physiological Integrity
Cognitive Level: Application
***Reference:** Ignatavicius, D., and Workman, M. (2012). Medical-Surgical Nursing: Patient-Centered Collaborative Care (7th ed.). St. Louis, MO: Saunders.*

11. **ANSWER: 4.**
Rationale:
1. The nurse's goal when teaching a pregnant adolescent should be to improve nutritional knowledge, meal planning, and food preparation skills, not to encourage the adolescent to eat foods she likes and is accustomed to eating. Adolescents are more likely than adults to have unhealthy dietary habits, such as eating nonnutritional snacks and ingesting inadequate amounts of nutrients.
2. Recommending the ingestion of low-calorie foods to restrict weight gain is an intervention, not a goal—and in this case, it would be an inappropriate intervention. Pregnant adolescents should be encouraged to select a weight-gain goal at the upper end of their body mass index range to reduce the incidence of low-birth-weight infants.
3. Identifying sources of peer pressure and eating habits is an assessment, not a goal. This assessment is necessary when evaluating the client's diet history to achieve the goal of improved nutritional knowledge, meal planning, and food preparation skills.
4. The nurse's goal when teaching a pregnant adolescent should be to improve nutritional knowledge, meal planning, and food preparation skills. Adolescents are more likely than adults to have unhealthy dietary habits, such as eating nonnutritional snacks and ingesting inadequate amounts of nutrients. In addition, they are highly susceptible to peer influence. Identifying these influences and eating habits is necessary when assessing the client's diet history to achieve the goal of improved nutritional knowledge, meal planning, and food preparation skills.
TEST-TAKING TIP: A *goal* is a broad statement about the client's status that a nurse hopes to achieve by implementing nursing interventions. Rule out options that are interventions (options 1 and 2) and assessments (option 3) to identify the nursing goal.
Content Area: Maternal Health
Integrated Processes: Nursing Process: Planning
Client Need: Physiological Integrity
Cognitive Level: Application
***Reference:** Perry, S., Hockenberry, M., Lowdermilk, D., and Wilson, D. (2010). Maternal Child Nursing Care (4th ed.). St. Louis, MO: Mosby.*

12. **ANSWER: 400.**
Rationale:
Use the following formula to calculate the dose:

Dosage on hand/Dosage unit = Desired dosage/Dose given
1 mEq/10 mL = 40 mEq/X mL (cross multiply) =
$1 \times X$ mL = 400 mL
$X = 400$

TEST-TAKING TIP: Potassium is a high-alert medication. Always double-check medication calculations and confirm the concentration of potassium-containing solutions with another registered nurse before administration.
Content Area: Adult Health
Integrated Processes: Nursing Process: Implementation
Client Need: Physiological Integrity
Cognitive Level: Application
***Reference:** Deglin, J. H., Vallerand, A. H., and Sanoski, C. A. (2013). Davis's Drug Guide for Nurses (13th ed.). Philadelphia, PA: F. A. Davis.*

13. **ANSWER: 1.**
Rationale:

60 mEq ÷ 3 doses = 20 mEq each dose
20 mEq = 1 tablet

TEST-TAKING TIP: Potassium is a high-alert medication. Always double-check medication calculations before administration.
Content Area: Adult Health
Integrated Processes: Nursing Process: Implementation
Client Need: Physiological Integrity
Cognitive Level: Application
***Reference:** Deglin, J. H., Vallerand, A. H., and Sanoski, C. A. (2013). Davis's Drug Guide for Nurses (13th ed.). Philadelphia, PA: F. A. Davis.*

14. **ANSWER: 50.**
Rationale:
Use the following formula to calculate the dose:

Volume × Drop factor/Time = Rate
100 mL × 60 gtt/60 min = 6,000/60 = 100 mL/hr ÷ 2 hr =
50 mL/hr

TEST-TAKING TIP: Read the question carefully. Note that the solution is to be infused over 2 hours.
Content Area: Adult Health
Integrated Processes: Nursing Process: Implementation
Client Need: Physiological Integrity
Cognitive Level: Application
***Reference:** Deglin, J. H., Vallerand, A. H., and Sanoski, C. A. (2013). Davis's Drug Guide for Nurses (13th ed.). Philadelphia, PA: F. A. Davis.*

15. **ANSWER: 3, 4.**
Rationale:
1. Sodium imbalances do not cause VT.
2. Sodium imbalances do not cause VT.
3. The nurse should associate nonsustained VT with the development of either hypokalemia or hyperkalemia. Hypokalemia increases the likelihood that the cardiac cells will depolarize spontaneously and cause PVCs, which may lead to VT.
4. The nurse should associate nonsustained VT with the development of either hypokalemia or hyperkalemia.

Hyperkalemia increases the excitability of the cardiac cell membrane and makes it more sensitive to stimuli (more irritable), increasing the likelihood of spontaneous depolarization leading to VT.
5. Fluid imbalances do not directly cause VT but may contribute to electrolyte imbalances that result in VT.
6. Fluid imbalances do not directly cause VT but may contribute to electrolyte imbalances that result in VT.
TEST-TAKING TIP: Recall that sodium imbalances do not cause cardiac dysrhythmias. Fluid imbalances contribute indirectly to cardiac dysrhythmias because they are associated with various electrolyte imbalances.
Content Area: Adult Health
Integrated Processes: Nursing Process: Analysis
Client Need: Physiological Integrity
Cognitive Level: Application
Reference: Ignatavicius, D., and Workman, M. (2012). Medical-Surgical Nursing: Patient-Centered Collaborative Care (7th ed.). St. Louis, MO: Saunders.

16. ANSWER: 4.
Rationale:
1. A history of corticosteroid use would predispose a client to hypokalemia, not hyperkalemia.
2. A history of diuretic use would predispose a client to hypokalemia, not hyperkalemia.
3. Urinary incontinence is not a risk factor for hyperkalemia or hypokalemia.
4. The nurse should associate a history of uncontrolled diabetes mellitus with the development of hyperkalemia. Uncontrolled diabetes mellitus causes a relative increase in potassium. Insulin increases the activity of the sodium-potassium pumps that move potassium out of the ECF and into the cell. Conversely, the lack of insulin decreases the activity of the sodium-potassium pumps, leaving potassium in the ECF and increasing serum potassium levels.
TEST-TAKING TIP: Review the pathophysiology associated with uncontrolled type 1 diabetes mellitus if you had difficulty answering this question.
Content Area: Adult Health
Integrated Processes: Nursing Process: Analysis
Client Need: Physiological Integrity
Cognitive Level: Application
Reference: Ignatavicius, D., and Workman, M. (2012). Medical-Surgical Nursing: Patient-Centered Collaborative Care (7th ed.). St. Louis, MO: Saunders.

17. ANSWER: 1, 2, 4.
Rationale:
1. A serum potassium level greater than 6.5 mEq/L is considered severe hyperkalemia that requires aggressive therapy. The nurse should anticipate that a health-care provider will order sodium polystyrene sulfonate by mouth as an adjunct to remove potassium via the gastrointestinal tract.
2. A serum potassium level greater than 6.5 mEq/L is considered severe hyperkalemia that requires aggressive therapy. The nurse should anticipate that a health-care provider will order regular insulin administered simultaneously with 50% glucose and albuterol inhalation to rapidly decrease the client's serum potassium level by shifting potassium back into the cells.
3. Because the client is not experiencing ECG changes, it is unlikely that calcium gluconate would be ordered because this medication antagonizes the effect of hyperkalemia on cardiac muscle.
4. A serum potassium level greater than 6.5 mEq/L is considered severe hyperkalemia that requires aggressive therapy. The nurse should anticipate that a health-care provider will order regular insulin administered simultaneously with 50% glucose and albuterol inhalation to rapidly decrease the client's serum potassium level by shifting potassium back into the cells.
TEST-TAKING TIP: Recognize that the client is experiencing severe hyperkalemia with no ECG changes. Review the emergency treatment for severe hyperkalemia if you had difficulty answering this question.
Content Area: Adult Health
Integrated Processes: Nursing Process: Planning
Client Need: Physiological Integrity
Cognitive Level: Application
Reference: Lewis, J. L., III (Reviewer). (2009). Disorders of potassium concentration. In The Merck Manuals Online Library. Retrieved from http://www.merckmanuals.com/professional/endocrine_and_metabolic_disorders/electrolyte_disorders/disorders_of_potassium_concentration.html?qt=&sc=&alt=.

18. ANSWER: 2, 5.
Rationale:
1. A serum potassium level of 2.5 mEq/L is below normal and is considered hypokalemia. Implementation of fall precautions is appropriate and should not be questioned. Fall precautions are necessary because hypokalemia causes muscle weakness, which increases the risk of falls.
2. A serum potassium level of 2.5 mEq/L is below normal and is considered hypokalemia. The nurse should question the order to implement seizure precautions because hypokalemia does not cause seizures, as hyponatremia would.
3. A serum potassium level of 2.5 mEq/L is below normal and is considered hypokalemia. Administration of IV potassium is appropriate and should not be questioned. Potassium replacement is required to correct hypokalemia.
4. A serum potassium level of 2.5 mEq/L is below normal and is considered hypokalemia. Continuous telemetry monitoring is appropriate and should not be questioned. Cardiac monitoring is important in clients with potassium imbalances because of the potential for dysrhythmias.
5. A serum potassium level of 2.5 mEq/L is below normal and is considered hypokalemia. The nurse should question the order to administer chlorothiazide (Diuril), which would further deplete the already low serum potassium level. The use of chlorothiazide or any other non–potassium-sparing diuretic would be contraindicated for this client.
TEST-TAKING TIP: Read the question carefully and select the incorrect options.
Content Area: Adult Health
Integrated Processes: Nursing Process: Analysis
Client Need: Safe and Effective Care Environment
Cognitive Level: Analysis
Reference: Ignatavicius, D., and Workman, M. (2012). Medical-Surgical Nursing: Patient-Centered Collaborative Care (7th ed.). St. Louis, MO: Saunders.

19. ANSWER: 4.

Rationale:

1. A blood pressure of 100/45 mm Hg may be present in a client admitted with a 2-day history of vomiting and diarrhea and at increased risk for hypokalemia, but respiratory alterations should be the priority.
2. Weakness and lightheadedness may be present in a client admitted with a 2-day history of vomiting and diarrhea and at increased risk for hypokalemia, but respiratory alterations should be the priority.
3. A pulse of 100 bpm may be present in a client admitted with a 2-day history of vomiting and diarrhea and at increased risk for hypokalemia, but respiratory alterations should be the priority.
4. **The nurse should investigate the client's shallow respirations and tachypnea first, because vomiting and diarrhea place the client at increased risk for hypokalemia. Respiratory changes are likely with hypokalemia because of weakness of the muscles needed for breathing.**

TEST-TAKING TIP: Remember the "ABCs" of assessment. Alterations in respiration should be the priority.

Content Area: Older Adult Health
Integrated Processes: Nursing Process: Implementation
Client Need: Safe and Effective Care Environment
Cognitive Level: Analysis
***Reference:** Ignatavicius, D., and Workman, M. (2012). Medical-Surgical Nursing: Patient-Centered Collaborative Care (7th ed.). St. Louis, MO: Saunders.*

20. ANSWER: 2.

Rationale:

1. Although the nurse should investigate mental confusion, this should not be the nurse's priority over cardiac dysrhythmias.
2. **The nurse should immediately intervene in the event of cardiac dysrhythmias. Cardiac dysrhythmias are life-threatening manifestations of potassium imbalances. Because this client has been taking furosemide (a non-potassium-sparing diuretic) for treatment of CHF, the client is most likely experiencing an actual loss of potassium.**
3. Although the nurse should investigate abdominal distention, this should not be the nurse's priority over cardiac dysrhythmias.
4. Although the nurse should investigate hypotension, this should not be the nurse's priority over cardiac dysrhythmias. Cardiac dysrhythmias may be the cause of hypotension.

TEST-TAKING TIP: The most life-threatening manifestation should always be the first priority.

Content Area: Adult Health
Integrated Processes: Nursing Process: Implementation
Client Need: Safe and Effective Care Environment
Cognitive Level: Analysis
***Reference:** Ignatavicius, D., and Workman, M. (2012). Medical-Surgical Nursing: Patient-Centered Collaborative Care (7th ed.). St. Louis, MO: Saunders.*

21. ANSWER: 2, 3, 4, 5.

Rationale:

1. Diarrhea related to Spastic Colonic Activity is associated with hyperkalemia, not hypokalemia.
2. **The nurse should assign the diagnosis Constipation Related to Smooth Muscle Atony to this client. The client is experiencing hypokalemia, which results in muscle weakness, smooth muscle atony, and cardiac dysrhythmias.**
3. **The nurse should assign the diagnosis Decreased Cardiac Output Related to Dysrhythmia to this client. The client is experiencing hypokalemia, which results in muscle weakness, smooth muscle atony, and cardiac dysrhythmias.**
4. **The nurse should assign the diagnosis Impaired Physical Mobility Related to Skeletal Muscle Weakness to this client. The client is experiencing hypokalemia, which results in muscle weakness, smooth muscle atony, and cardiac dysrhythmias.**
5. **The nurse should assign the diagnosis Potential for Respiratory Insufficiency Related to Muscle Weakness to this client. The client is experiencing hypokalemia, which results in muscle weakness, smooth muscle atony, and cardiac dysrhythmias.**

TEST-TAKING TIP: Become familiar with the similarities and differences in the signs and symptoms of hypokalemia and hyperkalemia.

Content Area: Adult Health
Integrated Processes: Nursing Process: Analysis
Client Need: Physiological Integrity
Cognitive Level: Analysis
***Reference:** Ignatavicius, D., and Workman, M. (2012). Medical-Surgical Nursing: Patient-Centered Collaborative Care (7th ed.). St. Louis, MO: Saunders.*

22. ANSWER: 2.

Rationale:

1. The nursing diagnosis Impaired Physical Mobility Related to Skeletal Muscle Weakness is appropriate for this client but should not be the nurse's first priority.
2. **The nurse should give priority to the nursing diagnosis Decreased Cardiac Output Related to Dysrhythmias because cardiac dysrhythmias are potentially life threatening.**
3. The nursing diagnosis Risk for Falls Related to Skeletal Muscle Weakness is appropriate for this client but should not be the nurse's first priority.
4. The nursing diagnosis Constipation Related to Smooth Muscle Atony is appropriate for this client but should not be the nurse's first priority.

TEST-TAKING TIP: The most life-threatening manifestation should always be the first priority.

Content Area: Adult Health
Integrated Processes: Nursing Process: Analysis
Client Need: Physiological Integrity
Cognitive Level: Analysis
***Reference:** Ignatavicius, D., and Workman, M. (2012). Medical-Surgical Nursing: Patient-Centered Collaborative Care (7th ed.). St. Louis, MO: Saunders.*

23. ANSWER: 2.

Rationale:

1. ECG strip 1 shows normal sinus rhythm, not a rhythm indicative of hypokalemia.
2. **The nurse should identify ECG strip 2 as indicative of hypokalemia because it displays a normal sinus rhythm with prominent U waves, which are a classic ECG change associated with serum potassium levels less than 3.5 mEq/L.**

3. ECG strip 3 shows sinus tachycardia (heart rate greater than 100 bpm), not a rhythm indicative of hypokalemia.
4. ECG strip 4 shows sinus bradycardia (heart rate less than 60 bpm), not a rhythm indicative of hypokalemia.

TEST-TAKING TIP: Review the effects of hypokalemia on the electrical conduction of the heart, and choose the option that reflects those effects.

Content Area: Older Adult Health
Integrated Processes: Nursing Process: Evaluation
Client Need: Physiological Integrity
Cognitive Level: Analysis
Reference: *Jones, S. (2010). ECG Notes: Interpretation and Management Guide (2nd ed.). Philadelphia, PA: F. A. Davis.*

24. ANSWER: 3.
Rationale:
1. ECG strip 1 shows the prominent U waves associated with hypokalemia, not hyperkalemia.
2. ECG strip 2 shows normal sinus rhythm, not a rhythm indicative of potassium imbalance.
3. The nurse should identify ECG strip 3 as indicative of hyperkalemia because it displays peaked, tented T waves, which are a classic ECG change associated with serum potassium levels greater than 5.0 mEq/L.
4. ECG strip 4 shows atrial fibrillation, which is not related to electrolyte imbalance.

TEST-TAKING TIP: Review the effects of hyperkalemia on the electrical conduction of the heart, and choose the option that reflects those effects.

Content Area: Adult Health
Integrated Processes: Nursing Process: Evaluation
Client Need: Physiological Integrity
Cognitive Level: Analysis
Reference: *Jones, S. (2010). ECG Notes: Interpretation and Management Guide (2nd ed.). Philadelphia, PA: F. A. Davis.*

25. ANSWER: 3.
Rationale:
1. Chlorothiazide is not an appropriate choice for this client. Chlorothiazide is a non–potassium-sparing diuretic that would increase the renal excretion of potassium and worsen the client's hypokalemia.
2. Bumetanide is not an appropriate choice for this client. Bumetanide is a non–potassium-sparing diuretic that would increase the renal excretion of potassium and worsen the client's hypokalemia.
3. The nurse should identify spironolactone, a potassium-sparing diuretic, as most appropriate for this client. Potassium-sparing diuretics increase urine output (decreasing fluid volume excess), without increasing potassium loss.
4. Furosemide is not an appropriate choice for this client. Furosemide is a non–potassium-sparing diuretic that would increase the renal excretion of potassium and worsen the client's hypokalemia.

TEST-TAKING TIP: Differentiate between potassium-sparing and non–potassium-sparing diuretics. A potassium-sparing diuretic should be administered to a client who needs to conserve potassium.

Content Area: Adult Health
Integrated Processes: Nursing Process: Analysis
Client Need: Physiological Integrity
Cognitive Level: Analysis
Reference: *Deglin, J. H., Vallerand, A. H., and Sanoski, C. A. (2013). Davis's Drug Guide for Nurses (13th ed.). Philadelphia, PA: F. A. Davis.*

Calcium Imbalances

KEY TERMS

Calcitonin—A hormone produced by the thyroid gland that helps regulate calcium levels in the body; involved in the process of building bone; acts to reduce blood calcium (Ca^{2+}), opposing the effects of parathyroid hormone (PTH).

Calcitriol—The active form of vitamin D; promotes calcium absorption in the intestines and inhibits calcium excretion by the kidneys; acts with PTH to maintain calcium balance.

Chvostek's sign—A spasm of the facial muscles following a tap on the facial nerve; seen in hypocalcemic tetany.

Hypercalcemia—Total serum calcium (Ca^{2+}) greater than 10.2 mg/dL or 2.55 mmol/L.

Hyperparathyroidism—A condition caused by excessive levels of parathyroid hormone (PTH) in the body; the most common cause of hypercalcemia.

Hypocalcemia—Total serum calcium (Ca^{2+}) less than 8.2 to 9 mg/dL or 2.05 mmol/L.

Milk-alkali syndrome—A disorder caused by the prolonged intake of excessive amounts of milk and soluble alkali; usually occurs as an undesired side effect of treating a peptic ulcer with calcium-containing antacids; also known as Burnett's syndrome.

Parathyroid hormone—A hormone produced by the parathyroid glands that stimulates bone cells to release calcium into the blood, enhances the absorption of calcium from the small intestine, and suppresses calcium loss in urine; the most important endocrine regulator of calcium and phosphorus concentration in extracellular fluid.

Trousseau's sign—A muscular spasm of the hand and wrist elicited by applying a blood pressure cuff and inflating it to 20 mm Hg above the client's normal systolic blood pressure for 3 minutes; a sign of hypocalcemia.

I. Description

Calcium (Ca^{2+}) is the most abundant cation in the human body, and the bones store approximately 99% of it. The small intestine absorbs calcium, and vitamin D is required for this absorption to take place. Magnesium, phosphorus, and vitamin K are also needed for the body to absorb and use calcium. Calcium is excreted by the kidneys. Intracellular calcium is essential for numerous cellular events, including muscle contraction, signaling, hormone secretion, glycogen metabolism, and cell division. Extracellular calcium provides a steady supply of calcium for intracellular use and also plays an important role in clotting and membrane integrity. Calcium performs the following primary functions:

1. Assists in building strong bones and teeth
2. Facilitates blood clotting
3. Is essential for nerve impulse transmission
4. Plays a key role in skeletal and cardiac muscle contraction and relaxation, making it important for normal heart and muscular functioning
5. Assists in the activation of certain enzymes

Normal Lab Value The normal total serum calcium level is 8.2 to 10.2 mg/dL for adults. The normal ionized serum calcium level is 4.6 to 5.3 mg/dL for adults.

A. Calcium balance

1. Serum calcium levels are regulated by a loop feedback system involving three major hormones (Fig. 5.1).
   a. **Parathyroid hormone (PTH)** is excreted by the chief cells of the parathyroid glands and acts to increase the concentration of calcium in the blood.
   b. **Calcitriol** is the hormonally active form of vitamin D that increases the level of calcium in the blood by (1) increasing the absorption of calcium in the small intestine, (2) decreasing the renal transfer of calcium from the blood to the kidneys, and (3) increasing the release of calcium from the bones into the bloodstream.
   c. **Calcitonin** is a hormone produced by the thyroid gland that acts to decrease the calcium concentration in the blood by increasing calcium absorption in the bones.

MAKING THE CONNECTION

Bound and Ionized Calcium

Calcium exists in the bloodstream in two forms: bound and unbound (or ionized). Bound calcium is attached to serum proteins, primarily albumin, so the amount of total calcium varies with the level of serum albumin. When a client's serum albumin level is normal, the total serum calcium level, which is a measure of both bound and unbound calcium in the blood, provides a relatively accurate measurement of the serum calcium level. Approximately 40% of calcium is bound to protein. Unbound calcium, also called ionized, active, or free calcium, is the active form of calcium and must be maintained within a narrow range. It is described as "ionized" because it has a positive electrical (ionic) charge. Ionized calcium circulates freely in the blood and other extracellular fluids and does not vary with the albumin level. Therefore, it is useful to measure the ionized calcium level when a client's serum albumin is abnormal or when a calcium disorder is suspected even though the total serum calcium level is normal. Approximately 50% of calcium is ionized and active.

II. Types of Calcium Imbalance

Calcium imbalances occur when there is a decrease or increase in the calcium content of the blood in relation to the amount of water in the body.

A. **Hypocalcemia**, or calcium deficit, is a total serum calcium level less than 8.2 mg/dL or an ionized serum calcium level less than 4.6 mg/dL.
   1. When serum calcium levels are too low, calcium is borrowed from the bones in response to the secretion of PTH and calcitriol, the active form of vitamin D (see Fig. 5.1).
   2. Hypocalcemia is frequently encountered in hospitalized clients, and the presentation can vary widely, from asymptomatic to life-threatening events.
   3. Mild calcium deficits are usually the result of a chronic disease.
   4. Mild or moderate decreases in serum calcium levels are more common than severe, symptomatic hypocalcemia.
   5. Prolonged low calcium levels can result in poor bone formation, which may lead to brittle bones that are prone to fracture.
   6. Depending on the cause, undiagnosed or poorly treated hypocalcemia can lead to significant morbidity or death.

(!) Acute hypocalcemia may result in the rapid onset of life-threatening symptoms such as seizures and respiratory distress, which are caused by neuromuscular irritability.

B. **Hypercalcemia**, or calcium excess, is a total serum calcium level greater than 10.2 mg/dL or an ionized serum calcium level greater than 5.3 mg/dL.
   1. When serum calcium levels are too high, PTH excretion is inhibited, and calcitonin is produced by the thyroid gland to increase the bones' reabsorption of calcium.
   2. Hypercalcemia most commonly results from malignancy or primary hyperparathyroidism.
   3. Between 20% and 40% of clients diagnosed with cancer will experience hypercalcemia at some point during their disease.
   4. Other causes of elevated calcium are less common and are usually not considered until malignancy and parathyroid disease have been ruled out.

(!) A total serum calcium level less than 7 mg/dL or greater than 12 mg/dL is a medical emergency and can lead to life-threatening cardiac dysrhythmias.

III. Causes of Calcium Imbalance

Calcium imbalance can be caused by the direct loss or gain of calcium, inadequate or excessive intake of calcium, and inadequate absorption or excessive retention of calcium. However, hormonal imbalances and increases or decreases in other electrolytes cause most calcium imbalances (Table 5.1).

A. Hypocalcemia may be caused by calcium loss, inadequate calcium intake, or inadequate calcium absorption.
   1. Hyperphosphatemia, or increased serum phosphate levels, also causes hypocalcemia because phosphate binds easily with calcium. Hyperphosphatemia may result from renal failure or excess tissue breakdown, such as rhabdomyolysis or tumor lysis, when phosphorus in the form of phosphate (the most abundant intracellular anion) is released from the cells into the extracellular fluid.

DID YOU KNOW?

Calcium and phosphorus have an inverse relationship in the body. When serum phosphorus levels are high, serum calcium levels are usually low because phosphorus binds with calcium, decreasing the availability of calcium in the bloodstream.

   2. Hypoalbuminemia, a common cause of hypocalcemia, is a decrease in serum albumin that may

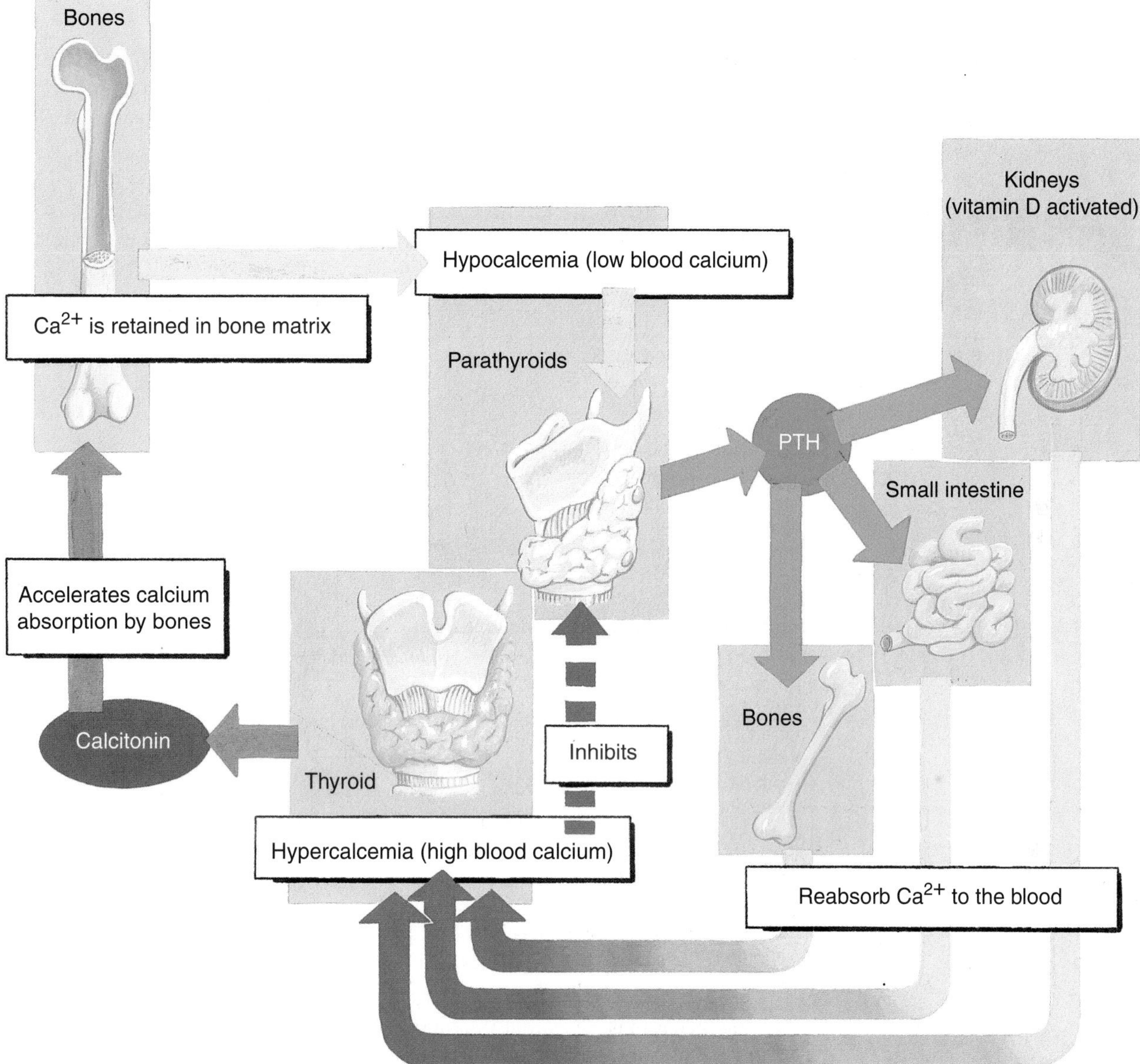

Fig 5.1 When serum calcium levels are too low, the parathyroid glands are stimulated to release PTH, which activates vitamin D in the kidneys (calcitriol), increases calcium absorption by the small intestine, and stimulates the bones to release calcium into the bloodstream to increase serum calcium levels. When serum calcium levels are too high, excretion of PTH by the parathyroid glands is inhibited, and the thyroid gland produces calcitonin to accelerate calcium absorption by the bones to decrease serum calcium levels.

occur as a result of liver cirrhosis, nephrosis, malnutrition, burns, chronic illness, or sepsis or in critically ill clients (see Table 5.1).

a. Because calcium binds with albumin in the blood, a lack of serum albumin results in a lack of circulating calcium.
b. Alkalosis, a condition in which the blood pH exceeds 7.45, causes ionized calcium to bind with albumin.
c. Remember that when serum albumin levels are abnormal, the serum ionized (active) calcium level should be measured to rule out the presence of another underlying disorder that is causing the hypocalcemia.

3. Hypoparathyroidism, either hereditary or acquired, is a deficiency of PTH.
   a. The causes of hypoparathyroidism vary, but all share the common feature of hypocalcemia.

b. Acute pancreatitis is characterized by inadequate PTH secretion; lack of PTH prevents the reuptake of calcium from the bones, resulting in hypocalcemia.

4. Severe hypomagnesemia, or magnesium deficiency, can lead to hypocalcemia that is resistant to the administration of calcium and vitamin D.
   a. Hypomagnesemia is usually caused by magnesium loss via the kidneys or the gastrointestinal tract.
   b. Clients with hypomagnesemia usually have low PTH levels and hypocalcemia.

Table 5.1 Causes of Calcium Imbalance

Imbalance	Causes and Risk Factors
Hypocalcemia	

Calcium loss	• Hyperphosphatemia, secondary to
	  • Renal failure
	  • Rhabdomyolysis
	  • Tumor lysis
	  • Excessive phosphate administration
	• Acute pancreatitis
	• Hungry bone syndrome
	• Chelation
	• Widespread bone metastases
	• Diarrhea, steatorrhea
	• Wound drainage
	• Immobility (promotes calcium loss from bones)

Inadequate calcium intake or absorption	• The most common cause of hypocalcemia is hypoalbuminemia caused by cirrhosis, nephrosis, malnutrition, burns, chronic illness, and sepsis
	• Inadequate dietary intake of calcium, vitamin D, or magnesium
	  • Rickets
	  • Vitamin D deficiency
	  • Nothing-by-mouth (NPO) status
	  • Lactose intolerance
	• Malabsorption of foods or calcium from gastrointestinal tract
	  • Celiac sprue
	  • Crohn's disease
	• Hypoparathyroidism (absence of PTH secretion)
	  • Postoperative parathyroidectomy
	  • Autoimmune
	  • Congenital
	  • Pseudohypoparathyroidism
	  • Hypomagnesemia, which induces PTH resistance and affects PTH production
	  • Severe hypermagnesemia (greater than 6 mg/dL), which can lead to hypocalcemia by inhibiting PTH secretion
	• Medications that inhibit absorption of calcium or promote calcium excretion
	  -anticonvulsants such as phenobarbital (Luminal) and phenytoin (Dilantin)
	  -cimetidine (Tagamet)
	  -drugs that lower serum magnesium, such as cisplatin and gentamicin
	  -furosemide (Lasix) and other loop diuretics
	  -phosphates, such as phosphate enemas (Fleet, OsmoPrep, Visicol)
	• Alkalosis
	• Massive transfusion of banked blood
	  • Citrate, which is added to banked blood as a preservative and to prevent clotting, binds with serum calcium and decreases the amount of ionized (active) calcium; this occurs when blood is administered faster than the liver can metabolize the citrate
	• Excessive alcohol ingestion (alcohol reduces intestinal absorption of calcium and interferes with other processes that regulate calcium balance)
	• Age (older adults have an increased risk, especially women because of decreased estrogen levels)

Hypercalcemia	
Calcium retention	• The main cause of hypercalcemia is hyperparathyroidism • Some cancers • Addison's disease • Obstructive uropathy • HIV/AIDS

Table 5.1 Causes of Calcium Imbalance—cont'd

Imbalance	Causes and Risk Factors

Excessive calcium intake	• Excessive dietary calcium intake
	• Excessive dietary vitamin A or D intake
	• Excessive calcium supplement intake
	• Addison's disease
	• Excessive vitamin D level
	• Certain cancers
	  • Metastatic bone cancer
	  • Multiple myeloma
	  • Tumors producing PTH-like substance
	  • Some types of breast, kidney, and lung cancer
	• Prolonged immobilization
	• Paget's disease
	• Sarcoidosis
	• Milk-alkali syndrome
	• Medications
	  -lithium may increase the release of PTH
	  -thiazide diuretics decrease the amount of calcium excreted in urine

DID YOU KNOW?

Serum calcium and magnesium levels usually move in the same direction. When serum calcium levels are low, serum magnesium levels may also be low, and vice versa.

5. Vitamin D deficiency
   a. Adequate vitamin D is necessary for PTH to be effective.
   b. Poor nutritional intake, chronic renal insufficiency, or reduced exposure to sunlight may cause vitamin D deficiency.
   c. Current federal guidelines recommend 800 to 1,000 IU of vitamin D per day for adults, depending on age.
   d. Research studies have shown that vitamin D deficiency can occur despite adequate intake, leading to increased PTH and eventual osteoporosis.
   e. Numerous conditions can impair the absorption of vitamin D, including diseases of the small intestines, such as celiac disease; pancreatic diseases; gastric bypass surgery; and steatorrhea (see Table 5.1).
6. Massive blood transfusion
   a. Citrate, a preservative added to blood products, acts as an anticoagulant, preventing the blood from clotting.
   b. Citrate also binds with ionized calcium, causing it to be inactive.
7. Certain medications can lead to the development of hypocalcemia.
   a. Antiseizure medications, such as phenytoin (Dilantin), carbamazepine, phenobarbitol, and primidone, may lower levels of calcium in the body. Vitamin D supplementation is recommended in clients taking antiseizure drugs to try to maintain calcium levels; because each interferes with the absorption of the other, they should be taken at least 2 hours apart.
   b. Loop diuretics, such as furosemide (Lasix), promote the excretion of calcium by the kidneys.
   c. Corticosteroids, when administered in large doses or over a prolonged period, can reduce calcium absorption and increase calcium excretion.
   d. When calcium citrate is taken with aluminum-containing antacids, the amount of aluminum absorbed by the blood may be increased significantly. In people with kidney disease, this absorbed aluminum may reach toxic levels.
   e. Cholesterol-lowering medications such as cholestyramine, colestipol, and colesevelam (bile acid sequestrants) interfere with normal calcium absorption and increase the loss of calcium in the urine.
   f. Phosphates, such as Fleet enemas and OsmoPrep, increase serum phosphorus levels, resulting in decreased serum calcium levels.

B. Hypercalcemia, which is much less common than hypocalcemia, may be caused by the excessive release of calcium from bone, increased intestinal absorption, excessive calcium intake, or decreased calcium excretion (retention) by the kidneys.
   1. Primary hyperthyroidism, or an increase in the production of thyroid hormone, is a common cause of hypercalcemia.
   2. Primary **hyperparathyroidism,** or an overactive parathyroid gland, is a condition in which too

much PTH is produced, causing calcium to be released from the bones into the bloodstream.

3. Cancer cells can secrete substances that dissolve osteoclasts (bone cells), increasing serum calcium levels.
4. Paget's disease of the bone is a chronic disorder characterized by the excessive breakdown and formation of bone tissue, resulting in enlarged, misshapen bones and hypercalcemia. Although there is no known cure, medications such as bisphosphonates and calcitonin can help control the disorder.
5. Excessive ingestion of vitamin D may result in hypercalcemia because vitamin D enhances the absorption of calcium in the small intestine.
6. **Milk-alkali syndrome,** also known as Burnett's syndrome, is characterized by hypercalcemia caused by the excessive ingestion of calcium and an absorbable alkali.
   a. This syndrome may occur in clients ingesting excessive calcium carbonate (Tums) or milk and sodium bicarbonate (excess calcium with an excess base) to control dyspepsia.
   b. The ingestion of more than 2 gm of calcium daily may produce this disorder in susceptible individuals.
7. Medications such as lithium and thiazide diuretics may lead to the development of hypercalcemia (see Table 5.1).

IV. Nursing Assessment for Calcium Imbalance

The nurse should conduct a focused nursing assessment for calcium imbalance, beginning with a thorough nursing history. Interview the client and family members to identify any risk factors or preexisting conditions that would contribute to calcium imbalance, such as pancreatitis, anxiety disorders, renal or liver failure, gastrointestinal disorders, bowel surgery, hyperthyroidism, or hyperparathyroidism. Previous neck surgery or trauma may place the client at risk for hypoparathyroidism. A history of seizures may suggest hypocalcemia secondary to anticonvulsant therapy. The nurse should also assess the client's ability to drink and tolerate oral fluids. Include a current dietary history, inquiring about the intake of vitamin D, calcium supplements, and antacids that contain calcium or magnesium (Table 5.2). The nursing history should also include current medications, focusing on the use of diuretics, bisphosphonates, antibiotics, and anticonvulsants. A thorough physical assessment is necessary because calcium imbalances affect many body systems. Assess each body system, observing for signs and symptoms of calcium imbalance. Assess the client for signs of tetany, if hypocalcemia is suspected, by eliciting **Chvostek's sign** and **Trousseau's sign** (Figs. 5.2 and 5.3). Measure and record the client's vital signs, and review the client's laboratory data to assess for the presence of hypo- or hypercalcemia (see Table 5.2).

V. Electrocardiogram Changes and Calcium Imbalance

Electrocardiogram (ECG) changes occur when serum calcium levels are either too low or too high. Although calcium does not affect the heart rate, it does influence how hard the heart contracts (inotropic effect).

A. If serum calcium levels are too low, the heart will not contract as it should.
   1. Acute hypocalcemia is characterized by prolongation of the Q-T interval and a prolonged ST segment.
   2. As hypocalcemia worsens, ventricular tachycardia (VT) and decreased myocardial contractility may

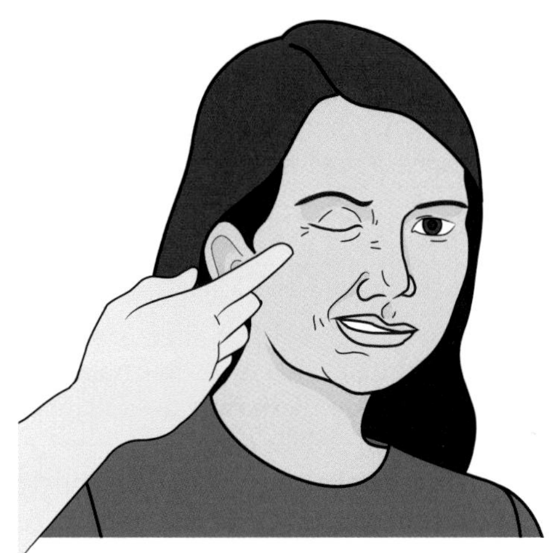

Fig 5.2

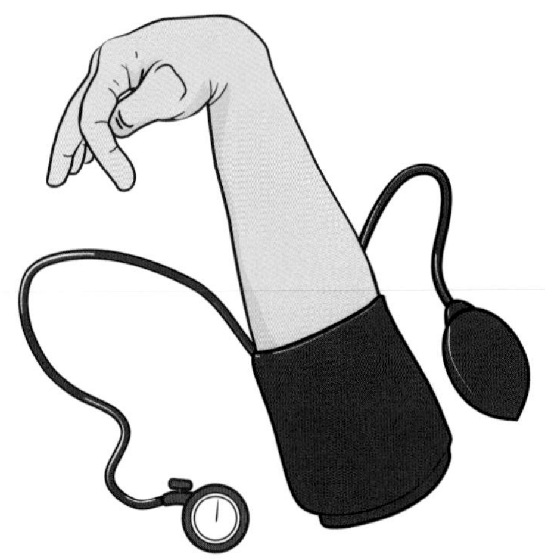

Fig 5.3

Table 5.2 Signs and Symptoms of Calcium Imbalance

Vital Signs

	Hypocalcemia	*Hypercalcemia*
Blood pressure	Hypotension	Mild: increased
Heart rate	Increased or decreased	Mild: increased Severe or prolonged: decreased
Respiratory rate	Increased	Increased
Temperature	Within normal limits	Within normal limits

Signs and Symptoms by Body System

	Hypocalcemia	*Hypercalcemia (Mild or Chronic May Produce No Symptoms)*
Cardiovascular	• Bradycardia or tachycardia • Prolonged Q-T interval • Weak, thready pulse • Irregular heartbeat • Hypotension	• Increased blood clotting times • Excessive clotting, especially in lower legs and pelvic region
Cerebral	• Confusion • Irritability • Anxiety • Lethargy • Altered mental status	• Confusion • Fatigue • Lethargy to unresponsiveness • Altered mental status
ECG changes	• Prolonged Q-T interval • Prolonged ST segment	• Shortened Q-T interval
Gastrointestinal	• Hyperactive bowel sounds • Abdominal cramping • Steatorrhea • Diarrhea	• Hypoactive or absent bowel sounds • Abdominal distention • Constipation • Nausea and vomiting • Anorexia

Musculoskeletal	• Skeletal changes
	  • Osteoporosis
	  • Frequent fractures
	  • Pathological fractures
	• Spinal curvature secondary to fractured vertebrae
		• Muscle and joint aches

Neuromuscular	• Seizures (all types) • Paresthesias and numbness of fingertips and perioral area • Positive Chvostek's sign • Positive Trousseau's sign • Myalgia • Muscle stiffness and frequent, painful cramping (charleyhorse) • Tetany	• Severe muscle weakness • Decreased DTRs without paresthesias
Respiratory	• Stridor caused by prolonged contraction of respiratory and laryngeal muscles • Respiratory distress	*None*

Laboratory Values

	Hypocalcemia	*Hypercalcemia*
Total serum calcium	Less than 8.2 mg/dL	Greater than 10.2 mg/dL
Ionized serum calcium	Less than 4.6 mg/dL	Greater than 5.3 mg/dL

develop, which can lead to hypotension, angina, and heart failure.

B. If serum calcium levels are too high, rapid repolarization occurs, resulting in spastic contractions of the heart muscle.
   1. In the presence of mild hypercalcemia, broad-based, peaking T waves may be seen.
   2. In severe hypercalcemia, the QT interval becomes extremely short in addition to the presence of widened T waves (Fig. 5.4).

VI. Nursing Interventions for Clients with Calcium Imbalance

A. Identify high-risk clients.
   1. Postmenopausal women who are not taking estrogen (hypocalcemia)
   2. Clients diagnosed with osteoporosis or osteopenia (hypocalcemia)
   3. Clients who have had the thyroid and/or parathyroid glands removed (hypocalcemia)
   4. Clients with a history of Crohn's disease or other small bowel disorders (hypocalcemia)
   5. Clients with cancer (hypercalcemia)
   6. Clients with renal impairment (hypercalcemia)
   7. Clients who are hospitalized or immobile (hypocalcemia or hypercalcemia)
   8. Clients who frequently take antacids (hypocalcemia or hypercalcemia, depending on the antacid taken)

B. Implement the health-care provider's orders to treat the underlying cause of the imbalance.
   1. The health-care provider's orders may include oral or IV fluid administration, oral or IV calcium administration, vitamin D supplementation or restriction, oral or IV magnesium replacement, oral or IV phosphorus replacement, medication administration, and dialysis (in clients with severe renal dysfunction) (Table 5.3).

C. Monitor the client and the client's serum calcium levels.
   1. Monitor the client's serum calcium levels as ordered by the health-care provider.
   2. Monitor other laboratory values associated with calcium imbalance.
      a. Vitamin D: 15 to 60 pg/mL
      b. PTH: 10 to 65 pg/mL (adult)
      c. Albumin: 3.2 to 5.1 g/dL (adults younger than 90 years)
      d. Serum magnesium: 1.6 to 2.6 mg/dL (adult)
      e. Serum phosphorus: 2.5 to 4.5 mg/dL (adult)
      f. Serum digoxin levels (because hypercalcemia enhances the effects of digoxin): 0.8 to 2 ng/mL
      g. 24-hour urine calcium levels (useful to identify parathyroid gland disorders):
         1) Low-calcium diet: less than 150 mg/24 hr
         2) Average-calcium diet: 150 to 250 mg/24 hr
         3) High-calcium diet: 250 to 300 mg/24 hr
   3. Monitor for cardiovascular changes.
      a. Auscultate the apical pulse.
      b. Assess for alterations in blood pressure.
      c. Observe for bleeding or bruising related to decreased blood clotting secondary to hypocalcemia.
      d. Observe the ECG for abnormal heart rhythms.

DID YOU KNOW?

Cardiac monitoring is essential to identify and treat dysrhythmias.

   4. Monitor for neuromuscular changes.
      a. Establish a baseline for the client's deep tendon reflexes, muscle strength, and tone.
      b. Monitor the client for muscle weakness, muscle twitching, or irregular muscle contractions during each nursing shift.
      c. Assess the client for positive Chvostek's sign and Trousseau's sign (tetany related to hypocalcemia).

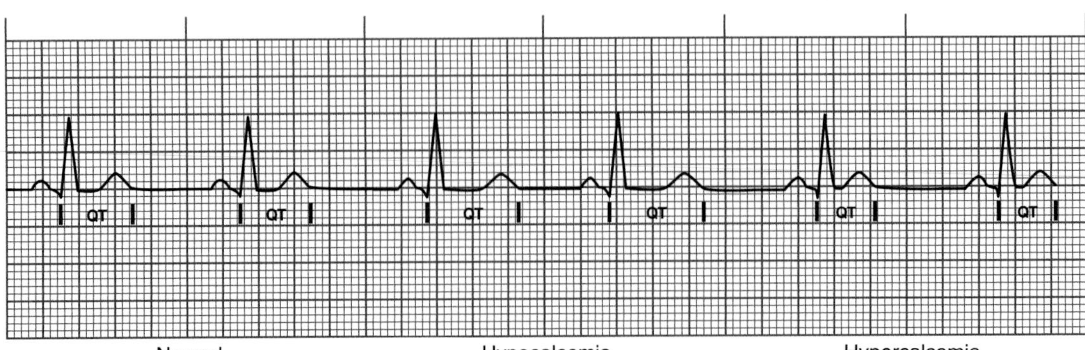

Fig 5.4 ECG changes associated with calcium imbalances. Notice that the Q-T interval gets wider in the presence of hypocalcemia and shorter in the presence of hypercalcemia.

Table 5.3 Nursing Interventions to Control Serum Calcium Levels

Hypocalcemia	Hypercalcemia

Increase calcium level
• Administer oral supplements, as ordered, to clients with mild hypocalcemia who are asymptomatic
• Administer IV replacement therapy, as ordered, for clients with moderate to severe hypocalcemia who are symptomatic
  • Monitor client's ECG and cardiovascular status during IV infusion
• Administer aluminum hydroxide and vitamin D to enhance calcium absorption
• Increase dietary calcium intake by providing a high-calcium diet
	Decrease calcium level
	• Assist in removal of parathyroid gland if appropriate
	• Limit dietary calcium
	• Discontinue or decrease calcium supplements, as ordered
	• Administer IV normal (0.9%) saline solution to replace fluids, dilute serum calcium, and increase the kidneys' excretion of calcium
	• Avoid the administration of lactated Ringer's solution or other IV solutions containing calcium or vitamin D
	• Hospitalize client if symptomatic
	Severe hypercalcemia
	• Treat in acute care facility with cardiac monitoring capabilities
	• Decrease serum calcium by direct removal (especially if renal failure is a cause)
	  • Hemodialysis
	  • Continuous venovenous hemofiltration
	  • Continuous renal replacement therapy

Administer medications as ordered
• Bisphosphonates to inhibit bone destruction, preserve bone mass, and increase bone density in the spine and hip, reducing risk of fractures; IV or PO administration, depending on drug
  -alendronate (Fosamax)
  -etidronate (Didronel)
  -ibandronate (Boniva)
  -pamidronate (Aredia)
  -risedronate (Actonel)
  -zoledronate (Zometa)
  -zoledronic acid (Reclast)
• Calcitonin to reduce bone resorption and slow bone loss
  -calcitonin (Calcimar)
• Oral calcium supplements to increase serum calcium levels
  -calcium carbonate (generic only)
  -calcium citrate (Citracal + D)
  -calcium glubionate (Calcionate)
  -calcium gluconate (generic only)
  -calcium lactate (Ridactate)
  -calcium with vitamin D (Caltrate 600 + D)
  -tribasic calcium phosphate (Ascocid, Cal-C-Caps, Cal-G, Cal-Lac, Citracal, PhosLo, Posture, Prelief, Rolaids)
• PTH, or an analogue of PTH, to stimulate new bone growth
  -teriparatide (Fortéo)
• Selective estrogen receptor modulators to mimic the beneficial effects of estrogen on bone density in postmenopausal women, without the associated risks
  -raloxifene (Evista); approved only for women with osteoporosis; not currently approved for use in men
  -tamoxifen (Soltamox, Nolvadex); reduces risk of fractures
	Administer medications as ordered
	• Bisphosphonates to inhibit calcium resorption
	  -clodronate (Bonefos)
	  -pamidronate (Aredia)
	  -zoledronate (Zometa)
	• Calcitonin to reduce bone resorption and slow bone loss
	  -calcitonin (Calcimar)
	• Calcium chelating agents to bind calcium for removal via the gastrointestinal tract
	  -penicillamine (Cuprimine, Pendramine)
	  -plicamycin (Mithracin)
	• Corticosteroids to counter effects of excess vitamin D
	  -prednisolone or prednisone
	• Loop diuretics to promote excretion of calcium
	  -furosemide (Lasix)

5. Monitor for gastrointestinal changes.
   a. Auscultate bowel sounds in all four quadrants.
   b. Observe the frequency and consistency of bowel movements.

D. Ensure client safety

1. Monitor cardiac function to identify and treat dysrhythmias.
   a. Continuous ECG monitoring is essential to identify and treat potentially fatal dysrhythmias, especially if the client is receiving IV calcium replacement.
2. Reduce environmental stimuli for a client with hypocalcemia.
   a. Provide a quiet room.
   b. Limit the client's visitors.
   c. Darken the client's room.
   d. Speak in soft tones.
3. Implement seizure precautions for a client with hypocalcemia.
   a. Pad side rails.
   b. Have oxygen and suction equipment available.
   c. Ensure the patency of IV access devices.

d. Administer emergency medications as ordered.
e. Prepare for possible endotracheal intubation.
f. Prepare for cardiac defibrillation if necessary.

4. Implement fall precautions related to muscle weakness caused by hypocalcemia or hypercalcemia.
   a. Perform a fall risk assessment.
   b. Maintain the bed in a low position with locked wheels.
   c. Remove all obstacles from pathways, especially to the toilet.
   d. Monitor the environment for safety hazards (e.g., torn carpet, liquid spills on floors).
   e. Place assistive devices (walkers, canes) within the client's reach.
   f. Use nightlights.
   g. Instruct the client to request assistance to ambulate.
   h. Ensure availability of the call light.
   i. Assess the client's footwear and provide appropriate footwear if necessary; clients must use antiskid soles.
   j. Keep items such as the telephone and fluids close to the client.
   k. Request that family members remain with the client if necessary.
   l. Position the client to allow close observation by staff members.
   m. Communicate the client's fall risk during the shift report and as necessary.

E. Educate the client

1. Hypocalcemia
   a. Teach the client or caregiver the causes of calcium deficit.
   b. Provide specific information regarding the client's medical diagnosis and related interventions and treatments.
   c. Teach the client how to identify the signs and symptoms of calcium deficiency.
   d. Instruct the client and family to notify the primary health-care provider if the client exhibits signs or symptoms of hypocalcemia or if they have any other specific concerns.
   e. Teach the client how to prevent calcium deficiency.
   f. Advise the client to exercise to prevent osteoporosis.
      1) A 30-minute walk three to five times per week is the most effective exercise for osteoporosis prevention.
      2) General weight-bearing exercises should be implemented in collaboration with the primary health-care provider; weight-bearing exercises include walking, jogging, hiking, climbing stairs, dancing, and weight training.
   g. Teach the client about foods that contain calcium (Table 5.4).
      1) Milk, yogurt, and cheese are rich sources of calcium.
      2) Nondairy sources of calcium include vegetables such as Chinese cabbage, kale, and broccoli.
      3) Most grains do not have high amounts of calcium unless they are fortified.
      4) Foods fortified with calcium include many fruit juices and drinks, tofu, and cereals.
      5) Inform the client that the recommended intake of calcium varies by age (Table 5.5).

Table 5.4 Foods High in Calcium

Food (Standard Amount)	Calcium (mg)	% Daily Value
Yogurt, plain, low-fat, 8 oz	415	42
Sardines, canned in oil, with bones, 3 oz	324	32
Cheddar cheese, 1.5 oz	306	31
Milk, nonfat, 8 oz	302	30
Milk, reduced-fat (2% milk fat), 8 oz	297	30
Milk, lactose-reduced, 8 oz	285–302	29–30
Milk, whole (3.25% milk fat), 8 oz	291	29
Buttermilk, 8 oz	285	29
Mozzarella, part-skim, 1.5 oz	275	28
Yogurt, fruit, low-fat, 8 oz	245–384	25–38
Orange juice, *calcium-fortified*, 6 oz	200–260	20–26
Tofu, firm, made with calcium sulfate, ½ cup	204	20
Salmon, pink, canned, solids with bones, 3 oz	181	18
Chocolate pudding, instant, made with 2% milk, ½ cup	153	15
Ready-to-eat cereal, *calcium-fortified*, 1 cup	100–1,000	10–100
Instant breakfast drink, powdered, various flavors and brands, prepared with water, 8 oz	105–250	10–25
Soy beverage, *calcium-fortified*, 8 oz	80–500	8–50
Chinese cabbage, raw, 1 cup	74	7
Tortilla, corn, ready-to-bake/fry, 1 medium	42	4
Sour cream, reduced-fat, cultured, 2 tbsp	32	3

Source: National Institutes of Health, Office of Dietary Supplements. (Reviewed 2012). Dietary supplement fact sheet: calcium. http://ods.od.nih.gov/factsheets/Calcium-HealthProfessional/.

Table 5.5 Recommended Daily Intake of Calcium

Age	Male	Female	Pregnant	Lactating
Birth to 6 months	200 mg	200 mg		
7 to 12 months	260 mg	260 mg		
1 to 3 years	700 mg	700 mg		
4 to 8 years	1,000 mg	1,000 mg		
9 to 13 years	1,300 mg	1,300 mg		
14 to 18 years	1,300 mg	1,300 mg	1,300 mg	1,300 mg
19 to 50 years	1,000 mg	1,000 mg	1,000 mg	1,000 mg
51 to 70 years	1,000 mg	1,200 mg		
70+ years	1,200	1,200		

Source: National Institutes of Health, Office of Dietary Supplements. (Reviewed 2012). Dietary supplement fact sheet: calcium. http://ods.od.nih.gov/factsheets/Calcium-HealthProfessional/.

h. Teach the client how to take oral calcium supplements.
   1) Use only as directed; do not take a greater amount or more often than instructed.
   2) Do not take other medications within 1 to 2 hours of calcium ingestion; calcium may interfere with the absorption of other medications.
   3) Take calcium supplements 1 to 1½ hours after meals, unless otherwise directed.
   4) Clients taking the syrup form should be instructed to take the syrup before meals, which allows the supplement to work faster. Mix the syrup in water or fruit juice for infants or children.
   5) If supplements contain calcium carbonate, they should be taken with meals because gastric acid enhances the absorption of calcium carbonate.
   6) Calcium is absorbed most efficiently when it is taken in amounts of 500 mg or less; recommend that the client split the daily dose into two or three separate portions, if necessary.
   7) Chew the chewable tablet form completely before swallowing.
   8) Ensure that effervescent tablets are completely dissolved before drinking; dissolve in a glass of water or juice, and drink slowly.
   9) Take all supplements with a large glass of water.
   10) Do not take calcium supplements within 1 to 2 hours of eating large amounts of fiber-containing foods, such as bran and whole-grain cereals or breads.
   11) Do not drink large amounts of alcohol or caffeine-containing beverages (usually more than 8 cups of coffee a day) or use tobacco.
   12) Monitor for adverse effects of supplementation and for overdose; calcium supplements are generally well tolerated.
   13) Report any adverse effects to the primary health-care provider; the most common side effects include dizziness, flushing sensation, irregular heart rhythm, nausea or vomiting, skin rash, diaphoresis, and paresthesias.
   14) Early signs of overdose include constipation, dry mouth, unremitting headache, polydipsia, irritability, anorexia, depression, metallic taste, and unusual fatigue or weakness.
   15) Later signs of overdose include confusion, severe drowsiness, hypertension, photophobia, cardiac dysrhythmias, and polyuria.

i. Ensure that client or caregiver understands the specifics, rationale, potential side effects, and desired effects of the treatment regimen.

j. Include medication administration, nutrition, and hydration in client teaching; adequate protein, magnesium, vitamin K, calcium, and vitamin D are necessary for bone health.

k. Teach the client how to prevent falls in the home environment.
   1) Avoid the use of throw rugs; use slip-proof underpads if throw rugs are used.
   2) Maintain a clutter-free environment.
   3) Avoid wet or slippery floors, and repair floors as necessary.
   4) Ensure adequate lighting in the home.
   5) Install handrails on stairs and grab bars in bathrooms.
   6) Use nonslip bath mats.
   7) Use raised toilet seats.
   8) Evaluate visual acuity, and treat as necessary.

9) Evaluate hearing, and treat as necessary.
10) Evaluate mobility, and recommend assistive devices as necessary.

2. Hypercalcemia
   a. Teach the client or caregiver the causes of calcium excess.
   b. Provide specific information regarding the client's medical diagnosis and related interventions and treatments.
   c. Teach the client how to identify the signs and symptoms of calcium excess.
   d. Instruct the client and family to notify the primary health-care provider if the client exhibits signs or symptoms of hypercalcemia or if they have any other specific concerns.
   e. Teach the client how to prevent calcium excess.
      1) Avoid foods high in calcium during the acute phase. Avoid or limit dark green leafy vegetables, edible bones of fish, calcium-fortified foods, and dairy products (see Table 5.4).
      2) Drink more fluids, especially water, because dehydration may exacerbate hypercalcemia and kidney stone formation.
      3) Teach the client to read labels on food packages to determine calcium content.
   f. Ensure that the client or caregiver understands the specifics, rationale, potential side effects, and desired effects of the treatment regimen.
   g. Include medication administration, nutrition, hydration, dietary restrictions, and foods high in calcium in client teaching.

F. Evaluate and document
1. Document all assessment findings and interventions per institution policy.
2. Evaluate and document the client's response to interventions and education.
   a. Total and ionized serum calcium levels should return to the normal reference ranges.
   b. Other laboratory values should return to the normal reference ranges.
   c. Vital signs should return to baseline.
   d. Underlying cause of calcium imbalance should be resolved.
   e. Heart rate and rhythm should return to baseline.

CASE STUDY: Putting It All Together

Subjective Data

A postoperative client who had a thyroidectomy 2 days ago reports fatigue and anxiety. The client states, "My hands are asleep and I feel prickly pins around my mouth." The client has a history of goiter, hypertension, and anxiety. The client's current medications are:

- atenolol (Tenormin) 50 mg by mouth (PO) daily
- aspirin 81 mg PO daily
- hydrochlorothiazide/triamterene (Dyazide) 1 capsule daily
- potassium chloride (K-Lor) 20 mEq PO daily

Objective Data

Nursing Assessment

1. Alert; irritable; anxious; oriented to person, place, and time
2. Heart sounds S_1 and S_2 regular, slow
3. Hypotensive
4. Trousseau's sign and Chvostek's sign present
5. Deep tendon reflexes 3+ bilaterally
6. Pedal and radial pulses regular, 1+, and weak bilaterally
7. Bowel sounds hyperactive in all four quadrants

Vital Signs	
Temperature:	97.8°F (36.6°C) orally
Blood pressure:	90/60 mm Hg
Heart rate:	58 bpm
Respiratory rate:	20
O_2 saturation:	97% on room air

Laboratory Results	
Serum calcium:	7.4 mg/dL
Ionized calcium:	3.2 mg/dL
Serum albumin:	2.5 g/dL
Serum phosphate:	4.9 mg/dL
Serum magnesium:	1.3 mEq/L
Serum potassium:	3.5 mEq/L
Vitamin D:	8 pg/mL

Health-Care Provider Orders

1. O_2 2 L/min via nasal cannula.
2. 0.9% saline solution IV 1,000 mL at 125 mL/hr.
3. Start telemetry and monitor closely during calcium administration.

CASE STUDY: Putting It All Together *cont'd*

4. Vital signs every 15 minutes × 1 hour and every 30 minutes × 1 hour, then every 4 hours if stable.
5. Administer 10% calcium gluconate IV 30 mL over no less than 15 minutes now and every 6 hours × 2 doses.
6. Hold atenolol (Tenormin) and hydrochlorothiazide/triamterene (Dyazide).
7. Implement seizure precautions and fall precautions.
8. Monitor intake and output.
9. Reevaluate clinical signs and symptoms; repeat ECG, serum calcium, ionized calcium, magnesium, phosphate, and potassium in 6 hours; notify health-care provider of results.

Case Study Questions

A. What *subjective* assessment findings indicate that the client is experiencing a health alteration?

1. ______
2. ______
3. ______
4. ______

B. What *objective* assessment findings indicate that the client is experiencing a health alteration?

1. ______
2. ______
3. ______
4. ______
5. ______
6. ______
7. ______
8. ______
9. ______
10. ______
11. ______
12. ______
13. ______

C. After analyzing the data collected, what **primary** nursing diagnosis should the nurse assign to this client?

______

Continued

CASE STUDY: Putting It All Together *cont'd*

Case Study Questions

D. What interventions should the nurse plan and/or implement to meet this client's needs?

1. ______
2. ______
3. ______
4. ______
5. ______
6. ______
7. ______
8. ______
9. ______

E. What client outcomes should the nurse plan to evaluate the effectiveness of the nursing interventions?

1. ______
2. ______
3. ______
4. ______
5. ______
6. ______
7. ______

REVIEW QUESTIONS

1. A nurse is assessing a client for signs of hypocalcemia. Which action should the nurse perform to assess for the presence of Chvostek's sign?
   1. Apply a blood pressure cuff to the upper arm, inflate the cuff to a reading higher than the client's systolic blood pressure for 1 to 4 minutes, and observe for carpopedal spasm.
   2. Tap the facial nerve anterior to the earlobe and just below the zygomatic arch, and observe for facial twitching on the same side as the stimulus.
   3. Assess the biceps, triceps, and brachioradialis reflexes of the arm and wrist, and observe for hyperstimulation.
   4. Instruct the client to hyperventilate, and observe for muscle spasms of the hands or feet.

2. Which dietary modification should a nurse instruct a postmenopausal client who is at risk for hypocalcemia to make?
   1. Drink tea daily.
   2. Eat a high-fiber diet.
   3. Use a salt substitute when cooking.
   4. Limit the intake of high-oxalate foods.

3. Which condition, when noted in a client's health history, should a nurse associate with the development of hypercalcemia?
   1. Crohn's disease
   2. Hypoparathyroidism
   3. Metastatic cancer
   4. Lactose intolerance

4. Which findings should a nurse associate with the development of a calcium imbalance when assessing a client diagnosed with hyperparathyroidism? **Select all that apply.**
   1. Impaired blood flow
   2. Hyperactive bowel sounds
   3. Prolonged Q-T interval
   4. Decreased deep tendon reflexes
   5. Confusion

5. Which factors in a client's health history should a nurse identify as contributing to a diagnosis of hypocalcemia? **Select all that apply.**
   1. Excess PTH
   2. Vitamin D deficiency
   3. Hypophosphatemia
   4. Osteoporosis
   5. Acute pancreatitis

6. A nurse is instructing a client who is at risk for hypocalcemia. Which snack should the nurse advise the client to choose to prevent the development of this imbalance?
   1. Nonfat milk (8 oz) and part-skim mozzarella (1.5 oz)
   2. Calcium-fortified orange juice (6 oz) and canned pink salmon, solids with bone (3 oz)
   3. Reduced-fat (2%) milk (8 oz) and white-bread toast (1 slice)
   4. Powdered instant breakfast drink prepared with water (8 oz) and low-fat (1%) cottage cheese (1 cup)

Calcium Amounts in Various Foods

Food	Calcium (mg) per Serving	% Daily Value
Yogurt, plain, low-fat, 8 oz	415	42
Orange juice, calcium-fortified, 6 oz	200–260	20–26
Yogurt, fruit, low-fat, 8 oz	245–384	25–38
Mozzarella, part-skim, 1.5 oz	275	28
Sardines, canned in oil, with bones, 3 oz	325	33
Milk, nonfat, 8 oz	302	30
Milk, reduced-fat (2% milk fat), 8 oz	293	29
Salmon, pink, canned (solids with bones), 3 oz	181	18
Cottage cheese, low-fat (1% milk fat), 1 cup	138	14
Instant breakfast drink, powdered (various flavors and brands), prepared with water, 8 oz	105–250	10–25
Bread, white, 1 slice	73	7

Source: National Institutes of Health, Office of Dietary Supplements. (Reviewed 2012). Dietary supplement fact sheet: calcium. http://ods.od.nih.gov/factsheets/Calcium-HealthProfessional/.

7. A nurse is admitting a client with suspected hypocalcemia. Which actions should the nurse take to assess the client for Trousseau's sign? Place each nursing action in the correct sequence (1–7).

   ________ Monitor for spasm of the client's hand and forearm muscles.

   ________ Observe palmar flexion and adduction of the client's fingers.

   ________ Place a blood pressure cuff around the client's upper arm.

   ________ Remove the blood pressure cuff.

   ________ Report and document the findings.

   ________ Inflate the blood pressure cuff 20 mm Hg higher than the client's systolic blood pressure.

   ________ Hold the inflated blood pressure cuff in place for 1 to 4 minutes.

8. A nurse is teaching the parents of a 3-month-old client who was diagnosed with inherited hypoparathyroidism. Which instruction should the nurse include when teaching the parents how to care for this infant?
   1. Decrease milk and vitamin D intake.
   2. Monitor for constipation, abdominal distention, and flaccidity.
   3. Feed the infant a formula that has a high phosphate-to-calcium ratio.
   4. Monitor for muscle stiffness, nausea, vomiting, and diarrhea.

9. A nurse assesses a client with suspected hypocalcemia. To confirm this suspicion, the nurse attempts to elicit Chvostek's sign. Which actions should the nurse take to assess for this sign? Place each nursing action in the correct sequence (1–5).

   ________ Report and document the findings.
   ________ Tap the client's face just below the zygomatic arch.
   ________ Place a finger just below and in front of the client's ear.
   ________ Monitor twitching of the mouth, nose, or cheek.
   ________ Observe for the appearance of facial twitching on the ipsilateral side.

10. A nurse is instructing an elderly client in calcium supplementation. The nurse notes that, based on the National Institutes of Health chart, the client requires 1,200 mg of elemental calcium per day. How many tablets of the preparation shown in the exhibit should the nurse instruct the client to take daily? Record your answer as a whole number.

    ____

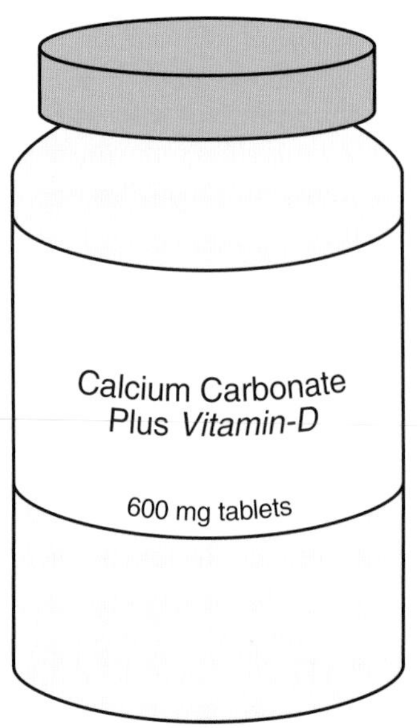

11. A nurse is preparing to administer IV calcium gluconate 10% to a child weighing 45 lb who has acute hypocalcemia. A physician orders 0.7 mEq/kg three times per day. The dose on hand is 0.45 mEq/mL. How many milliliters of this medication should the nurse administer at each dose? Record your answer using one decimal point.

    ____

12. A nurse plans to administer calcium gluconate to an elderly client for the treatment of hypocalcemia. Which routes of administration should the nurse identify as appropriate when giving this medication? **Select all that apply.**
    1. PO route
    2. Subcutaneous route
    3. Intramuscular (IM) route
    4. IV route
    5. Intradermal route
    6. Rectal route

13. A nurse is caring for a client diagnosed with end-stage renal disease. The client reports muscle cramping and tingling of the hands and feet. Suspecting that the client may be experiencing hypocalcemia, the nurse should elicit Chvostek's sign by tapping on which area of the client's face?

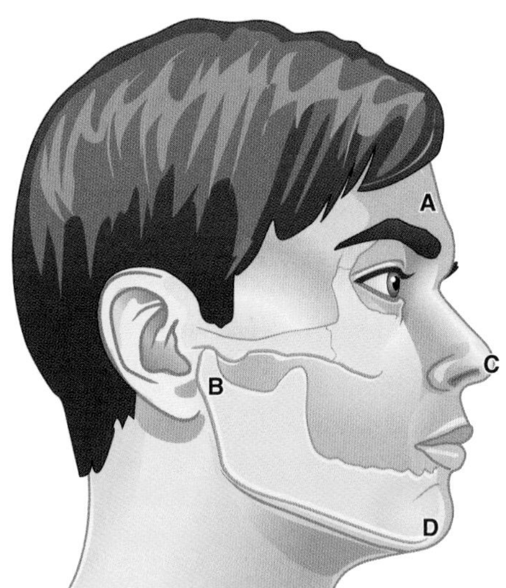

    1. Site A
    2. Site B
    3. Site C
    4. Site D

14. A nurse is infusing IV calcium chloride 10% for a client with a serum calcium level of 6.8 mg/dL. Which nursing intervention should be the nurse's *first* priority when infusing this medication?
    1. Check the patency of the client's IV line every hour.
    2. Monitor the client's blood pressure, pulse, and ECG throughout.
    3. Draw blood to assess the client's serum calcium level.
    4. Monitor the client for signs and symptoms of hypercalcemia.

15. A pregnant client with Graves' disease presents to an obstetrical clinic reporting a "racing heart," recent weight loss, nausea, and constipation. A nurse assesses the client and notes that her heart rate is greater than 100 bpm and that she has a widening pulse pressure and decreased deep tendon reflexes (DTRs). Serum laboratory tests are ordered by the physician. Which serum calcium level should the nurse anticipate?
    1. 7.8 mg/dL
    2. 8.8 mg/dL
    3. 9.8 mg/dL
    4. 10.8 mg/dL

16. A nurse is caring for a hospitalized adolescent client who has been diagnosed with metastatic testicular cancer and has a serum calcium level of 11.2 mg/dL. Which orders should the nurse anticipate for this client? **Select all that apply.**
    1. IV normal (0.9%) saline solution at 125 mL/hr
    2. IV furosemide (Lasix) 40 mg twice daily
    3. Vitamin D 400 IU PO daily
    4. IV plicamycin (Mithracin) 25 mcg/kg daily × 3 days
    5. IV morphine sulfate 20 mg every 4 to 6 hours

17. A school nurse counsels a 16-year-old client about the need for adequate calcium in the diet. According to the National Institutes of Health, how much calcium should the nurse instruct the client to ingest daily?
    1. 500 mg
    2. 800 mg
    3. 1,000 mg
    4. 1,300 mg

18. An emergency department nurse assesses multiple clients for fluid and electrolyte imbalances. Which factors in the medical histories of the clients should the nurse associate with the development of hypercalcemia? **Select all that apply.**
    1. Hypoparathyroidism
    2. Hyperparathyroidism
    3. Hypothyroidism
    4. Hyperthyroidism
    5. Hypophosphatemia
    6. Hyperphosphatemia

19. Which manifestation should a nurse associate with the development of hypocalcemia if it is noted during the assessment of a client who is status post-thyroidectomy?
    1. Tetany
    2. Muscle weakness
    3. Hypoactive bowel sounds
    4. Decreased DTRs

20. Which finding should a nurse report to a health-care provider immediately if it is identified in a client who has received multiple blood transfusions to treat lower gastrointestinal bleeding?
    1. Positive Chvostek's sign
    2. Hemoglobin 10.3 mg/dL
    3. Dark, red stool
    4. Abdominal pain

21. A nurse is developing a plan of care with a client who has a nursing diagnosis of Decreased Cardiac Output Related to Cardiac Dysrhythmias Secondary to Hypocalcemia. Which outcome should receive priority in the plan of care?
    1. Cardiac rhythm will be monitored continuously.
    2. Client will consume adequate dietary calcium.
    3. Client will remain free from injury.
    4. Client will maintain blood pressure within the normal range.

22. A nurse assesses an infant who is brought to a pediatric office. The nurse observes that the infant has rigid muscles, abdominal distention, and brief episodes of apnea that are causing irregular cyanosis. The infant's mother reports that the infant has been extremely irritable for the past several days. Which condition should the nurse suspect?
    1. Hypocalcemia secondary to hyperparathyroidism
    2. Hypocalcemia secondary to hypoparathyroidism
    3. Hypercalcemia secondary to hyperparathyroidism
    4. Hypercalcemia secondary to hypoparathyroidism

23. An elderly client is receiving an IV infusion of calcium gluconate for severe hypocalcemia. Which ECG finding should a nurse expect to see when monitoring this client's rhythm strip?

1.

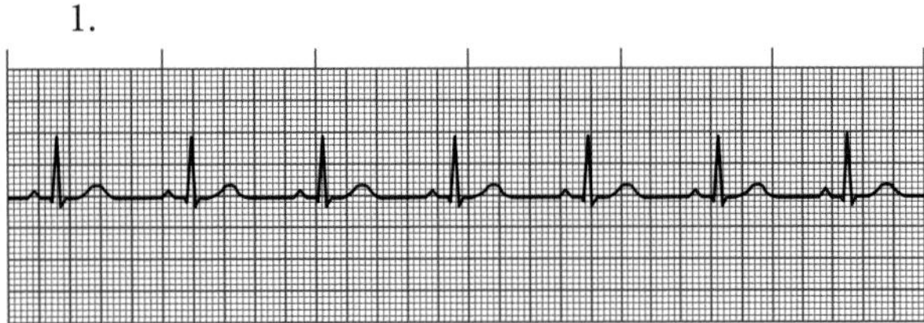

2.

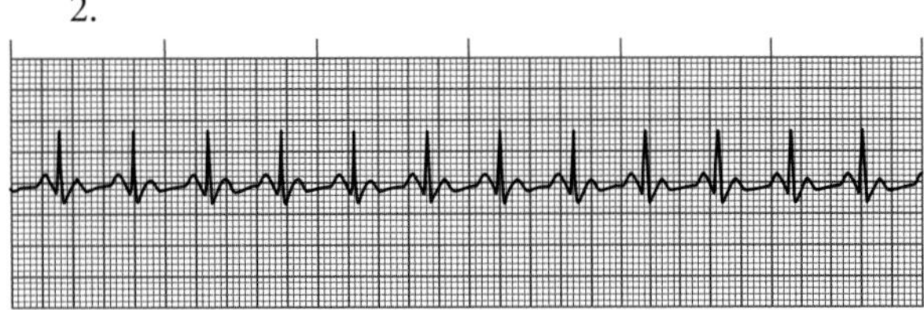

3.

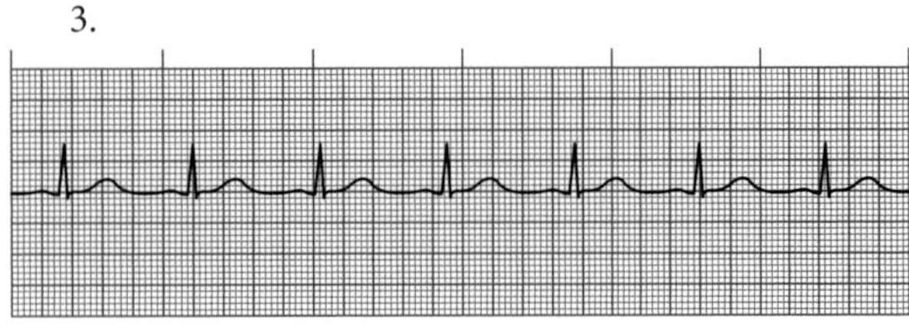

4.

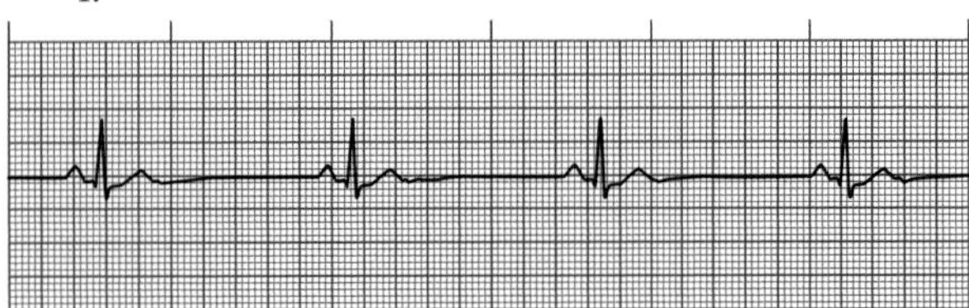

24. A client with chronic kidney disease presents to the emergency department reporting severe muscle weakness, constipation, and abdominal pain. The client is diagnosed with hypercalcemia. Which ECG finding should a nurse identify as indicative of hypercalcemia?

1.

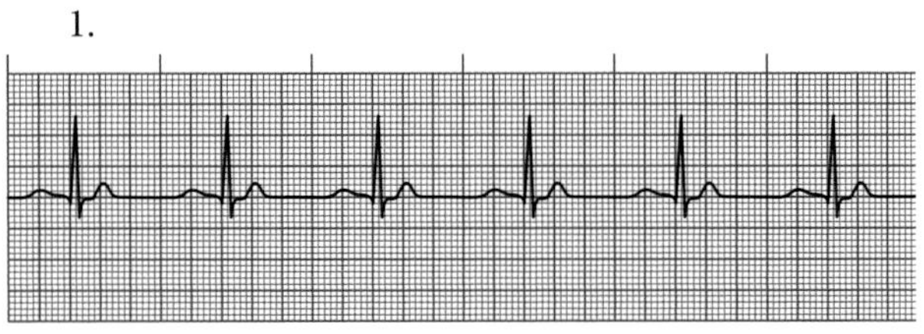

2.

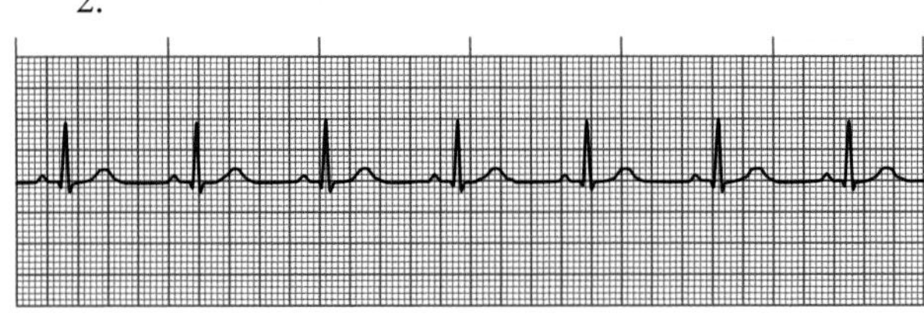

3.

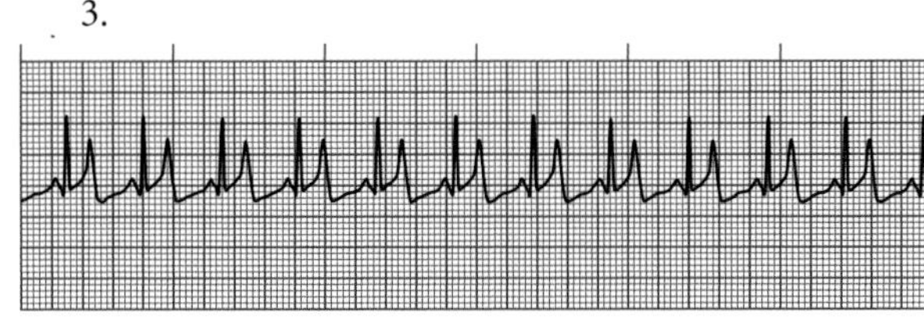

4.

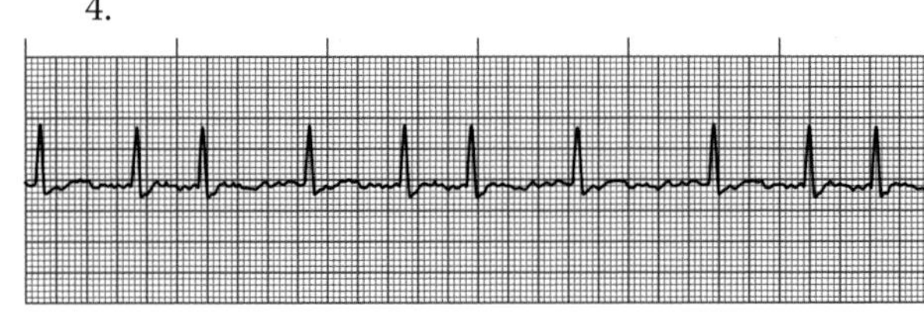

25. A physician writes orders for a client diagnosed with hypocalcemia. Which order should the nurse question?

1. IV calcium chloride 10% 10 mEq × 1
2. Calcium citrate (Citracal) 1,000 mg PO twice daily
3. IM calcium glubionate 10% (Calcionate) 8 mEq × 1
4. Calcium acetate (PhosLo) 1,000 mg PO twice daily

REVIEW ANSWERS

1. ANSWER: 2.

Rationale:

1. Inflating a blood pressure cuff on the upper arm is used to elicit Trousseau's sign, not Chvostek's sign. Trousseau's sign is also a sign of hypocalcemia.

2. The nurse assessing a client for hypocalcemia should elicit Chvostek's sign by tapping the client's facial nerve anterior to the earlobe and just below the zygomatic arch and observing for facial twitching of the mouth, nose, or cheek on the same side as the stimulus. Twitching in response to this stimulus is considered a positive Chvostek's sign and indicates the presence of hypocalcemia. Hypocalcemia increases neuromuscular irritability and results in cells that depolarize more easily and at inappropriate times.

3. Assessing deep tendon reflexes is important in a client with calcium imbalance, but this does not assess for the presence of Chvostek's sign.

4. Instructing the client to hyperventilate and observing for muscle spasms is not an appropriate assessment to conduct on any client.

TEST-TAKING TIP: Know how to elicit both Chvostek's sign and Trousseau's sign for the NCLEX examination.

Content Area: Adult Health

Integrated Processes: Nursing Process: Assessment

Client Need: Physiological Integrity

Cognitive Level: Knowledge

Reference: Ignatavicius, D., and Workman, M. (2012). Medical-Surgical Nursing: Patient-Centered Collaborative Care (7th ed.). St. Louis, MO: Saunders.

2. ANSWER: 4.

Rationale:

1. Tea interferes with calcium absorption and should be limited. Increasing tea consumption would not be an appropriate dietary modification for a postmenopausal client at risk for hypocalcemia.

2. A high-fiber diet may interfere with calcium absorption and would not be an appropriate dietary modification for a postmenopausal client at risk for hypocalcemia.

3. Salt substitutes are high in phosphorus and would not be an appropriate dietary modification for a postmenopausal client at risk for hypocalcemia.

4. The nurse should instruct the postmenopausal client to limit the intake of high-oxalate foods. Foods high in oxalic acid decrease calcium absorption and should be avoided in clients at risk for hypocalcemia. High-oxalate foods include dark or "robust" beer, black tea, chocolate milk, cocoa, instant coffee, hot chocolate, Ovaltine, soy drinks, soy cheese, soy yogurt, nuts, blackberries, blueberries, figs, collards, dandelion greens, eggplant, escarole, kale, leeks, okra, and olives.

TEST-TAKING TIP: Key words are "at risk for hypocalcemia." Select the option that would reduce the client's risk.

Content Area: Older Adult Health

Integrated Processes: Nursing Process: Implementation

Client Need: Health Promotion and Maintenance

Cognitive Level: Application

Reference: Nix, C. (2009). Williams' Basic Nutrition and Diet Therapy (13th ed.). St. Louis, MO: Mosby.

3. ANSWER: 3.

Rationale:

1. Crohn's disease is associated with hypocalcemia, not hypercalcemia.

2. Hypoparathyroidism is associated with hypocalcemia, not hypercalcemia.

3. The nurse should associate metastatic cancer with the development of hypercalcemia because of increased osteoclastic activity in the bone, which causes calcium to be released into the bloodstream and increases serum calcium levels.

4. Lactose intolerance is associated with hypocalcemia, not hypercalcemia.

TEST-TAKING TIP: Consider the pathophysiology of each condition. Recall that metastatic means that the cancer has spread throughout the body. Metastases to the bone would cause it to break down, releasing calcium.

Content Area: Adult Health

Integrated Processes: Nursing Process: Analysis

Client Need: Physiological Integrity

Cognitive Level: Application

Reference: Ignatavicius, D., and Workman, M. (2012). Medical-Surgical Nursing: Patient-Centered Collaborative Care (7th ed.). St. Louis, MO: Saunders.

4. ANSWER: 1, 4, 5.

Rationale:

1. A nurse assessing a client who has hyperparathyroidism should associate impaired blood flow with the development of hypercalcemia, a complication of hyperparathyroidism.

2. A client who has hyperparathyroidism is at risk for the development of hypercalcemia, and a client with hypercalcemia would display hypoactive, not hyperactive, bowel sounds.

3. A client who has hyperparathyroidism is at risk for the development of hypercalcemia, and a client with hypercalcemia would display a shortened, rather than a prolonged, Q-T interval.

4. A nurse assessing a client who has hyperparathyroidism should associate decreased deep tendon reflexes with the development of hypercalcemia, a complication of hyperparathyroidism.

5. A nurse assessing a client who has hyperparathyroidism should associate confusion with the development of hypercalcemia, a complication of hyperparathyroidism.

TEST-TAKING TIP: Recall that hyperparathyroidism results in hypercalcemia, and select options that are signs or symptoms of this imbalance.

Content Area: Adult Health

Integrated Processes: Nursing Process: Assessment

Client Need: Physiological Integrity

Cognitive Level: Application

Reference: Ignatavicius, D., and Workman, M. (2012). Medical-Surgical Nursing: Patient-Centered Collaborative Care (7th ed.). St. Louis, MO: Saunders.

5. ANSWER: 2, 5.

Rationale:

1. Hypocalcemia is most often caused by hypoparathyroidism (a deficiency of PTH) resulting from surgery, not excess PTH. Additional causes of hypocalcemia include acute pancreatitis, hyperphosphatemia, hypomagnesemia, alkalosis, and malabsorption disorders.

2. A nurse obtaining a client's health history should identify vitamin D deficiency as a factor that would contribute to the development of hypocalcemia.
3. Hypocalcemia may be caused by hyperphosphatemia, not hypophosphatemia. Hyperphosphatemia often occurs in clients with acute renal failure.
4. Osteoporosis may occur as a result of chronic hypocalcemia; it is not a cause of hypocalcemia.
5. A nurse obtaining a client's health history should identify acute pancreatitis as a factor that would contribute to the development of hypocalcemia. Additional causes of hypocalcemia include hypoparathyroidism, hyperphosphatemia, hypomagnesemia, alkalosis, and malabsorption disorders.
TEST-TAKING TIP: Read the question carefully. Use the process of elimination to rule out options that are *not* risk factors for hypocalcemia.
Content Area: Adult Health
Integrated Processes: Nursing Process: Analysis
Client Need: Physiological Integrity
Cognitive Level: Application
***Reference:** Lemone, P., and Burke, K. (2010). Medical-Surgical Nursing: Critical Thinking in Client Care (5th ed.). Upper Saddle River, NJ: Pearson Prentice Hall.*

6. ANSWER: 1.
Rationale:
1. A nurse instructing a client who is at risk for hypocalcemia should advise the client to choose the option that provides the most calcium. Nonfat milk (8 oz) and part-skim mozzarella (1.5 oz) provide the most calcium: 632 mg.
2. A nurse instructing a client who is at risk for hypocalcemia should advise the client to choose the option that provides the most calcium. Calcium-fortified orange juice (6 oz) and canned salmon (3 oz) provide 556 mg of calcium—not the option with the most calcium.
3. A nurse instructing a client who is at risk for hypocalcemia should advise the client to choose the option that provides the most calcium. Reduced-fat (2%) milk (8 oz) and white-bread toast (1 oz) provide 366 mg of calcium—not the option with the most calcium.
4. A nurse instructing a client who is at risk for hypocalcemia should advise the client to choose the option that provides the most calcium. Instant breakfast drink (8 oz) and cottage cheese (1 cup) provide 243 to 388 mg of calcium—not the option with the most calcium.
TEST-TAKING TIP: Use the table provided to add the calcium content of each combination of food choices. Select the combination with the highest calcium content.
Content Area: Adult Health
Integrated Processes: Nursing Process: Analysis
Client Need: Physiological Integrity
Cognitive Level: Application
***Reference:** National Institutes of Health. (Reviewed 2012). Dietary supplement fact sheet: calcium. Office of Dietary Supplements. http://ods.od.nih.gov/factsheets/Calcium-HealthProfessional/.*

7. ANSWER: 4, 5, 1, 6, 7, 2, 3.
Rationale:
A nurse assessing for the presence of Trousseau's sign should first place a blood pressure cuff around the client's upper arm and inflate the cuff 20 mm Hg higher than the client's systolic blood pressure. The inflated blood pressure cuff should remain in place for 1 to 4 minutes, while the nurse monitors for spasm of the client's hand and forearm muscles, specifically observing for palmar flexion and adduction of the fingers. Finally, the nurse should remove the blood pressure cuff and report and document the findings.
TEST-TAKING TIP: Review the details of assessing for hypocalcemia using Trousseau's sign. Envision the technique in your mind's eye, placing each action in the correct sequence from first to last.
Content Area: Adult Health
Integrated Processes: Nursing Process: Assessment
Client Need: Health Promotion and Maintenance
Cognitive Level: Application
***Reference:** Ignatavicius, D., and Workman, M. (2012). Medical-Surgical Nursing: Patient-Centered Collaborative Care (7th ed.). St. Louis, MO: Saunders.*

8. ANSWER: 4.
Rationale:
1. Hypoparathyroidism causes decreased serum calcium levels (hypocalcemia). Decreasing the milk and vitamin D intake would worsen hypocalcemia and would not be appropriate instructions for the parents of this infant.
2. Teaching parents to recognize the signs of hypocalcemia is a primary objective in the ongoing management of hypoparathyroidism. Constipation, abdominal distention, and muscle weakness are signs of hypercalcemia, not hypocalcemia.
3. Feeding a formula with a high phosphate-to-calcium ratio is a cause of hypoparathyroidism and would not be appropriate instructions for the parents of this infant.
4. The nurse should teach the parents of an infant diagnosed with hypoparathyroidism to monitor for muscle stiffness, nausea, vomiting, and diarrhea because these signs indicate the development of hypocalcemia. Teaching parents to recognize the signs of hypocalcemia is a primary objective in the ongoing management of hypoparathyroidism. Decreased serum calcium levels occur because there is a lack of parathyroid hormone (PTH), which, along with vitamin D and calcitonin, regulates serum calcium levels.
TEST-TAKING TIP: Recall that hypoparathyroidism results in hypocalcemia. Review the signs of hypocalcemia if you had difficulty answering this question.
Content Area: Child Health
Integrated Processes: Teaching/Learning
Client Need: Physiological Integrity
Cognitive Level: Application
***Reference:** Perry, S., Hockenberry, M., Lowdermilk, D., and Wilson, D. (2010). Maternal Child Nursing Care (4th ed.). St. Louis, MO: Mosby.*

9. ANSWER: 5, 2, 1, 3, 4.
Rationale:
A nurse assessing a client with suspected hypocalcemia should attempt to elicit Chvostek's sign by first placing a finger just below and in front of the client's ear and tapping the client's face just below the zygomatic arch. The nurse should monitor for twitching of the mouth, nose, or cheek and observe for the appearance of facial twitching on the ipsilateral side. Finally, the nurse should report and document the findings.

TEST-TAKING TIP: Envision the procedure in your mind's eye, and select the appropriate actions from first to last.
Content Area: Adult Health
Integrated Processes: Nursing Process: Assessment
Client Need: Physiological Integrity
Cognitive Level: Application
Reference: Ignatavicius, D., and Workman, M. (2012). Medical-Surgical Nursing: Patient-Centered Collaborative Care (7th ed.). St. Louis, MO: Saunders.

10. ANSWER: 2.
Rationale:
The nurse should calculate that a client requiring 1,200 mg of elemental calcium per day would need to take 2 tablets of the preparation shown in the figure. This preparation supplies 600 mg of elemental calcium per tablet: 1,200 mg ÷ 600 mg = 2 tablets per day.
TEST-TAKING TIP: Read the product label when calculating dosages.
Content Area: Adult Health
Integrated Processes: Nursing Process: Implementation
Client Need: Physiological Integrity
Cognitive Level: Application
Reference: National Institutes of Health, Office of Dietary Supplements. (Reviewed 2012). Dietary supplement fact sheet: calcium. http://ods.od.nih.gov/factsheets/Calcium-HealthProfessional/.

11. ANSWER: 31.8.
Rationale:

$$45 \text{ lb} \div 2.2 \text{ lb/kg} = 20.45 \text{ kg}$$

$$20.45 \text{ kg} \times 0.7 \text{ mEq/kg} = 14.3 \text{ mEq}$$

$$14.3 \text{ mEq} \div 0.45 \text{ mEq/mL} = 31.77 \text{ mL} = 31.8 \text{ mL}$$

(rounded to one decimal point) in each dose

TEST-TAKING TIP: Always double-check medication calculations: confusion can occur with milligram doses of calcium gluconate, which are *not* equal to milliequivalent doses.
Content Area: Child Health
Integrated Processes: Nursing Process: Analysis
Client Need: Physiological Integrity
Cognitive Level: Application
Reference: Deglin, J. H., Vallerand, A. H., and Sanoski, C. A. (2013). Davis's Drug Guide for Nurses (13th ed.). Philadelphia, PA: F. A. Davis.

12. ANSWER: 1, 4.
Rationale:
1. The nurse should identify PO as an appropriate route for the administration of calcium gluconate. Calcium is usually administered PO to prevent the development of hypocalcemia and osteoporosis or to treat mild hypocalcemia.
2. The subcutaneous route is an unacceptable method of administering calcium gluconate.
3. The IM route is an unacceptable method of administering calcium gluconate.
4. The nurse should identify the IV route as appropriate for the administration of calcium gluconate. The IV route is used to treat acute hypocalcemia. IV calcium gluconate should be administered with great care because extravasation may cause cellulitis, necrosis, and sloughing.
5. The intradermal route is an unacceptable method of administering calcium gluconate.
6. The rectal route is an unacceptable method of administering calcium gluconate.
TEST-TAKING TIP: Recall that calcium may be administered only by PO and IV routes.
Content Area: Older Adult Health
Integrated Processes: Nursing Process: Planning
Client Need: Physiological Integrity
Cognitive Level: Application
Reference: Deglin, J. H., Vallerand, A. H., and Sanoski, C. A. (2013). Davis's Drug Guide for Nurses (13th ed.). Philadelphia, PA: F. A. Davis.

13. ANSWER: 2.
Rationale:
1. Tapping the client's forehead would not elicit Chvostek's sign.
2. When attempting to elicit Chvostek's sign, the nurse should tap the client's face just in front of and below the ear, below the zygomatic arch, and observe for facial twitching on the same side of the face. A positive Chvostek's sign indicates hypocalcemia.
3. Tapping the tip of the client's nose would not elicit Chvostek's sign.
4. Tapping the client's chin would not elicit Chvostek's sign.
TEST-TAKING TIP: Review the technique for assessing Chvostek's sign if you had difficulty answering this question.
Content Area: Adult Health
Integrated Processes: Nursing Process: Implementation
Client Need: Physiological Integrity
Cognitive Level: Application
Reference: Williams, L., and Hopper, P. (2010). Understanding Medical-Surgical Nursing (4th ed.). Philadelphia, PA: F. A. Davis.

14. ANSWER: 2.
Rationale:
1. Checking the patency of the client's IV line is important when infusing calcium chloride because extravasation may cause cellulitis, necrosis, and sloughing; however, this should not be the nurse's first priority.
2. The nurse's first priority when infusing calcium chloride should be to monitor the client's blood pressure, pulse rate, and ECG rhythm throughout the infusion because IV calcium may cause vasodilation, resulting in hypotension, bradycardia, arrhythmias, and cardiac arrest.
3. Although drawing blood to assess the client's serum calcium level is an appropriate intervention when infusing calcium chloride, it is not the first priority.
4. Although monitoring for signs of hypercalcemia is an appropriate intervention when infusing calcium chloride, it is not the first priority.
TEST-TAKING TIP: Use the "ABCs" when establishing priority. Select the most immediate problem when prioritizing interventions.
Content Area: Adult Health
Integrated Processes: Nursing Process: Implementation
Client Need: Physiological Integrity
Cognitive Level: Application
Reference: Deglin, J. H., Vallerand, A. H., and Sanoski, C. A. (2013). Davis's Drug Guide for Nurses (13th ed.). Philadelphia, PA: F. A. Davis.

15. ANSWER: 4.

Rationale:

1. The nurse should anticipate that a pregnant client with Graves' disease who presents with a "racing heart," recent weight loss, nausea, and constipation; a heart rate greater than 100 bpm; a widening pulse pressure; and decreased DTRs is most likely to have a serum calcium level of 10.8 mg/dL or greater. A serum calcium level of 7.8 mg/dL is below normal limits. The normal reference range for serum calcium is 8.2 to 10.2 mg/dL.

2. The nurse should anticipate that a pregnant client with Graves' disease who presents with a "racing heart," recent weight loss, nausea, and constipation; a heart rate greater than 100 bpm; a widening pulse pressure; and decreased DTRs is most likely to have a serum calcium level of 10.8 mg/dL or greater. A serum calcium level of 8.8 mg/dL is within normal limits. The normal reference range for serum calcium is 8.2 to 10.2 mg/dL.

3. The nurse should anticipate that a pregnant client with Graves' disease who presents with a "racing heart," recent weight loss, nausea, and constipation; a heart rate greater than 100 bpm; a widening pulse pressure; and decreased DTRs is most likely to have a serum calcium level of 10.8 mg/dL or greater. A serum calcium level of 9.8 mg/dL is within normal limits. The normal reference range for serum calcium is 8.2 to 10.2 mg/dL.

4. The nurse should anticipate that a pregnant client with Graves' disease who presents with a "racing heart," recent weight loss, nausea, and constipation; a heart rate greater than 100 bpm; a widening pulse pressure; and decreased DTRs is most likely to have a serum calcium level of 10.8 mg/dL or greater. Clients with hyperthyroidism (Graves' disease) are at increased risk for developing hypercalcemia, especially during pregnancy. A racing heart, nausea, constipation, tachycardia, a widening pulse pressure, and decreased DTRs are manifestations of hypercalcemia. The normal reference range for serum calcium is 8.2 to 10.2 mg/dL.

TEST-TAKING TIP: Recall that hyperthyroidism (Graves' disease) may cause elevated serum calcium levels.

Content Area: Maternal Health

Integrated Processes: Nursing Process: Evaluation

Client Need: Physiological Integrity

Cognitive Level: Application

Reference: *Ward, S. L., and Hisley, S. M. (2011). Maternal-Child Nursing Care: Optimizing Outcomes for Mothers, Children and Families. Philadelphia, PA: F. A. Davis.*

16. ANSWER: 1, 2, 4.

Rationale:

1. The nurse caring for a hospitalized adolescent client with metastatic testicular cancer and a serum calcium level of 11.2 mg/dL should anticipate orders for IV normal saline and IV furosemide to increase the kidneys' excretion of calcium.

2. The nurse caring for a hospitalized adolescent client with metastatic testicular cancer and a serum calcium level of 11.2 mg/dL should anticipate orders for IV normal saline and IV furosemide to increase the kidneys' excretion of calcium.

3. Vitamin D is contraindicated for a client with a serum calcium level of 11.2 mg/dL because it would increase the serum calcium level.

4. The nurse caring for a hospitalized adolescent client with metastatic testicular cancer and a serum calcium level of 11.2 mg/dL should anticipate orders for plicamycin, a calcium-binding agent, to reduce the client's serum calcium level.

5. Morphine sulfate may be appropriate for this hospitalized adolescent client with metastatic testicular cancer and a serum calcium level of 11.2 mg/dL; however, the dosage is too high. The average dose of IV morphine sulfate is 4 to 10 mg every 3 to 4 hours.

TEST-TAKING TIP: Recognize that a serum calcium level greater than 10.5 mg/dL indicates hypercalcemia. Select the options that would decrease the serum calcium level.

Content Area: Child Health

Integrated Processes: Nursing Process: Analysis

Client Need: Physiological Integrity

Cognitive Level: Application

Reference: *Deglin, J. H., Vallerand, A. H., and Sanoski, C. A. (2013). Davis's Drug Guide for Nurses (13th ed.). Philadelphia, PA: F. A. Davis.; Ignatavicius, D., and Workman, M. (2012). Medical-Surgical Nursing: Patient-Centered Collaborative Care (7th ed.). St. Louis, MO: Saunders.*

17. ANSWER: 4.

Rationale:

1. Toddlers, 1 to 3 years old, need approximately 700 mg of calcium per day.

2. School-age children, 4 to 8 years old, need approximately 1,000 mg of calcium per day.

3. Adults, 19 to 50 years old, need 1,000 mg of calcium per day.

4. According to the recommendations of the National Institutes of Health, the nurse should instruct the 16-year-old client to ingest 1,300 mg of calcium per day.

TEST-TAKING TIP: Refer to Table 5.5 if you had difficulty answering this question.

Content Area: Child Health

Integrated Processes: Teaching/Learning

Client Need: Physiological Integrity

Cognitive Level: Application

Reference: *National Institutes of Health, Office of Dietary Supplements. (Reviewed 2012). Dietary supplement fact sheet: calcium. http://ods.od.nih.gov/factsheets/Calcium-HealthProfessional/.*

18. ANSWER: 2, 4, 5.

Rationale:

1. *Hypo*parathyroidism is associated with hypocalcemia, not hypercalcemia.

2. The nurse should associate the development of hypercalcemia with *hyper*parathyroidism. Hyperparathyroidism causes elevated serum calcium levels because PTH releases free calcium from bone storage sites and decreases the kidneys' excretion of calcium.

3. *Hypo*thyroidism is associated with hypocalcemia, not hypercalcemia.

4. The nurse should associate the development of hypercalcemia with *hyper*thyroidism. Hyperthyroidism causes elevated serum calcium levels because excess circulating thyroid hormone stimulates bone resorption and bone demineralization, resulting in hypercalcemia.

5. The nurse should associate the development of hypercalcemia with *hypo*phosphatemia. Hypophosphatemia causes hypercalcemia because a decrease in serum phosphorus levels results in an increase in serum calcium levels (an inverse relationship).
6. *Hyper*phosphatemia is associated with hypocalcemia, not hypercalcemia.
TEST-TAKING TIP: Recall that *resorption* is the process by which osteoclasts break down bone and release minerals into the bloodstream. In contrast, *reabsorption* is the process of "absorbing again," such as occurs in the kidneys when some materials filtered out of the blood by the glomerulus are reabsorbed as the filtrate passes through the nephron.
Content Area: Adult Health
Integrated Processes: Nursing Process: Analysis
Client Need: Physiological Integrity
Cognitive Level: Application
***Reference:** Ignatavicius, D., and Workman, M. (2012). Medical-Surgical Nursing: Patient-Centered Collaborative Care (7th ed.). St. Louis, MO: Saunders.*

19. ANSWER: 1.
Rationale:
1. The nurse should associate tetany with the development of hypocalcemia. Tetany is a combination of signs and symptoms caused by low ionic calcium in the extracellular fluid (between cells) and intracellular fluid (within cells). Tetany is characterized by sensory symptoms consisting of paresthesias (odd feelings) of the lips, tongue, fingers, and feet; generalized muscle pain; and spasms of the facial musculature.
2. Muscle weakness is a sign of hypercalcemia, not hypocalcemia.
3. Hypoactive bowel sounds are a sign of hypercalcemia, not hypocalcemia.
4. Decreased DTRs are a sign of hypercalcemia, not hypocalcemia.
TEST-TAKING TIP: Recall that calcium is an excitable membrane stabilizer. Lack of calcium allows depolarization to occur more easily, which increases the excitability of the cell membrane and results in physical manifestations such as tetany.
Content Area: Adult Health
Integrated Processes: Nursing Process: Assessment
Client Need: Physiological Integrity
Cognitive Level: Analysis
***Reference:** Ignatavicius, D., and Workman, M. (2012). Medical-Surgical Nursing: Patient-Centered Collaborative Care (7th ed.). St. Louis, MO: Saunders.*

20. ANSWER: 1.
Rationale:
1. The nurse should immediately report a positive Chvostek's sign to the health-care provider because this is an indication of hypocalcemia. Multiple transfusions pose a risk for hypocalcemia because citrate, a preservative used in units of blood, combines with and reduces serum calcium.
2. A hemoglobin of 10.3 mg/dL would not need to be reported immediately to the health-care provider if identified in a client who has received multiple blood transfusions to treat lower gastrointestinal bleeding. A decreased hemoglobin level is an expected manifestation of lower gastrointestinal bleeding.
3. Dark, red stool would not need to be reported immediately to the health-care provider if identified in a client who has received multiple blood transfusions to treat lower gastrointestinal bleeding. Dark, red stool is an expected manifestation of lower gastrointestinal bleeding.
4. Abdominal pain would not need to be reported immediately to the health-care provider if identified in a client who has received multiple blood transfusions to treat lower gastrointestinal bleeding. Abdominal pain is an expected manifestation of lower gastrointestinal bleeding.
TEST-TAKING TIP: Select the finding that would be least expected and most life threatening.
Content Area: Adult Health
Integrated Processes: Nursing Process: Analysis
Client Need: Physiological Integrity
Cognitive Level: Analysis
***Reference:** Ignatavicius, D., and Workman, M. (2012). Medical-Surgical Nursing: Patient-Centered Collaborative Care (7th ed.). St. Louis, MO: Saunders.*

21. ANSWER: 4.
Rationale:
1. "Monitoring cardiac rhythm" is an intervention, not an outcome.
2. "Consuming adequate dietary calcium" is an outcome for the nursing diagnosis Imbalanced Nutrition, not Decreased Cardiac Output Related to Cardiac Dysrhythmias Secondary to Hypocalcemia.
3. "Remaining free from injury" is an outcome for the nursing diagnosis Risk for Injury, not Decreased Cardiac Output Related to Cardiac Dysrhythmias Secondary to Hypocalcemia.
4. Maintaining blood pressure within the normal range should be the nurse's priority outcome in the plan of care for a client with a nursing diagnosis of Decreased Cardiac Output Related to Cardiac Dysrhythmias Secondary to Hypocalcemia. An appropriate outcome for decreased cardiac output relates to goals that establish hemodynamic stability, such as maintaining blood pressure within the normal range.
TEST-TAKING TIP: Key words are "Decreased Cardiac Output." Select the option that is related to cardiac output.
Content Area: Adult Health
Integrated Processes: Nursing Process: Planning
Client Need: Safe and Effective Care Environment
Cognitive Level: Analysis
***Reference:** Ignatavicius, D., and Workman, M. (2012). Medical-Surgical Nursing: Patient-Centered Collaborative Care (7th ed.). St. Louis, MO: Saunders.*

22. ANSWER: 2.
Rationale:
1. Hyperparathyroidism is associated with hypercalcemia, not hypocalcemia.
2. The nurse should suspect that the infant is experiencing hypocalcemia secondary to hypoparathyroidism. Hypoparathyroidism (deficiency of PTH) results in a decrease in the serum calcium level (hypocalcemia). Low calcium levels increase cell membrane irritability, caus-

ing the infant to exhibit muscular rigidity, abdominal distention (possibly with vomiting), brief periods of apnea and cyanosis, and irritability.
3. Muscular rigidity, abdominal distention (possibly with vomiting), brief periods of apnea and cyanosis, and irritability are signs of hypocalcemia, not hypercalcemia.
4. Muscular rigidity, abdominal distention (possibly with vomiting), brief periods of apnea and cyanosis, and irritability are signs of hypocalcemia, not hypercalcemia. Hypoparathyroidism is associated with hypocalcemia, not hypercalcemia.
TEST-TAKING TIP: When thinking about calcium imbalances, think opposites. *Decreased* calcium levels cause an *increase* in bowel motility (diarrhea), muscle spasms, twitching, hyperreflexia, and irritability. *Increased* calcium levels cause a *decrease* in bowel motility (constipation), severe muscle weakness, and fatigue.
Content Area: Child Health
Integrated Processes: Nursing Process: Analysis
Client Need: Physiological Integrity
Cognitive Level: Analysis
Reference: *Ward, S. L., and Hisley, S. M. (2011). Maternal-Child Nursing Care: Optimizing Outcomes for Mothers, Children and Families. Philadelphia, PA: F. A. Davis.*

23. ANSWER: 3.
Rationale:
1. ECG strip 1 shows normal sinus rhythm, which does not indicate any electrolyte abnormality.
2. ECG strip 2 shows sinus tachycardia (heart rate greater than 100 bpm), which does not indicate any calcium abnormality.
3. The nurse should identify ECG strip 3 as indicative of hypocalcemia because it shows a normal sinus rhythm with prolonged Q-T intervals, a classic ECG change associated with serum calcium levels less than 8.2 mg/dL.
4. ECG strip 4 shows sinus bradycardia (heart rate less than 60 bpm), which does not indicate any calcium abnormality.
TEST-TAKING TIP: Review the effects of hypocalcemia on the electrical conduction of the heart, and choose the answer that reflects those effects.
Content Area: Adult Health
Integrated Processes: Nursing Process: Evaluation
Client Need: Physiological Integrity
Cognitive Level: Analysis
References: *Ignatavicius, D., and Workman, M. (2012). Medical-Surgical Nursing: Patient-Centered Collaborative Care (7th ed.). St. Louis, MO: Saunders; Jones, S. (2010). ECG Notes: Interpretation and Management Guide (2nd ed.). Philadelphia, PA: F. A. Davis.*

24. ANSWER: 1.
Rationale:
1. The nurse should identify ECG strip 1 as indicative of hypercalcemia because it shows shortened Q-T intervals, a classic ECG change associated with serum calcium levels greater than 10.5 mg/dL.
2. ECG strip 2 shows a normal sinus rhythm, which does not indicate any electrolyte abnormality.
3. ECG strip 3 shows the peaked T waves associated with hyperkalemia, not a calcium imbalance.
4. ECG strip 4 shows atrial fibrillation, which is not related to electrolyte imbalance.
TEST-TAKING TIP: Review the effects of hypercalcemia on the electrical conduction of the heart, and choose the answer that illustrates those effects.
Content Area: Adult Health
Integrated Processes: Nursing Process: Evaluation
Client Need: Physiological Integrity
Cognitive Level: Analysis
Reference: *Ignatavicius, D., and Workman, M. (2012). Medical-Surgical Nursing: Patient-Centered Collaborative Care (7th ed.). St. Louis, MO: Saunders; Jones, S. (2010). ECG Notes: Interpretation and Management Guide (2nd ed.). Philadelphia, PA: F. A. Davis.*

25. ANSWER: 3.
Rationale:
1. The order for IV calcium chloride 10% 10 mEq × 1 is appropriate in both dosage and route for a client diagnosed with hypocalcemia.
2. The order for calcium citrate (Citracal) 1,000 mg PO twice daily is appropriate in both dosage and route for a client diagnosed with hypocalcemia.
3. The nurse should question the order for IM calcium glubionate (Calcionate). No calcium-containing solution should be given intramuscularly because the IM administration of calcium salts can cause severe necrosis and tissue sloughing.
4. The order for calcium acetate (PhosLo) 1,000 mg PO twice daily is appropriate in both dosage and route for a client diagnosed with hypocalcemia.
TEST-TAKING TIP: Recall that calcium should *never* be given by the IM route.
Content Area: Adult Health
Integrated Processes: Nursing Process: Analysis
Client Need: Physiological Integrity
Cognitive Level: Analysis
Reference: *Deglin, J. H., Vallerand, A. H., and Sanoski, C. A. (2013). Davis's Drug Guide for Nurses (13th ed.). Philadelphia, PA: F. A. Davis.*

Chapter 6

Magnesium Imbalances

KEY TERMS

Hypermagnesemia—Serum magnesium greater than 2.6 mg/dL; magnesium excess

Hypomagnesemia—Serum magnesium less than 1.6 mg/dL; magnesium deficit

Iatrogenic—Due to the action of a physician or a therapy prescribed by a physician.

Magnesium deficiency—Deficit of magnesium in the bones.

Nystagmus—Rapid, repetitious, rhythmic involuntary eye movements; can be horizontal, vertical, or rotary.

Torsades de pointes ("twisting of the points")—A type of ventricular tachycardia with a spiral-like appearance and complexes that look first positive and then negative on an electrocardiogram (ECG), precipitated by a long Q-T interval; indicative of hypomagnesemia.

I. Description

Magnesium (Mg^{2+}) is the second most abundant cation in the body and is required for muscle relaxation after contraction and for more than 300 biochemical reactions in the body. Approximately 50% to 65% of total body magnesium is found in bone, with the remainder found in the intracellular fluid (ICF) and in the intravascular system (approximately 1%). Because magnesium is stored primarily in the bones, measuring the blood level of magnesium is not adequate to establish the total amount of available magnesium. The primary source of magnesium is through the diet; the recommended daily intake for adults is 320 to 420 mg/day. Magnesium is plentiful in leafy green vegetables, grains, nuts, dried fruits, legumes, dairy products, meats, and seafood. It is absorbed in the ileum and excreted in stool and urine. The kidneys act as the main regulator of serum magnesium concentrations. It should be noted that urine magnesium levels reflect hypomagnesemia before serum levels do. Severe magnesium deficiency can result in low levels of calcium, potassium, and phosphate in the blood. Magnesium performs the following functions:

1. Maintains normal muscle function, nerve function, and heart rhythm
2. Supports a healthy immune system and aids in the regulation of blood coagulation
3. Powers the sodium-potassium pump and aids in converting adenosine triphosphate (ATP) to adenosine diphosphate (ADP) for energy release
4. Acts synergistically with calcium in hundreds of reactions in the body
5. Is required for calcium and vitamin B_{12} absorption
6. Stimulates parathyroid hormone (PTH) secretion, which regulates ICF calcium levels, and fights tooth decay by binding calcium to tooth enamel
7. Has a sedative effect on the neuromuscular junction, which decreases acetylcholine release, causing smooth muscle relaxation

Normal Lab Value The normal serum magnesium level is 1.6 to 2.6 mg/dL (1.32 to 2.14 mEq/L).

II. Types of Magnesium Imbalance

A. **Hypomagnesemia**, or magnesium deficit, is defined as a serum magnesium level less than 1.6 mg/dL (1.32 mEq/L).
   1. Hypomagnesemia is usually indicative of a systemic magnesium deficit.
   2. Magnesium deficiency, which is defined as low levels of magnesium in the bones, can exist even when serum magnesium levels are within normal limits.
   3. Hypomagnesemia can be present without an actual magnesium deficiency, and vice versa.
   4. Pregnant women may be magnesium depleted, especially those with preterm labor.
   5. Signs and symptoms are similar to those of hypocalcemia and hypokalemia because magnesium, calcium, and potassium are all cations.

6. Positive Chvostek's sign and Trousseau's sign can occur, associated with the related decrease in serum calcium levels.
7. Hypomagnesemia can cause the heart muscle to spasm and the heart to stop beating if there is not enough magnesium to relax the heart between contractions.

DID YOU KNOW?

Chronic alcoholism is the most common cause of hypomagnesemia.

B. **Hypermagnesemia**, or magnesium excess, is a serum magnesium level greater than 2.6 mg/dL (2.14 mEq/L).
   1. This relatively rare but potentially lethal electrolyte abnormality is found primarily in clients with renal impairment, because normal kidneys are able to eliminate excess magnesium by rapidly reducing tubular reabsorption.
   2. Hypermagnesemia is usually asymptomatic.

DID YOU KNOW?

Magnesium supplementation is the most frequent cause of magnesium excess.

A critical serum magnesium level less than 1.2 mg/dL or greater than 4.9 mg/dL can cause serious ECG changes and cardiac arrest.

III. Causes of Magnesium Imbalance

Magnesium imbalances may be caused by actual or relative increases or decreases in magnesium. An *actual* increase or decrease occurs as a direct result of magnesium gain or loss. A *relative* increase or decrease occurs when magnesium shifts back and forth between the intracellular and extracellular compartments. A relative increase in magnesium may also occur when the blood is concentrated (hemoconcentration) secondary to fluid volume deficit.

A. Actual hypomagnesemia may be caused by direct loss, inadequate intake, impaired absorption, or increased excretion of magnesium, resulting in *actual decreases* in serum magnesium (Table 6.1).
   1. Magnesium loss
      a. Diarrhea, draining intestinal fistulas, ileostomy (removal of the ileum), and prolonged gastric suctioning result in the direct loss of magnesium ions from the body.
      b. Excessive diaphoresis (profuse sweating) also results in direct magnesium loss.
      c. Diabetes causes osmotic diuresis, resulting in magnesium loss via increased renal excretion.
   2. Inadequate magnesium intake or impaired absorption
      a. Chronic lack of magnesium may be due to a diet low in fruits and vegetables; only about 50% of dietary magnesium is absorbed.

Table 6.1 Causes of Magnesium Imbalance

Imbalance	Causes
Hypomagnesemia	

Actual decrease in magnesium	Magnesium loss
	• Prolonged gastric suctioning
	• Diarrhea
	• Steatorrhea (presence of excess fat in feces)
	• Crohn's disease
	• Excessive diaphoresis
	• Massive burns
	• Medications (those that act on the kidneys to increase magnesium excretion)
	  • Aminoglycoside antibiotics such as tobramycin sulfate
	  • Antifungals such as amphotericin B (Amphotec)
	  • Antineoplastics such as cisplatin (Platinol)
	  • Immunosuppressants such as cyclosporine (Sandimmune)
	  • Loop diuretics such as furosemide (Lasix)
	  • Thiazide diuretics such as chlorothiazide (Diuril)
	• Rapid administration of citrated blood
	• Ethanol ingestion
	• Chronic kidney disease
	Inadequate intake or impaired absorption or excretion
	• Chronic alcoholism
	• Prolonged NPO status
	• Malnutrition
	• Celiac disease/sprue
	• Diabetic ketoacidosis
	  • Hyperglycemia causes osmotic diuresis and polyuria, which increases the excretion of magnesium in urine

Table 6.1 Causes of Magnesium Imbalance—cont'd

Imbalance	Causes
Hypomagnesemia	
Relative decrease in magnesium	Intracellular or extracellular shifts • Correction of acidosis • Acute pancreatitis • Massive burns • Hungry bone syndrome
Hypermagnesemia	

Actual increase in magnesium	Excessive magnesium intake
	• Ingestion of magnesium-containing antacids, vitamins, and laxatives
	• Excessive IV magnesium replacement during treatment for
	  • Preeclampsia or eclampsia
	  • Asthma
	  • Torsades de pointes or other cardiac dysrhythmias
	• Neonates at risk after maternal treatment with magnesium
	• Frequently iatrogenic
	Increased gastrointestinal absorption of magnesium
	• Hypomotility caused by
	  • Diabetic gastroparesis
	  • Postoperative status (anesthesia)
	  • Paralytic ileus
	  • Bowel obstruction
	  • Chronic constipation
	• Medications (those that induce hypomotility)
	-anticholinergics such as tolterodine (Detrol, Detrol LA)
	-narcotics such as morphine sulfate
	Magnesium retention or inability to excrete magnesium
	• Chronic kidney disease
	• Acute renal failure
	(!) Older adult clients are at increased risk for hypermagnesemia because of decreased renal function and increased use of over-the-counter laxatives and medications that contain magnesium

Relative increase in magnesium	Magnesium excess secondary to hemoconcentration
	• Intracellular-extracellular shifts
	  • Tumor lysis syndrome
	  • Rhabdomyolysis
	  • Hypoparathyroidism
	  • Hypothyroidism

b. Starvation and eating disorders, such as anorexia and bulimia, may lead to inadequate magnesium intake.

c. Decreased absorption of magnesium may be caused by gastrointestinal disorders such as inflammatory bowel disease, Crohn's disease, and chronic pancreatitis.

d. Magnesium absorption is also decreased when vitamin D and PTH levels are low (similar to calcium).

e. Certain medications, such as aminoglycoside antibiotics, antifungals, and proton pump inhibitors, may interfere with magnesium absorption in some individuals.

3. Increased excretion of magnesium

a. Alcohol dependence is a common cause of hypomagnesemia; alcohol acts as a magnesium diuretic, causing an increase in the urinary excretion of magnesium as well as other electrolytes. Chronic intake of alcohol causes the body stores of magnesium to become depleted.

b. Diuretics, such as furosemide (Lasix), cause increased renal excretion of water, sodium, potassium, and magnesium.

c. Loop and thiazide diuretics cause an increase in phosphate excretion as they act on the kidneys to increase urine output.

B. Relative hypomagnesemia may occur when magnesium shifts *into* the intracellular compartment.

1. Water gain

a. Excessive intake of water (water intoxication) causes the magnesium concentration in the blood to become diluted.

b. Excessive administration of IV solutions without magnesium supplementation may cause serum magnesium levels to become diluted, resulting in hypomagnesemia; lactated Ringer's solution contains numerous electrolytes but does not contain magnesium.
2. Shifts between intracellular and extracellular compartments
 a. Hungry bone syndrome occurs when magnesium is removed from the extracellular fluid (ECF) compartment and deposited in bone following parathyroidectomy or total thyroidectomy, resulting in decreased serum magnesium levels.
 b. Refeeding syndrome may occur when a severely malnourished client receives nourishment; serum insulin levels increase, causing potassium, magnesium, and phosphate to move into the cells. Cardiac dysrhythmias, heart failure, acute respiratory failure, paralysis, coma, and liver dysfunction may result.
 c. With insulin therapy for diabetic ketoacidosis, the anabolic effects of insulin can cause magnesium, potassium, and phosphorus to shift back into cells (see Table 6.1).

DID YOU KNOW?

Hypokalemia (low serum potassium) is common in clients with hypomagnesemia, occurring in 40% to 60% of cases.

C. Actual hypermagnesemia may be caused iatrogenically or by excessive magnesium intake, increased absorption of magnesium, magnesium retention, or inability of the kidneys to excrete magnesium, resulting in an *actual increase* in serum magnesium levels.

Hypermagnesemia usually results from a combination of excess magnesium intake and impairment of renal function (see Table 6.1).

1. Magnesium gain
 a. Excessive oral or IV administration of magnesium increase serum magnesium levels.
 b. Oral ingestion of magnesium-containing antacids, vitamins, and laxatives and the use of epsom salt enemas may result in an actual magnesium gain.
 c. Therapeutically induced hypermagnesemia, achieved by administering excessive IV magnesium, is used to treat severe asthma, to correct torsades de pointes or other dysrhythmias, and to prevent seizure activity in pregnant women with pre-eclampsia.
2. Increased absorption of magnesium in the intestines
 a. Anesthesia decreases bowel motility, allowing excess magnesium to be absorbed in the intestines.
 b. Diabetic gastroparesis, chronic constipation, bowel obstruction, and paralytic ileus also cause a decrease in bowel motility. Paralytic ileus is obstruction of the intestine due to paralysis of the intestinal muscles; this commonly occurs following some types of surgery, especially abdominal surgery; from the administration of certain drugs; following spinal injuries; or in the presence of inflammation in the abdomen.
 c. Certain medications, such as anticholinergics and narcotics, increase magnesium levels by inducing bowel hypomotility.

MAKING THE CONNECTION

Total Parenteral Nutrition and Magnesium Imbalance

Total parenteral nutrition (TPN) is a method of providing the body with nutrients while bypassing the digestive system. The nutrient solution is dripped directly into a vein, usually via a central catheter. TPN is used when the intestines are obstructed, when the small intestine is not absorbing nutrients properly, or when the bowels need to rest. Most TPN solutions do not contain magnesium, so the nurse should closely monitor a client receiving TPN for signs and symptoms of hypomagnesemia, such as mood changes, muscle twitching, tachycardia, and dysrhythmias. The addition of 4 to 12 mmol of magnesium per day to TPN is recommended to prevent hypomagnesemia.

MAKING THE CONNECTION

Eclampsia and Magnesium

Eclampsia is the most serious complication of pregnancy-induced hypertension and preeclampsia. It is characterized by grand mal seizures, coma, hypertension, proteinuria, and edema. Eclampsia most often occurs during or after the 20th week of gestation or in the postpartum period, with 80% of eclamptic seizures occurring in the intrapartum period or within 48 hours of delivery. Although delivery of the infant is the only definitive treatment for eclampsia, IV magnesium sulfate is administered to terminate seizures, lower the blood pressure, and increase perfusion to the organs, especially the kidneys. Thus, hypermagnesemia is deliberately induced to prevent seizure activity. Extreme caution must be used when administering magnesium. Magnesium toxicity can cause coma and death.

3. Inadequate excretion of magnesium
    a. Acute renal failure and chronic kidney disease render the kidneys unable to excrete magnesium adequately.

DID YOU KNOW?
The most common cause of hypermagnesemia is renal failure.

D. Relative hypermagnesemia occurs when magnesium shifts out of the cells and *into* the extracellular compartment.
    1. Water loss
        a. Dehydration produced by diabetic ketoacidosis causes relative hypermagnesemia secondary to hemoconcentration until insulin is administered, which results in hypomagnesemia.
    2. Shifts between intracellular and extracellular compartments
        a. Soft tissue damage resulting from tumor lysis, rhabdomyolysis, sepsis, severe burns, and myocardial infarction can cause large amounts of magnesium, phosphorus, and potassium to rapidly shift out of the ICF and into the ECF; this is especially dangerous in clients with renal failure because the kidneys are unable to excrete these excess electrolytes.
        b. Hypothyroidism is associated with elevated magnesium and calcium levels.
        c. Hypoparathyroidism may be caused by low serum magnesium levels; magnesium is required for PTH secretion.

DID YOU KNOW?
Symptom-producing hypermagnesemia is uncommon. It occurs most often in clients with renal failure after the ingestion of magnesium-containing drugs.

IV. Nursing Assessment for Magnesium Imbalance

The nurse should conduct a focused nursing assessment for magnesium imbalance, beginning with a thorough nursing history. Interview the client and family members to identify any risk factors or preexisting conditions that would contribute to magnesium imbalance, such as vomiting, nasogastric suctioning, diarrhea, acute kidney injury, chronic kidney disease, or other conditions associated with magnesium loss or gain. The nurse should also assess the client's ability to drink and tolerate oral fluids. Include a current dietary history, inquiring about dietary habits. The nursing history should include lifestyle factors, such as long-standing alcohol use and chronic malnutrition, and current medications, including excessive antacids or the use of glucocorticoids or chemotherapeutic agents. A thorough physical assessment is necessary. Specifically, the client should be asked about recent muscle cramps (Fig. 6.1). Assess each body system, observing for signs and symptoms of magnesium imbalance as well as related calcium imbalances. Measure and record the client's vital signs, and review the client's laboratory data to assess for the presence of hypo- or hypermagnesemia (Table 6.2).

V. Nursing Interventions for Clients with Magnesium Imbalance

A. Identify high-risk clients.
    1. Clients with chronic alcoholism
    2. Clients with gastrointestinal disorders or malabsorption syndromes
    3. Clients with diabetes
    4. Clients taking medications, such as diuretics, that increase urine excretion
B. Implement the health-care provider's orders to treat the underlying cause of the imbalance.
    1. The health-care provider's orders may include oral or IV fluid administration, oral or IV magnesium administration, and medication administration.
C. Monitor the client and the client's serum magnesium levels.
    1. Monitor the client's serum magnesium level as ordered by the health-care provider (Table 6.3).
        a. Normal reference range for serum magnesium is 1.6 to 2.6 mg/dL.
        b. Observe for rebound hypermagnesemia when administering IV magnesium.
    2. Monitor other laboratory values associated with magnesium imbalance.
        a. Serum potassium: normal reference range is 3.5 to 5.0 mEq/L.

Normal Muscle Cell

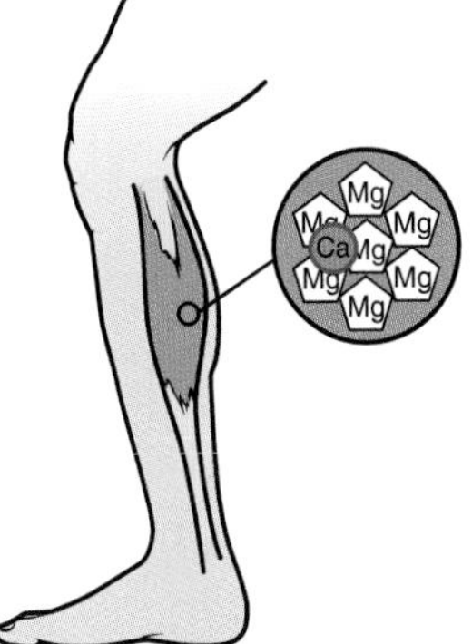

A normal muscle cell has 10,000 times as much magnesium inside the cell than the amount of calcium.

Cramping Muscle Cell

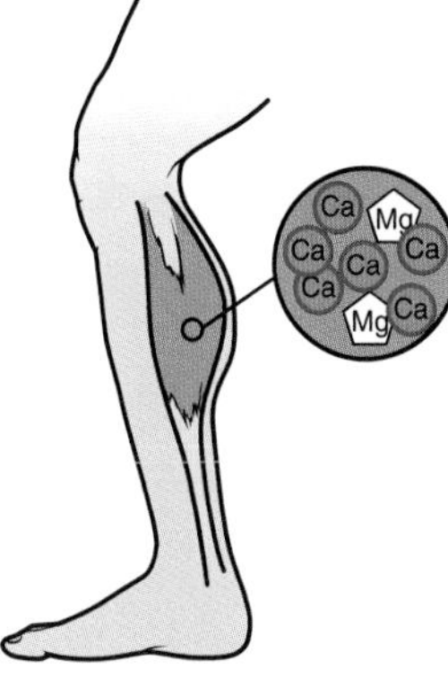

A cramping muscle cell is low on magnesium, thus allowing too much calcium inside, which produces muscle contractions.

Fig 6.1 Why muscles cramp.

Table 6.2 Signs and Symptoms of Magnesium Imbalance

Vital Signs		
	Hypomagnesemia	*Hypermagnesemia*
Blood pressure	Elevated	Decreased
Heart rate	Increased	Decreased
Respiratory rate	Decreased	Decreased; severe hypermagnesemia may result in respiratory arrest
Temperature	Within normal limits	Within normal limits
Signs and Symptoms by Body System		
	Hypomagnesemia	*Hypermagnesemia*
Cardiovascular	• Elevated blood pressure • Tachycardia (!) Causes life-threatening cardiac dysrhythmias • Torsades de pointes • Premature ventricular contractions (PVCs) • Ventricular tachycardia • Ventricular fibrillation • Cardiac arrest	• Hypotension (!) Causes life-threatening cardiac dysrhythmias • Complete heart block • Bradycardia • Asystole • Cardiac arrest
Cerebral	• Disorientation, confusion • Mood changes (apathy, depression, agitation) • Vertigo	(!) Central nervous system depression increases as the magnesium level increases • Lethargy, drowsiness, sleepiness • Lightheadedness • Hallucinations • Decreased level of consciousness to coma
ECG changes	• Similar if not identical to changes seen with hypokalemia • Prolonged P-R interval • Widened QRS complex • Prolonged Q-T interval • Depressed ST segment • Flattened T waves • Possibly prominent U wave	• Prolonged P-R interval • Widened QRS complex • Increased T wave amplitude
Gastrointestinal	• Anorexia • Nausea • Vomiting • Abdominal distention • Hypoactive bowel sounds • Constipation	• Nausea • Vomiting
Integumentary	None	• Facial flushing • Diaphoresis • Feeling of warmth
Neuromuscular	Characterized by irritability and hyperexcitability • Weakness (generalized) • Paresthesias • Increased (hyperactive) DTRs to tetany • Muscle spasm or cramps, twitching, tremors • Possibly nystagmus • Seizures (usually seen at levels less than 1 mEq/L) • Positive Chvostek's sign and Trousseau's sign (see Chapter 5, page 124)	• Weakness (!) Decreased to absent DTRs are a primary sign of hypermagnesemia
Respiratory	• Hypoventilation • Bradypnea	• Depression because of respiratory muscle weakness • Severe depression may produce respiratory arrest
Laboratory Values		
	Hypomagnesemia	*Hypermagnesemia*
Serum magnesium	Less than 1.6 mg/dL (1.32 mEq/L)	Greater than 2.6 mg/dL (2.14 mEq/L)

Table 6.3 Nursing Interventions to Control Serum Magnesium Levels

Hypomagnesemia

Increase magnesium level

Asymptomatic hypomagnesemia

- Administer oral supplements, as ordered, to a client who can tolerate oral medications
- Usual dose
  - *-magnesium hydroxide (Phillips' Milk of Magnesia, Maalox): 10 mL 1–2 times per day*
  - *-magnesium oxide: 400–800 mg 3 times per day*
  - *-magnesium chloride (Slow-Mag) may be used; it causes fewer diarrhea stools but also delivers less magnesium*

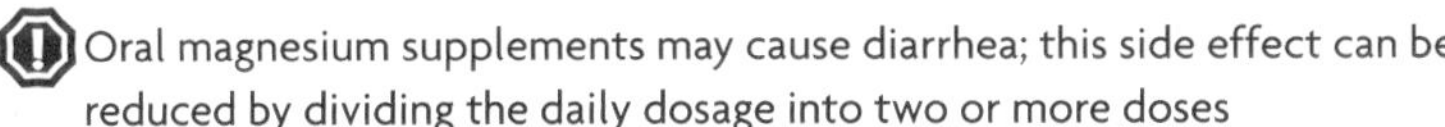
Oral magnesium supplements may cause diarrhea; this side effect can be reduced by dividing the daily dosage into two or more doses

Severe hypomagnesemia

- Administer IV magnesium sulfate as ordered
  - IV magnesium sulfate is used to treat severe hypomagnesemia in adults and older children, especially if the client is experiencing neurological changes or cardiac dysrhythmias
  - Magnesium should be administered very slowly: 1–4 gm magnesium sulfate can be given intravenously in 10%–20% solution with extreme caution; the rate should not exceed 1.5 mL of 10% solution or equivalent per minute until relaxation is obtained
  - Monitor blood pressure, pulse, respiratory rate, and ECG frequently throughout administration
  - Respirations should be at least 16 breaths/min before each dose
  - Monitor neurological status, and implement seizure precautions
  - Monitor intake and output to ensure adequate renal clearance
  - Monitor a newborn for hypotension, hyporeflexia, and respiratory depression if the mother has received magnesium sulfate
  - Assess DTRs before each dose

Hold magnesium and notify the health-care provider if DTRs become hypoactive or absent

- Administer IM magnesium sulfate as ordered
  - Intramuscular magnesium sulfate is often used to treat severe hypomagnesemia in young children and in pregnant women with uterine tetany (eclampsia), as it is a myometrial relaxant; although magnesium sulfate can be given intramuscularly, the injection can be very painful
  - Intramuscular doses greater than 1 gm must be divided and given at different injection sites
- Magnesium replacement must be given with extreme caution to a client with impaired renal function because of the increased risk of hypermagnesemia
- Decreased dosing and more frequent laboratory and clinical monitoring are indicated in a client with any degree of renal impairment

Hypermagnesemia

Decrease magnesium level

Mild to moderate hypermagnesemia

- Discontinue medications or preparations that contain magnesium
  - *-antacids such as magnesium hydroxide/aluminum hydroxide (Maalox)*
  - *-laxatives such as magnesium citrate or magnesium hydroxide (Phillips' Milk of Magnesia)*
  - *-mineral or electrolyte supplements such as magnesium chloride (Slow-Mag) or magnesium oxide Mag-Ox 400)*

Severe hypermagnesemia

- Treat in an acute care facility with cardiac monitoring capabilities
- Decrease serum magnesium by direct removal (especially if renal failure is a cause)
  - Hemodialysis
  - Continuous venovenous hemofiltration
  - Continuous renal replacement therapy
- Administer IV calcium gluconate, as ordered, to treat the cardiac muscle effects of hypermagnesemia
- Administer medications as ordered
  - Loop diuretics decrease total serum magnesium by increasing excretion by the kidneys
    - *-bumetanide (Bumex)*
    - *-ethacrynic acid (Edecrin)*
    - *-furosemide (Lasix)*
    - *-torsemide (Demadex)*

   b. Serum calcium: normal reference range is 8.2 to 10.2 mg/dL (adults).
3. Monitor for neuromuscular changes.
   a. Establish a baseline for the client's deep tendon reflexes (DTRs), muscle strength, and tone (Box 6.1).
   b. Monitor the client for muscle weakness, tetany, or seizure activity during each nursing shift; monitor more frequently if administering IV magnesium.
4. Monitor for neurological changes.
   a. Establish the client's usual cognitive and behavioral pattern.
   b. Observe the client's behavior, level of consciousness, and mental status.
   c. Monitor for seizure activity.
5. Monitor for cardiovascular changes.
   a. Auscultate the client's apical pulse.
   b. Monitor for ECG changes, particularly torsades de pointes (Fig. 6.2).
   c. Check orthostatic blood pressures.
6. Monitor for gastrointestinal changes.
   a. Auscultate bowel sounds in all four quadrants.
   b. Observe the frequency and consistency of bowel movements.

Box 6.1 Assessing Deep Tendon Reflexes

1. Assess the biceps reflex by resting the client's elbow in your nondominant hand, with your thumb over the client's biceps tendon. Strike the percussion hammer to your thumb.

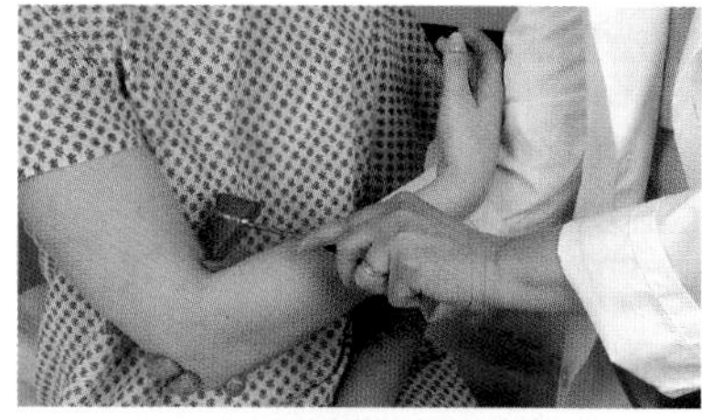

2. Assess the patellar reflex by having the client sit with legs dangling. Strike the tendon directly below the patella.

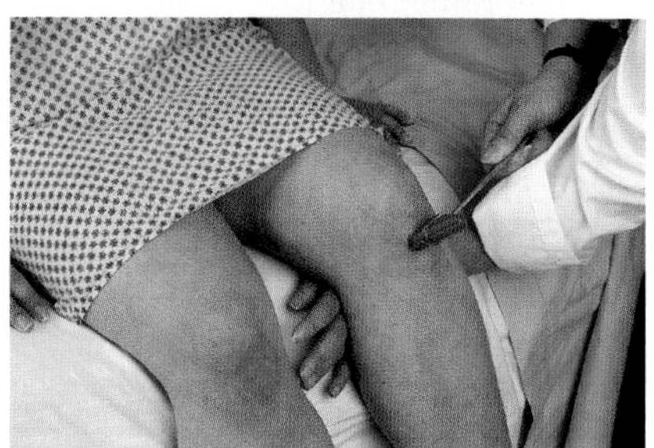

3. Grade the response:
   - 0 No response detected
   - +1 Diminished response
   - +2 Normal response
   - +3 Stronger than normal response
   - +4 Hyperactive response
4. Document your findings.

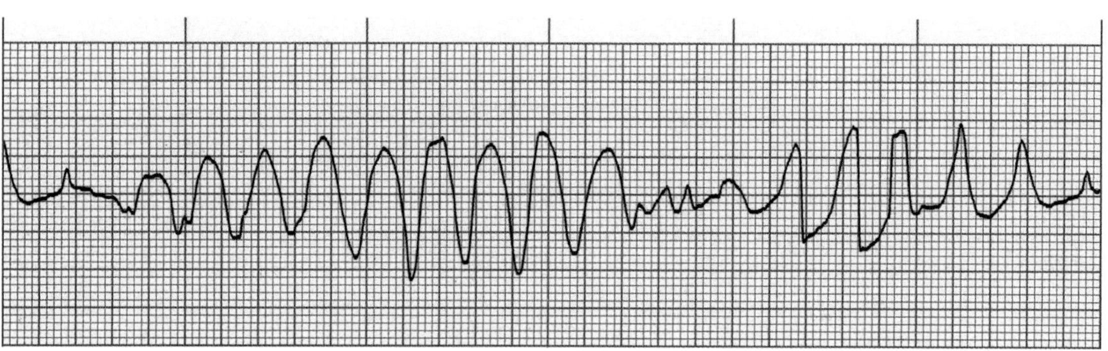

Fig 6.2 Torsades de pointes is a life-threatening type of ventricular tachycardia associated with hypomagnesemia.

D. Ensure client safety.
1. Reduce environmental stimuli.
   a. Provide a quiet room.
   b. Limit visitors.
   c. Darken the room.
   d. Speak in soft tones.
2. Implement seizure precautions.
   a. Pad side rails.
   b. Have oxygen and suction equipment available.
   c. Ensure the patency of IV access devices.
3. Administer emergency medications as ordered.
   a. Prepare for possible endotracheal intubation.
   b. Prepare for cardiac defibrillation if necessary.

E. Implement fall precautions related to muscle weakness caused by magnesium imbalances.
1. Perform a fall risk assessment.
2. Maintain the bed in a low position with locked wheels.
3. Remove all obstacles from pathways, especially to the toilet.
4. Monitor the environment for safety hazards, such as torn carpet, liquid spills on floors.
5. Place assistive devices (walkers, canes) within the client's reach.
6. Use nightlights.
7. Instruct the client to request assistance to ambulate.

8. Ensure availability of the call light.
9. Assess footwear, and provide appropriate footwear if necessary; clients must use antiskid soles.
10. Keep items such as the telephone and fluids close to the client.
11. Request that family members remain with the client if necessary.
12. Position the client to allow close observation by staff members.
13. Communicate the client's fall risk during the shift report and as necessary.

F. Educate the client.

1. Hypomagnesemia
   a. Teach the client or caregiver the causes of magnesium deficit.
   b. Provide specific information regarding the client's medical diagnosis and related interventions and treatments.
   c. Teach the client how to identify the signs and symptoms of magnesium deficiency.
   d. Instruct the client and family to notify the primary health-care provider if the client exhibits signs or symptoms of hypomagnesemia or if they have any other specific concerns.
   e. Teach the client how to prevent magnesium deficiency by consuming foods high in magnesium (Table 6.4).
   f. Teach the client how to take oral magnesium supplements.
      1) Magnesium supplements should be taken with meals. Taking them on an empty stomach may cause diarrhea.
      2) Instruct a client who is also taking an iron supplement to take the magnesium and iron supplements at least 2 to 3 hours apart.
      3) Teach a client who is taking an extended-release form of magnesium to:
         a) Swallow the tablets whole; do not chew or suck on them.
         b) Ask the health-care provider whether tablets can be broken or crushed and sprinkled on applesauce or another soft food. This is acceptable for some tablets, but most tablets should not be broken or crushed.
      4) Teach a client who is taking the powder form of magnesium to pour the powder into a glass, add water, and stir well.
      5) Instruct the client to report adverse effects, such as nausea, vomiting, diarrhea, and abdominal cramping, to the primary health-care provider.
      6) Encourage the client to keep appointments for laboratory studies to evaluate serum magnesium levels.
   g. Ensure that the client or caregiver understands the specifics, rationale, potential side effects, and desired effects of the treatment regimen.
   h. Include medication administration, nutrition, hydration, dietary restrictions, and foods high in magnesium (see Table 6.4) in client teaching.
2. Hypermagnesemia
   a. Teach the client or caregiver the causes of magnesium excess.
   b. Provide specific information regarding the client's medical diagnosis and related interventions and treatments.
   c. Teach the client how to identify the signs and symptoms of magnesium excess.
   d. Instruct the client and family to notify the primary health-care provider if the client exhibits signs or symptoms of hypermagnesemia or if they have any other specific concerns.
   e. Teach the client how to prevent magnesium excess.
      1) Advise the client to avoid high-magnesium foods.
      2) Teach the client and caregivers how to read food labels that list the amount of magnesium in each serving.

Table 6.4 Foods High in Magnesium

Food (Standard Amount)	Magnesium (mg)
Halibut, cooked, 3 oz	90
Almonds, dry roasted, 1 oz	80
Cashews, dry roasted, 1 oz	75
Soybeans, mature, cooked, ½ cup	75
Spinach, frozen, cooked, ½ cup	75
Nuts, mixed, dry roasted, 1 oz	65
Cereal, shredded wheat, 2 rectangular biscuits	55
Oatmeal, instant (fortified), prepared with water, 1 cup	55
Potato, baked with skin, 1 medium	50
Peanuts, dry roasted, 1 oz	50
Peanut butter, smooth, 2 tbsp	50
Wheat bran, crude, 2 tbsp	45
Black-eyed peas, cooked, ½ cup	45
Yogurt, plain, nonfat, 8 oz	45
Bran flakes, ½ cup	40
Vegetarian baked beans, ½ cup	40
Brown rice, long-grain, cooked, ½ cup	40
Lentils, mature seeds, cooked, ½ cup	35
Avocado, California, ½ cup pureed	35
Kidney beans, canned, ½ cup	35

f. Ensure that the client or caregiver understands the specifics, rationale, potential side effects, and desired effects of the treatment regimen.
g. Include medication administration, nutrition, hydration, dietary restrictions, and foods high in magnesium (see Table 6.4) in client teaching.

G. Evaluate and document
1. Document all assessment findings and interventions per institution policy.
2. Evaluate and document the client's response to interventions and education.
    a. Serum magnesium level should return to the normal reference range of 1.6 to 2.6 mg/dL.
    b. Other laboratory values should return to the normal reference range.
    c. Vital signs should return to baseline.
    d. Underlying cause of magnesium imbalance should be resolved.
    e. Level of consciousness should return to baseline.

CASE STUDY: Putting It All Together

Subjective Data

A 35-year-old client presents to an emergency department after a motor vehicle collision. The client shows no signs of traumatic injury but reports dizziness, nausea, generalized weakness, and leg twitching bilaterally. The client has a history of chronic alcohol abuse and hypertension. The client has no known allergies, and the only medication he currently takes is metoprolol (Lopressor) 25 mg by mouth (PO) twice a day.

Objective Data

Nursing Assessment

1. Lethargic
2. Oriented to person but not to place or time
3. Generalized weakness, muscle twitching
4. Heart sounds S_1 and S_2 irregular, rapid
5. Cardiac monitor reveals a 30-beat run of ventricular tachycardia with torsades de pointes configuration
6. Pedal and radial pulses irregular, 1+, and weak bilaterally
7. DTRs 3+ bilaterally
8. Bowel sounds hyperactive in all four quadrants
9. Incontinent of moderate amount of liquid brown stool

Vital Signs	
Temperature:	99°F (37.2°C) orally
Blood pressure:	168/94 mm Hg
Heart rate:	134 bpm
Respiratory rate:	10
O_2 saturation:	93% on room air

Laboratory Results	
Serum magnesium:	1 mEq/L
Serum calcium:	7.8 mg/dL
Serum potassium:	3.1 mEq/L
Blood alcohol level:	0.11%
Lactate dehydrogenase:	162 units/L
Serum alkaline phosphatase:	190 units/L
Serum aspartate aminotransferase:	52 units/L
Serum alanine aminotransferase:	64 units/L
ECG:	sinus tachycardia with occasional multifocal premature ventricular contractions (PVCs)

Health-Care Provider Orders

1. Assess vital signs every 15 minutes × 4, hourly × 2, then every 4 hours.
2. Administer O_2 2 L/min via nasal cannula.
3. Start telemetry.
4. Implement seizure precautions.
5. Initiate alcohol withdrawal protocol.
6. Perform neurological checks every hour × 4, then every 4 hours.
7. Administer magnesium sulfate 2 gm IV push now.
8. Add 2 gm magnesium sulfate to 1,000 mL normal (0.9%) saline solution at 100 mL/hr daily.
9. Start magnesium chloride (Slow-Mag) 2 tablets PO daily.
10. Administer IV metoprolol (Lopressor) now; increase PO dose to 50 mg twice a day.

CASE STUDY: Putting It All Together *cont'd*

11. Initiate fall precautions.
12. Monitor intake and output.
13. Reevaluate clinical signs and symptoms; repeat ECG and serum magnesium, calcium, and potassium levels in 6 hours.
14. Notify the health-care provider of results.
15. Initiate alcohol cessation counseling when client is stable.

Case Study Questions

A. What *subjective* assessment findings indicate that the client is experiencing a health alteration?

1. ___
2. ___
3. ___
4. ___
5. ___

B. What *objective* assessment findings indicate that the client is experiencing a health alteration?

1. ___
2. ___
3. ___
4. ___
5. ___
6. ___
7. ___
8. ___
9. ___
10. ___
11. ___
12. ___
13. ___
14. ___
15. ___
16. ___

C. After analyzing the data collected, what **primary** nursing diagnosis should the nurse assign to this client?

___

Continued

CASE STUDY: Putting It All Together *cont'd*

Case Study Questions

D. What interventions should the nurse plan and/or implement to meet this client's needs?

1. ______
2. ______
3. ______
4. ______
5. ______
6. ______
7. ______
8. ______
9. ______
10. ______
11. ______
12. ______
13. ______
14. ______

E. What client outcomes should the nurse plan to evaluate the effectiveness of the nursing interventions?

1. ______
2. ______
3. ______
4. ______
5. ______
6. ______

REVIEW QUESTIONS

1. A nurse assesses the DTRs of a pregnant client who is diagnosed with preeclampsia. The nurse documents that the client's DTRs are "more brisk than expected." Which grade should the nurse assign to this client's DTR response?
   1. Grade 0
   2. Grade 1
   3. Grade 2
   4. Grade 3
   5. Grade 4

2. Which clinical manifestations should a nurse associate with the development of hypomagnesemia if observed in a newly admitted client? **Select all that apply.**
   1. Diarrhea
   2. Excessive drowsiness
   3. Positive Chvostek's sign
   4. Positive Trousseau's sign
   5. Hyperactive DTRs

3. Which nursing diagnoses should a nurse assign to a client who has a serum magnesium level of 4.8 mg/dL? **Select all that apply.**
   1. Risk for Injury Related to Seizure Activity
   2. Risk for Falls Related to Muscle Weakness
   3. Constipation Related to Decreased Smooth Muscle Contraction
   4. Decreased Cardiac Output Related to Dysrhythmia
   5. Ineffective Breathing Pattern Related to Muscle Weakness

4. Which assessment should be performed by a nurse to identify whether an older adult client is developing a potentially dangerous side effect of the medication magnesium oxide (Mag-Ox 400)?
   1. Nutritional status
   2. Presence of constipation
   3. Input and output
   4. Deep tendon reflexes (DTRs)

5. A nurse is monitoring a client with a serum magnesium level of 1 mEq/L who is receiving magnesium sulfate 2 gm IV piggyback. Which finding, if present, should indicate to the nurse that the client's hypomagnesemia is improving?
   1. Regular ECG rhythm
   2. Widened QRS complexes on ECG
   3. DTRs 3+ bilaterally
   4. Presence of torsades de pointes on ECG

6. A nurse is reviewing the ECG strip of a client diagnosed with a fluid and electrolyte imbalance. Based on the exhibit provided, which imbalance should the nurse suspect?

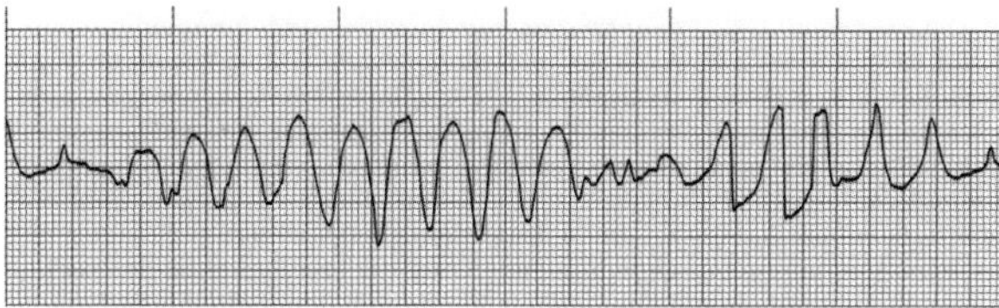

   1. Hypokalemia
   2. Hyperkalemia
   3. Hypomagnesemia
   4. Hypermagnesemia

7. A nurse is caring for an older adult client who is at risk for seizures secondary to neuromuscular irritability associated with hypomagnesemia. Which actions should the nurse take when implementing seizure precautions for this client? **Select all that apply.**
   1. Assess the functioning of suction equipment.
   2. Maintain the bed in a low position with the wheels locked.
   3. Place a tongue blade at the head of the client's bed.
   4. Pad the side rails and headboard of the client's bed.
   5. Ensure that the client's room is bright during daylight hours.

8. An older adult client who has been abusing laxatives is being discharged from the hospital. Which manifestations should the nurse instruct the client to report immediately?
   1. Muscle twitches and constipation
   2. Fatigue and hypertension
   3. Bradycardia and hypotension
   4. Anorexia and abdominal distention

9. Which serum magnesium level should a nurse anticipate when evaluating the laboratory data of a client admitted with diabetic ketoacidosis?
   1. 1.32 mg/dL
   2. 1.6 mg/dL
   3. 2.14 mg/dL
   4. 2.7 mg/dL

10. A nurse is providing discharge instructions to a client diagnosed with hypomagnesemia secondary to chronic alcohol abuse. The client reports frequent acid reflux. Which antacid should the nurse instruct the client to take?
    1. Tums
    2. Titralac
    3. Alka-Seltzer
    4. Maalox

11. A nurse is caring for a client who has been diagnosed with severe hypomagnesemia. Which medication would be most appropriate for this client?
 1. furosemide (Lasix)
 2. magnesium sulfate
 3. acetazolamide (Diamox)
 4. magnesium hydroxide (Phillips' Milk of Magnesia)

12. A nurse prepares to administer magnesium to a client diagnosed with hypomagnesemia. Which actions by the nurse are appropriate for this client? **Select all that apply.**
 1. Administer magnesium sulfate intramuscularly.
 2. Initiate seizure precautions.
 3. Monitor for decreased DTRs.
 4. Administer magnesium hydroxide by mouth.
 5. Monitor the client's serum calcium level.

13. A nurse admits a client with numerous electrolyte imbalances. Which nursing interventions should the nurse implement to ensure client safety? **Select all that apply.**
 1. Encourage the client to increase fluid intake.
 2. Assess the client's fall risk.
 3. Weigh the client daily.
 4. Use a pump to deliver IV fluids.
 5. Use a gait belt when assisting the client to ambulate.

14. A nurse assesses a newly admitted client and finds that the client has hyperactive DTRs. Which potential electrolyte imbalances should the nurse suspect? **Select all that apply.**
 1. Hypermagnesemia
 2. Hypomagnesemia
 3. Hypercalcemia
 4. Hypocalcemia
 5. Hyperkalemia
 6. Hypokalemia

15. A nurse assesses a pregnant client diagnosed with preeclampsia. The client's serum magnesium level is within the normal reference range, but she is receiving IV magnesium sulfate to prevent seizure activity. To monitor for hypermagnesemia, the nurse attempts to elicit the client's DTRs. Which actions should the nurse take to assess the biceps reflex? Place each nursing action in the correct sequence (1–7).

 ________ Report and document the findings.

 ________ Rest the client's elbow in the nurse's nondominant hand.

 ________ Place the thumb of the nurse's nondominant hand over the client's biceps tendon.

 ________ Strike the percussion hammer to the nurse's thumb.

 ________ Observe for slight flexion of the elbow.

 ________ Feel for contraction of the biceps muscle.

 ________ Explain the procedure to the client.

16. Which nursing diagnosis should a nurse assign to an adult client who has a serum magnesium level of 1.32 mg/dL? **Select all that apply.**
 1. Disturbed Sleep Pattern Related to Polyuria
 2. Fatigue Related to Muscle Weakness
 3. Diarrhea Related to Spastic Colonic Activity
 4. Constipation Related to Reduced Gastrointestinal Motility
 5. Decreased Cardiac Output Related to Dysrhythmia

17. A nurse is administering magnesium sulfate intravenously to a client diagnosed with hypomagnesemia. Which medication should the nurse keep readily available and why?
 1. Furosemide to increase the serum magnesium level
 2. Albuterol to increase gas exchange
 3. Calcium gluconate to decrease the effects of magnesium
 4. Digoxin to decrease cardiac output

18. Which outcome would be most appropriate for a nurse to establish when caring for a client with a nursing diagnosis of Risk for Falls Related to Skeletal Muscle Weakness Secondary to Hypomagnesemia?
 1. The client's DTRs will increase to within normal limits.
 2. The client will remain free from injury throughout the hospital stay.
 3. The nurse will promote oral fluid intake as appropriate.
 4. The dietitian will teach the client how to decrease dietary magnesium intake.

19. A nurse is preparing to administer IV magnesium sulfate 30 mg/kg as ordered to a 2-year-old child who has been diagnosed with torsades de pointes secondary to hypomagnesemia. The client weighs 22 lb. The dose on hand is 500 mg/mL. How many milliliters should the nurse administer? Record your answer using one decimal place.

 ____

20. A nurse is preparing to administer calcium gluconate 10% 7 mEq IV bolus to a postpartum client diagnosed with magnesium toxicity. Calcium gluconate 10% contains 0.45 mEq/mL. How many milliliters should the nurse administer to this client? Record your answer using one decimal place.

 ____

21. A nurse is caring for an older adult client who is at risk for falls secondary to muscle weakness associated with a magnesium imbalance. Which action should the nurse take when implementing fall precautions for this client?
    1. Perform a fall risk assessment.
    2. Maintain the bed in the Trendelenburg position.
    3. Place assistive devices (walkers, canes) at the end of the client's bed.
    4. Instruct the client to hold on to the side rail when getting out of bed.

22. A nurse is caring for a client whose serum magnesium level is 1.2 mEq/L. Based on this information, which physician orders should the nurse question? **Select all that apply.**
    1. Implement fall precautions.
    2. Implement seizure precautions.
    3. Administer IV magnesium chloride (Slow-Mag) 400 mg daily.
    4. Perform continuous telemetry monitoring.
    5. Administer IV furosemide (Lasix) 40 mg daily.

23. Which manifestation should a nurse investigate *first* when assessing a client admitted with severe preeclampsia that is being treated with a continuous infusion of IV magnesium sulfate?
    1. Pulse 100 bpm
    2. Blood pressure 164/100 mm Hg
    3. Respiratory rate 10 breaths/min
    4. Oral temperature 99.6°F

24. A nurse assesses that an adolescent diagnosed with anorexia nervosa has a serum magnesium level of 1.1 mg/dL. Which nursing intervention should the nurse implement *first*?
    1. Administer oxygen at 2 L/min via nasal cannula.
    2. Implement seizure precautions immediately.
    3. Administer magnesium sulfate 2 gm IV bolus.
    4. Place the client on continuous telemetry.

25. A nurse is administering magnesium sulfate intravenously to a client. The client begins vomiting and sweating, exhibits facial flushing, and is becoming extremely lethargic. The nurse immediately notifies the client's health-care provider and evaluates the client's ECG strip. Which cardiac rhythm is the nurse most likely to observe?
    1.

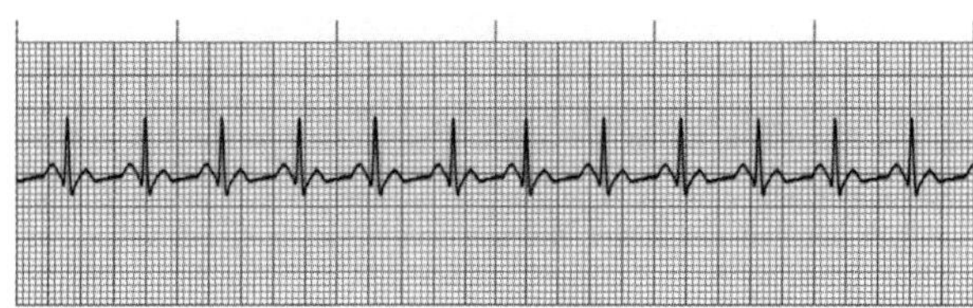

    2.

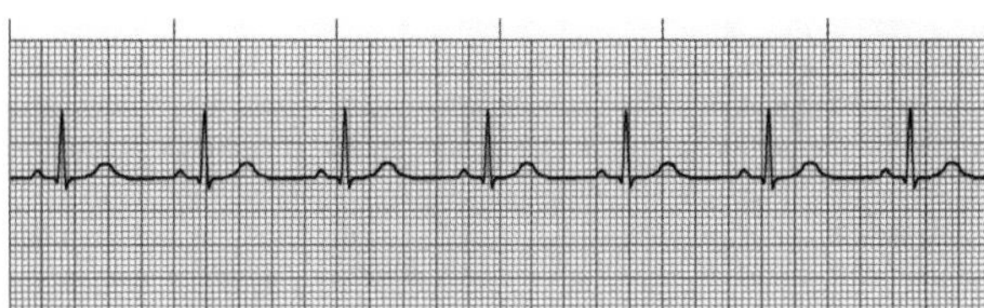

    3.

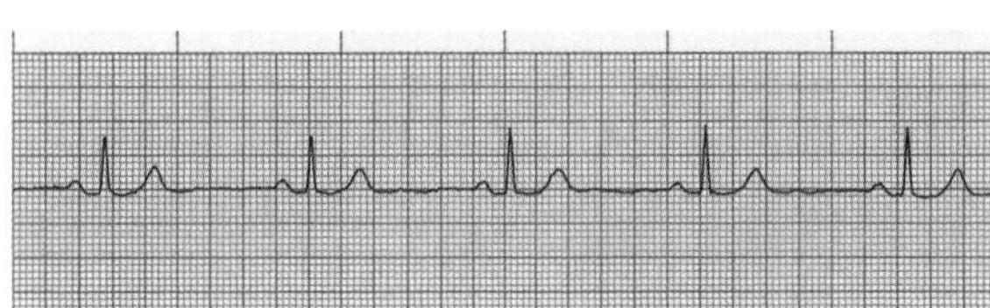

    4.

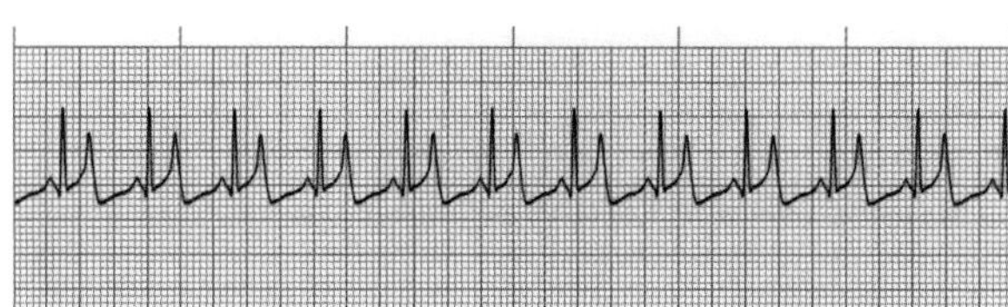

REVIEW ANSWERS

1. ANSWER: 4.

Rationale:

1. Grade 0 indicates no response.
2. Grade 1 indicates a weaker response than normal (hypoactive).
3. Grade 2 indicates a normal or expected response.
4. **When the client's DTRs are "more brisk than expected," the nurse should document that they are grade 3.**
5. Grade 4 indicates a brisk, hyperactive response with intermittent or transient clonus—a sudden, brief, jerking contraction of a muscle or muscle group that is often seen in seizures.

TEST-TAKING TIP: The key words are "more brisk than expected." Select the grade that is just above normal. Recall that a normal response is classified as grade 2.

Content Area: Maternal Health
Integrated Processes: Nursing Process: Assessment
Client Need: Health Promotion and Maintenance
Cognitive Level: Comprehension
Reference: Ignatavicius, D., and Workman, M. (2012). Medical-Surgical Nursing: Patient-Centered Collaborative Care (7th ed.). St. Louis, MO: Saunders.

2. ANSWER: 3, 4, 5.

Rationale:

1. Constipation, not diarrhea, is associated with hypomagnesemia because low magnesium levels result in a decrease in intestinal smooth muscle contraction.
2. Excessive drowsiness is a sign of hypermagnesemia because high magnesium levels result in depressed nerve impulse transmission.
3. **The nurse should associate a positive Chvostek's sign with hypomagnesemia because hypocalcemia usually accompanies hypomagnesemia.**
4. **The nurse should associate a positive Trousseau's sign with hypomagnesemia because hypocalcemia usually accompanies hypomagnesemia.**
5. **Hyperactive DTRs, also a sign of hypomagnesemia, occur because a lack of magnesium increases cellular excitability.**

TEST-TAKING TIP: Recall that magnesium is needed for neuromuscular relaxation. Select options related to the neuromuscular irritability caused by a low serum magnesium level. Remember that magnesium levels usually parallel calcium levels.

Content Area: Adult Health
Integrated Processes: Nursing Process: Assessment
Client Need: Physiological Integrity
Cognitive Level: Application
Reference: Ignatavicius, D., and Workman, M. (2012). Medical-Surgical Nursing: Patient-Centered Collaborative Care (7th ed.). St. Louis, MO: Saunders.

3. ANSWER: 2, 4, 5.

Rationale:

1. This client is experiencing hypermagnesemia. Hypermagnesemia does not cause seizures because magnesium is a membrane stabilizer.
2. **Hypermagnesemia causes muscle weakness, placing the client at risk for falls.**
3. Constipation is associated with hypomagnesemia because low magnesium levels result in a decrease in intestinal smooth muscle contraction.
4. **Hypermagnesemia causes bradycardia and decreased cardiac output, resulting in possible dysrhythmias.**
5. **Hypermagnesemia may weaken the respiratory muscles, resulting in ineffective breathing patterns.**

TEST-TAKING TIP: Recall that the normal reference range for serum magnesium is 1.6 to 2.6 mg/dL. The client is experiencing hypermagnesemia, so options 1 and 3 can be ruled out because seizure activity and constipation are signs of hypomagnesemia.

Content Area: Adult Health
Integrated Processes: Nursing Process: Analysis
Client Need: Physiological Integrity
Cognitive Level: Application
Reference: Ignatavicius, D., and Workman, M. (2012). Medical-Surgical Nursing: Patient-Centered Collaborative Care (7th ed.). St. Louis, MO: Saunders.

4. ANSWER: 4.

Rationale:

1. The client's overall nutritional status would not be affected by magnesium supplementation.
2. Constipation is associated with hypomagnesemia, not hypermagnesemia.
3. Increased urine output would be the desired effect of IV magnesium sulfate when treating severe preeclampsia in a pregnant client.
4. **When a client is taking magnesium oxide (Mag-Ox 400), the nurse should assess for deep tendon hyporeflexia because magnesium supplementation may cause hypermagnesemia, especially in an older adult client. An older adult client is at increased risk for electrolyte imbalances because of decreased renal function.**

TEST-TAKING TIP: The key words are "older adult client." Recall that clients receiving magnesium supplementation are at risk for hypermagnesemia, especially older adult clients with decreased renal excretion.

Content Area: Older Adult Health
Integrated Processes: Nursing Process: Assessment
Client Need: Physiological Integrity
Cognitive Level: Application
Reference: Deglin, J. H., Vallerand, A. H., and Sanoski, C. A. (2013). Davis's Drug Guide for Nurses (13th ed.). Philadelphia, PA: F. A. Davis.

5. ANSWER: 1.

Rationale:

1. **A nurse monitoring a client with a serum magnesium level of 1 mEq/L who is receiving IV magnesium sulfate should determine that a regular cardiac rhythm indicates that the client's hypomagnesemia is improving. Hypomagnesemia causes tachycardia and dysrhythmias.**
2. A widened QRS complex is a sign of hypomagnesemia.
3. Hyperactive DTRs are a sign of hypomagnesemia.
4. The presence of torsades de pointes on the ECG would indicate continued or worsened hypomagnesemia.

TEST-TAKING TIP: Select option 1 because this finding is within normal limits, indicating resolution of the client's hypomagnesemia.

Content Area: Adult Health
Integrated Processes: Nursing Process: Evaluation

Client Need: Physiological Integrity
Cognitive Level: Application
Reference: *Berman, A., Snyder, S., Kozier, B., and Erb, G. (2012). Kozier & Erb's Fundamentals of Nursing: Concepts, Process, and Practice (9th ed.). Upper Saddle River, NJ: Pearson.*

6. ANSWER: 3.
Rationale:
1. Hypokalemia may cause an irregular heartbeat (dysrhythmia).
2. Hyperkalemia may cause peaked T waves, widened QRS complexes, and, if severe, ventricular fibrillation and asystole.
3. The nurse should suspect that this client is experiencing hypomagnesemia because the ECG strip shows torsades de pointes, an unusual variant of ventricular tachycardia. Hypomagnesemia is the usual cause of torsades de pointes.
4. Hypermagnesemia may cause bradycardia, a prolonged P-R interval, and a widened QRS complex.
TEST-TAKING TIP: Associate the appearance of torsades de pointes on an ECG with hypomagnesemia. Be able to differentiate between ventricular tachycardia and torsades de pointes ventricular tachycardia.
Content Area: Adult Health
Integrated Processes: Nursing Process: Evaluation
Client Need: Physiological Integrity
Cognitive Level: Application
Reference: *Jones, S. (2010). ECG Notes: Interpretation and Management Guide (2nd ed.). Philadelphia, PA: F. A. Davis.*

7. ANSWER: 1, 2, 4.
Rationale:
1. When implementing seizure precautions for this client, the nurse should assess the functioning of suction equipment, which may be needed to keep the client's airway clear.
2. The nurse should maintain the bed in a low position with the wheels locked to maintain client safety during a seizure.
3. Placing a tongue blade at the head of the client's bed is inappropriate because one should never place anything in the mouth of a client who is having a seizure.
4. The nurse should pad the side rails and headboard of the client's bed to maintain client safety during a seizure.
5. The nurse should decrease environmental stimuli by darkening the room for a client who is at risk for seizures.
TEST-TAKING TIP: Consider each option, and select those that would prevent the client from being injured during a seizure.
Content Area: Older Adult Health
Integrated Processes: Nursing Process: Implementation
Client Need: Safe and Effective Care Environment
Cognitive Level: Application
Reference: *Ignatavicius, D., and Workman, M. (2012). Medical-Surgical Nursing: Patient-Centered Collaborative Care (7th ed.). St. Louis, MO: Saunders.*

8. ANSWER: 3.
Rationale:
1. Muscle twitches and constipation are associated with hypomagnesemia. This client is at risk for hypermagnesemia secondary to laxative abuse.
2. Fatigue and hypertension are not manifestations of hypermagnesemia.
3. Magnesium is an active ingredient in many over-the-counter laxatives. The nurse should instruct the client to report bradycardia and hypotension immediately to a health-care provider because these are signs of hypermagnesemia that require prompt intervention.
4. Anorexia and abdominal distention may be associated with hypomagnesemia or other disorders and are not signs of hypermagnesemia.
TEST-TAKING TIP: The key words are "abusing laxatives" and "report immediately." Select option 3 because these are signs of hypermagnesemia and are potentially life threatening.
Content Area: Older Adult Health
Integrated Processes: Teaching/Learning
Client Need: Physiological Integrity
Cognitive Level: Application
Reference: *Berman, A., Snyder, S., Kozier, B., and Erb, G. (2012). Kozier & Erb's Fundamentals of Nursing: Concepts, Process, and Practice (9th ed.). Upper Saddle River, NJ: Pearson.*

9. ANSWER: 1.
Rationale:
1. When evaluating the laboratory data of a client admitted with diabetic ketoacidosis, the nurse should anticipate a serum magnesium level of less than 1.6 mg/dL (hypomagnesemia) because hyperglycemia causes osmotic diuresis and polyuria, resulting in excess urinary excretion of magnesium. A serum magnesium level less than 1.2 mg/dL is considered a critical value and may result in cardiac arrest.
2. A serum magnesium level of 1.6 mg/dL is within the normal range.
3. A serum magnesium level of 2.14 mg/dL is within the normal range.
4. A serum magnesium level of 2.7 mg/dL is elevated, indicating hypermagnesemia.
TEST-TAKING TIP: The key words are "diabetic ketoacidosis." Recall that hyperglycemia causes diuresis and polyuria, which lead to hypomagnesemia. Select the serum magnesium level that is less than the normal reference range of 1.6 to 2.6 mg/dL.
Content Area: Adult Health
Integrated Processes: Nursing Process: Evaluation
Client Need: Physiological Integrity
Cognitive Level: Application
Reference: *Ignatavicius, D., and Workman, M. (2012). Medical-Surgical Nursing: Patient-Centered Collaborative Care (7th ed.). St. Louis, MO: Saunders.*

10. ANSWER: 4.
Rationale:
1. Tums contains calcium carbonate, which would not help increase the client's serum magnesium level.
2. Titralac (calcium carbonate) would be an appropriate choice for a client who is experiencing hypocalcemia but would not increase the serum magnesium level.
3. Alka-Seltzer contains sodium bicarbonate, citric acid, and aspirin, which neutralize stomach acid but do not increase the magnesium level.
4. The nurse should instruct the client to consume Maalox for acid reflux because it neutralizes stomach acid and contains magnesium hydroxide/aluminum hydroxide, which increases the client's magnesium intake.

TEST-TAKING TIP: Rule out the antacids that do not contain magnesium.
Content Area: Adult Health
Integrated Processes: Teaching/Learning
Client Need: Physiological Integrity
Cognitive Level: Application
Reference: Deglin, J. H., Vallerand, A. H., and Sanoski, C. A. (2013). Davis's Drug Guide for Nurses (13th ed.). Philadelphia, PA: F. A. Davis.

11. ANSWER: 2.
Rationale:
1. Furosemide is a loop diuretic that would promote magnesium loss through the urine.
2. Magnesium sulfate is the most appropriate medication for this client because it is administered intravenously to increase serum magnesium levels in clients diagnosed with severe hypomagnesemia.
3. Acetazolamide is an osmotic diuretic that would promote magnesium loss through the urine.
4. Magnesium hydroxide is contraindicated for this client because it is a laxative that may cause diarrhea when administered in high doses, resulting in additional magnesium loss.
TEST-TAKING TIP: Recall that IV magnesium sulfate is most often used to correct moderate to severe hypomagnesemia. Rule out options that would promote magnesium loss.
Content Area: Adult Health
Integrated Processes: Nursing Process: Analysis
Client Need: Physiological Integrity
Cognitive Level: Application
Reference: Ignatavicius, D., and Workman, M. (2012). Medical-Surgical Nursing: Patient-Centered Collaborative Care (7th ed.). St. Louis, MO: Saunders.

12. ANSWER: 2, 3, 5.
Rationale:
1. Magnesium sulfate should be administered intravenously because IM injections cause pain and tissue damage.
2. A nurse preparing to administer magnesium to a client should initiate seizure precautions because the magnesium may cause rebound hypermagnesemia, resulting in a seizure.
3. Clients receiving magnesium replacement should be monitored for decreased DTRs, which may indicate rebound hypermagnesemia.
4. Oral preparations of magnesium may cause diarrhea and increase magnesium loss.
5. The client's serum calcium level should be monitored because hypocalcemia frequently accompanies hypomagnesemia.
TEST-TAKING TIP: The key words are "prepares to administer magnesium." Rule out options 1 and 4 because these actions are contraindicated. Select nursing actions that are appropriate during magnesium administration.
Content Area: Adult Health
Integrated Processes: Nursing Process: Planning
Client Need: Physiological Integrity
Cognitive Level: Application
Reference: Ignatavicius, D., and Workman, M. (2012). Medical-Surgical Nursing: Patient-Centered Collaborative Care (7th ed.). St. Louis, MO: Saunders.

13. ANSWER: 2, 4, 5.
Rationale:
1. Encouraging the client to increase fluid intake is not a safety-related intervention.
2. The nurse should assess the client's fall risk because many electrolyte imbalances can cause muscle weakness.
3. Weighing the client daily is not a safety-related intervention.
4. The nurse should use a pump to administer IV fluids carefully to avoid fluid overload and prevent further electrolyte imbalances.
5. The nurse should use a gait belt when assisting a client with weak muscles to ambulate to prevent the client from falling.
TEST-TAKING TIP: The key words are "to ensure client safety." Rule out options that are not related to client safety.
Content Area: Adult Health
Integrated Processes: Nursing Process: Implementation
Client Need: Safe and Effective Care Environment
Cognitive Level: Application
Reference: Ignatavicius, D., and Workman, M. (2012). Medical-Surgical Nursing: Patient-Centered Collaborative Care (7th ed.). St. Louis, MO: Saunders.

14. ANSWER: 2, 4, 5.
Rationale:
1. Hypermagnesemia may result in hypoactive or absent DTRs because magnesium decreases nerve impulse transmission.
2. Serum magnesium levels less than 1.32 mEq/L (hypomagnesemia) increase membrane excitability, which could result in hyperactive DTRs.
3. Hypercalcemia may result in hypoactive DTRs and muscle weakness.
4. Serum calcium levels less than 8.5 mg/dL (hypocalcemia) increase nerve cell membrane excitability, causing the cells to depolarize spontaneously, which results in hyperactive DTRs.
5. Serum potassium levels greater than 5.0 mg/dL (hyperkalemia) result in hyperactive DTRs and increase a client's risk for life-threatening cardiac dysrhythmias.
6. Hypokalemia may result in hypoactive DTRs and skeletal muscle weakness.
TEST-TAKING TIP: Remember which electrolyte imbalances cause hyperactive DTRs—*hypo*magnesemia and *hypo*calcemia (which occur together) and *hyper*kalemia.
Content Area: Adult Health
Integrated Processes: Nursing Process: Assessment
Client Need: Physiological Integrity
Cognitive Level: Application
Reference: Ignatavicius, D., and Workman, M. (2012). Medical-Surgical Nursing: Patient-Centered Collaborative Care (7th ed.). St. Louis, MO: Saunders.

15. ANSWER: 7, 2, 3, 4, 6, 5, 1.
Rationale: A nurse assessing a client's biceps reflex should first explain the procedure to the client, then rest the client's elbow in the nurse's nondominant hand, place the thumb of the nurse's nondominant hand over the client's biceps tendon, strike the percussion hammer to the nurse's

thumb, feel for contraction of the biceps muscle, and observe for slight flexion of the elbow. Finally, the nurse should report and document the findings.

TEST-TAKING TIP: Envision the procedure in your mind's eye, and select the actions the nurse should perform from first to last.

Content Area: *Maternal Health*
Integrated Processes: *Nursing Process: Assessment*
Client Need: *Health Promotion and Maintenance*
Cognitive Level: *Application*
Reference: *Wilkinson, J., and Treas, L. (2010). Fundamentals of Nursing: Theory, Concepts & Applications (2nd ed.). Philadelphia, PA: F. A. Davis.*

16. ANSWER: 2, 4, 5.

Rationale:

1. The client is experiencing hypomagnesemia, which does not cause polyuria.
2. **Hypomagnesemia results in fatigue and muscle weakness.**
3. The client is experiencing hypomagnesemia, which causes reduced gastrointestinal motility, not spastic colonic activity.
4. **Hypomagnesemia causes decreased gastrointestinal motility, resulting in constipation.**
5. **Hypomagnesemia decreases the transmission of nerve impulses to cardiac muscle, causing cardiac dysrhythmias such as torsades de pointes and ventricular tachycardia.**

TEST-TAKING TIP: Think about how a low serum magnesium level affects the body. Rule out options 1 and 3 because these nursing diagnoses are not related to hypomagnesemia.

Content Area: *Adult Health*
Integrated Processes: *Nursing Process: Analysis*
Client Need: *Physiological Integrity*
Cognitive Level: *Application*
Reference: *Ignatavicius, D., and Workman, M. (2012). Medical-Surgical Nursing: Patient-Centered Collaborative Care (7th ed.). St. Louis, MO: Saunders.*

17. ANSWER: 3.

Rationale:

1. Furosemide is a loop diuretic that promotes magnesium loss.
2. Albuterol is a bronchodilator used to treat asthma and chronic obstructive pulmonary disease (COPD). Impaired gas exchange is not related to magnesium administration.
3. **The nurse should keep calcium gluconate readily available to reverse the cardiac effects of potential hypermagnesemia caused by excess administration of IV magnesium sulfate.**
4. Digoxin is contraindicated in a client with hypomagnesemia because it may potentiate digoxin toxicity.

TEST-TAKING TIP: Recall the action of each drug and what impact it would have on a client's magnesium level.

Content Area: *Adult Health*
Integrated Processes: *Nursing Process: Implementation*
Client Need: *Physiological Integrity*
Cognitive Level: *Application*
Reference: *Novello, N. P., and Blumstein, H. A. (2010). Hypermagnesemia: treatment and medication. http://emedicine.medscape.com/article/766604-treatment.*

18. ANSWER: 2.

Rationale:

1. Hypomagnesemia increases the client's DTRs. The desired outcome for this client would be a decrease in DTRs to within normal limits.
2. **The most appropriate outcome for a client with a nursing diagnosis of Risk for Falls Related to Skeletal Muscle Weakness Secondary to Hypomagnesemia is to remain free from injury throughout the hospital stay.**
3. Increasing oral fluid intake does not pertain to client safety.
4. Teaching about dietary magnesium intake does not pertain to client safety, and the dietitian should teach this client how to increase dietary magnesium.

TEST-TAKING TIP: Rule out the options that do not pertain to client safety.

Content Area: *Adult Health*
Integrated Processes: *Nursing Process: Analysis*
Client Need: *Safe and Effective Care Environment*
Cognitive Level: *Application*
Reference: *Ignatavicius, D., and Workman, M. (2012). Medical-Surgical Nursing: Patient-Centered Collaborative Care (7th ed.). St. Louis, MO: Saunders.*

19. ANSWER: 0.6.

Rationale:

$$22 \text{ lb} \div 2.2 \text{ lb/kg} = 10 \text{ kg}$$
$$10 \text{ kg} \times 30 \text{ mg/kg} = 300 \text{ mg}$$
$$300 \text{ mg}/X \times 500 \text{ mg}/1 \text{ mL} = 500X = 300 = 300/500 = 0.6 \text{ mL}$$

TEST-TAKING TIP: Remember to convert pounds to kilograms before setting up the equation.

Content Area: *Child Health*
Integrated Processes: *Nursing Process: Implementation*
Client Need: *Physiological Integrity*
Cognitive Level: *Application*
Reference: *Deglin, J. H., Vallerand, A. H., and Sanoski, C. A. (2013). Davis's Drug Guide for Nurses (13th ed.). Philadelphia, PA: F. A. Davis.*

20. ANSWER: 15.6.

Rationale:

$$0.45 \text{ mEq}/1 \text{ mL} \times 7 \text{ mEq}/X = 0.45X = 7 = 7/0.45 = 15.55 \text{ mL} = 15.6 \text{ mL (rounded to one decimal place)}$$

TEST-TAKING TIP: Always double-check your calculations before administering a medication to a client and before providing your answer on the NCLEX-RN examination.

Content Area: *Maternal Health*
Integrated Processes: *Nursing Process: Implementation*
Client Need: *Physiological Integrity*
Cognitive Level: *Application*
Reference: *Deglin, J. H., Vallerand, A. H., and Sanoski, C. A. (2013). Davis's Drug Guide for Nurses (13th ed.). Philadelphia, PA: F. A. Davis.*

21. ANSWER: 1.

Rationale:

1. **When implementing fall precautions for this client, the nurse should initially perform a fall risk assessment to determine the client's fall risk.**

2. The client's bed should be maintained in the lowest position with the wheels locked. In the Trendelenburg position, the client lies flat on the back (supine) with the feet higher than the head. This was once the standard position for treating shock, but it has fallen out of favor.
3. Assistive devices should be placed within reach beside the client's bed.
4. The client should be instructed to call for assistance before getting out of bed.
TEST-TAKING TIP: A fall risk assessment should be performed because both hypomagnesemia and hypermagnesemia cause muscle weakness.
Content Area: Older Adult Health
Integrated Processes: Nursing Process: Implementation
Client Need: Safe and Effective Care Environment
Cognitive Level: Application
Reference: *Ignatavicius, D., and Workman, M. (2012). Medical-Surgical Nursing: Patient-Centered Collaborative Care (7th ed.). St. Louis, MO: Saunders.*

22. ANSWER: 3, 5.
Rationale:
1. Fall precautions should be implemented because hypomagnesemia causes muscle weakness.
2. Hypomagnesemia may cause tetany and seizures because the lack of magnesium causes neuromuscular irritability.
3. The nurse should question the order to administer IV magnesium chloride because this medication should be administered—and is available—only in oral form. Oral magnesium should be given in divided doses, not once daily.
4. Cardiac monitoring is important in clients with magnesium imbalances because of the potential for dysrhythmias.
5. The nurse should question the order for furosemide because a loop diuretic would reduce the serum magnesium level further.
TEST-TAKING TIP: Remember that magnesium chloride (Slow-Mag) is given only *orally* and should be administered in divided doses. Rule out options 1, 2, and 4 because these are appropriate nursing actions.
Content Area: Adult Health
Integrated Processes: Nursing Process: Analysis
Client Need: Safe and Effective Care Environment
Cognitive Level: Analysis
References: *Deglin, J. H., Vallerand, A. H., and Sanoski, C. A. (2013). Davis's Drug Guide for Nurses (13th ed.). Philadelphia, PA: F. A. Davis; Ignatavicius, D., and Workman, M. (2012). Medical-Surgical Nursing: Patient-Centered Collaborative Care (7th ed.). St. Louis, MO: Saunders.*

23. ANSWER: 3.
Rationale:
1. The client's heart rate may be slightly elevated, but respiratory alterations should be the priority.
2. The client may be hypertensive, but respiratory alterations should be the priority.
3. The nurse should investigate the client's bradypnea, because the administration of IV magnesium sulfate places the client at increased risk for hypermagnesemia and magnesium toxicity. Loss of patellar reflexes, respiratory and neuromuscular depression, oliguria, and decreased level of consciousness are signs of magnesium toxicity.
4. The client may have a low-grade temperature, but respiratory alterations should be the priority.
TEST-TAKING TIP: Remember that the desired effect of magnesium sulfate also increases the client's risk of central nervous system depression. Use the "ABCs" to assist in prioritizing nursing interventions.
Content Area: Maternal Health
Integrated Processes: Nursing Process: Implementation
Client Need: Safe and Effective Care Environment
Cognitive Level: Analysis
Reference: *Perry, S., Hockenberry, M., Lowdermilk, D., and Wilson, D. (2010). Maternal Child Nursing Care (4th ed.). St. Louis, MO: Mosby.*

24. ANSWER: 4.
Rationale:
1. Administering oxygen is important for this client but should not be the first priority.
2. Implementing seizure precautions is important for this client but should not be the first priority.
3. Magnesium should be administered to reduce the client's risk of dysrhythmias, but this should not be the nurse's first priority.
4. The nurse's *first* intervention should be to place the client on continuous telemetry because the client is experiencing severe hypomagnesemia. A low serum magnesium level may predispose the client to life-threatening cardiac dysrhythmias.
TEST-TAKING TIP: Use the nursing process. Assess first, and then implement. Placing the client on continuous telemetry is part of the nursing assessment.
Content Area: Child Health
Integrated Processes: Nursing Process: Implementation
Client Need: Safe and Effective Care Environment
Cognitive Level: Analysis
Reference: *Ignatavicius, D., and Workman, M. (2012). Medical-Surgical Nursing: Patient-Centered Collaborative Care (7th ed.). St. Louis, MO: Saunders.*

25. ANSWER: 3.
Rationale:
1. ECG strip 1 shows sinus tachycardia, which is associated with hypomagnesemia.
2. ECG strip 2 shows a normal sinus rhythm.
3. The nurse is most likely to observe sinus bradycardia because the client is exhibiting signs of hypermagnesemia.
4. ECG strip 4 shows peaked T waves associated with hyperkalemia.
TEST-TAKING TIP: Review the effects of hypermagnesemia on the electrical conduction of the heart, and select the option that illustrates those effects.
Content Area: Adult Health
Integrated Processes: Nursing Process: Analysis
Client Need: Physiological Integrity
Cognitive Level: Analysis
References: *Jones, S. (2010). ECG Notes: Interpretation and Management Guide (2nd ed.). Philadelphia, PA: F. A. Davis; Williams, L., and Hopper, P. (2011). Understanding Medical-Surgical Nursing (4th ed.). Philadelphia, PA: F. A. Davis.*

Chapter 7

Phosphate Imbalances

KEY TERMS

Catecholamines—Water-soluble hormones, including epinephrine, norepinephrine, and dopamine, that are produced by the adrenal glands and increased in times of stress.

Hyperphosphatemia—Serum phosphorus greater than 4.5 mg/dL (4.5 mEq/L); phosphate excess.

Hypophosphatemia—Serum phosphorus less than 2.5 mg/dL (3.0 mEq/L); phosphate deficit.

Phosphate—A compound of phosphorus and oxygen that occurs in many forms and is usually combined with other elements, such as sodium, potassium, calcium, and aluminum; required to support life; phosphorus is found in the blood, and phosphate is found in all other body fluids and tissues.

Phosphorus—A mineral found in meats, milk, and whole grains that is present in every cell of the body but predominantly in the bones and teeth; important for the maintenance and repair of cells and tissues; serum phosphorus levels are measured in the blood.

Refeeding syndrome—A disorder in which metabolic disturbances result when nourishment is provided to a malnourished or starved client; usually occurs within 4 days of refeeding; causes fluid and electrolyte disturbances, especially hypophosphatemia.

Tetany—A combination of signs and symptoms, usually due to low calcium; these can include hyperreflexia (overactive neurological reflexes), carpopedal spasms (spasms of the hands and feet), cramps, and laryngospasm (spasm of the larynx).

Total parenteral nutrition (TPN)—Intravenous administration of all nutritional needs; used for clients who cannot tolerate adequate feedings via the enteral route; usually administered via central line.

Vitamin D—A fat-soluble vitamin needed for the absorption and metabolism of calcium and phosphorus; calcitriol is the active form of vitamin D.

I. Description

Phosphate (PO_4^-) is the major anion in the intracellular fluid (ICF). Although elemental **phosphorus** (P) is an essential mineral, it is never found as a free element in nature because of its high reactivity. Phosphorus is found in the body in combination with oxygen, as phosphate. The average American diet is high in phosphorus (1 to 2 gm/day); it is plentiful in meats, fish, poultry, milk products, and legumes. Although the terms "phosphorus" and "phosphate" are often used interchangeably, laboratory tests actually measure the amount of elemental phosphorus, not phosphate, in the blood, which may be confusing. Phosphate is excreted from the body in urine and stool. Approximately 85% of the phosphate in the body is bound with calcium in the teeth and bones (Fig. 7.1). The remainder is located primarily inside the cells. Phosphate performs the following functions:

1. Is essential in the formation of teeth and bones
2. Helps regulate calcium levels
3. Assists in muscle contraction, maintenance of heart rhythm, and kidney function
4. Aids in nerve conduction and cell membrane integrity
5. Sustains the functioning of red blood cells and is needed for the release of oxygen from hemoglobin molecules
6. Is an integral component of the nucleic acids that constitute DNA and RNA; phosphate bonds of adenosine triphosphate (ATP) carry the energy required for all cellular functions
7. Acts as a buffer to maintain acid-base balance
8. Is involved in protein, fat, and carbohydrate metabolism

Normal Lab Value The normal serum phosphorus level in adults is 2.5 to 4.5 mg/dL (3.0 to 4.5 mEq/L).

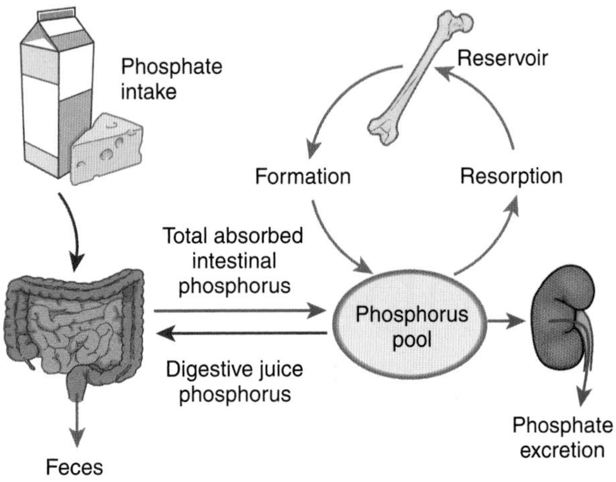

Fig 7.1 Phosphate homeostasis. When phosphorus is consumed, it is absorbed by the intestines; attaches to and detaches from different molecules, forming a constantly shifting phosphate pool; is stored in the bones and teeth until needed; and is excreted by the kidneys via urine or in the feces as part of the digestive juices.

DID YOU KNOW?

Children have higher serum phosphorus levels than adults because of their growing skeletons. Newborns' serum phosphorus levels are about twice as high as adults'.

II. Types of Phosphate Imbalance

Phosphate imbalances occur when there is an increase or decrease in the phosphorus content of the blood. Calcium imbalances almost always accompany phosphorus imbalances (Box 7.1).

A. **Hypophosphatemia**, or phosphate deficit, is a serum phosphorus level less than 2.5 mg/dL (3.0 mEq/L).
   1. Signs and symptoms of hypophosphatemia may not be apparent unless serum levels decrease to about 1 mg/dL.
   2. Manifestations are seen more often in chronic hypophosphatemia.

(!) The most dangerous problems associated with hypophosphatemia are related to *hypercalcemia,* which can lead to severe cardiovascular and neuromuscular problems.

B. **Hyperphosphatemia**, or phosphate excess, is a serum phosphorus level greater than 4.5 mg/dL (4.5 mEq/L).
   1. Hyperphosphatemia is relatively rare, except in clients with severe renal dysfunction; dialysis does not reduce the client's risk of hyperphosphatemia because dialysis does not remove phosphate efficiently.
   2. High phosphate levels are usually well tolerated, but the accompanying hypocalcemia causes problems.
   3. Hyperphosphatemia does not routinely produce signs and symptoms; manifestations are most often due to the underlying disorder causing the imbalance and other associated electrolyte abnormalities.

Box 7.1 Phosphorus and Calcium Balance: An Inverse Relationship

Phosphorus and calcium have an inverse relationship in the body. When serum phosphorus levels are elevated, serum calcium levels are decreased, and vice versa. High serum phosphorus levels decrease the movement of calcium from bones, causing hypocalcemia. Low serum phosphorus levels increase the movement of calcium from bones, causing hypercalcemia. Both phosphorus and calcium are regulated by parathyroid hormone (PTH) and calcitriol, the active form of **vitamin D**. PTH is secreted by the parathyroid glands when serum calcium levels are low. PTH *increases* serum calcium levels and *decreases* serum phosphorus levels to maintain the calcium-phosphorus balance in the body. Calcitriol is needed for gastrointestinal absorption and renal resorption of both calcium and phosphorus. Thus, vitamin D deficiency results in a decrease of both calcium and phosphorus in the body.

III. Causes of Phosphate Imbalance

Phosphate imbalances may be caused by actual or relative increases or decreases in phosphorus. An *actual* increase or decrease may be caused by phosphorus gain or loss, excessive or inadequate intake or absorption, and increased or decreased renal excretion. A *relative* increase or decrease occurs when phosphate shifts back and forth between intracellular and extracellular compartments. When phosphate shifts into the intracellular compartment, hypophosphatemia occurs; when phosphate shifts out of the cells and into the extracellular fluid (ECF), hyperphosphatemia occurs (Table 7.1).

A. Actual hypophosphatemia
   1. Phosphorus loss
      a. Vomiting, diarrhea, steatorrhea, and prolonged gastric suctioning can cause hypophosphatemia.
      b. Severe burns, and the associated release of catecholamines, decrease serum phosphorus levels; the maximal loss occurs between days two and five after the burn. Despite aggressive phosphorus supplementation, serum phosphorus levels rarely return to normal before day 10.
   2. Inadequate intake of phosphorus
      a. Malnutrition, starvation, prolonged NPO status
      b. Administration of total parenteral nutrition (TPN) in the absence of adequate serum phosphorus levels or phosphorus supplementation
      c. Alcohol abuse, which results in poor nutritional intake of phosphorus and other minerals, as well as vomiting, diarrhea, and antacid use

Table 7.1 Causes of Phosphate Imbalance

Imbalance	Causes
Hypophosphatemia	
Actual decrease in phosphate	Phosphate loss • Vomiting • Diarrhea • Steatorrhea (excess fat in feces) • Prolonged gastric suctioning • Severe burns • Excessive calcium supplementation • Hyperparathyroidism Inadequate intake • Malnutrition • Starvation • Prolonged NPO status • Administration of total parenteral nutrition (TPN) • Alcohol abuse Impaired absorption • Primary hyperthyroidism • Vitamin D deficiency (decreases renal reabsorption of phosphate) • Malabsorption syndromes, such as celiac disease or Crohn's disease • Medications (excessive intake) *-antacids and phosphate binders such as aluminum hydroxide (Amphojel), calcium carbonate (Tums), and magnesium hydroxide/aluminum hydroxide (Mylanta)* Increased excretion • Medications (those that act on the kidneys to increase phosphate excretion) *-corticosteroids such as prednisolone (Orapred) and dexamethasone (DexPak)* *-loop diuretics such as furosemide (Lasix)* *-thiazide diuretics such as chlorothiazide (Diuril)* • Hyperglycemia • Renal transplantation • Chronic kidney disease
Relative decrease in phosphate	Shift from extracellular compartments • FVE • Glucose and insulin administration • Refeeding syndrome (when previously malnourished clients are fed high-carbohydrate loads, the result is a rapid decrease in serum phosphorus, magnesium, and potassium levels) • Hungry bone syndrome • Acid-base imbalances (respiratory alkalosis, metabolic acidosis) • Alcohol withdrawal • Medications (hormonal effects cause phosphate to shift into cells) *-catecholamines such as epinephrine (Primatene, EpiPen) and dopamine (Intropin), terbutaline, albuterol (Proventil HFA, Ventolin HFA)* *-hormones such as glucagon (GlucaGen) and calcitonin (Fortical)* *-insulins such as regular insulin*
Hyperphosphatemia	
Actual increase in phosphate	Phosphate gain • IV phosphorus infusion • Excessive dietary ingestion of phosphorus • Feeding infants cow's milk • Vitamin D intoxication • Excessive use of phosphate-containing laxatives or enemas Increased absorption or retention • Vitamin D excess • Acute renal failure • Chronic kidney disease • Hypoparathyroidism • Vitamin D intoxication • Bisphosphonate therapy • Calcium or magnesium deficiency

Continued

Table 7.1 Causes of Phosphate Imbalance—cont'd

Imbalance	Causes
Relative increase in phosphate	Shift from intracellular compartment • Hemolysis • Chemotherapy for malignant tumors • Tumor lysis syndrome • Rhabdomyolysis • Hypoparathyroidism • Acid-base disorders (lactic acidosis, DKA, respiratory acidosis) • Sepsis or severe infection • Crush injuries or tissue trauma

3. Impaired absorption of phosphorus
   a. Primary hyperparathyroidism, caused by the oversecretion of parathyroid hormone (PTH), is the most common cause of increased renal phosphate excretion resulting in hypophosphatemia.
   b. Vitamin D and vitamin E deficiencies can contribute to hypophosphatemia by failing to stimulate phosphate absorption.
   c. Malabsorption syndromes, such as celiac disease or Crohn's disease, also result in hypophosphatemia.
   d. Antacids, such as magnesium- and aluminum-containing antacids, bind with phosphorus, inhibiting absorption.

DID YOU KNOW?

Celiac disease, also known as celiac sprue, is a genetic autoimmune disorder of the small intestine. It is caused by an inflammatory reaction to gluten that adversely affects the absorption of nutrients in the intestine and is characterized by chronic diarrhea, fatigue, and failure to thrive (in children). The only effective treatment is a lifelong gluten-free diet.

4. Increased excretion of phosphorus
   a. Certain medications, such as corticosteroids, loop diuretics, and thiazide diuretics, cause an increase in phosphate excretion as they act on the kidneys to increase urine output.
   b. Hyperglycemia causes an increase in the urinary loss of phosphorus.

B. Relative hypophosphatemia
1. Water gain
   a. Fluid volume excess (FVE) results in the dilution of phosphorus ions without an actual decrease in the amount of phosphorus in the body.
2. Phosphate shift into the intracellular compartment
   a. In **refeeding syndrome**, the administration of concentrated glucose solutions results in the release of insulin, causing glucose and phosphorus to move into the cells.
   b. Hungry bone syndrome occurs most often in postsurgical clients with bone disease caused by increased levels of PTH; severe hypocalcemia develops, which causes serum phosphorus levels to become elevated.
   c. Insulin administration, as in the treatment of diabetic ketoacidosis, also causes phosphorus to shift into the cells.
   d. Acute respiratory alkalosis, only caused by hyperventilation, causes phosphorus to move out of the cells and into the ECF.
   e. **Catecholamines,** such as epinephrine and dopamine, and hormones, such as glucagon and calcitonin, also cause phosphate to shift into the cells, resulting in a relative decrease in serum phosphorus levels.

C. Actual hyperphosphatemia
1. Phosphate gain
   a. Excessive IV phosphorus infusion
   b. Excessive dietary intake or supplements
   c. Feeding infants cow's milk (940 mg phosphorus) instead of breast milk (150 mg phosphorus)
   d. Excessive use of phosphate-containing laxatives or enemas, such as Phospho-Soda.

MAKING THE CONNECTION

Refeeding Syndrome and Phosphorus

Refeeding syndrome occurs when malnourished clients are fed high-carbohydrate diets, causing hyperglycemia. The sudden increase in the serum glucose level decreases the urinary excretion of phosphorus and stimulates the release of insulin, which causes phosphorus to shift into the cells. Hypokalemia and hypomagnesemia may also exist. One of the earliest reports of refeeding syndrome involved starved prisoners of war during World War II. Today, clients with anorexia nervosa, on prolonged NPO status, or receiving parenteral or enteral feedings after major surgery are at greatest risk for refeeding syndrome.

MAKING THE CONNECTION

Hypoparathyroidism and Phosphorus

Hypoparathyroidism is caused by the inadequate secretion of PTH by the parathyroid glands, which lie directly beneath the thyroid gland. Damage to or removal of one or more parathyroid glands, usually because of a surgical error during thyroidectomy, leads to decreased serum calcium levels and increased serum phosphorus levels—an inverse relationship. The symptoms of hypoparathyroidism are caused by hypocalcemia and can range from mild paresthesias (tingling in the hands, fingers, and around the mouth) to severe muscle cramping of the entire body (**tetany**).

2. Increased phosphate absorption or retention
   a. Low PTH levels (hypoparathyroidism) and high vitamin D levels enhance phosphate absorption in the renal proximal tubules, resulting in the retention of phosphorus.
3. Decreased excretion of phosphate
   a. Chronic glomerulonephritis, renal insufficiency, acute kidney injury, and chronic kidney disease decrease the kidneys' ability to excrete phosphorus.

D. Relative hyperphosphatemia
1. Water loss
   a. Fluid volume deficit (FVD) results in the hemoconcentration of phosphorus and other electrolytes, without an actual increase in the amount of phosphorus in the body.
2. Phosphate shift into the extracellular compartment
   a. Cell damage (lysis), crush injuries, tissue trauma, and severe infection cause phosphate to shift out of the cells.
   b. Rhabdomyolysis, the breakdown of muscle, results in the release of muscle fiber contents (myoglobin) into the bloodstream; this frequently results in kidney damage or failure.

IV. Nursing Assessment for Phosphate Imbalance

The nurse should conduct a focused nursing assessment for phosphate imbalance, beginning with a thorough nursing history. However, because most clients with hypophosphatemia are asymptomatic, the history alone rarely indicates the possibility of hypophosphatemia. Interview the client and family members to identify any risk factors or preexisting conditions that would contribute to phosphate imbalance, such as vomiting, nasogastric suctioning, diarrhea, acute kidney injury, chronic kidney disease, or other conditions associated with phosphorus loss or gain. The nurse should also assess the client's ability to drink and tolerate oral fluids. Include a current dietary history, inquiring about dietary habits. The nursing history should also include lifestyle factors, such as long-standing alcohol use and chronic malnutrition, and current medications, including excessive antacid use or the intake of glucocorticoids or chemotherapeutic agents. A thorough physical assessment is necessary because hyperphosphatemia is associated with hypocalcemia; thus, the client should be asked about recent muscle cramps, bone pain, or fractures. Assess each body system, observing for signs and symptoms of phosphorus imbalance as well as related calcium imbalances. Measure and record the client's vital signs, and review the client's laboratory data to assess for the presence of hypo- or hyperphosphatemia (Table 7.2).

V. Nursing Interventions for Clients with Phosphate Imbalance

A. Implement the health-care provider's orders to treat the underlying cause of the imbalance.
1. The health-care provider's orders may include the administration of IV fluids, phosphate and/or calcium supplementation, correction of related electrolyte or acid-base imbalances, and treatment of the underlying conditions (Table 7.3).

B. Monitor the client and the client's serum phosphorus level.
1. Monitor the client's serum phosphorus level as ordered by the health-care provider.
   a. Normal reference range for serum phosphorus is 2.5 to 4.5 mg/dL.
2. Monitor other laboratory values associated with phosphate imbalances.
   a. Calcium: normal reference range is 8.2 to 10.2 mg/dL.
   b. Blood urea nitrogen (BUN): normal reference range is 8 to 21 mg/dL.
   c. Creatinine: normal reference range is 0.5 to 1.2 mg/dL.
3. Monitor for cerebral changes.
   a. Establish the client's usual cognitive and behavioral pattern.
   b. Observe the client's behavior, level of consciousness, and mental status.
   c. Monitor for seizure activity.
4. Monitor for cardiovascular changes.
   a. Auscultate the apical pulse.
   b. Palpate peripheral pulses.
   c. Check orthostatic blood pressure.
   d. Observe for ECG changes.
5. Monitor for neuromuscular changes.
   a. Establish a baseline for the client's deep tendon reflexes (DTRs) and muscle strength and tone.

Table 7.2 Signs and Symptoms of Phosphate Imbalance

Vital Signs		
	Hypophosphatemia	*Hyperphosphatemia*
Blood pressure	Possibly decreased	Possibly decreased
Heart rate	Decreased	Possibly decreased
Respiratory rate	Decreased	Possibly decreased; depends on degree of accompanying hypocalcemia
Temperature	Within normal limits	Within normal limits
Signs and Symptoms by Body System		
	Hypophosphatemia	*Hyperphosphatemia*
Cardiovascular	• Decreased stroke volume • Decreased cardiac output • Weak peripheral pulses • Bradycardia • Bruising, bleeding, and anemia (secondary to increased fragility of red blood cells from low ATP levels)	• In the setting of severe renal dysfunction, calcium combines with phosphate to form crystals and calcifications in arteries, producing severe arteriosclerosis • Hypotension • Heart failure
Cerebral	Severe hypophosphatemia only: • Irritability • Change in level of consciousness • Possibly seizures • Coma	• Altered mental status • Confusion, irritability, anxiety • Obtundation • Coma • Seizures
ECG changes	None	• Prolongation of Q-T interval
Integumentary	None	• Crystals can form in the skin, causing severe itching
Neuromuscular	• Generalized muscle weakness; may progress to acute rhabdomyolysis • Paresthesias usually not present	• Paresthesias, especially circumoral and distal extremities • Muscle spasms, cramping, or tetany (positive Chvostek's sign and Trousseau's sign)
Respiratory	• Hypoventilation to respiratory failure as muscles weaken • Bradypnea	• Respiratory depression secondary to respiratory muscle weakness • Severe hyperphosphatemia may produce respiratory arrest
Skeletal	Chronic hypophosphatemia: • Decreased bone density • Fractures • Changes in bone shape	None
Laboratory Values		
	Hypophosphatemia	*Hyperphosphatemia*
Serum phosphorus level	Less than 2.5 mg/dL	Greater than 4.5 mg/dL

Table 7.3 Nursing Interventions to Control Serum Phosphorus Levels

Hypophosphatemia	**Hyperphosphatemia**
Increase serum phosphorus level	Decrease serum phosphorus level; increase serum calcium level
• Dietary management includes increasing phosphorus intake and decreasing calcium intake • Discontinue use of all medications or preparations that promote phosphate loss *-antacids such as magnesium hydroxide/aluminum hydroxide (Maalox)* *-calcium supplements such as calcium carbonate (Caltrate, Os-Cal, Tums)* *-osmotic diuretics such as mannitol (Osmitrol)*	• Discontinue medications or preparations that contain phosphorus • Decrease dietary intake of phosphorus • Saline diuresis can assist in dilution and increase the excretion of phosphate Administer medications as ordered • Diuretics that act on the proximal renal tubules to decrease total serum phosphorus by increasing excretion by the kidneys *-acetazolamide (Diamox)* • Phosphate binders to decrease serum phosphorus levels by reducing the absorption of phosphorus

Continued

Table 7.3 Nursing Interventions to Control Serum Phosphorus Levels—cont'd

Hypophosphatemia	Hyperphosphatemia
Administer medications as ordered • Oral or IV phosphate supplements to increase serum phosphorus levels *-potassium phosphate PO (Neutra-Phos-K)* *-potassium/sodium phosphate PO (Neutra-Phos)* *-sodium phosphate IV* 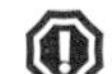 IV phosphorus infusions should not exceed 10 mEq/hr • Supplement with vitamin D to promote the absorption of calcium and phosphorus	*-aluminum hydroxide (ALternaGEL, Alu-Cap, Alu-Tab, Amphojel)* *-calcium acetate (PhosLo)* *-calcium carbonate—the medication most commonly prescribed for hyperphosphatemia (Alka-Mints, Caltrate 600, Chooz, Os-Cal 500, Calcium-Rich Rolaids, Titralac, Tums)* *-lanthanum carbonate (Fosrenol)* *-sevelamer hydrochloride (Renagel)*

b. Monitor the client for paresthesias, muscle weakness, muscle twitching, and irregular muscle contractions during each nursing shift.

6. Monitor for respiratory changes.
   a. Auscultate lung sounds.
   b. Observe the frequency and character of respirations.

C. Ensure client safety.

1. Reduce environmental stimuli.
   a. Provide a quiet room.
   b. Limit the client's visitors.
   c. Darken the client's room.
   d. Speak in soft tones.
2. Implement seizure precautions related to hyperphosphatemia and hypocalcemia.
   a. Pad the side rails.
   b. Have oxygen and suction equipment available.
   c. Ensure the patency of IV access devices.
   d. Administer emergency medications as ordered.
   e. Prepare for possible endotracheal intubation.
   f. Prepare for cardiac defibrillation if necessary.
3. Implement fall precautions related to muscle weakness caused by hypophosphatemia and hypercalcemia.
   a. Perform a fall risk assessment.
   b. Maintain the bed in a low position with locked wheels.
   c. Remove all obstacles from pathways, especially to the toilet.
   d. Monitor the environment for safety hazards (e.g., torn carpet, liquid spills on floors).
   e. Place assistive devices (walkers, canes) within the client's reach.
   f. Use nightlights.
   g. Instruct the client to request assistance to ambulate.
   h. Ensure the availability of the call light.
   i. Assess the client's footwear and provide appropriate footwear if necessary; clients must use antiskid soles.
   j. Keep items such as the telephone and fluids close to the client.
   k. Request that family members remain with the client if necessary.
   l. Position the client to allow close observation by staff members.
   m. Communicate the client's fall risk during the shift report and as necessary.

D. Educate the client.

1. Hypophosphatemia
   a. Teach the client or caregiver the causes of phosphate deficiency.
   b. Provide specific information regarding the client's medical diagnosis and related interventions or treatments.
   c. Teach the client how to identify the signs and symptoms of phosphate deficiency.
   d. Instruct the client and family to notify the primary health-care provider if the client exhibits signs or symptoms of hypophosphatemia or if they have any other specific concerns.
   e. Teach the client how to prevent phosphate deficiency.
      1) Teach the client about foods that contain phosphorus.
      2) Instruct the client to decrease calcium intake by avoiding high-calcium foods, such as milk, cheese, yogurt, collard greens, and rhubarb.
   f. Teach the client how to take oral phosphate supplements.
      1) Instruct the client to report adverse effects, such as nausea, vomiting, diarrhea, and abdominal cramping, to the primary health-care provider.
      2) Encourage the client to keep appointments for laboratory studies to evaluate serum phosphorus levels.
   g. Ensure that the client or caregiver understands the specifics, rationale, potential side effects, and desired effects of the treatment regimen.
   h. Include medication administration, nutrition, hydration, dietary restrictions, and foods high in phosphorus in client teaching.

2. Hyperphosphatemia
   a. Teach the client or caregiver the causes of phosphate excess.
   b. Provide specific information regarding the client's medical diagnosis and related interventions or treatments.
   c. Teach the client how to identify the signs and symptoms of phosphate excess.
   d. Instruct the client and family to notify the primary health-care provider if the client exhibits signs or symptoms of hyperphosphatemia or if they have any other specific concerns.
   e. Teach the client how to prevent phosphate excess.
      1) Avoid foods that are high in phosphorus: meats, organ meats, nuts, whole-grain breads, cereals.
      2) Avoid processed foods, many of which are "hidden sources" of phosphorus.
      3) Increase calcium intake.
      4) Teach the client and family how to read food labels, which list the amount of phosphorus contained in each serving.
      5) Encourage the client to keep appointments for laboratory studies to evaluate serum phosphorus levels.
   f. Ensure that the client or caregiver understands the specifics, rationale, potential side effects, and desired effects of the treatment regimen.
   g. Include medication administration, nutrition, hydration, dietary restrictions, and foods high in phosphorus in client teaching.

E. Evaluate and document.
1. Document all assessment findings and interventions per institution policy.
2. Evaluate and document the client's response to interventions and education.

CASE STUDY: Putting It All Together

Subjective Data

An older adult client who has been diagnosed with end-stage renal disease presents to the emergency department after missing a scheduled dialysis appointment 2 days ago. The client reports fatigue, muscle aches, itching, weakness, and severe cramping for 1 day. The client has a history of congestive heart failure, chronic kidney disease, and hypertension. The client has no known allergies. Current medications are:

- metoprolol (Toprol-XL) 100 mg by mouth (PO) daily
- lisinopril (Zestril) 5 mg PO daily
- digoxin (Lanoxin) 0.25 mg PO daily
- aspirin 81 mg PO daily
- furosemide (Lasix) 40 mg PO daily
- sevelamer hydrochloride (Renagel) 2 800-mg tablets three times per day with meals
- calcium carbonate (Caltrate 600) 1 tablet per day

Objective Data

Nursing Assessment

1. Alert, oriented to person, place, and time
2. Heart sounds S_1, S_2, and S_3 are present, irregular; no murmur
3. Crackles in lung bases bilaterally
4. Jugular venous distention (JVD)
5. Pedal and radial pulses irregular, 3+, and bounding bilaterally
6. DTRs 3+ (hyperactive) bilaterally
7. Positive Chvostek's sign and Trousseau's sign
8. Bowel sounds hyperactive in all four quadrants

Vital Signs	
Temperature:	97.8°F (36.6°C) orally
Blood pressure:	142/98 mm Hg
Heart rate:	58 bpm, irregular
Respiratory rate:	24
O_2 saturation:	91%

Laboratory Results	
Serum sodium:	140 mEq/L
Serum potassium:	6.7 mEq/L
Serum calcium:	6.2 mg/dL
Serum phosphorus:	8.2 mg/dL
Blood glucose:	80 mg/dL
Serum BUN:	68 mg/dL
Serum creatinine:	15.4 mg/dL
Chest x-ray:	cardiomegaly
ECG:	sinus bradycardia with prolonged Q-T interval, prolonged ST segment, occasional premature ventricular contractions (PVCs)

Health-Care Provider Orders

1. O_2 2 L/min via nasal cannula.
2. Place on telemetry; report any changes to health-care provider.
3. Prepare for emergent dialysis; check patency of dialysis site.

CASE STUDY: Putting It All Together *cont'd*

4. Vital signs every 15 minutes × 2 hours, every 30 minutes × 2 hours, every 1 hour × 2 hours, then every 4 hours × 24 hours.
5. Hold Lasix.
6. Begin 0.9% saline solution at 200 mL/hr × 2 hours and then decrease to 100 mL/hr.
7. Monitor for fluid volume excess.
8. Recheck serum sodium, potassium, phosphorus, calcium, glucose, and creatinine levels at the end of dialysis; repeat every 6 hours.
9. Check PTH, digoxin, thyroid-stimulating hormone (TSH), bicarbonate, chloride, and vitamin D levels; call health-care provider with results.
10. Implement a low-phosphate diet.
11. If the phosphorus level remains greater than 5.5 mg/dL after dialysis, increase Renagel to 4 tablets 30 minutes to 1 hour before each meal. When the phosphorus level is 3.5 to 5.5 mg/dL, keep at the current dose. If the phosphorus level is less than 3.5 mg/dL, decrease Renagel by 1 tablet at each meal.
12. Increase Caltrate 600 to 1 tablet PO with each meal.
13. Monitor bowel function for constipation; give docusate and senna (Senna-S) 2 tablets at bedtime as needed if no bowel movement in 3 days.
14. Obtain palliative care consultation for goals of care and code status.

Case Study Questions

A. What *subjective* assessment findings indicate that the client is experiencing a health alteration?

1. ______
2. ______
3. ______
4. ______
5. ______
6. ______
7. ______

B. What *objective* assessment findings indicate that the client is experiencing a health alteration?

1. ______
2. ______
3. ______
4. ______
5. ______
6. ______
7. ______
8. ______
9. ______
10. ______
11. ______
12. ______

C. After analyzing the data collected, what **primary** nursing diagnosis should the nurse assign to this client?

______

Continued

CASE STUDY: Putting It All Together *cont'd*

Case Study Questions

D. What interventions should the nurse plan and/or implement to meet this client's needs?

1. ______
2. ______
3. ______
4. ______
5. ______
6. ______
7. ______
8. ______
9. ______
10. ______
11. ______
12. ______
13. ______
14. ______

E. What client outcomes should the nurse plan to evaluate the effectiveness of the nursing interventions?

1. ______
2. ______
3. ______
4. ______
5. ______
6. ______

REVIEW QUESTIONS

1. Which laboratory value should a nurse anticipate when caring for a client diagnosed with hypophosphatemia?
   1. Serum phosphorus level 2.5 mg/dL
   2. Serum phosphorus level 4.7 mg/dL
   3. Serum calcium level 9 mg/dL
   4. Serum calcium level 11 mg/dL

2. A client diagnosed with chronic kidney disease is scheduled to start taking sevelamer hydrochloride (Renagel). A nurse should teach the client to observe for which side effects of this medication? **Select all that apply.**
   1. Constipation
   2. Hypophosphatemia
   3. Hyperphosphatemia
   4. Diarrhea
   5. Hypocalcemia
   6. Hypercalcemia

3. Which clinical manifestations should a nurse associate with chronic hyperphosphatemia if assessed in a newly admitted client?
   1. Paresthesias
   2. Weak peripheral pulses
   3. Weak skeletal muscles
   4. Positive Trousseau's sign

4. A nurse is admitting a client who is experiencing abdominal cramping, diarrhea, muscle spasms, and tingling around the mouth. Which electrolyte imbalance should the nurse associate with these signs?
   1. Hypercalcemia
   2. Hypermagnesemia
   3. Hyperphosphatemia
   4. Hyperchloremia

5. Which intervention should be a nurse's *priority* in the care of an older adult client with a serum phosphorus level of 1.9 mg/dL?
   1. Implementing seizure precautions
   2. Administering calcium carbonate (Tums)
   3. Completing a thorough diet history
   4. Administering acetazolamide (Diamox)

6. Which factor should a nurse associate with an increased risk for hypophosphatemia if identified in the medical history of a client with a serum phosphorus level of 2 mg/dL?
   1. Hypoparathyroidism
   2. Acute renal failure
   3. Rhabdomyolysis
   4. Diabetic ketoacidosis (DKA)

7. Which foods should a nurse teach a client to include in the diet to promote an increase in the client's daily intake of phosphorus?
   1. Collard greens and milk
   2. Pork and nuts
   3. Fresh and dried fruits
   4. Canned vegetables and soups

8. A nurse is caring for a client who has a serum phosphorus level of 2.1 mg/dL. Which medication should the nurse anticipate being ordered to correct the client's imbalance?
   1. IV potassium phosphate 15 mmol daily
   2. Vitamin D 1,400 IU by mouth daily
   3. Calcium carbonate (Caltrate) 1 tablet twice a day with meals
   4. Magnesium hydroxide/aluminum hydroxide (Maalox) PO three times a day with meals

9. Which food should a nurse, who is providing discharge instructions to a client diagnosed with hypophosphatemia, advise the client to *avoid*?
   1. Potato chips
   2. Yogurt
   3. Walnuts
   4. Liver

10. A nurse is preparing to administer IV potassium phosphate to a client diagnosed with severe hypophosphatemia. A health-care provider orders IV potassium phosphate 21 mmol over 4 hours. The dose on hand is 21 mmol/250 mL normal saline solution. How many milliliters of this medication should the nurse administer each hour? Record your answer as a whole number.

    ____

11. A nurse is instructing an older adult client who has been diagnosed with chronic kidney disease how to maintain a normal serum phosphorus level. In addition to dietary instructions, the client is being treated with calcium acetate (PhosLo) 2,000 mg PO three times per day with meals. How many tablets of the preparation shown in the exhibit should the nurse instruct the client to take with each meal? Record your answer as a whole number.

____

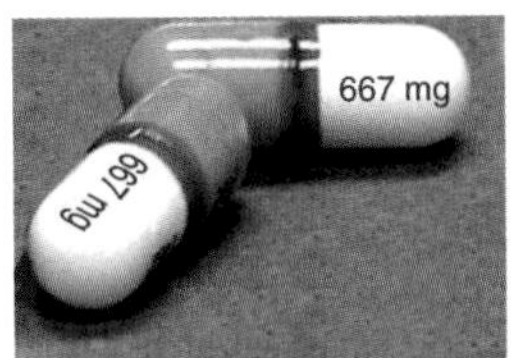

12. A nurse is preparing to administer IV potassium phosphate to a client diagnosed with severe hypophosphatemia. A health-care provider orders IV potassium phosphate 15 mmol at 3 mmol/hr. The dose on hand is 15 mmol/250 mL normal saline. How many milliliters of this medication should the nurse administer each hour? Record your answer as a whole number.

____

13. Which nursing diagnoses should a nurse assign to a client who is experiencing chronic hypophosphatemia? **Select all that apply.**
 1. Diarrhea Related to Spastic Colonic Activity
 2. Risk for Injury Related to Muscle Weakness
 3. Decreased Cardiac Output Related to Dysrhythmia
 4. Impaired Physical Mobility Related to Skeletal Muscle Weakness
 5. Potential for Respiratory Insufficiency Related to Muscle Weakness

14. Which clinical manifestation should a nurse associate with the development of hyperphosphatemia if it is observed in a client diagnosed with kidney disease?
 1. Itchy skin
 2. Muscle weakness
 3. Diarrhea
 4. Peaked T waves

15. A nurse is developing a plan of care with a client who has a nursing diagnosis of Risk for Injury Related to Muscle Weakness Secondary to Hypophosphatemia. Which outcome should receive priority in the plan of care?
 1. Cardiac rhythm will be monitored continuously.
 2. Client will decrease dietary intake of calcium.
 3. Client will remain free from injury.
 4. Client will maintain blood pressure within the normal range.

16. Which client should a nurse identify as being at greatest risk for developing hyperphosphatemia?
 1. A 20-year-old client with diabetic ketoacidosis
 2. A 45-year-old client with hypoparathyroidism
 3. A 55-year-old client who has been abusing alcohol
 4. A 75-year-old client who is taking sucralfate (Carafate) to treat an ulcer

17. An adolescent client presents to a clinic reporting numbness and tingling of the fingertips, muscle cramps, and weakness. Other findings include a body mass index of 17, blood pressure of 90/56 mm Hg, and serum phosphorus level of 2.3 mg/dL. Which additional information should the nurse obtain? **Select all that apply.**
 1. Alcohol use
 2. Laxative use
 3. Amount of exercise
 4. Detailed nutrition assessment
 5. Serum magnesium level
 6. Serum PTH level

18. A student nurse has been given instructions about the prevention of hypophosphatemia. Which statement, if made by the student, should indicate to the nursing instructor that the student has an adequate understanding of the role of phosphate in muscle functioning?
 1. "Phosphate is necessary for DNA production."
 2. "The sodium-potassium pump does not involve phosphate."
 3. "The formation of energy uses phosphate."
 4. "Phosphate affects how calcium works on muscles."

19. A client diagnosed with chronic kidney disease presents to the emergency department reporting severe muscle cramping and numbness and tingling of the mouth and hands. The client is diagnosed with hyperphosphatemia and hypocalcemia. Which ECG finding should a nurse identify as indicative of hypocalcemia?

1.

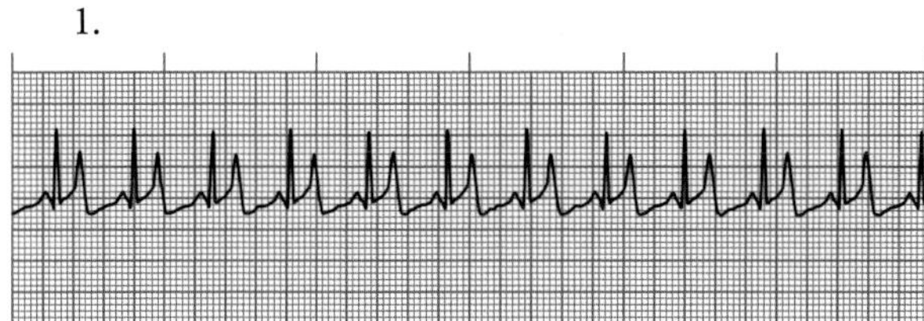

2.

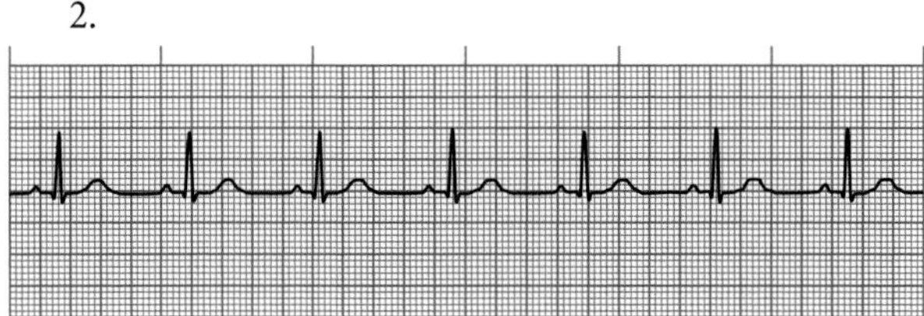

3.

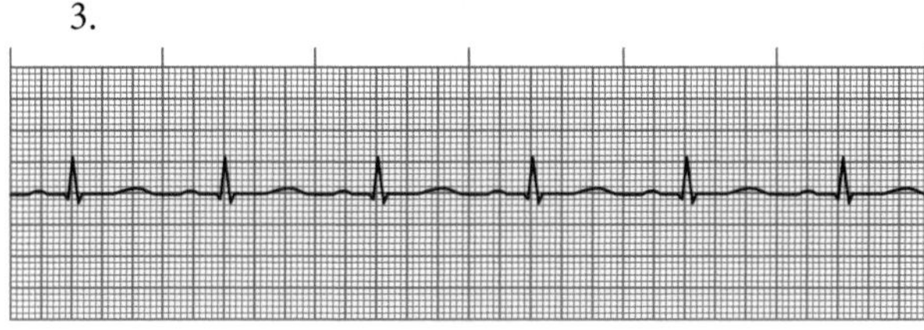

4.

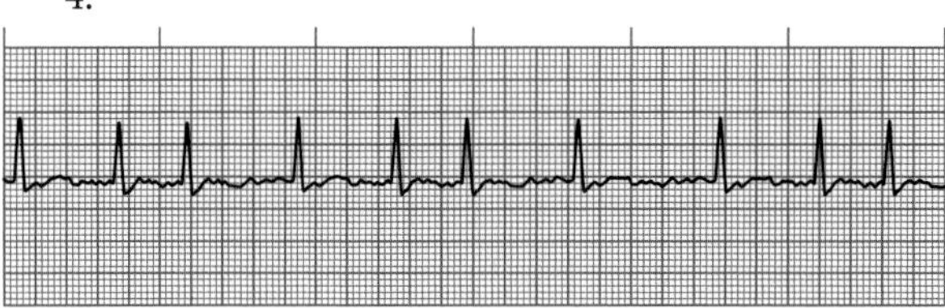

20. Which findings should a nurse associate with the development of a phosphate imbalance when assessing a client diagnosed with hyperparathyroidism? **Select all that apply.**

1. Weak peripheral pulses
2. Hyperactive DTRs
3. Prolonged Q-T interval
4. Generalized muscle weakness
5. Irritability

REVIEW ANSWERS

1. ANSWER: 4.

Rationale:

1. A serum phosphorus level of 2.5 mg/dL is within the normal reference range.
2. A serum phosphorus level of 4.7 mg/dL is elevated (hyperphosphatemia).
3. A serum calcium level of 9 mg/dL is within the normal reference range.
4. **When caring for a client diagnosed with hypophosphatemia, the nurse should anticipate a serum calcium level of 11 mg/dL (hypercalcemia). Because of the inverse relationship between phosphorus and calcium, a *decrease* in serum phosphorus results in an *increase* in the serum calcium.**

TEST-TAKING TIP: Recall that serum phosphorus and serum calcium levels are inversely proportionate. The normal reference range for serum phosphorus is 2.5 to 4.5 mg/dL. The normal reference range for calcium is 8.2 to 10.2 mg/dL.

Content Area: Adult Health
Integrated Processes: Nursing Process: Analysis
Client Need: Physiological Integrity
Cognitive Level: Comprehension
Reference: Ignatavicius, D., and Workman, M. (2012). Medical-Surgical Nursing: Patient-Centered Collaborative Care (7th ed.). St. Louis, MO: Saunders.

2. ANSWER: 1, 2, 4, 6.

Rationale:

1. **The nurse should instruct a client taking sevelamer hydrochloride (Renagel) to observe for constipation. Renagel is a phosphate binding agent that may cause constipation.**
2. **The nurse should instruct a client taking Renagel to observe for signs and symptoms of hypophosphatemia. Renagel binds with phosphorus obtained from foods and prevents it from being absorbed into the bloodstream.**
3. Renagel is used to *reduce* high levels of phosphorus in clients with chronic kidney disease who are on dialysis.
4. **Renagel may cause diarrhea and vomiting in some clients.**
5. When serum phosphorus levels decrease, serum calcium levels increase—that is, they are inversely proportional.
6. **The nurse should instruct a client taking Renagel to observe for signs and symptoms of hypercalcemia. As serum phosphorus levels decrease, serum calcium levels increase and can lead to hypercalcemia.**

TEST-TAKING TIP: Clients with chronic kidney disease frequently need treatment to decrease serum phosphorus levels. Be aware of the potential side effects of medications commonly prescribed in the management of chronic diseases. Remember that phosphorus and calcium levels are inversely proportional.

Content Area: Adult Health
Integrated Processes: Nursing Process: Assessment
Client Need: Physiological Integrity
Cognitive Level: Comprehension
Reference: Deglin, J. H., Vallerand, A. H., and Sanoski, C. A.(2013). Davis's Drug Guide for Nurses (13th ed.). Philadelphia, PA: F. A. Davis.

3. ANSWER: 4.

Rationale:

1. Paresthesia, a sensation of numbing or tingling of the skin, is a sign of hypercalcemia that often accompanies hypophosphatemia.
2. Weak peripheral pulses are a sign of hypophosphatemia and hypercalcemia.
3. Weak skeletal muscles are a sign of hypophosphatemia and hypercalcemia.
4. **The nurse should associate a positive Trousseau's sign with hypocalcemia, which would be related to hyperphosphatemia. A positive Trousseau's sign results from neuromuscular irritability caused by hypocalcemia, inducing spasms of the hand and forearm.**

TEST-TAKING TIP: Recall that *hyper*phosphatemia occurs with *hypo*calcemia. Select option 4 because it is a sign of hypocalcemia.

Content Area: Adult Health
Integrated Processes: Nursing Process: Assessment
Client Need: Physiological Integrity
Cognitive Level: Application
Reference: Berman, A., Snyder, S., Kozier, B., and Erb, G. (2012). Kozier & Erb's Fundamentals of Nursing: Concepts, Process, and Practice (9th ed.). Upper Saddle River, NJ: Pearson.

4. ANSWER: 3.

Rationale:

1. Hypocalcemia, not hypercalcemia, would elicit these signs and symptoms.
2. The most common signs of hypermagnesemia are cardiovascular changes, such as bradycardia and hypotension. Neuromuscular manifestations include decreased deep tendon reflexes and muscle weakness.
3. **The nurse should associate abdominal cramping, diarrhea, muscle spasms, and tingling around the mouth with hyperphosphatemia and hypocalcemia. Common signs and symptoms of hyperphosphatemia include circumoral and distal extremity numbness and tingling, muscle spasms, and tetany from increased serum phosphorus and corresponding decreased serum calcium levels.**
4. Chloride imbalances usually occur as a result of other electrolyte imbalances, most often sodium. Hyperchloremia usually produces signs and symptoms of hypernatremia.

TEST-TAKING TIP: Associate the signs and symptoms of potential phosphate imbalances with the corresponding signs and symptoms of potential calcium imbalances: hypophosphatemia with hypercalcemia, and hyperphosphatemia with hypocalcemia. Select option 3 because it is a sign of hypocalcemia with hyperphosphatemia.

Content Area: Adult Health
Integrated Processes: Nursing Process: Analysis
Client Need: Physiological Integrity
Cognitive Level: Application
Reference: Ignatavicius, D., and Workman, M. (2012). Medical-Surgical Nursing: Patient-Centered Collaborative Care (7th ed.). St. Louis, MO: Saunders.

5. ANSWER: 1.

Rationale:

1. **The nurse should place priority on the implementation of seizure precautions for a client with a serum phosphorus level of 1.9 mg/dL (severe hypophosphatemia) because the client has an increased risk of seizure activity.**

2. The administration of calcium carbonate is contraindicated because this client's severe hypophosphatemia indicates an elevated serum calcium level. Calcium replacement therapy could potentially worsen the client's hypophosphatemia.
3. Completion of a thorough diet history is important in determining the etiology of the client's phosphate deficiency, but it is not the priority intervention for this client.
4. The administration of acetazolamide is also contraindicated for this client because diuretics that act on the proximal renal tubules increase the renal excretion of phosphate, worsening the client's severe hypophosphatemia.
TEST-TAKING TIP: The key word is "priority." Recognize that the client's serum phosphorus level is low; recall the signs and symptoms of hypophosphatemia.
Content Area: Older Adult Health
Integrated Processes: Nursing Process: Planning
Client Need: Physiological Integrity
Cognitive Level: Application
Reference: *Ignatavicius, D., and Workman, M. (2012). Medical-Surgical Nursing: Patient-Centered Collaborative Care (7th ed.). St. Louis, MO: Saunders.*

6. ANSWER: 4.
Rationale:
1. Hypoparathyroidism places a client at risk for hypocalcemia and hyperphosphatemia.
2. Acute renal failure places a client at risk for hypocalcemia and hyperphosphatemia.
3. Rhabdomyolysis places a client at risk for hyperphosphatemia as muscle fibers break down and phosphate is released into the intravascular space.
4. The nurse should identify DKA as a factor that would contribute to the development of hypophosphatemia because DKA causes phosphate to shift *out* of the ECF and *into* the cells.
TEST-TAKING TIP: Recall that clients diagnosed with DKA initially exhibit signs of hypophosphatemia and hypercalcemia. Rule out option 1 because hypoparathyroidism results in decreased serum calcium and increased serum phosphorus levels (inversely proportional). Rule out option 2 because the kidneys are unable to excrete phosphate. Eliminate option 3 because when cells break down, electrolytes are released into the bloodstream.
Content Area: Adult Health
Integrated Processes: Nursing Process: Planning
Client Need: Physiological Integrity
Cognitive Level: Application
Reference: *Ignatavicius, D., and Workman, M. (2012). Medical-Surgical Nursing: Patient-Centered Collaborative Care (7th ed.). St. Louis, MO: Saunders.*

7. ANSWER: 2
Rationale:
1. Collard greens and milk should be avoided by this client because they contain high amounts of calcium.
2. The nurse should teach a client who is attempting to increase the amount of phosphorus in the diet to include pork and nuts because they have a high phosphorus content.
3. Fresh and dried fruits are a good source of potassium.
4. Canned vegetables and soups provide high levels of dietary sodium and chloride.
TEST-TAKING TIP: Recall that clients with decreased serum phosphorus levels have increased serum calcium levels. Do not recommend foods that are high in calcium to these clients.
Content Area: Adult Health
Integrated Processes: Teaching/Learning
Client Need: Health Promotion and Maintenance: Health Promotion/Disease Prevention
Cognitive Level: Application
Reference: *Ignatavicius, D., and Workman, M. (2012). Medical-Surgical Nursing: Patient-Centered Collaborative Care (7th ed.). St. Louis, MO: Saunders.*

8. ANSWER: 2.
Rationale:
1. IV phosphorus should be given only when a client's serum phosphorus level is less than 1 mg/dL.
2. A nurse caring for a client with mild to moderate hypophosphatemia should anticipate an order for the *oral* replacement of phosphorus along with vitamin D. Vitamin D promotes the absorption of phosphorus from the gastrointestinal tract.
3. Daily calcium supplements promote phosphate loss because of the inverse relationship between calcium and phosphorus.
4. Antacids that contain aluminum salts, such as Maalox, promote phosphate loss.
TEST-TAKING TIP: Recall that only a critical serum phosphorus level less than 1 mg/dL requires IV phosphorus replacement, eliminating option 1. Rule out options 3 and 4 because they would worsen hypophosphatemia.
Content Area: Adult Health
Integrated Processes: Nursing Process: Planning
Client Need: Physiological Integrity
Cognitive Level: Application
Reference: *Ignatavicius, D., and Workman, M. (2012). Medical-Surgical Nursing: Patient-Centered Collaborative Care (7th ed.). St. Louis, MO: Saunders.*

9. ANSWER: 2.
Rationale:
1. Potato chips contain excessive sodium but are not a food this client must avoid.
2. A nurse providing discharge instructions to a client diagnosed with hypophosphatemia should advise the client to avoid yogurt and other foods that are high in calcium because an increased calcium intake would worsen the client's hypophosphatemia.
3. Walnuts should be included in this client's diet to increase phosphorus intake.
4. Liver should be included in this client's diet to increase phosphorus intake.
TEST-TAKING TIP: The key word is "avoid." Foods that increase calcium decrease phosphorus and would be contraindicated for a client with a low serum phosphorus level.
Content Area: Adult Health
Integrated Processes: Teaching/Learning
Client Need: Health Promotion and Maintenance
Cognitive Level: Application
Reference: *Ignatavicius, D., and Workman, M. (2012). Medical-Surgical Nursing: Patient-Centered Collaborative Care (7th ed.). St. Louis, MO: Saunders.*

10. **ANSWER: 63.**
Rationale:

250 mL/4 hr = X/1 hr = 250 ÷ 4X = 62.5 mL = 63 mL (rounded to nearest whole number)

TEST-TAKING TIP: When calculating this type of preparation, make sure the amount and rate of infusion of the combination substance (either potassium or sodium with phosphate) do not exceed the maximum for either substance.
Content Area: Adult Health
Integrated Processes: Nursing Process: Implementation
Client Need: Physiological Integrity
Cognitive Level: Application
Reference: *Deglin, J. H., Vallerand, A. H., and Sanoski, C. A.(2013). Davis's Drug Guide for Nurses (13th ed.). Philadelphia, PA: F. A. Davis.*

11. **ANSWER: 3.**
Rationale:

2,000 mg/X = 667 mg/1 tab= 2,000/667X= 2.99 tabs = 3 tabs

TEST-TAKING TIP: The key words are "with each meal." Read the question carefully to answer correctly.
Content Area: Adult Health
Integrated Processes: Nursing Process: Implementation
Client Need: Physiological Integrity
Cognitive Level: Application
Reference: *Deglin, J. H., Vallerand, A. H., and Sanoski, C. A.(2013). Davis's Drug Guide for Nurses (13th ed.). Philadelphia, PA: F. A. Davis.*

12. **ANSWER: 50.**
Rationale:

15 mmol/250 mL = 3 mmol/X = 750/15= 50 mL

TEST-TAKING TIP: Potassium is part of the potassium phosphate solution being administered. Potassium is a high-alert medication. *Always* double-check calculations, especially when administering high-alert medications.
Content Area: Adult Health
Integrated Processes: Nursing Process: Implementation
Client Need: Physiological Integrity; Pharmacological and Parenteral Therapies: Dosage Calculation
Cognitive Level: Application
Reference: *Deglin, J. H., Vallerand, A. H., and Sanoski, C. A.(2013). Davis's Drug Guide for Nurses (13th ed.). Philadelphia, PA: F. A. Davis.*

13. **ANSWER: 2, 3, 4, 5.**
Rationale:
1. Diarrhea related to spastic colonic activity is not associated with hypophosphatemia.
2. The client is experiencing hypophosphatemia, which results in muscle weakness.
3. The client is experiencing hypophosphatemia, which results in cardiac dysrhythmias. Dysrhythmias are caused by low stores of intracellular energy in the myocardial cells, rendering the contractions weak and ineffective.
4. The client is experiencing hypophosphatemia, which results in muscle weakness that may impair the client's physical mobility.
5. The client is experiencing hypophosphatemia, which results in muscle weakness that may impair the client's ability to breathe.

TEST-TAKING TIP: Rule out nursing diagnoses that are not related to manifestations caused by a low serum phosphorus level.
Content Area: Adult Health
Integrated Processes: Nursing Process: Analysis
Client Need: Physiological Integrity
Cognitive Level: Application
Reference: *Ignatavicius, D., and Workman, M. (2012). Medical-Surgical Nursing: Patient-Centered Collaborative Care (7th ed.). St. Louis, MO: Saunders.*

14. **ANSWER: 1.**
Rationale:
1. The nurse should associate itchy skin with the development of hyperphosphatemia. Manifestations of hyperphosphatemia and hypophosphatemia are similar, with the exceptions of itchiness, ECG changes, and muscle spasms, cramping, or tetany in hyperphosphatemia and the presence of muscle weakness in hypophosphatemia.
2. Muscle weakness is associated with hypophosphatemia and other electrolyte imbalances.
3. Diarrhea is associated with hypophosphatemia, not hyperphosphatemia.
4. Peaked T waves may indicate hyperkalemia.
TEST-TAKING TIP: Recall that clients with chronic kidney disease frequently report itchy skin secondary to excessive serum phosphorus levels.
Content Area: Adult Health
Integrated Processes: Nursing Process: Assessment
Client Need: Physiological Integrity
Cognitive Level: Application
Reference: *Ignatavicius, D., and Workman, M. (2012). Medical-Surgical Nursing: Patient-Centered Collaborative Care (7th ed.). St. Louis, MO: Saunders.*

15. **ANSWER: 3.**
Rationale:
1. Monitoring cardiac rhythm is an intervention, not an outcome.
2. Decreasing the dietary intake of calcium is an intervention directed at the resulting hypercalcemia and imbalanced nutrition.
3. The nurse's priority outcome in the plan of care for a client with a nursing diagnosis of Risk for Injury Related to Muscle Weakness Secondary to Hypophosphatemia should be that the client will remain free from injury. An appropriate outcome for a Risk for Injury diagnosis is a goal that establishes the client's safety.
4. Maintaining blood pressure within the normal range is an outcome for the nursing diagnosis Decreased Cardiac Output.
TEST-TAKING TIP: Key words are "Risk for Injury Related to Muscle Weakness." Choose the option that specifically addresses the issue in the question.
Content Area: Adult Health
Integrated Processes: Nursing Process: Planning
Client Need: Safe and Effective Care Environment; Management of Care: Establishing Priorities
Cognitive Level: Application
Reference: *Ignatavicius, D., and Workman, M. (2012). Medical-Surgical Nursing: Patient-Centered Collaborative Care (7th ed.). St. Louis, MO: Saunders.*

16. ANSWER: 2.

Rationale:

1. Clients who are diagnosed with DKA develop hypophosphatemia when given insulin because insulin causes phosphate to shift *from* the ECF *into* the ICF, decreasing serum phosphorus levels.

2. The nurse should identify that a 45-year-old client diagnosed with hypoparathyroidism is at greatest risk for developing hyperphosphatemia. A decrease in parathyroid function or lack of PTH results in increased phosphate reabsorption, leading to hyperphosphatemia. This client would also have hypocalcemia because of reduced bone resorption of calcium.

3. Alcohol impairs the absorption of phosphate, resulting in hypophosphatemia.

4. Sucralfate, which is commonly used to prevent and treat gastrointestinal ulcers, binds with phosphate and decreases serum phosphorus levels.

TEST-TAKING TIP: The key word is "*hyper*phosphatemia." Consider the effect of each condition on serum phosphorus levels, and rule out conditions that would cause a decrease in serum phosphorus levels.

Content Area: Adult Health

Integrated Processes: Nursing Process: Analysis

Client Need: Physiological Integrity

Cognitive Level: Analysis

Reference: Ignatavicius, D., and Workman, M. (2012). Medical-Surgical Nursing: Patient-Centered Collaborative Care (7th ed.). St. Louis, MO: Saunders.

17. ANSWER: 1, 2, 3, 4, 6.

Rationale:

1. The nurse should obtain information that would help determine the cause of the client's hypophosphatemia, including the client's alcohol use.

2. Laxative use may cause diarrhea, which results in the loss of phosphorus.

3. Excessive exercise can contribute to electrolyte imbalances if nutrient intake does not meet the demand.

4. This client is at increased risk for an eating disorder because of the age group and as evidenced by the client's body mass index of 17.

5. It would be important to obtain serum calcium levels, not serum magnesium levels, because calcium has an inverse relationship with phosphorus.

6. The serum PTH level should be assessed because hyperparathyroidism may result in decreased serum phosphorus levels.

TEST-TAKING TIP: Recognize that the client is displaying signs and symptoms of chronic hypophosphatemia, and select the options that would contribute to hypophosphatemia. Recall that calcium and phosphorus have an inverse relationship and that the magnesium level parallels the potassium level.

Content Area: Child Health

Integrated Processes: Nursing Process: Assessment

Client Need: Physiological Integrity

Cognitive Level: Analysis

Reference: Ignatavicius, D., and Workman, M. (2012). Medical-Surgical Nursing: Patient-Centered Collaborative Care (7th ed.). St. Louis, MO: Saunders.

18. ANSWER: 3.

Rationale:

1. Although phosphate is a component of DNA, this does not affect muscle functioning.

2. Phosphate *is* involved in the mechanisms of the sodium-potassium pump.

3. The statement "The formation of energy uses phosphate" should indicate to the instructor that the student has an adequate understanding of the role of phosphate in muscle functioning. Phosphate is needed to form ATP to make energy.

4. Although phosphorus and calcium have an inversely proportional relationship, phosphate does not directly affect how calcium works on muscles.

TEST-TAKING TIP: The key words are "the role of phosphate in muscle functioning." Recall the actions of phosphate on various body systems. Note that options 1 and 3 are similar; if two options are similar, it is likely that one of them is correct.

Content Area: Adult Health

Integrated Processes: Teaching/Learning

Client Need: Physiological Integrity

Cognitive Level: Analysis

Reference: Ignatavicius, D., and Workman, M. (2012). Medical-Surgical Nursing: Patient-Centered Collaborative Care (7th ed.). St. Louis, MO: Saunders.

19. ANSWER: 3.

Rationale:

1. ECG strip 1 shows peaked T waves, associated with hyperkalemia.

2. ECG strip 2 shows a normal sinus rhythm.

3. The nurse should identify ECG strip 3 as indicative of hyperphosphatemia and hypocalcemia because it shows a prolonged Q-T interval, which is a classic ECG change associated with hypocalcemia accompanied by hyperphosphatemia.

4. ECG strip 4 shows atrial fibrillation, which is not related to electrolyte imbalances.

TEST-TAKING TIP: Select the option that illustrates the effects of hypocalcemia on the electrical conduction of the heart.

Content Area: Adult Health

Integrated Processes: Nursing Process: Evaluation

Client Need: Physiological Integrity

Cognitive Level: Analysis

References: Ignatavicius, D., and Workman, M. (2012). Medical-Surgical Nursing: Patient-Centered Collaborative Care (7th ed.). St. Louis, MO: Saunders; Jones, S. (2010). ECG Notes: Interpretation and Management Guide (2nd ed.). Philadelphia, PA: F. A. Davis.

20. ANSWER: 1, 4, 5.

Rationale:

1. A nurse who is assessing a client with hyperparathyroidism should associate weak peripheral pulses with the development of hypophosphatemia.

2. A client with hypophosphatemia and hypercalcemia would display hypoactive DTRs.

3. A client with hypophosphatemia and hypercalcemia would display a shortened Q-T interval.

4. A nurse who is assessing a client with hyperparathyroidism should associate generalized muscle weakness with the development of hypophosphatemia (and hypercalcemia), a complication of hyperparathyroidism.
5. A nurse who is assessing a client with hyperparathyroidism should associate irritability with the development of hypophosphatemia.
TEST-TAKING TIP: First recall that hyperparathyroidism results in hypophosphatemia and hypercalcemia. Then select the options that are signs or symptoms of these imbalances.
Content Area: Adult Health
Integrated Processes: Nursing Process: Assessment
Client Need: Physiological Integrity
Cognitive Level: Analysis
Reference: *Ignatavicius, D., and Workman, M. (2012). Medical-Surgical Nursing: Patient-Centered Collaborative Care (7th ed.). St. Louis, MO: Saunders.*

UNIT III

Acid-Base Imbalances

Acidosis and Alkalosis

KEY TERMS

Acid—A substance that releases hydrogen ions when dissolved in water, increasing the concentration of hydrogen ions and lowering pH.

Acidosis—Blood and body tissue pH less than 7.35.

Alkalosis—Blood and body tissue pH greater than 7.45.

Anion gap—The difference between the concentrations of serum cations and anions; it is estimated by subtracting the combined value of chloride and bicarbonate from that of sodium: anion gap = serum Na^+ minus (serum Cl^- plus serum HCO_3^-). The normal anion gap is 8 to 16 mEq/L.

Arterial blood gas (ABG)—A laboratory test that measures the pH and levels of oxygen (PaO_2), carbon dioxide ($PaCO_2$), and bicarbonate (HCO_3^-) in arterial blood.

Base—A substances that binds free hydrogen ions in water, reducing the concentration of hydrogen ions and increasing pH.

Bicarbonate (HCO_3^-)—The principal alkaline substance (base) in the body; itresponds slowly to changes in pH.

Buffer—A weak acid or base that is capable of minimizing changes in pH by accepting or releasing hydrogen.

Compensation—The body's attempt to return the pH of blood and body fluids to within the normal range of 7.35 to 7.45; involves primarily the lungs and kidneys.

Kussmaul respirations—An abnormal respiratory pattern characterized by rapid, deep breathing, often seen in patients with metabolic acidosis.

Metabolic acidosis—A gain of hydrogen ions and/or a loss of bicarbonate ions; pH decreases, and bicarbonate (HCO_3^-) decreases.

Metabolic alkalosis—A loss of hydrogen ions and/or a gain in bicarbonate ions; pH increases, and bicarbonate increases.

pH—The measure of hydrogen ion concentration in a fluid; an increase in hydrogen ions may result in acidosis, and a decrease in hydrogen ions may result in alkalosis.

Respiratory acidosis—An acid-base imbalance caused by hypoventilation; carbon dioxide is retained, and pH decreases.

Respiratory alkalosis—An acid-base imbalance caused by hyperventilation; excess carbon dioxide is lost, and pH increases.

Venous blood gas (VBG)—A laboratory test that measures the pH and levels of carbon dioxide (PCO_2) and bicarbonate (HCO_3^-) in venous blood.

I. Description

Acid-base imbalances are changes in the concentration of hydrogen ions (H^+) in the blood that alter its pH. Acid-base imbalances impair the functioning of many organs, reduce the activity of hormones and enzymes, affect the distribution of electrolytes, and decrease the effectiveness of many drugs. Acid-base imbalances occur when the pH of the body is outside the normal range, resulting in acidosis or alkalosis. **Acidosis** is an increase in the concentration of free hydrogen ions in the blood, resulting in an arterial blood pH less than 7.35 (Fig. 8.1). **Alkalosis** is a decrease in the concentration of free hydrogen ions in the blood, resulting in an arterial blood pH greater than 7.45 (Fig. 8.2).Both acidosis and alkalosis are conditions caused by underlying disorders; they are not disease processes.

Normal Lab Value The normal reference range for the pH of arterial blood is 7.35 to 7.45.

II. Types of Acid-Base Imbalance

Acid-base imbalances are classified as either respiratory or metabolic, depending on the underlying cause of the alteration. Some acid-base imbalances are caused by a combination of both respiratory and metabolic alterations. The two main types of respiratory acid-base imbalance are

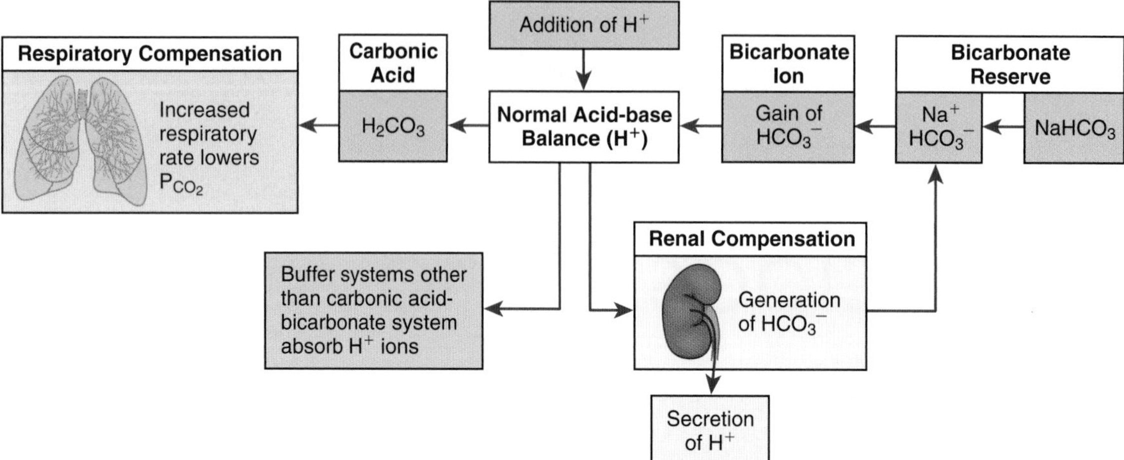

Fig 8.1 The body's response to respiratory acidosis. When the pH of the blood falls below 7.35, the respiratory system responds by increasing the respiratory rate to "blow off" carbon dioxide in an attempt to increase blood pH. The kidneys generate bicarbonate to bind with and eliminate hydrogen ions from the body to increase blood pH.

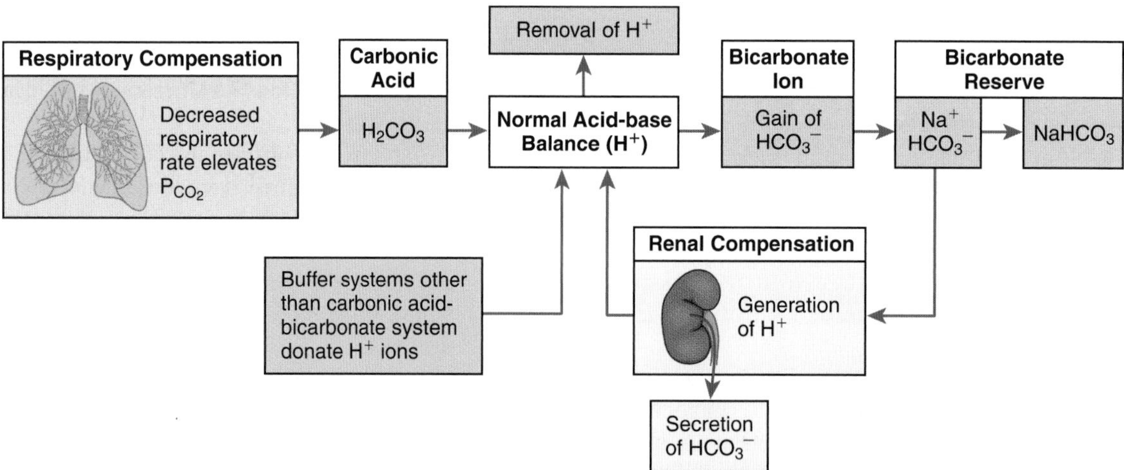

Fig 8.2 The body's response to respiratory alkalosis. When the pH of the blood rises above 7.45, the respiratory system responds by decreasing the respiratory rate to retain carbon dioxide in an attempt to decrease blood pH. The kidneys retain hydrogen ions and secrete bicarbonate to decrease blood pH.

respiratory acidosis and respiratory alkalosis; the two main types of metabolic acid-base imbalance are metabolic acidosis and metabolic alkalosis.

A. **Respiratory acidosis** is a blood pH less than 7.35 caused by the retention of carbon dioxide (CO_2) or by conditions that impair gas exchange, such as hypoventilation and chronic lung disease.
   1. Uncompensated respiratory acidosis may be associated with a normal or slightly increased bicarbonate (HCO_3^-) level, an increased $PaCO_2$ level, an increased serum potassium level (hyperkalemia), and either an increased or decreased serum calcium level (Table 8.1).

B. **Respiratory alkalosis** is a blood pH greater than 7.45 caused by excessive loss of carbon dioxide.
   1. The only cause of respiratory alkalosis is mechanical or spontaneous hyperventilation.
   2. Uncompensated respiratory alkalosis may be associated with a normal or slightly decreased HCO_3^- level, a decreased $PaCO_2$ level, a decreased serum potassium level (hypokalemia), and a normal serum calcium level (see Table 8.1).

C. **Metabolic acidosis** is a blood pH less than 7.35 caused by the overproduction of hydrogen ions, inadequate elimination of hydrogen ions, underproduction of bicarbonate (HCO_3^-), or excessive elimination of

Table 8.1 Acid-Base Laboratory Value Changes in Acidosis and Alkalosis (Uncompensated)

Imbalance	pH	HCO_3^-	$PaCO_2$	K^+	Ca^{2+}	Cl^-
Respiratory acidosis	↓	↑ or normal	↑	↑	↑ or ↓	Normal
Respiratory alkalosis	↑	↓ or normal	↓	↓	Normal	↑
Metabolic acidosis	↓	↓	↓ or normal	↑	Normal	↑ or normal
Metabolic alkalosis	↑	↑	↑ or normal	↓	↓	↓

bicarbonate, as occurs in chronic renal disease or poorly controlled diabetes.

1. Uncompensated metabolic acidosis may be associated with a normal or slightly decreased $PaCO_2$ level, an increased serum potassium level (hyperkalemia), and a normal serum calcium level (see Table 8.1).
2. Metabolic acidosis may be identified by the presence of a high anion gap (Box 8.1).

D. **Metabolic alkalosis** is a blood pH greater than 7.45 caused by a base excess or an acid deficit, which may be caused by the excessive ingestion of antacids or prolonged vomiting.

1. Uncompensated metabolic alkalosis may be associated with an increased HCO_3^- level, a normal or slightly increased $PaCO_2$ level, a decreased serum potassium level (hypokalemia), and a decreased serum calcium level (hypocalcemia) (see Table 8.1).

III. Causes of Acid-Base Imbalance

A. Respiratory acidosis is caused by the retention of carbon dioxide due to a decreased respiratory rate or depth. This causes body fluids, especially the blood, to become too acidic. In acute respiratory acidosis, carbon dioxide builds up very quickly, and the kidneys do not have time to compensate for the imbalance. Chronic respiratory acidosis, which occurs over a long period, is usually a more stable condition because the kidneys have time to compensate for the carbon dioxide retention (Table 8.2).

1. Hypoventilation may be caused by abnormalities in central nervous system functioning, overdose of narcotics, chest trauma, or neuromuscular diseases such as multiple sclerosis (MS) and amyotrophic lateral sclerosis (ALS).
   a. MS is an autoimmune disease that affects the brain and spinal cord and damages the myelin sheath, the protective covering of the nerve cells; this damage slows or stops nerve signals to every muscle in the body, including the respiratory muscles.
   b. ALS, also called Lou Gehrig's disease, is a disease of the nerve cells in the brain and spinal cord that control voluntary and involuntary muscle movement.
2. Respiratory disorders impair gas exchange in the lungs. When gas exchange is impaired, adequate amounts of oxygen fail to enter the bloodstream, and carbon dioxide (CO_2) is not "blown off" (is retained), causing the blood to become acidic.
   a. Chronic obstructive pulmonary disease (COPD) is one of the most common lung diseases. The two main forms of COPD are chronic bronchitis (long-term cough with mucus) and emphysema (destruction of the lungs over time); most clients have a combination of both conditions.
   b. Pneumonia is caused by infection in the lungs; it may be community acquired or hospital acquired.
   c. Asthma is caused by inflammation in the airways, causing the breathing passages to swell and narrow and leading to wheezing, shortness of breath, chest tightness, and coughing. Asthma symptoms can be triggered by breathing in allergens; common asthma triggers include animal dander, dust, mold spores, chemicals, cold weather, and exercise. Many (but not all) people with asthma have a personal or family history of allergies.
   d. Near drowning refers to suffocation by submersion in water; this prevents the lungs from eliminating carbon dioxide, resulting in the

Box 8.1 What Is an Anion Gap?

Sodium, potassium, chloride, and bicarbonate are routinely measured to evaluate electrolyte balance. This leaves several cations (calcium and magnesium) and anions (phosphate, sulfate, organic acids, and proteins) unmeasured. The **anion gap** is the difference between the measured cation (sodium) and the measured anions (chloride and bicarbonate) in serum, plasma, or urine. It normally ranges from 8 to 16 mEq/L.

$$Na^+ - (Cl^- + HCO_3^-) = \text{anion gap}$$

The anion gap can be classified as high, normal, or, in rare cases, low. A high anion gap indicates the presence of *metabolic acidosis*.

Table 8.2 Causes of Acid-Base Imbalance

Respiratory

Acidosis	*Alkalosis*

Retention of carbon dioxide
• *Hypoventilation* secondary to:
  • Central nervous system dysfunction
  • Overdose of narcotics or sedatives
  • Brain injury that affects the respiratory center
  • Chest trauma
  • Neuromuscular disease
• Respiratory disorders
  • Chronic obstructive pulmonary disease (COPD)
  • Chronic lung disease
  • Acute pulmonary edema
  • Pneumonia
  • Near drowning
• Airway obstruction or aspiration of foreign body
• Drugs that suppress breathing
• Severe obesity
	Excessive loss of carbon dioxide
	• *Hyperventilation* secondary to:
	  • Anxiety
	  • Stress
	  • Fear
	  • Pain
	  • Head injury
	  • Stroke
	  • Asthma
	  • Pneumonia
	  • Pulmonary edema
	  • Sepsis
	  • Thyrotoxicosis
	  • Salicylate overdose
	  • Progesterone during pregnancy
	  • Increased basal metabolic rate
	  • Excessive mechanical ventilation

Metabolic

Acidosis	*Alkalosis*

Excessive production of hydrogen ions
• Sepsis
• Poorly controlled diabetes
• Diabetic ketoacidosis
• Starvation
• Cardiac arrest
Excessive acid intake
• Alcohol (also causes respiratory acidosis)
• Salicylate (aspirin) overdose or toxicity
• Excessive infusion of chloride-containing IV fluids (NaCl)
Retention of hydrogenions
• Renal insufficiency
• Acute kidney injury
• Chronic kidney disease
Excessive elimination of bicarbonate
• Vomiting
• Diarrhea
Underproduction of bicarbonate
• Pancreatitis
• Liver failure
Potassium shift
• Hyperkalemia
  • When extracellular potassium levels are high, potassium shifts into the cells and hydrogen ions shift out of the cells, decreasing blood pH (metabolic acidosis)
	Excessive loss of hydrogen ions
	• Excessive gastrointestinal loss
	  • Prolonged vomiting
	  • Gastric suctioning
	• Renal losses via urine
	Excessive bicarbonate intake
	• Excessive intake of bicarbonate-containing antacids or non-absorbable antacids
	• Excessive administration of IV sodium bicarbonate ($NaHCO_3$)
	Decreased excretion of bicarbonate
	• Cushing's syndrome
	• Chloride depletion
	Potassium shift
	• Primary hyperaldosteronism (Conn's syndrome)
	• Hypokalemia
	  • Use of potassium-depleting diuretics
	  • When extracellular potassium levels are low, potassium shifts out of the cells and hydrogen ions shift into the cells, increasing blood pH (metabolic alkalosis)

retention of hydrogen ions and a decrease in serum pH (acidosis).

e. Drugs that suppress breathing, such as narcotics and benzodiazepines, may cause respiratory depression and acidosis, especially when combined with alcohol.

f. Severe obesity, which can restrict lung expansion, may impair gas exchange, resulting in carbon dioxide retention and respiratory acidosis.

B. Respiratory alkalosis is caused by an excessive loss of CO_2 through spontaneous or mechanical hyperventilation; hyperventilation is characterized by an increased respiratory rate and depth (see Table 8.2).

1. Hyperventilation is the act of breathing faster or deeper than normal, resulting in the excessive exhalation of carbon dioxide; spontaneous hyperventilation can be caused by extreme stress or panic attack or in response to increased carbon dioxide levels or metabolic acidosis.

2. Mechanical hyperventilation, when a client's ventilation is being assisted or controlled by a mechanical device, may occur accidentally when attempting to correct acidosis or as a therapeutic treatment to decrease intracranial pressure and cerebral edema.

C. Metabolic acidosis occurs when the body produces too much acid or when the kidneys do not remove enough acid from the body. There are several types of metabolic acidosis: diabetic ketoacidosis (DKA) develops when acidic ketone bodies build up in clients with uncontrolled type 1 diabetes; hyperchloremic acidosis results from excessive loss of sodium bicarbonate from the body; and lactic acidosis, a buildup of lactic acid, is caused by prolonged exercise, alcohol consumption, lack of oxygen, and many other reasons (see Table 8.2).

DID YOU KNOW?

Infection and new-onset diabetes are the most common causes of DKA.

1. Excessive production of hydrogen ions
   a. Sepsis is a life-threatening condition in which the blood is overwhelmed with bacteria, causing inflammation and decreased perfusion to the organs and resulting in the production of lactic acid.
   b. Diabetic ketoacidosis is a dangerous complication of diabetes mellitus caused by a total or partial lack of insulin that produces severe hyperglycemia. Hyperglycemia results in dehydration and electrolyte loss; ketones then build up in the blood, causing the blood pH to decrease (Box 8.2).
2. Excessive intake of acidic substances
   a. Excessive alcohol intake, such as during binge drinking, may cause metabolic acidosis when a client has eaten little or no food and has persistent vomiting; it is also called *alcoholic ketoacidosis.*
   b. Overdose of aspirin (acetylsalicylic acid) occurs when excessive amounts are ingested or absorbed; this results in both respiratory alkalosis and metabolic acidosis. The earliest signs of salicylate toxicity include nausea, vomiting, and hyperventilation; late signs include convulsions, lethargy, stupor, coma, or death; hyperthermia is an indication of severe toxicity in young children (Box 8.3).
   c. Excessive infusion of IV solutions that contain chloride, such as 0.9% saline solution (normal saline) and hypertonic solutions containing sodium chloride, can cause metabolic acidosis.
3. Retention of hydrogen ions
   a. Renal insufficiency, acute kidney injury, and chronic kidney disease decrease the kidneys' ability to filter waste from the blood, resulting in the retention of hydrogen ions; the kidneys maintain acid-base balance by bicarbonate reclamation and acid excretion.
4. Excessive elimination or underproduction of bicarbonate
   a. Diarrhea is the most common cause of the external loss of alkaline body fluids, especially bicarbonate; loose, watery stools and increased stool volume may result in the loss of several liters of water per day. Because diarrheal stools have a higher bicarbonate concentration than plasma, the net result is metabolic acidosis with volume depletion.

DID YOU KNOW?

When vomiting and diarrhea occur at the same time, both hydrochloric acid and bicarbonate (base) are lost. If these losses occur in relatively equal proportions, acid-base homeostasis is usually maintained even though a large amount of fluid is lost.

Box 8.2 DKA and Metabolic Acidosis

Diabetic ketoacidosis is an acute, life-threatening complication of diabetes that requires emergency treatment with insulin and IV fluids. It occurs mainly in clients with type 1 diabetes but may also be seen in some older adults with type 2 diabetes. The most common causes are underlying infection (40%), disruption of insulin treatment (25%), and new onset of diabetes (15%).

The absence of insulin means that glucose cannot be broken down and used for energy, so the body begins to use fat for energy instead. When fats (triglycerides) are broken down into free fatty acids, gluconeogenesis (the synthesis of glucose from noncarbohydrate sources) occurs, resulting in extremely elevated serum glucose levels (much greater than 250 mg/dL) and an increase in the formation of ketone bodies. Serum ketone levels increase to greater than 5 mEq/L, and the serum pH decreases to less than 7.3 (ketoacidosis) as extracellular and intracellular buffers, such as bicarbonate, become depleted, resulting in hyperchloremic acidosis.

Increasing serum glucose levels (hyperglycemia) eventually exceed the renal threshold of glucose absorption, and glucose spills into the urine (glycosuria), causing water loss of approximately 6 L via the urine due to osmotic diuresis, resulting in profound dehydration. Dehydration then leads to a decrease in tissue perfusion and possibly lactic acid buildup in the body (lactic acidosis).

Because clients with DKA are dehydrated and acidotic and have low serum potassium levels, great care must be taken when insulin and fluids are administered. Serum potassium levels may appear normal or even elevated due to the extracellular shift in potassium that occurs in the presence of acidosis, but these values do not accurately reflect the client's true potassium stores. Insulin administration causes potassium to move back into the cells, worsening hypokalemia, and IV fluids dilute the potassium molecules circulating in the blood. It is imperative that the blood levels of potassium and other electrolytes be monitored repeatedly so that these imbalances can be corrected.

Box 8.3 How Aspirin Overdose Affects Acid-Base Balance

Aspirin, a salicylate, is used as an analgesic agent for mild to moderate pain and as an anti-inflammatory agent for soft tissue and joint inflammation. Aspirin overdose, or salicylate toxicity, adversely affects every organ system of the body. The acid-base, fluid, and electrolyte imbalances caused by salicylate toxicity occur in two main phases:

- The first phase is characterized by increases in respiratory rate (tachypnea) and depth (hyperpnea) caused by the drug's toxic effects on the respiratory system. Hyperventilation causes respiratory alkalosis (increased serum pH) as the lungs "blow off" too much carbon dioxide. The increase in serum pH causes the urine pH to increase as well (alkaluria), which causes the kidneys to excrete potassium (a buffer) and bicarbonate (a base) in an attempt to lower the blood pH. This phase begins within hours of salicylate overdose and continues until sufficient amounts of potassium have been lost by the kidneys (12 to 24 hours in adults).
- The second phase begins about 24 hours after overdose and is characterized by dehydration caused by vomiting and insensible fluid loss resulting from hyperventilation. Dehydration leads to renal insufficiency, which results in the retention of salicylate and the accumulation of phosphoric and sulfuric acids, causing metabolic acidosis. The presence of acidosis increases the amount of salicylate that crosses the blood-brain barrier, resulting in central nervous system toxicity. Severe toxicity can progress to disorientation, seizures, cerebral edema, coma, respiratory depression, cardiac dysrhythmias, and, eventually, death.

b. Pancreatitis, or inflammation of the pancreas, may cause digestive juices (enzymes and bicarbonate) and digestive hormones (mainly insulin and glucagon) to become trapped and start "digesting" the pancreas itself. Pancreatitis can be either acute or chronic, but either type can result in serious complications and may even be life threatening.

5. Electrolyte shift
   a. Hyperkalemia is a serum potassium level greater than 5.0 mEq/L; when extracellular potassium levels are elevated, potassium shifts into the cells, causing hydrogen ions to move out of the cells and decreasing blood pH; this is called a "potassium shift."

D. Metabolic alkalosis is caused by a loss of hydrogen ions from the body, a shift of hydrogen ions into the cells, or a gain in bicarbonate. The most common causes of metabolic alkalosis are the use of diuretics and the external loss of gastric secretions. Metabolic alkalosis is characterized by an elevation in the serum bicarbonate level. Remember that an elevated serum bicarbonate level may also be the result of compensation for respiratory acidosis. A serum bicarbonate level greater than 35 mEq/L is almost always caused by metabolic alkalosis (see Table 8.2).

1. Excessive loss of hydrogen ions
   a. Prolonged vomiting and nasogastric suctioning cause metabolic alkalosis through the loss of gastric secretions, which are rich in hydrochloric acid (HCl); whenever a hydrogen ion is excreted, a bicarbonate ion is gained in the extracellular space.
   b. Renal losses of hydrogen ions occur whenever the kidneys reabsorb too much sodium, such as in the presence of excess aldosterone; sodium retention leads to the secretion of hydrogen ions and potassium ions in the urine.
2. Excessive bicarbonate intake
   a. Excessive intake of bicarbonate-containing antacids or nonabsorbable antacids, such as magnesium hydroxide, calcium hydroxide, or aluminum hydroxide, can cause metabolic alkalosis because the hydroxide anion buffers hydrogen ions in the stomach.
   b. Administration of IV sodium bicarbonate, used in the treatment of acidosis, may exceed the kidneys' capacity to excrete the excess bicarbonate, resulting in metabolic alkalosis.
3. Decreased excretion of bicarbonate
   a. Cushing's syndrome, a hormonal disorder caused by high levels of cortisol in the blood, can result from the administration of glucocorticoid drugs or from tumors that produce cortisol. Excess cortisol impairs the kidneys' ability to excrete bicarbonate; thus bicarbonate is retained, increasing the pH of the blood.
   b. Chloride depletion may occur through the loss of gastric secretions, which are rich in chloride ions as well as hydrogen ions; chloride depletion, even without volume depletion, enhances bicarbonate reabsorption, which may result in metabolic alkalosis. Thiazide and loop diuretic therapy causes metabolic alkalosis by depleting chloride and increasing water, potassium, and hydrogen ion secretions.
4. Electrolyte shift
   a. Primary hyperaldosteronism, also known as Conn's syndrome, is caused by a benign tumor on the adrenal gland that results in the overproduction of aldosterone; increased aldosterone levels cause the kidneys to increase sodium reabsorption and excrete potassium and hydrogen ions, increasing blood pH.
   b. Hypokalemia, or low serum potassium, causes potassium to shift *out of* the cells and *into* the extracellular fluid (ECF) and hydrogen ions to move *out of* the ECF and *into* the cells; the loss of hydrogen ions from the ECF causes the

blood pH to increase, resulting in metabolic alkalosis.

IV. Nursing Assessment of Clients with Acid-Base Imbalance

The nurse should conduct a focused nursing assessment for acid-base imbalances, beginning with a thorough nursing history. Interview the client and family members to identify any risk factors or preexisting conditions that would contribute to acid-base imbalance, such as vomiting, respiratory disorders, kidney injury or failure, diabetes, and other conditions associated with acidosis or alkalosis. The nursing history should also include lifestyle factors, such as the consumption of bicarbonate-containing antacids, alcohol, narcotics, sedatives, or illicit substances and current medication use. A thorough physical assessment is necessary because acid-base imbalances affect many body systems. Assess each body system, observing for signs and symptoms of acid-base and electrolyte imbalances. Measure and record the client's vital signs, and review the client's laboratory data, including arterial or venous blood gas values, to assess for the presence of acid-base imbalances and associated electrolyte imbalances (Table 8.3).

Table 8.3 Signs and Symptoms of Acid-Base Imbalance

Arterial Blood Gases

	Respiratory Acidosis	*Metabolic Acidosis*	*Respiratory Alkalosis*	*Metabolic Alkalosis*
pH	Less than 7.35	Less than 7.35	Greater than 7.45	Greater than 7.45
$PaCO_2$	Greater than 45 mm Hg	Normal or less than 35 mm Hg (CO_2 decreases to compensate)	Less than 35 mm Hg	Greater than 45 mm Hg (CO_2 increases to compensate)
HCO_3^-	*Acute:* normal or slightly elevated *Chronic:* greater than 26 mEq/L (HCO_3^- increases to compensate)	Less than 21 mEq/L	Normal or less than 21 mEq/L (HCO_3^- is excreted by the kidneys to compensate)	Greater than 28 mEq/L

Signs and Symptoms by Body System

	Respiratory and Metabolic Acidosis	*Respiratory and Metabolic Alkalosis*
Cardiovascular	• Tachycardia (mild) • Bradycardia (severe) • Weak peripheral pulses • Hypotension (result of peripheral dilation)	• Increased heart rate • Thready pulse • Normal or low blood pressure • Increased digoxin toxicity
Cerebral	• Lethargy • Confusion • Headache • Stupor or coma (severe)	• Confusion • Lightheadedness • Headache • Dizziness • Anxiety • Irritability • Tetany • Seizures
Integumentary	• Warm, flushed skin (metabolic acidosis) • Pale or cyanotic mucous membranes (respiratory acidosis)	
Neuromuscular	• Hyporeflexia • Hypotonia • Muscle twitching to seizures (acute) • Generalized weakness (chronic) • Flaccid paralysis (severe)	• Hyperreflexia • Muscle cramping and twitching • Tetany • Skeletal muscle weakness • Circumoral paresthesia • Numbness and tingling of extremities • Positive Chvostek's sign • Positive Trousseau's sign
Respiratory	• Tachypnea • ***Kussmaul respirations***: abnormal respiratory pattern characterized by deep, rapid breaths that are not under the client's voluntary control(metabolic acidosis) • Shallow respirations (respiratory acidosis)	• Increased rate and depth of ventilation (respiratory alkalosis) • Decreased respiratory effort related to skeletal muscle weakness (metabolic alkalosis)

V. Nursing Interventions for Clients with Acid-Base Imbalance

A. Implement the health-care provider's orders to treat the underlying cause of the imbalance.
1. The health-care provider's orders may include oral or IV fluid administration, oral or IV bicarbonate or potassium administration, and medication administration.
2. Review the client's initial laboratory values and try to determine which acid-base disorder(s) the client is experiencing (Fig. 8.3).

B. Monitor the client and the client's arterial or venous blood gas values.
1. Monitor the client's vital signs as ordered by the health-care provider.
2. Monitor the client's arterial blood gas (ABG) or venous blood gas (VBG) values as ordered by the health-care provider, and identify alterations in these values (Table 8.4).
3. Monitor other laboratory values associated with acid-base imbalance.
   a. Serum potassium: normal reference range is 3.5 to 5.0mEq/L.
   b. Serum calcium: normal reference range is 8.2 to 10.2 mg/dL (adult).
   c. Serum chloride: normal reference range is 97 to 107 mEq/L.
   d. Hemoglobin: normal reference ranges are 13.2 to 17.3 g/dL (adult male) and 11.7 to 15.5 g/dL (adult female).
4. Monitor for cerebral changes.
   a. Establish the client's usual cognitive and behavioral pattern.
   b. Observe the client's behavior, level of consciousness, and mental status.
   c. Monitor for seizure activity.
5. Monitor for cardiovascular changes.
   a. Auscultate the apical pulse.
   b. Monitor for peripheral vasodilation.
   c. Check orthostatic blood pressures.

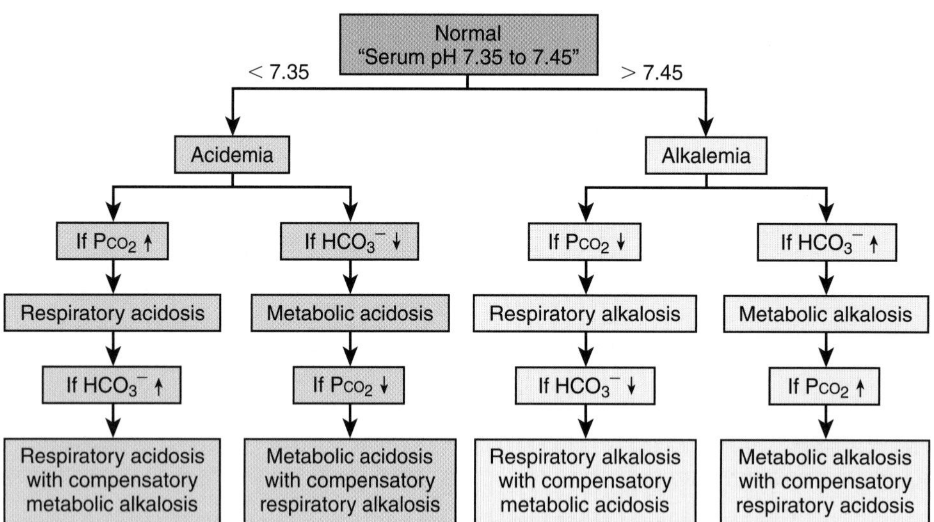

Fig 8.3 Algorithm for classifying simple acid-base imbalances.

Table 8.4 Normal Arterial and Venous Blood Gas Values

	Arterial	Venous
pH	7.35–7.45	7.32–7.43
Oxygen	PaO_2: 80–95 mm Hg	PO_2: 20–49 mm Hg
Carbon dioxide	$PaCO_2$: 35–45 mm Hg	PCO_2: 41–51 mm Hg
Bicarbonate (HCO_3^-)	21–28 mEq/L	24–28 mEq/L
Base excess	−2 to +3 mEq/L	N/A
Arterial oxygen saturation (SaO_2)	95%–99%	N/A

6. Monitor for neuromuscular changes.
   a. Establish a baseline for the client's muscle strength and tone.
   b. Monitor the client for muscle weakness, muscle twitching, or irregular muscle contractions during each nursing shift.
   c. Monitor for circumoral paresthesia and numbness and tingling of the extremities.
7. Monitor for respiratory changes.
   a. Establish a baseline for the client's respiratory rate and depth.
   b. Monitor for tachypnea and Kussmaul respirations.
8. Document observations, and notify the health-care provider as ordered.

C. Measure intake and output.
1. Measure intake.
   a. Record the type and amount of all fluids received at least every 8 hours and describe the route as oral, parenteral, rectal, or by enteric tube.
   b. Record ice chips as fluid at approximately one-half their volume.
   c. Compare the client's intake with the intake of an average adult.
2. Measure output.
   a. Record the type and amount of all fluids the client has lost and the route; describe output as urine, liquid stool, vomitus, tube drainage (including from chest, closed wound drainage, and nasogastric tubes), and any fluid aspirated from a body cavity.
   b. Measure the amount of irrigation fluid instilled when irrigating a nasogastric or other tube or the bladder; subtract it from total output.
   c. Measure drainage in a calibrated container. Observe it at eye level, and record the reading at the bottom of the meniscus.
   d. Compare the client's output to that of an average adult; intake and output should be relatively equivalent.

VI. Perform Imbalance-Specific Interventions

A. Respiratory acidosis
1. Implement the health-care provider's orders to treat the underlying cause of the imbalance.
   a. Assess the client's respiratory status and auscultate lung sounds at least every 2 hours.
      1) Assess the client's nail beds and oral membranes for cyanosis.
   b. Maintain a patent airway.
      1) Reverse hypoventilation.
      2) Provide supplemental oxygen as needed.
      3) Implement pulmonary hygiene measures to improve gas exchange: chest percussion and physiotherapy, postural drainage.
      4) Place the client in a mid to high Fowler's position to increase lung expansion.
      5) Prepare for mechanical ventilation as necessary.

(!) Use oxygen with caution in clients with COPD or chronic lung disease; supplemental oxygen may result in respiratory arrest.

   c. Maintain adequate hydration by providing 2 to 3 L of fluid per day.
   d. Discontinue central nervous system depressants, as ordered by the health-care provider.
      1) Barbiturates
      2) Benzodiazepines
      3) Muscle relaxants
      4) Opioid analgesics
      5) Sedatives
      6) Tranquilizers
2. Administer medications as ordered.
   a. Bronchodilators to increase the diameter of the upper airways
      1) albuterol (Ventolin, Proventil)
      2) aminophylline (Phyllocontin)
   b. Corticosteroids to decrease inflammation and increase the diameter of the upper airways
      1) hydrocortisone (Solu-Cortef)—short acting
      2) methylprednisolone (Solu-Medrol)—intermediate acting
      3) dexamethasone (DexPak)—long acting
   c. Mucolytics to thin pulmonary secretions
      1) acetylcysteine solution (Mucomyst)
   d. Narcotic or benzodiazepine antagonists to reduce respiratory depression
      1) flumazenil (Romazicon)
      2) naloxone hydrochloride (Narcan)
   e. System alkalinizer to increase blood pH, only if serum bicarbonate levels are low
      1) sodium bicarbonate (Neut)

B. Metabolic acidosis
1. Implement the health-care provider's orders to treat the underlying cause of the imbalance.
   a. Monitor for loss of bicarbonate through the gastrointestinal tract as appropriate.
      1) Diarrhea
      2) External small bowel fistula; a dressing may be adequate for a fistula draining a small amount, but for a fistula draining more than 150 mL in 24 hours, a pouching system is better
   b. Maintain adequate hydration by providing 2 to 3 L of fluid per day.
   c. Prepare the client for dialysis as appropriate.

2. Administer medications as ordered.
   a. Antidiarrheals to prevent or decrease watery stools
      1) diphenoxylate/atropine (Lomotil)
      2) loperamide (Imodium, Kaopectate)
   b. Isotonic or hypotonic IV solutions to restore fluid balance
      1) IV 0.45% saline solution
      2) IV 0.9% saline solution (normal saline solution)
   c. System alkalinizer to increase blood pH
      1) sodium bicarbonate (Neut)
   d. Insulin to decrease serum glucose level when metabolic acidosis is caused by DKA. Be certain that you understand which insulin you are administering, and always double-check the dosage: insulin is a high-alert medication (Table 8.5).

C. Respiratory alkalosis
1. Implement the health-care provider's orders to treat the underlying cause of the imbalance.
   a. Maintain a patent airway.
      1) Reverse hyperventilation.
      2) Encourage the client to relax and breathe slowly.
      3) Assist the client to breathe into a paper bag, rebreather mask, or cupped hands to increase the retention of CO_2.
      4) Reduce mechanical ventilation by adjusting the respiratory rate and tidal volume.

D. Metabolic alkalosis
1. Implement the health-care provider's orders to treat the underlying cause of the imbalance.
   a. Plan for possible hemodialysis.
   b. Monitor for and treat associated hypokalemia, if indicated.
2. Administer medications as ordered.
   a. Antiemetics to prevent or decrease nausea or vomiting
      1) ondansetron (Zofran)
      2) promethazine (Phenergan)
   b. Electrolyte replacement as needed
      1) potassium chloride (K-Lor, K-Dur)
      2) potassium phosphate
   c. Isotonic IV solutions to restore fluid balance
      1) IV 0.9% saline solution (normal saline solution)
      2) IV lactated Ringer's solution

VII. Perform General Nursing Interventions

A. Ensure client safety
1. Reduce environmental stimuli.
   a. Provide a quiet room.
   b. Limit the client's visitors.
   c. Darken the client's room.
   d. Speak in soft tones.
2. Implement seizure precautions.
   a. Pad the side rails.
   b. Have oxygen and suction equipment available.

Table 8.5 Types of Insulin

Type	Agent	Onset	Peak	Duration
Rapid-acting insulin	Insulin lispro (Humalog)	5 min	60–90 min	4–6 hr
	Insulin aspart (NovoLog)	10–20 min	1–3 hr	3–5 hr
Short-acting insulin	Regular insulin (Humulin R) (!) Regular insulin is the only insulin that can be given by the IV route	Subcutaneous route: 30–60 min IV route: 10–30 min	Subcutaneous route: 2–4 hr IV route: 15–30 min	Subcutaneous route: 5–7 hr IV route: 30–60 min
	Concentrated insulin (Insulin U-500) (!) Do not give by the IV route	30–60 min	2–3 hr	5–7 hr
Intermediate-acting insulin	NPH (Humulin N, Novolin R)	1–2 hr	8–12 hr	18–24 hr
Long-acting insulin	Insulin glargine (Lantus) (!) Cannot be mixed with other insulins	3–4 hr	None	24 hr
	Insulin detemir (Levemir)	3–4 hr	3–14 hr	24 hr
Premixed insulin	NPH/regular (Humulin 50/50, Humulin 70/30, Novolin 70/30)	30 min	4–8 hr	24 hr
	Aspart protamine/aspart (NovoLog Mix 70/30)	15 min	1–4 hr	24 hr
	Lispro protamine/lispro (Humalog Mix 75/25)	15–30 min	2.8 hr	24 hr

c. Ensure the patency of IV access devices.
d. Administer emergency medications as ordered.
e. Prepare for possible endotracheal intubation.
f. Prepare for cardiac defibrillation if necessary.

3. Implement fall precautions because of muscle weakness secondary to acid-base imbalance.
   a. Perform a fall risk assessment.
   b. Maintain the bed in a low position with locked wheels.
   c. Remove all obstacles from pathways, especially to the toilet.
   d. Monitor the environment for safety hazards, such as torn carpet and liquid spills on floors.
   e. Place assistive devices, such as walkers and canes, within the client's reach.
   f. Use nightlights.
   g. Instruct the client to request assistance to ambulate.
   h. Ensure the availability of the call light.
   i. Assess the client's footwear and provide appropriate footwear if necessary; clients must use antiskid soles.
   j. Keep items such as telephone and fluids close to the client.
   k. Request that family members remain with the client if necessary.
   l. Position the client to allow close observation by staff members.
   m. Communicate the client's fall risk during the shift report and as necessary.

B. Educate the client

1. Acidosis
   a. Teach the client or caregiver the causes of acidosis.
   b. Provide specific information regarding the client's medical diagnosis and related interventions and treatments.
   c. Teach the client how to identify signs and symptoms of acid-base imbalances.
   d. Instruct the client and family to notify the primary health-care provider if the client exhibits signs or symptoms of acid-base imbalance or if they have any other specific concerns.
   e. Ensure that the client or caregiver understands the specifics, rationale, potential side effects, and desired effects of the treatment regimen.
   f. Include medication administration, nutrition, hydration, and any dietary restrictions in client teaching.
   g. Teach the client to adhere to the medication regimen, especially a client at risk for DKA.
   h. Encourage the client, especially one with COPD or chronic lung disease, to quit smoking and participate in a smoking cessation program.
2. Alkalosis
   a. Teach the client or caregiver the causes of alkalosis.
   b. Provide specific information regarding the client's medical diagnosis and related interventions and treatments.
   c. Teach the client how to identify the signs and symptoms of acid-base imbalances.
   d. Instruct the client and family to notify the primary health-care provider if the client exhibits signs or symptoms of acid-base imbalance or if they have any other specific concerns.
   e. Ensure that the client or caregiver understands the specifics, rationale, potential side effects, and desired effects of the treatment regimen.
   f. Include medication administration, nutrition, hydration, and any dietary restrictions in client teaching.
   g. Teach the client to adhere to the medication regimen.
   h. Instruct the client in stress management, especially controlled breathing, to decrease anxiety-induced hyperventilation.

C. Evaluate and document

1. Document all assessment findings and interventions per institution policy.
2. Evaluate and document the client's response to interventions and education.
   a. Arterial and venous blood gas values should be within the normal reference ranges.
   b. Fluid volume status should be within normal limits; urinary output should be a minimum of 30 mL/hr for adults.
   c. All laboratory values should be returned to baseline.
   d. Vital signs should be within normal limits.

CASE STUDY: Putting It All Together

Subjective Data

An adult client presents to the emergency department with a 4-day history of weakness, fever, nausea, vomiting, and abdominal pain. The client's family reports that the client, who has a history of type 2 diabetes mellitus and hypertension, has also been confused. The client reports extreme thirst and has been voiding large volumes of dilute urine for several days. The client has no known allergies, and the current medications are as follows:

- metformin (Glucophage) 500 mg by mouth (PO) twice a day, before breakfast and dinner
- lisinopril/hydrochlorothiazide (Zestoretic) 20/12.5 mg PO once a day
- multivitamin 1 tablet PO once a day

Objective Data

Nursing Assessment

1. Drowsy, easily arousable; oriented to person but not to place or time; occasionally restless; PERRLA (pupils equal, regular, react to light and accommodation)
2. Strong odor of ketones ("fruity" breath odor)
3. Skin flushed, warm, dry; mucous membranes pink, dry
4. Heart sounds S_1 and S_2 regular, rapid
5. Respirations deep, rapid, dry; lung sounds clear in all fields
6. Pedal and radial pulses regular, 1+, and weak bilaterally
7. Bowel sounds hypoactive in all four quadrants; abdomen soft, nontender

Vital Signs	
Temperature:	101.2°F (38.4°C) orally
Blood pressure:	86/54 mm Hg
Heart rate:	138 bpm
Respiratory rate:	38
O_2 saturation:	95% on room air

Laboratory Results	
Serum glucose:	440 mg/dL
Serum sodium:	132 mEq/L
Serum chloride:	113 mEq/L
Serum potassium:	3.0 mEq/L
Creatinine:	1.8 mg/dL
Blood urea nitrogen (BUN):	22 mg/dL
Anion gap:	20.8 mEq/L
Urinalysis:	cloudy, dark yellow; pH 6.0; specific gravity 1.045; 4+ glucose; 3+ ketones; leukocyte positive
White blood cell (WBC) count:	20 (× $10^3/mm^3$); with 60% neutrophils, 12% bands, 25% lymphocytes, 3% monocytes

Laboratory Results—cont'd	
ABG:	pH 7.16, $PaCO_2$ 20 mm Hg, HCO_3^- 6.2 mEq/L, PaO_2 90 mm Hg
ECG:	sinus tachycardia with left ventricular hypertrophy
Chest x-ray:	no evidence of pathology or infiltrate

Health-Care Provider Orders

1. Monitor oxygen (O_2) saturation continuously; provide O_2 at 2 L/min via nasal cannula as needed to maintain O_2 saturation greater than 95%.
2. Assess vital signs every 15 minutes × 2 hours, then hourly until stable, then every 4 hours.
3. Start telemetry.
4. Monitor strict intake and output hourly.
5. Hold oral medications until instructed to resume.
6. Monitor blood glucose level per insulin protocol (every 15 to 60 minutes).
7. Administer 10 to 20 units of regular insulin (as ordered), and begin an insulin drip per insulin protocol.
8. Administer IV 0.9% normal saline solution 1,000 mL over 30 minutes, then a second 1,000 mL over 60 minutes, while monitoring blood pressure tolerance.
9. Monitor for fluid volume excess (fluid deficit is usually 3 to 5 L).
10. Change IV fluid to dextrose 5% in normal saline when blood glucose level reaches 250 mg/dL.
11. Discontinue insulin drip and administer subcutaneous regular insulin per sliding scale when acidosis or ketosis is corrected and the client is tolerating oral intake.
12. Provide clear liquid diet as tolerated.
13. Obtain laboratory values hourly × 4, then every 4 hours: glucose, sodium, potassium, and creatinine levels and BUN. Obtain ABGs 2 hours after initiation of insulin therapy.
14. Obtain urine for culture and sensitivity, and report results to health-care provider.
15. Administer IV ciprofloxacin (Cipro) 400 mg every 12 hours.
16. Repeat ECG in 4 hours.
17. Implement fall precautions.
18. Provide client education, when the client is stable, regarding etiology, treatment, and prevention of DKA and associated fluid and electrolyte imbalances.

CASE STUDY: Putting It All Together *cont'd*

Case Study Questions

A. What *subjective* assessment findings indicate that the client is experiencing a health alteration?

1. ______
2. ______
3. ______
4. ______
5. ______
6. ______

B. What *objective* assessment findings indicate that the client is experiencing a health alteration?

1. ______
2. ______
3. ______
4. ______
5. ______
6. ______
7. ______
8. ______
9. ______
10. ______
11. ______
12. ______
13. ______

C. After analyzing the data collected, what **primary** nursing diagnosis should the nurse assign to this client?

______

Continued

CASE STUDY: Putting It All Together *cont'd*

Case Study Questions

D. What interventions should the nurse plan and/or implement to meet this client's needs?

1. ___
2. ___
3. ___
4. ___
5. ___
6. ___
7. ___
8. ___
9. ___
10. ___
11. ___
12. ___
13. ___
14. ___
15. ___
16. ___
17. ___

E. What client outcomes should the nurse plan to evaluate the effectiveness of the nursing interventions?

1. ___
2. ___
3. ___
4. ___
5. ___
6. ___
7. ___
8. ___

REVIEW QUESTIONS

1. When caring for a client with an acid-base imbalance, which serum electrolytes are essential for a nurse to monitor? **Select all that apply.**
   1. Potassium
   2. Sodium
   3. Calcium
   4. Chloride
   5. Magnesium

2. A student nurse is observing a specially trained registered nurse who is preparing to draw an ABG specimen from an adult client who has been diagnosed with pneumonia. Which statement by the student nurse is correct?
   1. "Arterial blood gases are used to evaluate a client's fluid and electrolyte status."
   2. "Venous blood and arterial blood provide the same information about a client's status."
   3. "It is important to apply pressure for 2 minutes after drawing an arterial blood gas."
   4. "Arterial blood gases may be drawn by a laboratory technician, respiratory therapist, or nurse with specialized training."

3. A nurse who is assessing a client diagnosed with DKA notes that the client is exhibiting Kussmaul respirations. The nurse should associate this respiratory pattern with which physiological goals?
   1. Increased CO_2 retention, decreased serum pH
   2. Decreased CO_2 retention, increased serum pH
   3. Increased CO_2 excretion, increased serum pH
   4. Decreased CO_2 excretion, decreased serum pH

4. A nurse prepares to interpret the ABG values of a client diagnosed with an acid-base imbalance. Which values are most important for the nurse to consider? **Select all that apply.**
   1. pH
   2. PaO_2
   3. $PaCO_2$
   4. SpO_2
   5. HCO_3^-

5. A client runs into an emergency department after witnessing a fatal automobile collision. The client is dizzy and breathing rapidly and is immediately assisted by a nurse. The nurse assesses that the client is hyperventilating and instructs the client to rebreathe into a paper bag. What is the nurse's rationale for this intervention?
   1. To increase the blood pH by rebreathing oxygen
   2. To decrease the blood pH by rebreathing oxygen
   3. To increase the blood pH by rebreathing CO_2
   4. To decrease the blood pH by rebreathing CO_2

6. A nurse calculates the anion gap of a client suspected of having metabolic acidosis. The client's serum sodium level is 158 mEq/L, serum chloride level is 105 mEq/L, and serum bicarbonate level is 28 mEq/L. What is the value of this client's anion gap in mEq/L? Record your answer as a whole number.

   ____

7. A nursing instructor is explaining acid-base imbalance to a group of nursing students. Which statements by the nursing instructor are correct regarding the body's attempt to restore acid-base balance? **Select all that apply.**
   1. Respiratory compensation is slow but very efficient.
   2. Renal compensation is slow and long lasting.
   3. Respiratory compensation is fast and long lasting.
   4. Renal compensation is fast but temporary.
   5. Respiratory compensation is fast but temporary.

8. A nurse is caring for a client who is at risk for metabolic acidosis. Which mechanism should the nurse identify as the first line of defense against changes in the pH of the blood?
   1. Acids
   2. Buffers
   3. Respiratory system
   4. Renal system

9. A nurse admits an older adult client with a history of COPD. The client's respirations are 24 breaths per minute and shallow, pulse oximetry is 86%, and circumoral cyanosis is noted. Which acid-base imbalance should the nurse identify in this client?
   1. Respiratory acidosis
   2. Metabolic acidosis
   3. Respiratory alkalosis
   4. Metabolic alkalosis

10. A nurse in the emergency department is planning care for a client who is inebriated. Which acid-base imbalance should the nurse anticipate when planning care for this client?
    1. Respiratory acidosis
    2. Metabolic acidosis
    3. Respiratory alkalosis
    4. Metabolic alkalosis

11. A nurse obtains the recent medical history of a newly admitted client. Which factors in the client's history should the nurse identify as placing the client at risk for respiratory acidosis? **Select all that apply.**
    1. Renal failure
    2. Fever
    3. Oxycodone use
    4. Dehydration
    5. Pneumonia

12. A nurse assesses an older adult client for the presence of an acid-base imbalance. Which questions should the nurse ask the client when performing this assessment? **Select all that apply.**
    1. "Did you get a flu shot this year?"
    2. "Has your urine changed color or odor?"
    3. "When was your last physical examination?"
    4. "Have you had any shortness of breath during activity or at rest?"
    5. "Have you noticed any changes in memory or difficulty concentrating?"

13. A nurse reviews the laboratory data of a client diagnosed with COPD. The nurse notes that the client's blood pH is within the normal reference range, although the client's respirations are shallow, labored, and at a rate of 11 breaths per minute. What should the nurse identify as the best explanation for this scenario?
    1. The client's lungs are partially compensating for respiratory acidosis.
    2. The client's lungs have fully compensated for respiratory acidosis.
    3. The client's kidneys have partially compensated for respiratory acidosis.
    4. The client's kidneys have fully compensated for respiratory acidosis.

14. A nurse analyzes the STAT laboratory data of a child admitted to the emergency department after inhaling a marble. Which laboratory results should the nurse expect to be abnormal? **Select all that apply.**
    1. Blood pH
    2. HCO_3^- level
    3. PaO_2 level
    4. $PaCO_2$ level
    5. Serum K^+ level

15. A nurse is caring for a client who is having a panic attack and begins to hyperventilate. The client reports dizziness and circumoral tingling and numbness. For which acid-base imbalance is the client most at risk?
    1. Respiratory acidosis
    2. Metabolic acidosis
    3. Respiratory alkalosis
    4. Metabolic alkalosis

16. A nurse assesses an older adult client in the emergency department. Which signs should the nurse associate with the development of respiratory or metabolic acidosis if observed in this client? **Select all that apply.**
    1. Hyperreflexia
    2. Paresthesias
    3. Positive Chvostek's sign
    4. Lethargy
    5. Muscle weakness
    6. Warm, flushed, dry skin

17. A nurse is caring for a critically ill client who begins exhibiting Kussmaul respirations. Which acid-base imbalance should the nurse associate with this type of respiration?
    1. Respiratory acidosis
    2. Metabolic acidosis
    3. Respiratory alkalosis
    4. Metabolic alkalosis

18. A nurse who is assessing an adolescent client who has just been injured in a motor vehicle collision finds that the client is anxious, has no memory of the accident, and is reporting dizziness, tingling hands, and headache. The client has a blood pressure of 136/76 mm Hg, a heart rate of 98 bpm, and a respiratory rate of 32 breaths per minute. Which acid-base imbalance should the nurse associate with these signs and symptoms?
    1. Metabolic acidosis
    2. Metabolic alkalosis
    3. Respiratory acidosis
    4. Respiratory alkalosis

19. A nurse is preparing to administer a continuous insulin infusion to a client diagnosed with DKA. A physician orders an initial IV infusion of 10 units of regular insulin per hour. The pharmacy supplies 50 units of regular insulin in 100 mL of 0.9% saline solution. How many milliliters of solution should the nurse infuse hourly? Record your answer as a whole number.

    ____

20. A nurse is preparing to administer an insulin drip to a client with a blood glucose level of 600 mg/dL and an arterial blood pH of 7.21. A physician orders an initial IV infusion of 20 units of regular insulin per hour. The pharmacy supplies 100 units of regular insulin in 500 mL of 0.9% saline solution. How many milliliters of solution should the nurse infuse hourly? Record your answer as a whole number.

    ____

21. A nurse is preparing to administer an IV sodium bicarbonate infusion to a client diagnosed with moderate metabolic acidosis. A physician orders 3 mEq/kg sodium bicarbonate over 4 hours. The client weighs 223 lb. How many milliequivalents of sodium bicarbonate should the nurse administer? Record your answer as a whole number.

    ____

22. A nurse is preparing to administer an IV sodium bicarbonate infusion to a client diagnosed with moderate metabolic acidosis. A physician orders 3 mEq/kg sodium bicarbonate 5% to be infused over 8 hours. The dose on hand is 0.6 mEq/mL in 500 mL of 0.9% saline solution. The client weighs 175 lb. How many milliliters of sodium bicarbonate 5% solution should the nurse administer? Record your answer as a whole number.

____

23. A nurse who is assessing a client admitted to the emergency department with a closed head injury notes that the client's respiratory rate is 8 breaths per minute. The nurse should associate this finding with which acid-base imbalance?
    1. Respiratory acidosis
    2. Metabolic acidosis
    3. Respiratory alkalosis
    4. Metabolic alkalosis

24. Which laboratory values should a nurse expect when evaluating the ABG values of a client diagnosed with partially compensated respiratory alkalosis?
    1. pH decreasing toward 7.45 and an increase in HCO_3^-
    2. pH decreasing toward 7.45 and a decrease in HCO_3^-
    3. pH increasing toward 7.35 and an increase in HCO_3^-
    4. pH increasing toward 7.35 and a decrease in HCO_3^-

25. A nurse is assessing a child who has a history of type 1 diabetes mellitus and is experiencing weakness, nausea, and anorexia of 4 days' duration. The child has not received the prescribed insulin during this illness and currently has a blood glucose level of 400 mg/dL. Which ABG pH is the nurse most likely to find?
    1. Greater than 7.45
    2. Less than 7.35
    3. Approximately 7.40
    4. Between 7.35 and 7.45

26. A nurse is assessing an adolescent client who reports numbness and tingling of the hands and face and increased stress related to school and peer relationships. The client's vital signs are temperature 98.8°F (37°C), blood pressure 116/72 mm Hg, heart rate 96 bpm, and respiratory rate 32 breaths per minute. Which acid-base imbalance should the nurse suspect that this client is experiencing?
    1. Respiratory acidosis
    2. Respiratory alkalosis
    3. Metabolic acidosis
    4. Metabolic alkalosis

27. A nurse assesses a pregnant client in her first trimester of pregnancy who has been vomiting for 3 days. The client is diagnosed with hyperemesis gravidarum. The nurse should correctly identify that the client is experiencing which fluid and acid-base imbalance?
    1. Fluid volume excess and respiratory acidosis
    2. Fluid volume deficit and metabolic acidosis
    3. Fluid volume excess and respiratory alkalosis
    4. Fluid volume deficit and metabolic alkalosis

28. A nurse assesses a client diagnosed with Cushing's disease. The client's ABG values are pH 7.42, $PaCO_2$ 48 mm Hg, and HCO_3^- 32 mEq/L. Which acid-base imbalance should the nurse identify in this client?
    1. Partially compensated respiratory acidosis
    2. Fully compensated respiratory alkalosis
    3. Partially compensated metabolic acidosis
    4. Fully compensated metabolic alkalosis

29. An emergency department nurse admits a client who has tried to commit suicide by taking an overdose of oxycodone (OxyContin). For which acid-base imbalance should the nurse assess this client?
    1. Respiratory acidosis
    2. Metabolic acidosis
    3. Respiratory alkalosis
    4. Metabolic alkalosis

30. A nurse comforts a pregnant client who is experiencing vaginal bleeding. The client has a panic attack and begins to hyperventilate. Which intervention should a nurse initiate *first* when caring for this client?
    1. Assist the client to breathe into cupped hands.
    2. Perform a vaginal examination.
    3. Position the client on her left side.
    4. Administer oxygen via nasal cannula.

31. A 2-year-old child is brought to an urgent care clinic after ingesting a bottle of baby aspirin. For which acid-base imbalances should a nurse assess this child?
    1. Respiratory acidosis and metabolic acidosis
    2. Respiratory acidosis and metabolic alkalosis
    3. Metabolic acidosis and respiratory alkalosis
    4. Metabolic acidosis and metabolic alkalosis

32. A psychiatric inpatient begins to hyperventilate for an extended period. A unit nurse applies a rebreather mask but is unable to calm the client. In addition to a physician's order to administer a sedative to this client, the nurse should anticipate an order for which intervention?
    1. 0.9% saline solution by IV bolus
    2. Epinephrine by IV push
    3. Sodium bicarbonate by IV push
    4. No additional treatment

33. A nurse admits to the emergency department a 3-year-old child who is experiencing a fluid volume deficit secondary to fever and diarrhea for 5 days. Based on this information, for which acid-base imbalance should the nurse assess this client?
1. Respiratory acidosis
2. Respiratory alkalosis
3. Metabolic acidosis
4. Metabolic alkalosis

34. A nurse is planning care for a client with a history of COPD who was recently diagnosed with pneumonia. Which interventions should the nurse include to prevent this client from developing respiratory acidosis? **Select all that apply.**
1. Provide pulmonary hygiene.
2. Instruct the client about the use of ordered bronchodilators.
3. Administer ordered IV sodium bicarbonate 5%.
4. Maintain hydration.
5. Increase dietary potassium intake.

35. A nurse prepares to interpret the ABG values of a client. Which steps should the nurse take to interpret the client's acid-base balance? Place each step in the correct sequence (1–5).
_______ Determine whether there is compensation.
_______ Examine the blood $PaCO_2$ and HCO_3^- values.
_______ Examine the blood pH value.
_______ Determine the degree of compensation.
_______ Compare the blood $PaCO_2$ and HCO_3^- values.

36. A nurse is evaluating the laboratory values of a client diagnosed with DKA. After reviewing the client's serum sodium, chloride, and bicarbonate levels, the nurse calculates that the client's anion gap is 25 mEq/L. How should the nurse interpret this value?
1. Confirmation of metabolic acidosis
2. Evidence of metabolic alkalosis
3. Verification of respiratory acidosis
4. Proof of respiratory alkalosis

37. Which interventions should a nurse include in the plan of care for a client with a history of COPD who is diagnosed with pneumonia and respiratory acidosis? **Select all that apply.**
1. Place the client in a mid to high Fowler's position.
2. Increase fluid intake, unless contraindicated.
3. Position the client supine with the head of the bed flat.
4. Administer 100% oxygen via a nonrebreather mask.
5. Auscultate breath sounds every 2 hours and as needed.

38. A nurse is preparing to administer a loading dose of aminophylline at 6 mg/kg (as ordered) to a client who has been diagnosed with respiratory acidosis related to acute exacerbation of emphysema. The client weighs 140 lb. The dose on hand is 25 mg/mL. How many milliliters should the nurse administer? Record your answer using one decimal place.

____

39. A nurse is preparing to administer a continuous infusion of aminophylline at 0.7 mg/kg/hr (as ordered) to a client who has been diagnosed with respiratory acidosis related to acute exacerbation of emphysema. The client weighs 180 lb. How many milligrams per hour should the nurse administer? Record your answer using one decimal place.

____

40. A newly diagnosed client with type 1 diabetes mellitus asks a nurse how much regular insulin he should expect to self-inject over the course of an entire day. The nurse reinforces that the client should follow his prescribed insulin schedule carefully and informs the client that the general calculation for the body's daily insulin requirement is the client's weight in pounds divided by 4. If the client weighs 150 lb, how many units of insulin should the client require each day? Record your answer as a whole number.

____

41. A nurse reviews the laboratory values of a newly admitted client. The nurse notes that the client has a serum calcium level of 7.6 mg/dL. Which possible blood pH should the nurse associate with the development of hypocalcemia?
   1. 7.25
   2. 7.35
   3. 7.45
   4. 7.55

42. A nurse interprets that a client's arterial blood pH of 7.50 is metabolic in origin. Which other abnormal laboratory finding should the nurse associate with this pH imbalance?
   1. Decreased serum potassium level
   2. Increased serum chloride level
   3. Decreased bicarbonate level
   4. Increased serum calcium level

43. Which acid-base imbalance should a nurse associate with chronic diarrhea in a client diagnosed with Crohn's disease?
   1. Respiratory acidosis
   2. Metabolic acidosis
   3. Respiratory alkalosis
   4. Metabolic alkalosis

44. A client's ABG report reveals a pH of 6.65. How should a nurse interpret this value?
   1. The pH is slightly decreased.
   2. The pH is within the normal reference range.
   3. The pH is extremely increased.
   4. The pH is incompatible with life.

45. A nurse is caring for a client diagnosed with uncompensated metabolic acidosis secondary to end-stage renal disease. When reviewing this client's laboratory data, which values should the nurse anticipate? **Select all that apply.**
   1. Increased pH
   2. Decreased pH
   3. Increased $PaCO_2$
   4. Normal $PaCO_2$
   5. Decreased $PaCO_2$
   6. Increased HCO_3^-
   7. Normal HCO_3^-
   8. Decreased HCO_3^-

46. A nurse is caring for a client diagnosed with uncompensated metabolic alkalosis secondary to prolonged vomiting. When reviewing this client's laboratory data, which values should the nurse anticipate? **Select all that apply.**
   1. Increased pH
   2. Decreased pH
   3. Increased $PaCO_2$
   4. Normal $PaCO_2$
   5. Decreased $PaCO_2$
   6. Increased HCO_3^-
   7. Normal HCO_3^-
   8. Decreased HCO_3^-

47. A nurse is caring for a client diagnosed with uncompensated respiratory acidosis secondary to hypoventilation related to a traumatic brain injury. When reviewing this client's laboratory data, which values should the nurse anticipate? **Select all that apply.**
   1. Increased pH
   2. Decreased pH
   3. Increased $PaCO_2$
   4. Normal $PaCO_2$
   5. Decreased $PaCO_2$
   6. Increased HCO_3^-
   7. Normal HCO_3^-
   8. Decreased HCO_3^-

48. A nurse is caring for a client diagnosed with uncompensated respiratory alkalosis secondary to hyperventilation related to an acute asthma attack. When reviewing this client's laboratory data, which values should the nurse anticipate? **Select all that apply.**
   1. Increased pH
   2. Decreased pH
   3. Increased $PaCO_2$
   4. Normal $PaCO_2$
   5. Decreased $PaCO_2$
   6. Increased HCO_3^-
   7. Normal HCO_3^-
   8. Decreased HCO_3^-

49. A nurse is assessing an older adult client suspected of having DKA. Which respiratory pattern should the nurse identify as indicative of DKA?

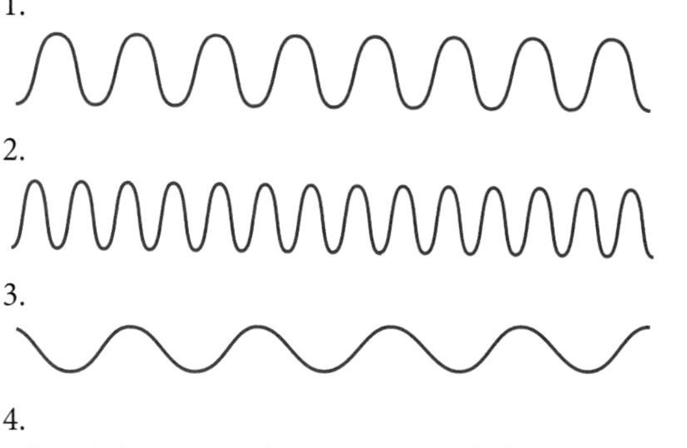

50. A home health nurse visits an older adult client diagnosed with type 2 diabetes mellitus. The client has signs and symptoms of a urinary tract infection and has been limiting fluid intake to avoid urination. The client's blood glucose level is 620 mg/dL, and the client's urine dipstick is negative for ketones. Which condition should the nurse associate with these manifestations?
   1. Diabetic ketoacidosis (DKA)
   2. End-stage renal disease
   3. Exocrine pancreatic insufficiency
   4. Hyperosmolar hyperglycemic state (HHS)

51. Which interventions are appropriate for a nurse to implement when caring for a client diagnosed with respiratory acidosis secondary to COPD? **Select all that apply.**
   1. Implement airborne precautions.
   2. Place the client in an upright position.
   3. Administer oxygen at 6 L/min via nasal cannula.
   4. Administer IV 0.45% saline solution as ordered.
   5. Administer methylprednisolone (Solu-Medrol) as ordered.

52. A nurse is preparing to administer insulin to a client diagnosed with DKA. Which agent should the nurse identify as the insulin of choice for this client?
   1. Humalog
   2. Humulin R
   3. Novolin R
   4. Lantus

53. A nurse is caring for a critically ill client in the intensive care unit. Which factors should the nurse identify as placing the client at risk for an acid-base imbalance? **Select all that apply.**
   1. Age
   2. Gender
   3. Cerebral edema
   4. Opioid administration
   5. Mechanical ventilation
   6. Administration of IV 0.9% saline solution

54. A nurse is assessing a client who may be experiencing metabolic alkalosis. Which signs and symptoms, if noted during the assessment, should the nurse associate with this particular acid-base imbalance? **Select all that apply.**
   1. Cyanosis
   2. Muscle cramping
   3. Lethargy
   4. Shallow respirations
   5. Deep respirations

55. A nurse is caring for a client diagnosed with pancreatitis. The client's blood pH is 7.20. When reviewing the client's laboratory data, which other abnormalities should the nurse anticipate? **Select all that apply.**
   1. Decreased bicarbonate (HCO_3^-) level
   2. Decreased partial pressure of oxygen (PaO_2) level
   3. Normal partial pressure of carbon dioxide ($PaCO_2$) level
   4. Increased serum potassium (K^+) level
   5. Increased serum calcium (Ca^{2+}) level

56. Which potential nursing diagnoses should a nurse assign to a client with a blood pH of 7.25 secondary to diarrhea lasting 4 days? **Select all that apply.**
   1. Risk for Falls Related to Skeletal Muscle Weakness
   2. Risk for Constipation Related to Decreased Bowel Motility
   3. Impaired Memory Related to Fluid and Electrolyte Imbalance
   4. Ineffective Breathing Pattern Related to Impaired Gas Exchange
   5. Deficient Fluid Volume Related to Dehydration

57. A nurse is managing the care of a client who was just admitted with a diagnosis of DKA. A physician writes orders for the client. Which physician orders should the nurse question? **Select all that apply.**
1. Monitor neurological status every hour.
2. Place the client on a potassium-restricted diet.
3. Check vital signs every 15 minutes until stable.
4. Administer regular insulin subcutaneously per sliding scale.
5. Administer IV 0.45% saline solution at 1,000 mL/hr.

58. A nurse analyzes a client's ABG values. The client's serum pH is 7.25, $PaCO_2$ is 47 mm Hg, and HCO_3^- is 24 mEq/L. Which acid-base imbalance should the nurse associate with these ABG values?
1. Uncompensated respiratory acidosis
2. Compensated respiratory acidosis
3. Uncompensated metabolic acidosis
4. Compensated metabolic acidosis

59. A nurse analyzes a client's ABG values. The client's serum pH is 7.51, $PaCO_2$ is 32 mm Hg, and HCO_3^- is 25 mEq/L. Which acid-base imbalance should the nurse associate with these ABG values?
1. Uncompensated metabolic alkalosis
2. Compensated metabolic alkalosis
3. Uncompensated respiratory alkalosis
4. Compensated respiratory alkalosis

60. A nurse analyzes a client's ABG values. The client's serum pH is 7.30, $PaCO_2$ is 38 mm Hg, and HCO_3^- is 20 mEq/L. Which acid-base imbalance should the nurse associate with these ABG values?
1. Uncompensated respiratory acidosis
2. Uncompensated metabolic acidosis
3. Compensated respiratory acidosis
4. Compensated metabolic acidosis

61. A nurse analyzes a client's ABG values. The client's serum pH is 7.49, $PaCO_2$ is 43 mm Hg, and HCO_3^- is 28 mEq/L. Which acid-base imbalance should the nurse associate with these ABG values?
1. Uncompensated metabolic alkalosis
2. Compensated metabolic alkalosis
3. Uncompensated respiratory alkalosis
4. Compensated respiratory alkalosis

62. A nurse analyzes a client's ABG values. The client's serum pH is 7.32, $PaCO_2$ is 46 mm Hg, and HCO_3^- is 29 mEq/L. Which acid-base imbalance should the nurse associate with these ABG values?
1. Fully compensated metabolic acidosis
2. Partially compensated metabolic acidosis
3. Fully compensated respiratory acidosis
4. Partially compensated respiratory acidosis

63. A nurse analyzes a client's ABG values. The client's serum pH is 7.37, $PaCO_2$ is 46 mm Hg, and HCO_3^- is 29 mEq/L. Which acid-base imbalance should the nurse associate with these ABG values?
1. Partially compensated metabolic acidosis
2. Fully compensated respiratory acidosis
3. Partially compensated metabolic alkalosis
4. Fully compensated respiratory alkalosis

64. A nurse analyzes a client's ABG values. The client's serum pH is 7.44, $PaCO_2$ is 34 mm Hg, and HCO_3^- is 19 mEq/L. Which acid-base imbalance should the nurse associate with these ABG values?
1. Partially compensated metabolic acidosis
2. Fully compensated respiratory acidosis
3. Partially compensated metabolic alkalosis
4. Fully compensated respiratory alkalosis

65. A nurse reviews the laboratory values of multiple clients on a medical-surgical unit. Which ABG values should the nurse associate with a client reporting surgical pain who has a blood pressure of 142/86 mm Hg, a heart rate of 104 bpm, and a respiratory rate of 34 breaths per minute?

1.

pH	7.30
$PaCO_2$	35 mm Hg
HCO_3^-	16 mEq/L

2.

pH	7.48
$PaCO_2$	45 mm Hg
HCO_3^-	32 mEq/L

3.

pH	7.32
$PaCO_2$	50 mm Hg
HCO_3^-	24 mEq/L

4.

pH	7.50
$PaCO_2$	28 mm Hg
HCO_3^-	22 mEq/L

66. A nurse in a postanesthesia care unit notes that a client recovering from surgery is lethargic and difficult to arouse. The client has been receiving IV morphine sulfate 4 mg for pain. The client's respiratory rate is 10 breaths per minute with a shallow pattern. Which ABG values should the nurse associate with this client's manifestations?

Lab Report A		Lab Report B		Lab Report C		Lab Report D	
pH	7.15	pH	7.30	pH	7.44	pH	7.50
$PaCO_2$	64mm Hg	$PaCO_2$	40mm Hg	$PaCO_2$	40mm Hg	$PaCO_2$	28 mm Hg
HCO_3^-	*22mEq/L*	HCO_3^-	14mEq/L	HCO_3^-	24 mEq/L	HCO_3^-	22 mEq/L

1. Lab Report A
2. Lab Report B
3. Lab Report C
4. Lab Report D

67. Which nursing diagnoses should a nurse assign to an adult client diagnosed with respiratory acidosis related to hypoventilation secondary to excessive narcotic effects? **Select all that apply.**
1. Ineffective Breathing Pattern Related to Reduced Gas Exchange
2. Fatigue Related to Inadequate Tissue Oxygenation
3. Diarrhea Related to Spastic Colonic Activity
4. Risk for Falls Related to Skeletal Muscle Weakness
5. Decreased Cardiac Output Related to Increased Heart Rate

68. A nurse is caring for multiple clients on a medical-surgical unit. Which client should the nurse identify as being at greatest risk for respiratory acidosis?
1. A client who is extremely anxious
2. A client with uncontrolled type 1 diabetes mellitus
3. A client with COPD
4. A client with gastroesophageal reflux disease

69. A nurse on an oncology unit notes that a client recently diagnosed with terminal cancer is reporting dizziness, weakness, and numbness and tingling of the face and hands. The client's respiratory rate is 38 breaths per minute with a shallow pattern. Which ABG values should the nurse associate with this client's manifestations?

Lab Report A		Lab Report B		Lab Report C		Lab Report D	
pH	7.28	pH	7.32	pH	7.43	pH	7.48
$PaCO_2$	60mm Hg	$PaCO_2$	42mm Hg	$PaCO_2$	41mm Hg	$PaCO_2$	27 mm Hg
HCO_3^-	*23mEq/L*	HCO_3^-	15mEq/L	HCO_3^-	23 mEq/L	HCO_3^-	24 mEq/L

1. Lab Report A
2. Lab Report B
3. Lab Report C
4. Lab Report D

70. A client is rushed to the emergency department after falling through thin ice into a partially frozen pond. The client's core body temperature is 86°F (30°C). A nurse assesses that the client is bluish gray in color, rigid, and unconscious; has no audible heartbeat; and has no apparent respirations. The client's condition remains unchanged after being placed on mechanical ventilation, receiving medical treatment, and being slowly rewarmed to 96.8°F (36°C). The client's ABG values are reviewed by the nurse: blood pH 6.7, $PaCO_2$ 48 mm Hg, and HCO_3^- 19 mEq/L. How should the nurse interpret the client's condition?
1. The client has a very good prognosis and should fully recover from the incident.
2. The client has a good prognosis and is slowly recovering from the incident.
3. The client has a fair prognosis and may recover from the incident in time.
4. The client has a poor prognosis and will not recover from the incident.

REVIEW ANSWERS

1. ANSWER: 1, 3, 4.

Rationale:

1. **When caring for a client with an acid-base imbalance, the nurse should monitor the client for related electrolyte imbalances, which include potassium, calcium, and chloride imbalances. ABG values are used to confirm acid-base imbalances, whereas serum electrolyte levels often reveal the underlying cause of the imbalance. Serum potassium levels are *increased in the presence of acidosis* as the body attempts to buffer the decrease in blood pH. Serum potassium levels are *decreased in the presence of alkalosis*, causing central nervous system, neuromuscular, cardiac, and respiratory changes.**
2. Sodium levels are not directly affected by acid-base imbalances.
3. **Serum calcium levels are *decreased in the presence of alkalosis*, causing central nervous system, neuromuscular, cardiac, and respiratory changes.**
4. **Serum chloride levels are *increased in the presence of acidosis* as the body attempts to buffer the decrease in blood pH.**
5. Magnesium levels are not directly affected by acid-base imbalances.

TEST-TAKING TIP: Recall that potassium, calcium, and chloride are directly affected by acid-base imbalances.

Content Area: Adult Health

Integrated Processes: Nursing Process: Implementation

Client Need: Physiological Integrity

Cognitive Level: Knowledge

Reference: *Ignatavicius, D., and Workman, M. (2012). Medical-Surgical Nursing: Patient-Centered Collaborative Care (7th ed.). St. Louis, MO: Saunders.*

2. ANSWER: 4.

Rationale:

1. ABGs are not used to evaluate fluid and electrolyte status; ABGs are used to assess oxygenation status and to detect acid-base imbalances.
2. Arterial blood and venous blood provide different information about the client's oxygenation. Venous blood is warmer than arterial blood and has a lower oxygen content, lower pH, lower concentrations of glucose and other nutrients, and higher concentrations of urea and other waste products.
3. Pressure must be applied for at least 5 minutes after drawing an ABG specimen.
4. **The statement "Arterial blood gases may be drawn by a laboratory technician, respiratory therapist, or nurse with specialized training" is correct. Specialized training is required to draw ABG specimens because of the increased risk of bleeding and damage to the artery.**

TEST-TAKING TIP: Use the process of elimination to rule out statements that are incorrect.

Content Area: Adult Health

Integrated Processes: Teaching/Learning

Client Need: Physiological Integrity

Cognitive Level: Comprehension

Reference: *Berman, A., Snyder, S., Kozier, B., and Erb, G. (2012). Kozier & Erb's Fundamentals of Nursing: Concepts, Process, and Practice (9th ed.). Upper Saddle River, NJ: Pearson.*

3. ANSWER: 3.

Rationale:

1. Increasing CO_2 retention would cause the client's serum pH to decrease, worsening the client's acidosis.
2. Although increasing the client's serum pH is the desired goal, decreasing CO_2 retention is not a goal because this client is experiencing metabolic, not respiratory, acidosis.
3. **The nurse should associate Kussmaul respirations with the body's need to increase CO_2 excretion and to increase serum pH. Kussmaul respirations are very deep, rapid respirations that attempt to correct acidosis by exhaling CO_2, increasing the blood pH.**
4. Decreasing CO_2 excretion would cause the client's serum pH to decrease (acidosis).

TEST-TAKING TIP: Picture in your mind what Kussmaul respirations look like, and envision CO_2 being exhaled with every deep, rapid breath.

Content Area: Adult Health

Integrated Processes: Nursing Process: Analysis

Client Need: Physiological Integrity

Cognitive Level: Comprehension

Reference: *Ignatavicius, D., and Workman, M. (2012). Medical-Surgical Nursing: Patient-Centered Collaborative Care (7th ed.). St. Louis, MO: Saunders.*

4. ANSWER: 1, 2, 3, 5.

Rationale:

1. **When interpreting a client's ABGs, it is most important for the nurse to consider the client's blood pH. An arterial blood pH below 7.35 indicates a state of acidosis. An arterial blood pH above 7.45 indicates a state of alkalosis.**
2. **The partial pressure of oxygen in arterial blood (PaO_2) is important for assessing the client's respiratory function. An arterial PaO_2 level less than 80 mm Hg (decreased) may indicate respiratory depression, decreased cardiac output, or carbon monoxide poisoning, which may result in an acid-base imbalance. An arterial PaO_2 level greater than 100 mm Hg (increased) may indicate an increased ventilation rate or excess oxygen administration, which may result in an acid-base imbalance.**
3. **When interpreting a client's ABGs, it is most important for the nurse to consider the client's partial pressure of carbon dioxide in arterial blood ($PaCO_2$). An arterial $PaCO_2$ level less than 35 mm Hg may indicate a state of respiratory alkalosis. An arterial $PaCO_2$ level greater than 45 mm Hg may indicate a state of respiratory acidosis.**
4. Although oxygen saturation measured by pulse oximetry (SpO_2) is important for assessing respiratory function, this values does not provide useful information about the client's acid-base balance.
5. **When interpreting a client's ABGs, it is most important for the nurse to consider the client's serum HCO_3^- level. An arterial HCO_3^- level less than 21 mEq/L (decreased) may indicate a state of metabolic acidosis. An arterial HCO_3^- level greater than 28 mEq/L (increased) may indicate a state of metabolic alkalosis.**

TEST-TAKING TIP: Recall that the free hydrogen ion level, not the oxygen level, determines blood pH. Rule out option 4 because it is a measurement of oxygen content in the blood.

Content Area: Adult Health
Integrated Processes: Nursing Process: Planning
Client Need: Physiological Integrity
Cognitive Level: Comprehension
Reference: *Berman, A., Snyder, S., Kozier, B., and Erb, G. (2012). Kozier & Erb's Fundamentals of Nursing: Concepts, Process, and Practice (9th ed.). Upper Saddle River, NJ: Pearson.*

5. ANSWER: 4.
Rationale:
1. Additional oxygen would worsen the client's alkalosis.
2. Additional oxygen would worsen the client's alkalosis.
3. By increasing the client's CO_2 level, the nurse would *decrease* the client's blood pH, causing it to become more acidic.
4. The nurse's rationale for instructing the client to rebreathe into a paper bag is to decrease the blood pH by rebreathing CO_2 because this client is hyperventilating and exhaling too much CO_2.
TEST-TAKING TIP: Recall that hyperventilation causes respiratory alkalosis. Choose the option that would decrease the client's blood pH.
Content Area: Adult Health
Integrated Processes: Nursing Process: Implementation
Client Need: Physiological Integrity
Cognitive Level: Comprehension
Reference: *Berman, A., Snyder, S., Kozier, B., and Erb, G. (2012). Kozier & Erb's Fundamentals of Nursing: Concepts, Process, and Practice (9th ed.). Upper Saddle River, NJ: Pearson.*

6. ANSWER: 25.
Rationale:

Anion gap = Serum sodium – (Serum chloride + Serum bicarbonate)
Anion gap = 158 mEq/L – (105 mEq/L + 28 mEq/L) = 158 – 133 = 25 mEq/L

TEST-TAKING TIP: When performing mathematical calculations, perform them in the correct order. To remember the correct order, use the phrase: Please Excuse My Dear Aunt Sally: Parentheses, Exponents, Multiply or Divide, Add or Subtract.
Content Area: Adult Health
Integrated Processes: Nursing Process: Planning
Client Need: Physiological Integrity
Cognitive Level: Comprehension
Reference: *Van Leeuwen, A. M., Poelhuis-Leth, D., and Bladh, M. (2011). Davis's Comprehensive Handbook of Laboratory and Diagnostic Tests With Nursing Implications (4th ed.). Philadelphia, PA: F. A. Davis.*

7. ANSWER: 2, 5.
Rationale:
1. The respiratory system responds rapidly to metabolic imbalances.
2. The statement that renal compensation is slow and long lasting is correct. The renal system is much slower to respond to metabolic imbalances than the respiratory system is, but the response is powerful, effective, and long lasting.
3. The respiratory system responds rapidly to metabolic imbalances, but the effects are easily overwhelmed and short-lived.
4. The renal system is slow to respond to metabolic imbalances, and the response is powerful, effective, and long lasting.
5. The statement that respiratory compensation is fast but temporary is correct. The respiratory system responds rapidly to metabolic imbalances, but the effects are easily overwhelmed and short-lived.
TEST-TAKING TIP: "Lungs are fast, but don't last. Kidneys are slow, but go and go."
Content Area: Adult Health
Integrated Processes: Teaching/Learning
Client Need: Physiological Integrity
Cognitive Level: Comprehension
Reference: *Williams, L., and Hopper, P. (2011). Understanding Medical-Surgical Nursing (4th ed.). Philadelphia, PA: F. A. Davis.*

8. ANSWER: 2.
Rationale:
1. Acids lower pH and would worsen the client's metabolic acidosis.
2. The nurse should identify buffers, such as bicarbonate, phosphate, and albumin, as the first line of defense against changes in the pH of the blood. Buffers bind with or release hydrogen ions to normalize blood pH.
3. The respiratory system is the second line of defense and responds to pH changes rapidly but has only a short-term effect.
4. The renal system is the third line of defense against pH changes; it responds slowly (24 to 48 hours) but has a long-lasting effect.
TEST-TAKING TIP: Recall that buffers can easily react to even subtle pH changes.
Content Area: Adult Health
Integrated Processes: Nursing Process: Analysis
Client Need: Physiological Integrity
Cognitive Level: Comprehension
Reference: *Ignatavicius, D., and Workman, M. (2012). Medical-Surgical Nursing: Patient-Centered Collaborative Care (7th ed.). St. Louis, MO: Saunders.*

9. ANSWER: 1.
Rationale:
1. The nurse should identify that the client is experiencing respiratory acidosis. Respiratory acidosis results when respiratory function is impaired. Oxygen and CO_2 exchange is reduced, causing CO_2 to be retained. An *increase in CO_2* increases the number of free hydrogen ions circulating in the blood, resulting in a *decrease in blood pH* (acidosis).
2. Metabolic acidosis is caused by the excessive breakdown of fatty acids, lactic acid production, or excessive intake of acids.
3. Alkalosis is a decrease in the number of free hydrogen ions circulating in the blood, which results in an increase in blood pH.
4. Alkalosis is a decrease in the number of free hydrogen ions circulating in the blood, which results in an increase in blood pH.
TEST-TAKING TIP: The key word is "COPD." Respiratory acidosis results whenever respiratory function is impaired.
Content Area: Older Adult Health
Integrated Processes: Nursing Process: Analysis
Client Need: Physiological Integrity
Cognitive Level: Application

Reference: *Ignatavicius, D., and Workman, M. (2012). Medical-Surgical Nursing: Patient-Centered Collaborative Care (7th ed.). St. Louis, MO: Saunders.*

10. ANSWER: 2.

Rationale:

1. The client's respiratory function is not impaired, ruling out respiratory acidosis.
2. The nurse should anticipate that this client will experience metabolic acidosis because the client has ingested excessive amounts of alcohol, which is an acid. Substances that cause acidosis when ingested include ethanol, methyl alcohol, and acetylsalicylic acid (aspirin).
3. Respiratory alkalosis is caused by hyperventilation or excessive oxygenation.
4. Excessive acid intake would cause acidosis, not alkalosis.

TEST-TAKING TIP: The key word is "inebriated," which means drunk or intoxicated by alcohol. Recall that ethanol (alcohol) intoxication causes acidosis, ruling out options 3 and 4.
Content Area: Adult Health
Integrated Processes: Nursing Process: Planning
Client Need: Physiological Integrity
Cognitive Level: Application
Reference: *Ignatavicius, D., and Workman, M. (2012). Medical-Surgical Nursing: Patient-Centered Collaborative Care (7th ed.). St. Louis, MO: Saunders.*

11. ANSWER: 3, 5.

Rationale:

1. Renal failure, fever, and dehydration are all risk factors for metabolic acidosis.
2. Renal failure, fever, and dehydration are all risk factors for metabolic acidosis.
3. The nurse should identify that the client's recent history of oxycodone use places the client at risk for respiratory acidosis. Oxycodone is an opioid, and opioids cause respiratory depression by decreasing the function of the brainstem neurons that trigger breathing movements.
4. Renal failure, fever, and dehydration are all risk factors for metabolic acidosis.
5. The nurse should identify that the client's recent history of pneumonia places the client at risk for respiratory acidosis. Pneumonia results in decreased alveolar-capillary diffusion, leading to poor gas exchange and CO_2 retention.

TEST-TAKING TIP: Select the options that would adversely affect the functioning of the respiratory system.
Content Area: Adult Health
Integrated Processes: Nursing Process: Assessment
Client Need: Physiological Integrity
Cognitive Level: Application
Reference: *Ignatavicius, D., and Workman, M. (2012). Medical-Surgical Nursing: Patient-Centered Collaborative Care (7th ed.). St. Louis, MO: Saunders.*

12. ANSWER: 2, 4, 5.

Rationale:

1. Asking the client about getting a flu shot would assess the client's risk for *developing* an acid-base imbalance; it does not help identify the *presence* of an acid-base imbalance.
2. The nurse should ask the client about changes in urine color or odor to assess for possible metabolic imbalances.
3. The date of the client's last physical examination is irrelevant in this instance.
4. Asking the client about shortness of breath assesses for the presence of respiratory acidosis.
5. Recent changes in memory or difficulty concentrating may also be indicative of acid-base imbalance.

TEST-TAKING TIP: The key words are "the presence of an acid-base imbalance." Select the options that indicate the client may be experiencing an acid-base imbalance.
Content Area: Adult Health
Integrated Processes: Nursing Process: Assessment
Client Need: Physiological Integrity
Cognitive Level: Application
Reference: *Ignatavicius, D., and Workman, M. (2012). Medical-Surgical Nursing: Patient-Centered Collaborative Care (7th ed.). St. Louis, MO: Saunders.*

13. ANSWER: 4.

Rationale:

1. Compensation via the lungs is impossible because the client's respiratory system is impaired by COPD.
2. Compensation via the lungs is impossible because the client's respiratory system is impaired by COPD.
3. If the client's blood pH was below the normal range, the client's acid-base imbalance would be *partially compensated*, not fully compensated.
4. The nurse should identify that the client's kidneys have fully compensated for the respiratory acidosis. Renal compensation occurs when the respiratory system is overwhelmed or diseased. In a client diagnosed with COPD, CO_2 is retained, causing the client's blood pH to decrease. To correct the pH level, the kidneys excrete more hydrogen ions via the urine and increase the reabsorption of bicarbonate back into the blood, increasing the blood pH. When this mechanism is completely effective, the acid-base imbalance is *fully compensated*, and the pH of the blood returns to normal even though the client's oxygen and bicarbonate levels are abnormal.

TEST-TAKING TIP: The key words are "the client's blood pH is within the normal reference range," indicating that the client's acid-base imbalance is *fully compensated*. Rule out options that indicate partial compensation, and recognize that the lungs cannot compensate for the imbalance because their function is impaired by COPD.
Content Area: Adult Health
Integrated Processes: Nursing Process: Evaluation
Client Need: Physiological Integrity
Cognitive Level: Application
Reference: *Ignatavicius, D., and Workman, M. (2012). Medical-Surgical Nursing: Patient-Centered Collaborative Care (7th ed.). St. Louis, MO: Saunders.*

14. ANSWER: 1, 3, 4, 5.

Rationale:

1. The nurse should expect the blood pH, PaO_2, $PaCO_2$, and serum K^+ levels to be abnormal in this child. The obstruction of the child's airway by the marble impairs gas exchange, resulting in respiratory acidosis. The blood pH would be decreased because CO_2 is being retained in the lungs.

2. A client with rapid-onset respiratory acidosis usually has a normal HCO_3^- level because compensation by the kidneys has not begun.
3. The PaO_2 level would be decreased because gas exchange is impaired.
4. The $PaCO_2$ level would be increased because gas exchange is impaired.
5. Serum K^+ levels are increased in acute respiratory acidosis.
TEST-TAKING TIP: Recognize that the marble would occlude the child's airway, resulting in respiratory acidosis. Rule out option 2 because the client's HCO_3^- level would remain normal in the presence of *respiratory* acidosis.
Content Area: Child Health
Integrated Processes: Nursing Process: Analysis
Client Need: Physiological Integrity
Cognitive Level: Application
Reference: Ignatavicius, D., and Workman, M. (2012). Medical-Surgical Nursing: Patient-Centered Collaborative Care (7th ed.). St. Louis, MO: Saunders.

15. ANSWER: 3.
Rationale:
1. Respiratory acidosis occurs when respiratory function is impaired and CO_2 is retained.
2. Metabolic acidosis is caused by an increase in hydrogen ions, a decrease in bicarbonate ions, or both.
3. The client is at risk for respiratory alkalosis caused by excessive loss of CO_2 through rapid respirations (hyperventilation) secondary to anxiety.
4. Metabolic alkalosis is caused by an increase in circulating bases and a decrease in circulating acids.
TEST-TAKING TIP: The key word is "hyperventilate," indicating the presence of respiratory alkalosis.
Content Area: Adult Health
Integrated Processes: Nursing Process: Implementation
Client Need: Physiological Integrity
Cognitive Level: Application
Reference: Ignatavicius, D., and Workman, M. (2012). Medical-Surgical Nursing: Patient-Centered Collaborative Care (7th ed.). St. Louis, MO: Saunders.

16. ANSWER: 1, 2, 3, 5.
Rationale:
1. The nurse should associate hyperreflexia with the development of acidosis. Hyperreflexia is caused by the hypocalcemia that may accompany acidosis.
2. The nurse should associate paresthesias with the development of acidosis. Paresthesias are caused by the hypocalcemia that may accompany acidosis.
3. The nurse should associate a positive Chvostek's sign with the development of acidosis. A positive Chvostek's sign results from the hypocalcemia that may accompany acidosis.
4. Lethargy is a sign of alkalosis.
5. The nurse should associate muscle weakness with the development of acidosis. Muscle weakness may be caused by the hypokalemia that may accompany acidosis.
6. Warm, flushed, dry skin is a sign of alkalosis.
TEST-TAKING TIP: Recall that acidosis (decreased blood pH) is related to *hypo*calcemia and *hypo*kalemia.
Content Area: Older Adult Health
Integrated Processes: Nursing Process: Assessment
Client Need: Physiological Integrity
Cognitive Level: Application
Reference: Ignatavicius, D., and Workman, M. (2012). Medical-Surgical Nursing: Patient-Centered Collaborative Care (7th ed.). St. Louis, MO: Saunders.

17. ANSWER: 2.
Rationale:
1. Kussmaul respirations are not associated with respiratory acidosis.
2. The nurse should associate the development of Kussmaul respirations with metabolic acidosis. Kussmaul respirations are very deep, rapid respirations that are not under the client's voluntary control. This type of breathing occurs when excess acids, caused by the absence of insulin, increase hydrogen ions and CO_2 levels in the blood, triggering the body to excrete more CO_2 by increasing the rate and depth of breathing (respiratory compensation).
3. Kussmaul respirations are not associated with respiratory alkalosis.
4. Kussmaul respirations are not associated with metabolic alkalosis.
TEST-TAKING TIP: Recall that Kussmaul respirations compensate for the metabolic acidosis most often caused by diabetic keto*acidosis*.
Content Area: Adult Health
Integrated Processes: Nursing Process: Implementation
Client Need: Physiological Integrity
Cognitive Level: Application
Reference: Ignatavicius, D., and Workman, M. (2012). Medical-Surgical Nursing: Patient-Centered Collaborative Care (7th ed.). St. Louis, MO: Saunders.

18. ANSWER: 4.
Rationale:
1. The client does not exhibit signs of metabolic acidosis.
2. The client does not exhibit signs of metabolic alkalosis.
3. The client does not exhibit signs of respiratory acidosis.
4. The nurse should associate respiratory alkalosis with these signs and symptoms. Anxiety, confusion, or loss of memory; tingling hands; and headache all are signs and symptoms of respiratory alkalosis. Hyperventilation (respiratory rate of 32 breaths per minute) is the cause of the imbalance.
TEST-TAKING TIP: Recall that hyperventilation (mechanical or spontaneous) is the *only* cause of respiratory alkalosis.
Content Area: Child Health
Integrated Processes: Nursing Process: Evaluation
Client Need: Physiological Integrity
Cognitive Level: Application
Reference: Williams, L., and Hopper, P. (2011). Understanding Medical-Surgical Nursing (4th ed.). Philadelphia, PA: F. A. Davis.

19. ANSWER: 20.
Rationale:

$$10 \text{ units}/X = 50 \text{ units}/100 \text{ mL} = 50X = 1{,}000 = 1{,}000 \div 50 = 20 \text{ mL/hr}$$

TEST-TAKING TIP: Practice medication calculations often to decrease the incidence of life-threatening medication errors. Insulin is a high-alert drug. Always ask another registered nurse to verify your calculation before administering an insulin infusion.

Content Area: Adult Health
Integrated Processes: Nursing Process: Analysis
Client Need: Physiological Integrity
Cognitive Level: Application
Reference: *Beaman, N. (2008). Pharmacology Clear and Simple: A Drug Classifications and Dosage Calculations Approach. Philadelphia, PA: F. A. Davis.*

20. ANSWER: 100.
Rationale:

$$20 \text{ units}/X = 100 \text{ units}/500 \text{ mL} = 100X = 10{,}000 = 10{,}000 \div 100 = 100 \text{ mL/hr}$$

TEST-TAKING TIP: Practice medication calculations often to decrease the incidence of life-threatening medication errors. Recall that errors in administering insulin can result in death.
Content Area: Adult Health
Integrated Processes: Nursing Process: Analysis
Client Need: Physiological Integrity
Cognitive Level: Application
Reference: *Beaman, N. (2008). Pharmacology Clear and Simple: A Drug Classifications and Dosage Calculations Approach. Philadelphia, PA: F. A. Davis.*

21. ANSWER: 304.
Rationale:

$$223 \text{ lb} \div 2.2 \text{ kg} = 101.36 \text{ kg}$$
$$101.36 \text{ kg} \times 3 \text{ mEq/kg} = 304.08 \text{ mEq} = 304 \text{ mEq}$$

TEST-TAKING TIP: Read the question carefully. In this scenario, the 4-hour administration period is irrelevant. Be sure to disregard extraneous information for success on the NCLEX-RN examination.
Content Area: Adult Health
Integrated Processes: Nursing Process: Analysis
Client Need: Physiological Integrity
Cognitive Level: Application
Reference: *Deglin, J. H., Vallerand, A. H., and Sanoski, C. A. (2013). Davis's Drug Guide for Nurses (13th ed.). Philadelphia, PA: F. A. Davis.*

22. ANSWER: 143.
Rationale:

$$175 \text{ lb} \div 2.2 \text{ kg} = 79.55 \text{ kg}$$
$$79.55 \text{ kg} \times 3 \text{ mEq/kg} = 238.65 \text{ mEq}$$
$$238.65 \text{ mEq} \times 0.6 \text{ mEq/mL} = 143.19 \text{ mL} = 143 \text{ mL}$$

TEST-TAKING TIP: Read the question carefully. In this scenario, the 8-hour administration period and the 500-mL diluent are irrelevant. Be sure to disregard extraneous information for success on the NCLEX-RN examination.
Content Area: Adult Health
Integrated Processes: Nursing Process: Analysis
Client Need: Physiological Integrity
Cognitive Level: Application
Reference: *Deglin, J. H., Vallerand, A. H., and Sanoski, C. A. (2013). Davis's Drug Guide for Nurses (13th ed.). Philadelphia, PA: F. A. Davis.*

23. ANSWER: 1.
Rationale:
1. The nurse should associate hypoventilation (respiratory rate of 8 breaths per minute) with an increased risk for respiratory acidosis because hypoventilation leads to the retention of CO_2, causing the increased production of free hydrogen ions.
2. The client's respiratory status would not produce metabolic acidosis or alkalosis.
3. An elevated (not decreased) respiratory rate would increase the client's risk for respiratory alkalosis.
4. The client's respiratory status would not produce metabolic acidosis or alkalosis.
TEST-TAKING TIP: Recall that the normal respiratory rate in adults is 12 to 20 breaths per minute. Associate hypoventilation with respiratory *acidosis*, and associate hyperventilation with respiratory *alkalosis*.
Content Area: Adult Health
Integrated Processes: Nursing Process: Analysis
Client Need: Physiological Integrity
Cognitive Level: Application
Reference: *Ignatavicius, D., and Workman, M. (2012). Medical-Surgical Nursing: Patient-Centered Collaborative Care (7th ed.). St. Louis, MO: Saunders.*

24. ANSWER: 2.
Rationale:
1. An increase in HCO_3^-would cause blood pH to increase (alkalosis).
2. A nurse evaluating the ABGs of a client diagnosed with partially compensated respiratory alkalosis should expect the client's pH to decrease toward 7.45, with a decrease in HCO_3^-. The kidneys excrete additional HCO_3^-, ridding the body of extra base and increasing the available hydrogen ions in an attempt to decrease the client's pH.
3. An increase in HCO_3^- would cause blood pH to increase (worsening alkalosis).
4. A decrease in HCO_3^- would worsen acidosis.
TEST-TAKING TIP: Associate a decrease in pH with the excretion of HCO_3^- or the retention of CO_2.
Content Area: Adult Health
Integrated Processes: Nursing Process: Analysis
Client Need: Physiological Integrity
Cognitive Level: Application
Reference: *Williams, L., and Hopper, P. (2011). Understanding Medical-Surgical Nursing (4th ed.). Philadelphia, PA: F. A. Davis.*

25. ANSWER: 2.
Rationale:
1. This client does not have any signs or symptoms of alkalosis (pH greater than 7.45).
2. The nurse should expect the client's ABG pH to be less than 7.35 because this client is experiencing DKA, a life-threatening complication caused by insulin deficiency. DKA may be precipitated by an acute illness or infection, or it may occur in a client who is noncompliant with insulin therapy.
3. This client would not have a normal pH value (7.35 to 7.45).
4. This client would not have a normal pH value (7.35 to 7.45).
TEST-TAKING TIP: Associate diabetes mellitus with an increased risk for metabolic acidosis; choose the pH value that reflects acidosis.
Content Area: Child Health
Integrated Processes: Nursing Process: Analysis
Client Need: Physiological Integrity
Cognitive Level: Application

Reference: *Ignatavicius, D., and Workman, M. (2012). Medical-Surgical Nursing: Patient-Centered Collaborative Care (7th ed.). St. Louis, MO: Saunders.*

26. ANSWER: 2.

Rationale:

1. Respiratory acidosis would be caused by hypoventilation, not hyperventilation.

2. The nurse should suspect that this client is experiencing respiratory alkalosis secondary to hyperventilation (respiratory rate 32 breaths per minute). Hyperventilation causes an excessive loss of CO_2, resulting in an increase in blood pH (alkalosis).

3. The client's respiratory system would not produce metabolic acidosis or alkalosis.

4. The client's respiratory system would not produce metabolic acidosis or alkalosis.

TEST-TAKING TIP: Associate conditions that cause hyperventilation with respiratory alkalosis.

Content Area: Child Health

Integrated Processes: Nursing Process: Analysis

Client Need: Physiological Integrity

Cognitive Level: Application

Reference: *Ignatavicius, D., and Workman, M. (2012). Medical-Surgical Nursing: Patient-Centered Collaborative Care (7th ed.). St. Louis, MO: Saunders.*

27. ANSWER: 4.

Rationale:

1. Vomiting would cause fluid volume deficit (FVD), not fluid volume excess (FVE). There is no indication that the client's respiratory status is impaired.

2. Vomiting would cause FVD and metabolic alkalosis because of gastric acid loss, not metabolic alkalosis.

3. Vomiting would cause FVD, not FVE. There is no indication that the client's respiratory status is impaired.

4. The nurse should correctly identify that this client is experiencing fluid volume deficit and metabolic alkalosis. The client has lost a significant amount of body fluid after vomiting for 3 days and has most likely been unable to tolerate oral fluid replacement. Gastric acid is also lost through vomitus, causing a decrease in circulating free hydrogen ions and resulting in an increase in blood pH (alkalosis) that is metabolic in origin.

TEST-TAKING TIP: Rule out options that include fluid volume excess because vomiting causes dehydration. Also rule out options that include respiratory-related imbalances because there is no mention of impaired respiratory function.

Content Area: Maternal Health

Integrated Processes: Nursing Process: Assessment

Client Need: Physiological Integrity

Cognitive Level: Application

Reference: *Perry, S., Hockenberry, M., Lowdermilk, D., and Wilson, D. (2010). Maternal Child Nursing Care (4th ed.). St. Louis, MO: Mosby.*

28. ANSWER: 4.

Rationale:

1. The client is experiencing *fully* compensated *metabolic alkalosis.*

2. The client is experiencing fully compensated *metabolic* alkalosis.

3. The client is experiencing *fully* compensated metabolic *alkalosis.*

4. The nurse should identify that this client is experiencing fully compensated metabolic alkalosis. In Cushing's disease, an excessive amount of the stress hormone cortisol is excreted by the adrenal cortex. The presence of excess cortisol reduces the kidneys' ability to excrete bicarbonate, causing serum pH levels to increase (alkalosis). The pH of 7.42 is within the normal reference range of 7.35 to 7.45, indicating that the primary imbalance has been fully compensated. CO_2 and HCO_3^- are increased, indicating that the respiratory system has compensated for the kidneys' inability to eliminate HCO_3^-.

TEST-TAKING TIP: Because a pH of 7.42 is within the normal reference range, that rules out a partially compensated imbalance. Recall that an elevated CO_2 level would cause the blood pH to decrease (acidosis), ruling out respiratory alkalosis.

Content Area: Adult Health

Integrated Processes: Nursing Process: Assessment

Client Need: Physiological Integrity

Cognitive Level: Application

Reference: *Ignatavicius, D., and Workman, M. (2012). Medical-Surgical Nursing: Patient-Centered Collaborative Care (7th ed.). St. Louis, MO: Saunders.*

29. ANSWER: 1.

Rationale:

1. The nurse should assess the client for respiratory acidosis because opioid analgesics cause respiratory depression, which increases CO_2 retention and leads to a decrease in blood pH (acidosis).

2. The nurse's primary concern should be respiratory depression resulting in respiratory acidosis. If the client had overdosed on oxycodone and acetaminophen (Percocet) or oxycodone and aspirin (Percodan), the nurse should also be concerned about metabolic acidosis, but OxyContin does not contain acetaminophen or aspirin.

3. An opioid overdose would cause respiratory depression resulting in respiratory acidosis, not respiratory alkalosis. The primary cause of respiratory alkalosis is hyperventilation.

4. An oxycodone overdose would not cause metabolic alkalosis.

TEST-TAKING TIP: Recall that narcotics may result in respiratory depression. Rule out alkalosis and metabolic etiologies because the imbalance was caused by the respiratory system.

Content Area: Adult Health

Integrated Processes: Nursing Process: Assessment

Client Need: Physiological Integrity

Cognitive Level: Application

Reference: *Berman, A., Snyder, S., Kozier, B., and Erb, G. (2012). Kozier & Erb's Fundamentals of Nursing: Concepts, Process, and Practice (9th ed.). Upper Saddle River, NJ: Pearson.*

30. ANSWER: 1.

Rationale:

1. The nurse's first intervention should be to assist the client to breathe into her cupped hands or a paper bag because this client is hyperventilating and exhaling too

much CO_2, potentially resulting in respiratory alkalosis. Breathing through pursed lips would also slow the client's rate of breathing.
2. Performing a vaginal examination is contraindicated because the client is bleeding.
3. Positioning the client on her left side may be appropriate to increase perfusion to the fetus, but this should not be the nurse's first priority.
4. Administering oxygen to this client would worsen the potential respiratory alkalosis.
TEST-TAKING TIP: Recall that hyperventilation causes respiratory alkalosis. Choose the option that would decrease the effects of hyperventilation.
Content Area: Maternal Health
Integrated Processes: Nursing Process: Implementation
Client Need: Physiological Integrity
Cognitive Level: Application
***Reference:** Perry, S., Hockenberry, M., Lowdermilk, D., and Wilson, D. (2010). Maternal Child Nursing Care (4th ed.). St. Louis, MO: Mosby.*

31. ANSWER: 3.
Rationale:
1. The nurse should assess the client for metabolic acidosis but not respiratory acidosis.
2. A salicylate overdose would not result in either respiratory acidosis or metabolic alkalosis.
3. The nurse should assess the client for metabolic acidosis and respiratory alkalosis because both occur with aspirin overdose. Aspirin, also known as acetylsalicylic acid, is a salicylate drug. A severe metabolic acidosis with compensatory respiratory alkalosis may develop with severe salicylate intoxication.
4. The client cannot have both metabolic acidosis and metabolic alkalosis at the same time.
TEST-TAKING TIP: The key words are "ingesting a bottle of baby aspirin." Recall that aspirin is acetylsalicylic acid; excess ingestion would increase the amount of acid in the body.
Content Area: Child Health
Integrated Processes: Nursing Process: Assessment
Client Need: Physiological Integrity
Cognitive Level: Application
***References:** Perry, S., Hockenberry, M., Lowdermilk, D., and Wilson, D. (2010). Maternal Child Nursing Care (4th ed.). St. Louis, MO: Mosby; Ignatavicius, D., and Workman, M. (2012). Medical-Surgical Nursing: Patient-Centered Collaborative Care (7th ed.). St. Louis, MO: Saunders.*

32. ANSWER: 4.
Rationale:
1. Administration of 0.9% saline solution would not have any effect on the client's respiratory rate.
2. Administration of epinephrine would increase the client's heart rate, not decrease the respiratory rate.
3. Administration of sodium bicarbonate is contraindicated because the client's hyperventilation increases the risk for respiratory alkalosis; sodium bicarbonate would worsen alkalosis.
4. The nurse should anticipate no additional treatment at this time. Sedation and attempts to assist the client to breathe more slowly are the appropriate treatments for this client.
TEST-TAKING TIP: Recall that the primary treatment of respiratory alkalosis is reversal of hyperventilation. Rule out options that do not affect the respiratory rate.
Content Area: Adult Health
Integrated Processes: Nursing Process: Implementation
Client Need: Physiological Integrity
Cognitive Level: Application
***Reference:** Berman, A., Snyder, S., Kozier, B., and Erb, G. (2012). Kozier & Erb's Fundamentals of Nursing: Concepts, Process, and Practice (9th ed.). Upper Saddle River, NJ: Pearson.*

33. ANSWER: 3.
Rationale:
1. There is no indication that the client's respiratory status is impaired.
2. The client's imbalance is metabolic in origin.
3. The nurse should assess the client for metabolic acidosis because prolonged diarrhea is a condition that causes excessive loss of HCO_3^-, resulting in a decrease in blood pH (acidosis).
4. Prolonged diarrhea would result in metabolic acidosis, not metabolic alkalosis.
TEST-TAKING TIP: Rule out options that include respiratory-related imbalances because there is no mention of impaired respiratory function.
Content Area: Child Health
Integrated Processes: Nursing Process: Assessment
Client Need: Physiological Integrity
Cognitive Level: Application
***Reference:** Berman, A., Snyder, S., Kozier, B., and Erb, G. (2012). Kozier & Erb's Fundamentals of Nursing: Concepts, Process, and Practice (9th ed.). Upper Saddle River, NJ: Pearson.*

34. ANSWER: 1, 2, 4.
Rationale:
1. The nurse should provide pulmonary hygiene to clear the airway, prevent CO_2 retention, and decrease the risk of developing respiratory acidosis.
2. Bronchodilators would improve gas exchange and help prevent respiratory acidosis.
3. IV sodium bicarbonate is not used to prevent acidosis and is administered only in cases of severe acidosis.
4. Adequate hydration would help decrease the viscosity of the client's mucous secretions, improving gas exchange and preventing respiratory acidosis.
5. Increasing dietary potassium intake would not affect the client's acid-base balance in this case.
TEST-TAKING TIP: Measures that help the client breathe more effectively will prevent the development of respiratory acidosis.
Content Area: Adult Health
Integrated Processes: Nursing Process: Planning
Client Need: Physiological Integrity
Cognitive Level: Application
***Reference:** Williams, L., and Hopper, P. (2011). Understanding Medical-Surgical Nursing (4th ed.). Philadelphia, PA: F. A. Davis.*

35. ANSWER: 4, 2, 1, 5, 3.
Rationale: To interpret the client's ABG values, the nurse should (1) examine the blood pH value to determine whether the blood is acidotic (pH less than 7.35) or alkalotic (pH greater than 7.45); (2) examine the blood $PaCO_2$

and HCO_3^- values to determine whether they are within the normal reference ranges, decreased, or increased; (3) compare the blood $PaCO_2$ and HCO_3^- to determine the etiology of the acid-base imbalance (in respiratory disorders, pH and $PaCO_2$ values move in opposite directions away from the normal range; in metabolic disorders, pH and HCO_3^- values move in the same direction); (4) determine whether there is compensation (in respiratory disorders, the renal system must compensate; in metabolic disorders, the respiratory system compensates: the lungs regulate CO_2, and the kidneys regulate HCO_3^-); and (5) determine the degree of compensation (if the pH is abnormal and only one ABG value is abnormal, no compensation has occurred; if the pH and one ABG value are abnormal and a second ABG value is beginning to change, partial compensation has occurred; complete compensation occurs when the second ABG value changes sufficiently to return the pH to normal).

TEST-TAKING TIP: Recall that the blood pH is always examined first when interpreting ABG values.

Content Area: Adult Health
Integrated Processes: Nursing Process: Analysis
Client Need: Physiological Integrity
Cognitive Level: Application
Reference: *Wilkinson, J., and Treas, L. (2011). Fundamentals of Nursing: Theory, Concepts & Applications (2nd ed.). Philadelphia, PA: F. A. Davis.*

36. ANSWER: 1.

Rationale:

1. The nurse should interpret an anion gap of 25 mEq/L as confirmation of the presence of metabolic acidosis. The normal range for the anion gap is 8 to 16 mEq/L; an anion gap greater than 16 mEq/L indicates the presence of metabolic acidosis. If metabolic acidosis is identified, the anion gap may be used to help monitor the effectiveness of treatment and the underlying condition.

2. An anion gap less than 8 mEq/L indicates the presence of metabolic alkalosis.

3. The anion gap is used to confirm a diagnosis of metabolic acidosis, not respiratory acidosis.

4. The anion gap is used to confirm a diagnosis of metabolic acidosis, not respiratory alkalosis.

TEST-TAKING TIP: Recall that the anion gap (normal reference range 8 to 16 mEq/L) is used to determine the presence of metabolic acidosis.

Content Area: Adult Health
Integrated Processes: Nursing Process: Planning
Client Need: Physiological Integrity
Cognitive Level: Application
Reference: *Van Leeuwen, A. M., Poelhuis-Leth, D., and Bladh, M. (2011). Davis's Comprehensive Handbook of Laboratory and Diagnostic Tests With Nursing Implications (4th ed.). Philadelphia, PA: F. A. Davis.*

37. ANSWER: 1, 2, 5.

Rationale:

1. The nurse should place the client in a mid to high Fowler's position to increase lung expansion.

2. The nurse should increase the client's fluid intake, unless contraindicated, to reduce the thickness of pulmonary secretions and aid in the expectoration of secretions.

3. Supine positioning interferes with lung expansion and causes pooling of secretions, which may exacerbate CO_2 retention.

4. Although oxygen therapy would most likely be indicated for this client, administration of 100% oxygen via a nonrebreather mask would decrease the client's respiratory drive and could lead to respiratory arrest.

5. The nurse should auscultate breath sounds every 2 hours and as needed to detect and prevent complications of the imbalance.

TEST-TAKING TIP: The key words are "a history of COPD." Choose interventions that would not adversely affect the chronic disease process and would improve the acid-base imbalance.

Content Area: Adult Health
Integrated Processes: Nursing Process: Planning
Client Need: Physiological Integrity
Cognitive Level: Application
Reference: *Ignatavicius, D., and Workman, M. (2012). Medical-Surgical Nursing: Patient-Centered Collaborative Care (7th ed.). St. Louis, MO: Saunders.*

38. ANSWER: 15.3.

Rationale:

140 lb ÷ 2.2 lb/kg = 63.64 kg
63.64 kg × 6 mg/kg = 381.84 mg
381.84 mg/*X*× 25 mg/1 mL= 25*X* = 381.84 = 381.84/25 = 15.27 mL = 15.3 mL (rounded to one decimal place)

TEST-TAKING TIP: Always double-check your calculations before providing your final answer on the NCLEX-RN examination *and* before administering medication to a client.

Content Area: Adult Health
Integrated Processes: Nursing Process: Implementation
Client Need: Physiological Integrity
Cognitive Level: Application
Reference: *Deglin, J. H., Vallerand, A. H., and Sanoski, C. A. (2013). Davis's Drug Guide for Nurses (13th ed.). Philadelphia, PA: F. A. Davis.*

39. ANSWER: 57.3.

Rationale:

180 lb ÷ 2.2 lb/kg = 81.8 kg
81.8 kg × 0.7 mg/kg/hr = 57.26 mg/hr = 57.3 mg/hr (rounded to one decimal place)

TEST-TAKING TIP: Read the question carefully; it is asking you to calculate how many milligrams per hour to administer.

Content Area: Adult Health
Integrated Processes: Nursing Process: Implementation
Client Need: Physiological Integrity
Cognitive Level: Application
Reference: *Deglin, J. H., Vallerand, A. H., and Sanoski, C. A. (2013). Davis's Drug Guide for Nurses (13th ed.). Philadelphia, PA: F. A. Davis.*

40. ANSWER: 38.

Rationale: Client education regarding glucose control is essential to prevent the development of DKA, which is the most serious complication of hyperglycemia.

Total daily insulin requirement (in units of insulin) = 150 lb ÷ 4 = 37.5 = 38 units

TEST-TAKING TIP: Double-check all medication calculations. Recall that insulin is a high-alert drug and should be administered in whole units, using only an insulin syringe for proper measurement.

Content Area: Adult Health
Integrated Processes: Teaching/Learning
Client Need: Physiological Integrity
Cognitive Level: Application
Reference: *Type 1 diabetes: diabetes treatment: calculating insulin dose.(2010). http://www.deo.ucsf.edu/type1/diabetes-treatment/medications-and-therapies/type-1-insulin-rx/calculating-insulin-dose.html.*

41. ANSWER: 4.
Rationale:
1. A blood pH of 7.25 indicates a state of acidosis.
2. Blood pH levels between 7.35 and 7.45 are within normal limits.
3. Blood pH levels between 7.35 and 7.45 are within normal limits.
4. The nurse should associate a low serum calcium level with a possible blood pH of 7.55 (alkalosis). A decrease in hydrogen ion concentration (increased pH) may cause a decrease in calcium concentration in the blood.
TEST-TAKING TIP: Recognize that hypocalcemia is related to alkalosis. Recall that the normal reference range for blood pH is 7.35 to 7.45.
Content Area: Adult Health
Integrated Processes: Nursing Process: Implementation
Client Need: Physiological Integrity
Cognitive Level: Application
Reference: *Van Leeuwen, A. M., Poelhuis-Leth, D., and Bladh, M. (2011). Davis's Comprehensive Handbook of Laboratory and Diagnostic Tests With Nursing Implications (4th ed.). Philadelphia, PA: F. A. Davis.*

42. ANSWER: 1.
Rationale:
1. The nurse should associate a blood pH of 7.5 that is metabolic in origin (metabolic alkalosis) with a decrease in the serum potassium level. When the body is in a state of metabolic alkalosis, potassium is shifted *into* the cells and hydrogen ions are shifted *out* of the cells in an attempt to decrease blood pH (compensation). The shift of potassium into the cell results in a decreased serum potassium level.
2. Alkalosis is associated with hypochloremia.
3. Alkalosis is associated with an increased bicarbonate level.
4. Alkalosis is associated with a decreased serum calcium level (hypocalcemia).
TEST-TAKING TIP: Recognize that a blood pH of 7.5 indicates alkalosis. Recall that hypokalemia and hypocalcemia are often associated with alkalosis.
Content Area: Adult Health
Integrated Processes: Nursing Process: Implementation
Client Need: Physiological Integrity
Cognitive Level: Application
Reference: *Ignatavicius, D., and Workman, M. (2012). Medical-Surgical Nursing: Patient-Centered Collaborative Care (7th ed.). St. Louis, MO: Saunders.*

43. ANSWER: 2.
Rationale:
1. Crohn's disease would cause metabolic acidosis, not respiratory acidosis.
2. The nurse should associate metabolic acidosis with severe diarrhea secondary to Crohn's disease. Crohn's disease is an inflammatory bowel disease characterized by abdominal pain, weight loss, and diarrhea. Chronic diarrhea results in the loss of HCO_3^- through the stool, resulting in metabolic acidosis.
3. Crohn's disease would cause metabolic acidosis, not respiratory alkalosis.
4. Crohn's disease would cause metabolic acidosis, not metabolic alkalosis. Prolonged vomiting, not diarrhea, may cause metabolic alkalosis.
TEST-TAKING TIP: Recall the signs and symptoms associated with Crohn's disease, and select the acid-base imbalance that would occur with chronic diarrhea.
Content Area: Adult Health
Integrated Processes: Nursing Process: Assessment
Client Need: Physiological Integrity
Cognitive Level: Application
Reference: *Williams, L., and Hopper, P. (2011). Understanding Medical-Surgical Nursing (4th ed.). Philadelphia, PA: F. A. Davis.*

44. ANSWER: 4.
Rationale:
1. The body's pH range is normally 7.35 to 7.45.
2. The body's pH range is normally 7.35 to 7.45.
3. The body's pH range is normally 7.35 to 7.45.
4. The nurse should interpret a blood pH of 6.65 as being incompatible with life. Values less than 6.9 or greater than 7.8 are generally considered incompatible with life. If the nurse assesses that this client is physiologically more stable than the results indicate, the possibility of a laboratory error should be considered.
TEST-TAKING TIP: Recall that the body's pH must be maintained within the narrow range of 7.35 to 7.45 to sustain life.
Content Area: Adult Health
Integrated Processes: Nursing Process: Evaluation
Client Need: Physiological Integrity
Cognitive Level: Application
Reference: *Williams, L., and Hopper, P. (2011). Understanding Medical-Surgical Nursing (4th ed.). Philadelphia, PA: F. A. Davis.*

45. ANSWER: 2, 4, 8.
Rationale: The nurse should anticipate that this client's laboratory values will show decreased pH (acidosis), normal $PaCO_2$ (no respiratory compensation yet), and decreased HCO_3^- (metabolic origin of pH alteration). If the client's respiratory system had begun to compensate, the client's $PaCO_2$ would be decreased in an attempt to increase pH to the normal reference range. End-stage renal disease causes an increase in acid in the body because of the kidneys' inability to filter and excrete waste products, resulting in metabolic acidosis.
TEST-TAKING TIP: Picture in your mind what must take place with regard to these three critical values to produce uncompensated metabolic acidosis.
Content Area: Adult Health
Integrated Processes: Nursing Process: Evaluation
Client Need: Physiological Integrity
Cognitive Level: Application
Reference: *Williams, L., and Hopper, P. (2011). Understanding Medical-Surgical Nursing (4th ed.). Philadelphia, PA: F. A. Davis.*

46. ANSWER: 1, 4, 6.
Rationale: The nurse should anticipate that the laboratory values for this client will show increased pH (alkalosis), normal $PaCO_2$ (no respiratory compensation yet), and

increased HCO_3^- (metabolic origin of pH alteration). If the client's respiratory system had begun to compensate, $PaCO_2$ would be increased in an attempt to decrease pH to the normal reference range. Prolonged vomiting causes excessive loss of hydrochloric acid from the stomach, resulting in metabolic alkalosis.

TEST-TAKING TIP: The key words are "metabolic alkalosis." Rule out decreased pH (acidosis), increased and decreased $PaCO_2$ (respiratory origin), and normal and decreased HCO_3^- (acidosis).

Content Area: Adult Health
Integrated Processes: Nursing Process: Evaluation
Client Need: Physiological Integrity
Cognitive Level: Application
Reference: *Williams, L., and Hopper, P. (2011). Understanding Medical-Surgical Nursing (4th ed.). Philadelphia, PA: F. A. Davis.*

47. ANSWER: 2, 3, 7.

Rationale: The nurse should anticipate that this client's laboratory values will show decreased pH (acidosis), increased $PaCO_2$ (respiratory origin of pH alteration), and normal HCO_3^- (no metabolic compensation yet). If the client's renal system had begun to compensate, the client's HCO_3^- would be increased in an attempt to increase pH to the normal reference range. Hypoventilation causes CO_2 retention, resulting in respiratory acidosis.

TEST-TAKING TIP: Recall that in a respiratory acid-base imbalance, the $PaCO_2$ value is abnormal; increased CO_2 equals increased acid, and decreased CO_2 equals decreased acid.

Content Area: Adult Health
Integrated Processes: Nursing Process: Evaluation
Client Need: Physiological Integrity
Cognitive Level: Application
Reference: *Williams, L., and Hopper, P. (2011). Understanding Medical-Surgical Nursing (4th ed.). Philadelphia, PA: F. A. Davis.*

48. ANSWER: 1, 5, 7.

Rationale: The nurse should anticipate that this client's laboratory values will show increased pH (alkalosis), decreased $PaCO_2$ (respiratory origin of pH alteration), and normal HCO_3^- (no metabolic compensation yet). If the client's renal system had begun to compensate, the HCO_3^- would be decreased in an attempt to decrease pH to the normal reference range. Hyperventilation causes excessive CO_2 loss, resulting in respiratory alkalosis.

TEST-TAKING TIP: Visualize what the client is experiencing during hyperventilation, picture the CO_2 molecules being rapidly exhaled with each breath.

Content Area: Adult Health
Integrated Processes: Nursing Process: Evaluation
Client Need: Physiological Integrity
Cognitive Level: Application
Reference: *Williams, L., and Hopper, P. (2011). Understanding Medical-Surgical Nursing (4th ed.). Philadelphia, PA: F. A. Davis.*

49. ANSWER: 4.

Rationale:

1. Respiratory pattern 1 displays a normal respiratory rate and depth.
2. Respiratory pattern 2 displays tachypnea, which is an increased respiratory rate of normal depth.
3. Respiratory pattern 3 displays bradypnea, which is characterized by slow but regular respirations.
4. **The nurse should identify respiratory pattern 4 as indicative of DKA because it displays fast, deep respirations without pauses, also known as Kussmaul respirations, which occur as the lungs attempt to compensate for acidosis by getting rid of extra CO_2.**

TEST-TAKING TIP: Kussmaul respirations are a classic compensatory mechanism for metabolic acidosis. Rule out normal or slow respirations. Select the respiratory pattern that would eliminate the most CO_2.

Content Area: Older Adult Health
Integrated Processes: Nursing Process: Assessment
Client Need: Physiological Integrity
Cognitive Level: Application
Reference: *Williams, L., and Hopper, P. (2011). Understanding Medical-Surgical Nursing (4th ed.). Philadelphia, PA: F. A. Davis.*

50. ANSWER: 4.

Rationale:

1. DKA occurs most frequently in younger clients and is characterized by a sudden onset, an inadequate insulin dose, the presence of infection, and a serum glucose level greater than 300 mg/dL, with positive serum or urine ketones.
2. The client's manifestations are not indicative of end-stage renal disease.
3. The client's manifestations are not indicative of exocrine pancreatic insufficiency.
4. **The nurse should associate hyperglycemic hyperosmolar syndrome (HHS) with this client's clinical manifestations. HHS occurs most often in older clients with type 2 diabetes mellitus and is characterized by a gradual onset, the presence of infection, poor fluid intake, and a serum glucose level greater than 600 mg/dL, without serum or urine ketones.**

TEST-TAKING TIP: The key words are "negative for ketones," which rules out DKA. Rule out the other options because they do not affect serum glucose levels.

Content Area: Older Adult Health
Integrated Processes: Nursing Process: Analysis
Client Need: Physiological Integrity
Cognitive Level: Application
Reference: *Ignatavicius, D., and Workman, M. (2012). Medical-Surgical Nursing: Patient-Centered Collaborative Care (7th ed.). St. Louis, MO: Saunders.*

51. ANSWER: 2, 4, 5.

Rationale:

1. COPD is not an infectious disease. Airborne precautions are unnecessary.
2. **The nurse should place the client in an upright position to increase lung expansion.**
3. Administration of oxygen at 6 L/min via nasal cannula is contraindicated for this client. Although supplemental oxygen may be needed, high amounts of delivered oxygen would decrease the client's respiratory drive, possibly leading to respiratory arrest.
4. **The nurse should administer 0.45% saline solution to restore fluid balance and to decrease the viscosity of pulmonary secretions.**

5. The nurse should administer methylprednisolone to decrease inflammation and increase the diameter of the upper airways.
TEST-TAKING TIP: The key term is "COPD." Rule out options that would harm or not benefit the client.
Content Area: *Adult Health*
Integrated Processes: *Nursing Process: Implementation*
Client Need: *Physiological Integrity*
Cognitive Level: *Application*
Reference: *Ignatavicius, D., and Workman, M. (2012). Medical-Surgical Nursing: Patient-Centered Collaborative Care (7th ed.). St. Louis, MO: Saunders.*

52. ANSWER: 2.
Rationale:
1. Humalog, also known as *insulin lispro*, is a rapid-acting insulin that is usually administered subcutaneously just before the client ingests carbohydrates.
2. The nurse should identify Humulin R as the insulin of choice for this client. Humulin R is regular insulin, which is the only insulin that can be administered intravenously to quickly correct the hyperglycemia associated with DKA.
3. Novolin R, also known as *NPH insulin*, is an intermediate-acting insulin that is administered subcutaneously, with a duration of 18 to 24 hours.
4. Lantus, also known as *insulin glargine*, is a long-acting insulin that is administered subcutaneously and provides a constant concentration over a 24-hour period.
TEST-TAKING TIP: Recall that DKA is a serious complication of diabetes mellitus that requires immediate treatment. Rule out insulins that cannot be given intravenously.
Content Area: *Adult Health*
Integrated Processes: *Nursing Process: Implementation*
Client Need: *Physiological Integrity*
Cognitive Level: *Application*
Reference: *Ignatavicius, D., and Workman, M. (2012). Medical-Surgical Nursing: Patient-Centered Collaborative Care (7th ed.). St. Louis, MO: Saunders.*

53. ANSWER: 1, 3, 4, 5.
Rationale:
1. The nurse should identify age as a risk factor for acid-base imbalances. Children and older adult clients are at higher risk for imbalances than adults.
2. There is no correlation between gender and the risk of acid-base imbalance.
3. Cerebral edema may cause respiratory depression, increasing the client's risk for respiratory acidosis.
4. Opioid administration may cause respiratory depression, increasing the client's risk for respiratory acidosis.
5. Inadequate or excessive mechanical ventilation places the client at risk for respiratory acidosis or alkalosis.
6. The administration of IV 0.9% saline solution would provide the client with the hydration needed to prevent or correct imbalances.
TEST-TAKING TIP: The key words are "at risk for an acid-base imbalance." Consider the effect of each option on acid-base balance, and rule out options that would have no significant effect.
Content Area: *Adult Health*
Integrated Processes: *Nursing Process: Implementation*
Client Need: *Physiological Integrity*
Cognitive Level: *Application*
Reference: *Ignatavicius, D., and Workman, M. (2012). Medical-Surgical Nursing: Patient-Centered Collaborative Care (7th ed.). St. Louis, MO: Saunders.*

54. ANSWER: 1, 2, 4.
Rationale:
1. The nurse should associate cyanosis with metabolic alkalosis; it a sign of inadequate oxygenation caused by slow, shallow respirations.
2. Muscle cramping is a sign of metabolic alkalosis resulting from the hypocalcemia and hypokalemia that accompany metabolic alkalosis.
3. Lethargy is a sign of metabolic acidosis, not metabolic alkalosis. Metabolic alkalosis results in irritability, twitching, and confusion.
4. Metabolic alkalosis is characterized by shallow respirations and a decreased respiratory effort secondary to skeletal muscle weakness.
5. Respiratory, not metabolic, alkalosis is characterized by an increased rate and depth of respirations. Manifestations of respiratory and metabolic alkalosis are similar, with the exception of respiratory patterns.
TEST-TAKING TIP: Recall that hypocalcemia and hypokalemia accompany metabolic alkalosis. Select options that are signs or symptoms of hypocalcemia and hypokalemia.
Content Area: *Adult Health*
Integrated Processes: *Nursing Process: Assessment*
Client Need: *Physiological Integrity*
Cognitive Level: *Application*
Reference: *Ignatavicius, D., and Workman, M. (2012). Medical-Surgical Nursing: Patient-Centered Collaborative Care (7th ed.). St. Louis, MO: Saunders.*

55. ANSWER: 1, 3, 4.
Rationale:
1. The nurse should anticipate that the client will have a decreased HCO_3^- level because the inflamed pancreas cannot produce enough bicarbonate ions to balance the free hydrogen ions in the blood.
2. The client's PaO_2 would be either normal or increased as the client's respiratory rate increases to "blow off" CO_2 (respiratory compensation).
3. The client's $PaCO_2$ level would be either normal or increased because the respiratory function is not impaired, and the client may be "blowing off" CO_2 to compensate for the acidotic state.
4. Serum K^+ levels are often increased in acidosis as the body attempts to buffer the blood pH by moving potassium out of the cells and into the bloodstream to counteract the hydrogen ions moving into the cells.
5. The client's serum Ca^{2+} level would not be affected by metabolic acidosis.
TEST-TAKING TIP: Identify that pancreatitis results in metabolic acidosis. Rule out laboratory values that would not occur in the presence of metabolic acidosis.
Content Area: *Adult Health*
Integrated Processes: *Nursing Process: Evaluation*
Client Need: *Physiological Integrity*
Cognitive Level: *Analysis*

Reference: Ignatavicius, D., and Workman, M. (2012). Medical-Surgical Nursing: Patient-Centered Collaborative Care (7th ed.). St. Louis, MO: Saunders.

56. ANSWER: 1, 3, 5.

Rationale:

1. The nurse should assign the nursing diagnosis Risk for Falls Related to Skeletal Muscle Weakness because hyperkalemia, which occurs with metabolic acidosis, results in skeletal muscle weakness.

2. The client is not at risk for constipation.

3. The nurse should assign the nursing diagnosis Impaired Memory Related to Fluid and Electrolyte Imbalance because memory function can be impaired by the fluid and electrolyte imbalances that occur with fluid volume deficit. Deficient fluid volume occurs as a result of fluid loss from prolonged diarrhea.

4. The client's respiratory function is not impaired. Common causes of metabolic acidosis include diarrhea, dehydration, renal failure, ethanol intoxication, starvation, and DKA.

5. The nurse should assign the nursing diagnosis Deficient Fluid Volume Related to Dehydration because the client is experiencing fluid volume deficit and metabolic acidosis as a result of prolonged diarrhea.

TEST-TAKING TIP: Recall that the normal reference range for blood pH is 7.35 to 7. 45—a very narrow range. Identify that the client is acidotic, and select the nursing diagnoses that would apply to acidosis and fluid volume deficit.

Content Area: Adult Health

Integrated Processes: Nursing Process: Analysis

Client Need: Physiological Integrity

Cognitive Level: Analysis

Reference: Ignatavicius, D., and Workman, M. (2012). Medical-Surgical Nursing: Patient-Centered Collaborative Care (7th ed.). St. Louis, MO: Saunders.

57. ANSWER: 2, 4.

Rationale:

1. The client's neurological status should be checked every hour when treating DKA.

2. The nurse should question the order to place the client on a potassium-restricted diet. Insulin administration causes serum potassium levels to decrease rapidly. The client should be assessed for signs of hypokalemia and should receive IV potassium replacement if needed.

3. Vital signs should be checked every 15 minutes until the client is stable.

4. The nurse should question the order to administer regular insulin subcutaneously per sliding scale. Regular insulin should initially be administered via IV bolus, followed by a continuous IV infusion of regular insulin to quickly decrease the client's serum glucose level. Subcutaneous insulin therapy is started when the client can take oral fluids and the ketosis has resolved.

5. The infusion of IV 0.45% saline solution at a rate of 1,000 mL/hr to replace fluids lost through excessive urination and vomiting is an appropriate intervention for this client.

TEST-TAKING TIP: DKA is a life-threatening medical emergency. Question orders that do not promptly address fluid replacement, glucose management, acid-base management, and prevention of hypokalemia.

Content Area: Adult Health

Integrated Processes: Nursing Process: Implementation

Client Need: Physiological Integrity

Cognitive Level: Analysis

Reference: Ignatavicius, D., and Workman, M. (2012). Medical-Surgical Nursing: Patient-Centered Collaborative Care (7th ed.). St. Louis, MO: Saunders.

58. ANSWER: 1.

Rationale:

1. The nurse should associate these ABG values with uncompensated respiratory acidosis. The pH of 7.25 reflects *uncompensated* acidosis because it remains below the normal reference range of 7.35 to 7.45; the *increased* $PaCO_2$ of 47 mm Hg indicates that CO_2 is being retained, making the respiratory system responsible for the acidosis; and the *normal* HCO_3^- of 24 mEq/L indicates that the kidneys have not yet begun reabsorbing or producing bicarbonate to compensate for the increased $PaCO_2$ level.

2. The client's serum pH would be at or near 7.35 if the client's kidneys were compensating for the respiratory acidosis.

3. The client's serum HCO_3^- level would be decreased in uncompensated metabolic acidosis.

4. The client's $PaCO_2$ level would be decreased and the HCO_3^- level would be increased in compensated metabolic acidosis.

TEST-TAKING TIP: Recall that in a compensated acid-base imbalance, the pH would be very near or within the normal reference range. Because the pH is significantly low, rule out all compensated acid-base imbalances.

Content Area: Adult Health

Integrated Processes: Nursing Process: Analysis

Client Need: Physiological Integrity

Cognitive Level: Analysis

Reference: Berman, A., Snyder, S., Kozier, B., and Erb, G. (2012). Kozier & Erb's Fundamentals of Nursing: Concepts, Process, and Practice (9th ed.). Upper Saddle River, NJ: Pearson.

59. ANSWER: 3.

Rationale:

1. These values are not indicative of uncompensated metabolic alkalosis.

2. These values are not indicative of compensated metabolic alkalosis.

3. The nurse should associate these ABG values with uncompensated respiratory alkalosis. The pH of 7.51 reflects *uncompensated* alkalosis because it remains greater than the normal reference range of 7.35 to 7.45; the *decreased* $PaCO_2$ of 32 mm Hg indicates that the client's lungs are "blowing off" too much CO_2, making the respiratory system the source of the alkalosis; and the *normal* HCO_3^- of 25 mEq/L indicates that the kidneys have not yet begun the process of compensation.

4. These values are not indicative of compensated respiratory alkalosis.

TEST-TAKING TIP: A decreased $PaCO_2$ level indicates that the client is most likely hyperventilating. Hyperventilation is the primary cause of respiratory alkalosis.

Content Area: Adult Health

Integrated Processes: Nursing Process: Analysis

Client Need: Physiological Integrity
Cognitive Level: Analysis
Reference: *Berman, A., Snyder, S., Kozier, B., and Erb, G. (2012). Kozier & Erb's Fundamentals of Nursing: Concepts, Process, and Practice (9th ed.). Upper Saddle River, NJ: Pearson.*

60. ANSWER: 2.
Rationale:
1. These ABG values are not indicative of uncompensated respiratory acidosis.
2. The nurse should associate these ABG values with uncompensated metabolic acidosis. The pH of 7.3 reflects *uncompensated* acidosis because it remains less than the normal reference range of 7.35 to 7.45; the *decreased* HCO_3^- of 20 mEq/L indicates that there is not enough bicarbonate in the blood, making the imbalance metabolic in origin; and the *normal* $PaCO_2$ of 38 mm Hg indicates that the lungs have not yet begun to "blow off" CO_2 to compensate for the acidosis.
3. These ABG values are not indicative of compensated respiratory acidosis.
4. These ABG values are not indicative of compensated metabolic acidosis.
TEST-TAKING TIP: After first analyzing the blood pH to identify the presence of acidosis or alkalosis, look for abnormalities in the other ABG values to determine the underlying cause of the acid-base imbalance.
Content Area: Adult Health
Integrated Processes: Nursing Process: Analysis
Client Need: Physiological Integrity
Cognitive Level: Analysis
Reference: *Berman, A., Snyder, S., Kozier, B., and Erb, G. (2012). Kozier & Erb's Fundamentals of Nursing: Concepts, Process, and Practice (9th ed.). Upper Saddle River, NJ: Pearson.*

61. ANSWER: 1.
Rationale:
1. The nurse should associate these ABG values with uncompensated metabolic alkalosis. The pH of 7.49 reflects *uncompensated* alkalosis because it remains greater than the normal reference range of 7.35 to 7.45; the *increased* HCO_3^- of 28 mEq/L indicates that there is too much bicarbonate in the blood, making the imbalance metabolic in origin; and the *normal* $PaCO_2$ of 43 mm Hg indicates that although the lungs have begun to compensate for the alkalotic state by retaining excess CO_2, they have not fully compensated for the imbalance.
2. These ABG values are not indicative of compensated metabolic alkalosis.
3. These ABG values are not indicative of uncompensated respiratory alkalosis.
4. These ABG values are not indicative of compensated respiratory alkalosis.
TEST-TAKING TIP: Recall that the normal reference range for $PaCO_2$ is 35 to 45 mm Hg. A $PaCO_2$ of 43 mm Hg is in the high-normal range, indicating that respiratory compensation is beginning, whereas the completely abnormal HCO_3^- level indicates that the imbalance is metabolic in origin.
Content Area: Adult Health
Integrated Processes: Nursing Process: Analysis
Client Need: Physiological Integrity
Cognitive Level: Analysis
Reference: *Berman, A., Snyder, S., Kozier, B., and Erb, G. (2012). Kozier & Erb's Fundamentals of Nursing: Concepts, Process, and Practice (9th ed.). Upper Saddle River, NJ: Pearson.*

62. ANSWER: 4.
Rationale:
1. These ABG values are not indicative of fully compensated metabolic acidosis.
2. These ABG values are not indicative of partially compensated metabolic acidosis.
3. These ABG values are not indicative of fully compensated respiratory acidosis.
4. The nurse should associate partially compensated respiratory acidosis with these ABG values. The pH of 7.32 reflects *partially compensated* acidosis because it remains below the normal reference range of 7.35 to 7.45. The *increased* $PaCO_2$ of 46 mm Hg indicates that the acidosis is respiratory in origin, whereas the *increased* HCO_3^- of 29 mEq/L (normal reference range is 21 to 28 mEq/L) indicates that the kidneys are attempting to minimize the imbalance but have not yet completed the process of compensation.
TEST-TAKING TIP: Remember to look at the pH value first. In this scenario, the pH is low (acidosis), and both the $PaCO_2$ and HCO_3^- values are elevated. An elevated bicarbonate level alone would cause *alkalosis,* not acidosis, ruling out imbalances that are metabolic in origin.
Content Area: Adult Health
Integrated Processes: Nursing Process: Analysis
Client Need: Physiological Integrity
Cognitive Level: Analysis
Reference: *Berman, A., Snyder, S., Kozier, B., and Erb, G. (2012). Kozier & Erb's Fundamentals of Nursing: Concepts, Process, and Practice (9th ed.). Upper Saddle River, NJ: Pearson.*

63. ANSWER: 2.
Rationale:
1. These ABG values are not indicative of partially compensated metabolic acidosis.
2. The nurse should associate fully compensated respiratory acidosis with these ABG values. The pH of 7.37 is within the normal reference range of 7.35 to 7.45, indicating full compensation. However, the pH is still on the lower (more acidotic) end of the normal reference range, and both $PaCO_2$ and HCO_3^- are elevated. An elevated $PaCO_2$ level would cause the blood to become acidotic (pH less than 7.35), but the elevated bicarbonate (HCO_3^-) level is pulling the pH up within the normal range, indicating that the kidneys are compensating for an imbalance that is respiratory in origin.
3. These ABG values are not indicative of partially compensated metabolic alkalosis.
4. These ABG values are not indicative of fully compensated respiratory alkalosis.
TEST-TAKING TIP: Look at the direction of the pH first, and then think about the other ABG values to determine the origin of the imbalance.
Content Area: Adult Health
Integrated Processes: Nursing Process: Analysis
Client Need: Physiological Integrity
Cognitive Level: Analysis
Reference: *Berman, A., Snyder, S., Kozier, B., and Erb, G. (2012). Kozier & Erb's Fundamentals of Nursing: Concepts, Process, and Practice (9th ed.). Upper Saddle River, NJ: Pearson.*

64. ANSWER: 4.

Rationale:

1. Theses ABG values are not indicative of partially compensated metabolic acidosis.
2. These ABG values are not indicative of fully compensated respiratory acidosis.
3. These ABG values are not indicative of partially compensated metabolic alkalosis.
4. **The nurse should associate fully compensated respiratory alkalosis with these ABG values. The pH of 7.44 is within the normal reference range of 7.35 to 7.45, indicating full compensation. However, the pH is still on the upper (more alkalotic) end of the normal reference range, and both $PaCO_2$ and HCO_3^- levels are decreased. A decreased $PaCO_2$ level would cause the blood to become alkalotic (pH greater than 7.45), but the decreased HCO_3^- level is pulling the pH down within the normal range, indicating that the kidneys are excreting HCO_3^- to compensate for an imbalance that is respiratory in origin.**

TEST-TAKING TIP: Look at the direction of the pH first, and then think about the other ABG values to determine the origin of the imbalance.

Content Area: Adult Health
Integrated Processes: Nursing Process: Analysis
Client Need: Physiological Integrity
Cognitive Level: Analysis
***Reference:** Berman, A., Snyder, S., Kozier, B., and Erb, G. (2012). Kozier & Erb's Fundamentals of Nursing: Concepts, Process, and Practice (9th ed.). Upper Saddle River, NJ: Pearson.*

65. ANSWER: 4.

Rationale:

1. These ABG values are indicative of metabolic acidosis.
2. These ABG values are indicative of metabolic alkalosis.
3. These ABG values are indicative of respiratory acidosis.
4. **The nurse should associate an arterial blood pH of 7.50, $PaCO_2$ of 28 mm Hg, and HCO_3^- of 22 mEq/L with a state of respiratory alkalosis. The client's hyperventilation (respiratory rate 34 breaths per minute) would cause the pH to become alkalotic (greater than 7.45) because CO_2 is being rapidly lost. The client's elevated blood pressure and heart rate are physiological signs of pain. A client with an increased respiratory rate of 34 breaths per minute would not have a normal or elevated $PaCO_2$ level.**

TEST-TAKING TIP: Recognize that the client is reporting pain, which can contribute to an increase in the respiratory rate and aloss of CO_2. An abnormal respiratory rate would have a significant effect on the client's CO_2 levels.

Content Area: Adult Health
Integrated Processes: Nursing Process: Evaluation
Client Need: Physiological Integrity
Cognitive Level: Analysis
***Reference:** Williams, L., and Hopper, P. (2010). Understanding Medical-Surgical Nursing (4th ed.). Philadelphia, PA: F. A. Davis.*

66. ANSWER: 1.

Rationale:

1. **The nurse should associate the client's manifestations with the development of respiratory acidosis secondary to hypoventilation (respiratory rate 10 breaths per minute). The client's ABG pH is less than 7.35 (7.15) and the $PaCO_2$ (64 mm Hg) is increased, indicating that the client is retaining CO_2. The normal HCO_3^- (22 mEq/L) indicates that the kidneys have not yet begun to compensate for the respiratory origin of the acidosis.**
2. Lab Report B indicates metabolic acidosis.
3. Lab Report C is within the normal reference range.
4. Lab Report D indicates respiratory alkalosis.

TEST-TAKING TIP: Recognize that the administration of morphine sulfate can cause respiratory depression, which results in respiratory acidosis.

Content Area: Adult Health
Integrated Processes: Nursing Process: Analysis
Client Need: Physiological Integrity
Cognitive Level: Analysis
***Reference:** Ignatavicius, D., and Workman, M. (2012). Medical-Surgical Nursing: Patient-Centered Collaborative Care (7th ed.). St. Louis, MO: Saunders.*

67. ANSWER: 1, 2, 4.

Rationale:

1. **The nurse should assign the nursing diagnosis Ineffective Breathing Pattern Related to Reduced Gas Exchange. This client is experiencing respiratory acidosis, which is caused by hypoventilation.**
2. **The nurse should assign the diagnosis Fatigue Related to Inadequate Tissue Oxygenation. This client is experiencing respiratory acidosis, which is caused by hypoventilation and results in further impairment of gas exchange and inadequate tissue oxygenation.**
3. The nursing diagnosis Diarrhea Related to Spastic Colonic Activity is associated with metabolic acidosis, not respiratory acidosis.
4. **The nurse should assign the diagnosis Risk for Falls Related to Skeletal Muscle Weakness. This client is experiencing respiratory acidosis, which is caused by hypoventilation and results in further impairment of gas exchange, inadequate tissue oxygenation, and skeletal muscle weakness.**
5. The nursing diagnosis Decreased Cardiac Output Related to Increased Heart Rate wouldbe appropriate for a client experiencing metabolic alkalosis.

TEST-TAKING TIP: The key words are "respiratory acidosis related to hypoventilation." Choose the options that are related to hypoventilation.

Content Area: Adult Health
Integrated Processes: Nursing Process: Analysis
Client Need: Physiological Integrity
Cognitive Level: Analysis
***Reference:** Ignatavicius, D., and Workman, M. (2012). Medical-Surgical Nursing: Patient-Centered Collaborative Care (7th ed.). St. Louis, MO: Saunders.*

68. ANSWER: 3.

Rationale:

1. The client who is extremely anxious is at risk for respiratory alkalosis secondary to possible hyperventilation.
2. The client with uncontrolled type 1 diabetes mellitus is at risk for metabolic acidosis.
3. **The nurse should identify that the client with COPD is at greatest risk for respiratory acidosis because this client's respiratory function is impaired; potential CO_2**

retention may decrease blood pH, resulting in respiratory acidosis.

4. The client with gastroesophageal reflux disease is at risk for metabolic alkalosis because these clients typically consume excessive antacids to control their reflux. Antacids contain HCO_3^-, which increases blood pH (alkalosis).

TEST-TAKING TIP: Use the process of elimination to rule out options that would cause a metabolic imbalance or an alkalosis.

Content Area: Adult Health
Integrated Processes: Nursing Process: Assessment
Client Need: Physiological Integrity
Cognitive Level: Analysis
Reference: *Williams, L. ,and Hopper, P. (2011). Understanding Medical-Surgical Nursing (4th ed.). Philadelphia, PA: F. A. Davis.*

69. ANSWER: 4.

Rationale:

1. Lab Report A indicates respiratory acidosis.
2. Lab Report B indicates metabolic acidosis.
3. Lab Report C is within the normal reference range.
4. **The nurse should associate the client's manifestations with the development of respiratory alkalosis secondary to hyperventilation (respiratory rate 38 breaths per minute). The client's arterial blood gas pH is greater than 7.45 (7.48), and $PaCO_2$ (27 mm Hg) is decreased, indicating that the client is losing CO_2. Normal HCO_3^- (24 mEq/L) indicates that the kidneys have not yet begun to compensate for the respiratory origin of the alkalosis.**

TEST-TAKING TIP: Recognize that hyperventilation results in respiratory alkalosis, indicated by a pH greater than 7.45, a decreased $PaCO_2$, and a normal (if uncompensated) HCO_3^-.

Content Area: Adult Health
Integrated Processes: Nursing Process: Analysis
Client Need: Physiological Integrity
Cognitive Level: Analysis
Reference: *Ignatavicius, D., and Workman, M. (2012). Medical-Surgical Nursing: Patient-Centered Collaborative Care (7th ed.). St. Louis, MO: Saunders.*

70. ANSWER: 4.

Rationale:

1. The client has a poor prognosis and will not recover from the incident.
2. The client has a poor prognosis and will not recover from the incident.
3. The client has a poor prognosis and will not recover from the incident.
4. **The nurse should interpret that the client has a poor prognosis and will not recover from the incident. After being rewarmed, the client's blood pH remains less than 6.9, which is usually fatal. The client's $PaCO_2$ is increased and HCO_3^- is decreased, indicating persistent respiratory and metabolic acidosis despite medical interventions. Most important, the client continues to have no audible heartbeat and no spontaneous respirations (on mechanical ventilation).**

TEST-TAKING TIP: The key words are "the client's condition remains unchanged." Although the client's ABG values indicate that death is imminent, the only certain criterion for death in hypothermia is irreversibility of cardiac arrest when the client is warm.

Content Area: Adult Health
Integrated Processes: Nursing Process: Evaluation
Client Need: Physiological Integrity
Cognitive Level: Analysis
Reference: *Ignatavicius, D., and Workman, M. (2012). Medical-Surgical Nursing: Patient-Centered Collaborative Care (7th ed.). St. Louis, MO: Saunders.*

UNIT IV

Comprehensive Tests

Chapter 9

Comprehensive Test I

REVIEW QUESTIONS

1. A client who has been diagnosed with acute renal failure has an intake of 2,000 mL and a urine output of 200 mL for the past 24 hours. Which assessment by the nurse is **most** important?
   1. Palpate peripheral pulses
   2. Auscultate breath sounds
   3. Check urine specific gravity
   4. Monitor blood urea nitrogen and creatinine

2. A nurse analyzes a client's arterial blood gas (ABG) values. The client's serum pH is 7.2, $PaCO_2$ is 48 mm Hg, and HCO_3^- is 25 mEq/L. Which acid-base imbalance should the nurse associate with these ABG values?
   1. Uncompensated respiratory acidosis
   2. Compensated respiratory acidosis
   3. Uncompensated metabolic acidosis
   4. Compensated metabolic acidosis

3. A nurse assesses the deep tendon reflexes (DTRs) of a pregnant client diagnosed with preeclampsia who is receiving IV magnesium sulfate. The nurse documents the client's DTRs as "less brisk than expected." Which grade should the nurse assign to this client's DTR response?
   1. Grade 0
   2. Grade 1
   3. Grade 2
   4. Grade 3
   5. Grade 4

4. A nurse assesses an adult client's laboratory values. The nurse should associate a serum sodium level of 122 mEq/L with which imbalance?
   1. Hyponatremia
   2. Hypernatremia
   3. Hypokalemia
   4. Hyperkalemia

5. An older adult client is admitted to the hospital with a history of intractable vomiting for 3 days. During the admission interview, the nurse notes that the client is confused. Which fluid, electrolyte, and acid-base imbalances are most likely affecting the client? **Select all that apply.**
   1. Hyponatremia
   2. Hypernatremia
   3. Respiratory acidosis
   4. Metabolic alkalosis
   5. Fluid volume excess
   6. Fluid volume deficit

6. Which assessments should a nurse perform to identify whether a client is developing potentially dangerous side effects of the medication captopril (Capoten)? **Select all that apply.**
   1. Apical pulse
   2. Breath sounds
   3. Intake and output
   4. Deep tendon reflexes
   5. 24-hour calorie count

7. A nurse is preparing to administer a continuous insulin infusion to a 250-lb client who has been diagnosed with diabetic ketoacidosis. A health-care provider orders an initial IV infusion of 0.1 unit/kg/hr of regular insulin. The pharmacy supplies 50 units of regular insulin in 100 mL of 0.9% normal saline solution. How many milliliters of solution should the nurse infuse hourly? Record your answer as a whole number.

____

8. A health-care provider orders hydrochlorothiazide oral solution 2 mg/kg/day every 8 hours for a 42-lb child with edema secondary to nephrotic syndrome. The dose on hand is 10 mg/mL. How many milliliters should a nurse administer to this child every 8 hours? Record your answer using one decimal place.

____

9. A nurse determines that a client's laboratory test reveals severe hyponatremia. Which nursing diagnosis should be the nurse's priority for this client?
   1. Risk for Falls
   2. Risk for Injury
   3. Acute Confusion
   4. Ineffective Breathing Pattern

10. A nurse is caring for a client diagnosed with ulcerative colitis and dehydration. Which finding should the nurse identify as the best indicator of fluid volume status in a client with ulcerative colitis?
    1. A 24-hour output of 1,000 mL
    2. Weight loss of 2 kg over 2 days
    3. Daily intake of 2,400 mL and output of 1,600 mL
    4. Stool count of eight episodes of diarrhea within 24 hours

11. A nurse assesses a newly admitted client and finds that the client has hyperactive deep tendon reflexes. Which potential electrolyte imbalance should the nurse suspect?
    1. Hypokalemia
    2. Hypercalcemia
    3. Hypernatremia
    4. Hypomagnesemia

12. A nurse analyzes a client's arterial blood gas (ABG) values. The client's serum pH is 7.42, $PaCO_2$ is 32 mm Hg, and HCO_3^- is 18 mEq/L. Which acid-base imbalance should the nurse associate with these ABG values?
    1. Partially compensated metabolic acidosis
    2. Fully compensated respiratory acidosis
    3. Partially compensated metabolic alkalosis
    4. Fully compensated respiratory alkalosis

13. A nurse assesses a newly admitted client with a serum sodium level of 118 mEq/L. For which clinical manifestations should the nurse observe? **Select all that apply.**
    1. Confusion
    2. Constipation
    3. Muscle spasms
    4. Tachypnea
    5. Headache

14. A client presents to a clinic reporting fatigue, shortness of breath, and restlessness. A nurse assesses the client, suspecting fluid volume excess (FVE). Which manifestations, if identified during assessment, should the nurse associate with FVE? **Select all that apply.**
    1. Oliguria
    2. Weak pulse
    3. Weight loss
    4. Crackles in lungs
    5. Decreased respirations

15. A nurse is caring for a critically ill client in the intensive care unit. Which factors should the nurse identify as placing the client at risk for hypophosphatemia? **Select all that apply.**
    1. Renal failure
    2. Acid-base imbalance
    3. Chemotherapy
    4. Insulin administration
    5. Total parenteral nutrition administration

16. Which laboratory values, if noted in a client's medical record, should a nurse associate with the development of hypocalcemia? **Select all that apply.**
    1. Decreased serum albumin level
    2. Increased serum phosphorus level
    3. Serum pH less than 7.35
    4. Serum ethanol level of 100 mg/dL
    5. Increased serum vitamin D level

17. A child is admitted to a hospital after experiencing severe vomiting and diarrhea for 18 hours. The child weighs 66 lb. Oral rehydration therapy is ordered. How much fluid should a nurse administer to this child daily? Record your answer using a whole number.

____

18. A nurse is preparing to administer IV hydrochloric acid 0.3 mEq/kg × (desired HCO_3^- minus measured HCO_3^-), as ordered, for a client who has been diagnosed with severe metabolic alkalosis. The client weighs 150 lb. The client's measured HCO_3^- is 12 mEq/L; the desired HCO_3^- is 18 mEq/L. How many milliequivalents should the nurse administer? Record your answer using one decimal place.

____

19. A 250-lb male client with moderate fluid volume excess gains 5% of his total body weight over a 3-day period. How many kilograms of weight did the client gain? Record your answer using one decimal place.

____

20. A nurse admits an older adult client who has been diagnosed with acute renal failure and has a serum potassium level of 6.4 mEq/L. Which medication should the nurse anticipate administering to help lower the client's potassium level?
1. furosemide (Lasix)
2. sodium bicarbonate (Neut)
3. regular insulin (Humulin R)
4. sodium polystyrene sulfonate (Kayexalate)

21. A nurse reviews the laboratory report of an adult client who has been taking furosemide (Lasix) for the treatment of fluid volume excess. Which serum potassium level should the nurse anticipate?
1. 2.5 mEq/L
2. 4.0 mEq/L
3. 5.0 mEq/L
4. 6.5 mEq/L

22. A nurse is monitoring a client with a serum magnesium level of 1.0 mEq/L who is receiving magnesium sulfate 2 gm IV piggyback. Which electrocardiogram (ECG) finding, if present, should indicate to the nurse that the client's electrolyte imbalance is improving?
1. Sinus rhythm
2. Torsades de pointes
3. Prominent U waves
4. Widened QRS complexes

23. A young child is receiving fluid replacement following a partial-thickness burn covering more than 15% of the client's total body surface area. Which indicator should the nurse use to determine the adequacy of fluid resuscitation?
1. Adequate urine output
2. Normal blood pressure
3. Normal capillary refill time
4. Improvement in level of consciousness

24. A nurse is assessing a client for signs of hypocalcemia. Which action should the nurse perform to assess for the presence of Trousseau's sign?
1. Apply a blood pressure cuff to the upper arm, inflate the cuff to a reading higher than the client's systolic blood pressure for 1 to 4 minutes, and observe for carpopedal spasm.
2. Tap the facial nerve anterior to the earlobe and just below the zygomatic arch, and observe for facial twitching on the same side as the stimulus.
3. Assess the biceps, triceps, and brachioradialis reflexes of the arm and wrist, and observe for hyperstimulation.
4. Instruct the client to hyperventilate, and observe for muscle spasms of the hands or feet.

25. A nurse is providing discharge teaching to a client who was admitted with heat exhaustion after working outdoors. What instructions should be included in the nurse's teaching? **Select all that apply.**
1. Wear close-fitting clothing when working in a hot environment.
2. Gradually increase the amount of activity.
3. Limit activity on hot or humid days.
4. Drink plenty of fluids before, during, and after working.
5. Take salt tablets if perspiring heavily.

26. A nurse is caring for a client who has been diagnosed with acute renal failure. The client's blood pH is 7.0. When reviewing the client's laboratory data, what other abnormalities should the nurse anticipate? **Select all that apply.**
1. Decreased bicarbonate (HCO_3^-) level
2. Increased serum potassium (K^+) level
3. Increased serum calcium (Ca^{2+}) level
4. Decreased partial pressure of arterial oxygen (PaO_2)
5. Normal partial pressure of arterial carbon dioxide ($PaCO_2$)

27. A nurse administers digoxin and a loop diuretic to an older adult client diagnosed with fluid volume excess related to congestive heart failure. The nurse is concerned that this client is at risk for developing digoxin toxicity. Which factor, if identified in this client, should the nurse associate with the development of digoxin toxicity?
1. Hyperkalemia
2. Premature ventricular contractions
3. Hypocalcemia
4. Hypermagnesemia

28. A nurse analyzes a client's arterial blood gas (ABG) values. The client's serum pH is 7.31, $PaCO_2$ is 39 mm Hg, and HCO_3^- is 18 mEq/L. Which acid-base imbalance should the nurse associate with these ABG values?
1. Uncompensated respiratory acidosis
2. Uncompensated metabolic acidosis
3. Compensated respiratory acidosis
4. Compensated metabolic acidosis

29. Which manifestation, if identified in a newborn diagnosed with viral gastroenteritis, should a nurse associate with the development of hypokalemia?
1. Oliguria
2. Diarrhea
3. Muscle weakness
4. Hyperactive bowel sounds

30. A client who is taking digoxin (Lanoxin) and furosemide (Lasix) for congestive heart failure is admitted to the emergency department. The client is disoriented and has an apical pulse rate of 49 bpm. Which action should the nurse take *first*?
 1. Place the client on telemetry.
 2. Administer oxygen at 2 L/min via nasal cannula.
 3. Assess the client for signs of hypokalemia.
 4. Notify the health-care provider immediately.

31. A nurse is preparing to administer an IV sodium bicarbonate infusion to a client diagnosed with moderate metabolic acidosis. A health-care provider orders 3 mEq/kg of sodium bicarbonate over 4 hours. The client weighs 150 lb. How many milliequivalents of sodium bicarbonate should the nurse administer? Record your answer as a whole number.

 ____

32. A nurse is preparing to administer 80 mEq of potassium by mouth in four divided doses. The dose on hand is 20 mEq/tablet. How many tablets should the nurse plan to administer at each dose? Record your answer as a whole number.

 ____

33. A toddler is brought to the emergency department after ingesting a bottle of baby aspirin. For which acid-base imbalances should a nurse assess this child?
 1. Metabolic acidosis and respiratory alkalosis
 2. Metabolic acidosis and metabolic alkalosis
 3. Respiratory acidosis and metabolic acidosis
 4. Respiratory acidosis and metabolic alkalosis

34. A nurse collects data from an older adult client who is receiving digoxin as treatment for fluid volume excess. Which manifestations, if reported by the client, should the nurse associate with the development of digoxin toxicity?
 1. Nausea, vomiting, and confusion
 2. Increased appetite, muscle weakness, and tinnitus
 3. Lethargy, hemoptysis, and diarrhea
 4. Euphoria, headache, and productive cough

35. A nurse is caring for a client who is receiving an amount of IV fluid that equals the client's urine output. Despite fluid replacement, the client is losing weight. What is the best explanation for the client's weight loss?
 1. Perspiration accounts for fluid loss greater than 1,000 mL/day.
 2. Approximately 1,000 mL of fluid is lost through the gastrointestinal tract.
 3. Insensible loss accounts for approximately 1,000 mL/day.
 4. Total fluid loss, other than urine, can exceed 1,000 mL/day.

36. A nurse is evaluating the laboratory values of a client diagnosed with diabetic ketoacidosis. After reviewing the client's serum sodium, chloride, and bicarbonate levels, the nurse calculates that the client's anion gap is 19 mEq/L. How should the nurse interpret this value?
 1. Confirmation of metabolic acidosis
 2. Evidence of metabolic alkalosis
 3. Verification of respiratory acidosis
 4. Proof of respiratory alkalosis

37. A nurse is providing discharge teaching to a client who developed iatrogenic hypoparathyroidism after total thyroidectomy. Which instruction should the nurse include in the teaching?
 1. Decrease milk and vitamin D intake.
 2. Monitor for tingling and numbness around the mouth.
 3. Consume foods that are high in phosphorus.
 4. Monitor for anorexia, nausea, vomiting, and constipation.

38. Which electrocardiogram rhythm strip, if recorded from a client who has been diagnosed with pulmonary edema and is receiving aggressive diuretic therapy, should a nurse identify as indicative of hypokalemia?

 1.

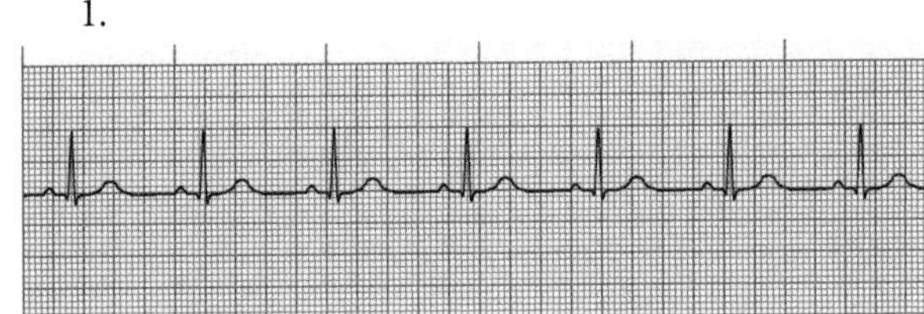

 2.

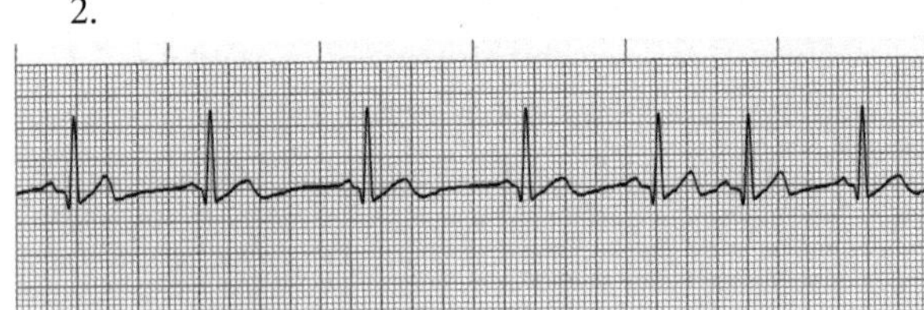

 3.

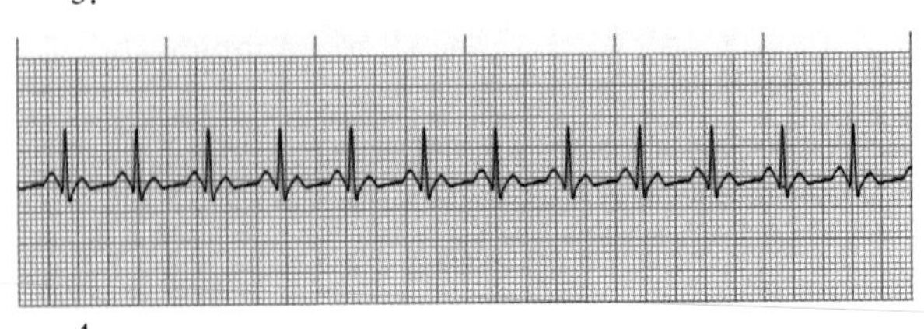

 4.

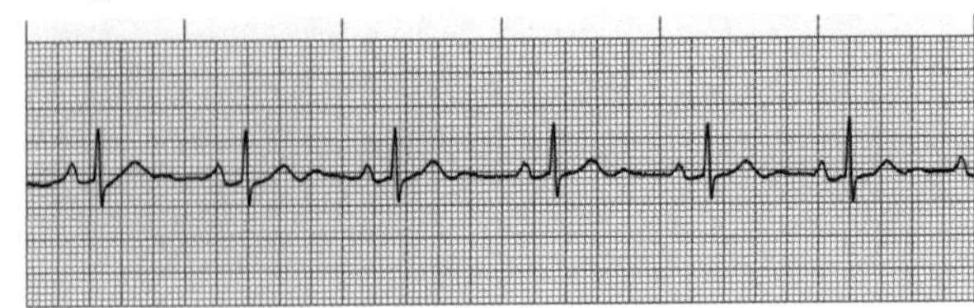

39. A nurse is caring for a client who has been diagnosed with diabetic ketoacidosis. Which health-care provider orders should a nurse question during the first 24 hours of treatment for this client? **Select all that apply.**
 1. 0.9% saline solution at 50 mL/hr
 2. 0.9% saline solution at 1,000 mL/hr × 2
 3. 3% saline solution at 125 mL/hr
 4. Dextrose 5% in 0.45% saline solution at 125 mL/hr when blood glucose reaches 250 mg/dL
 5. Dextrose 5% in lactated Ringer's solution at 125 mL/hr when blood glucose reaches 500 mg/dL

40. A nurse in the emergency department is planning care for a client who is experiencing ethanol intoxication. Which acid-base imbalances should the nurse anticipate when planning care for this client? **Select all that apply.**
 1. Metabolic acidosis
 2. Metabolic alkalosis
 3. Respiratory acidosis
 4. Respiratory alkalosis

41. A nurse who is caring for a client admitted with a serum potassium level of 2.5 mEq/L should question which orders for potassium replacement? **Select all that apply.**
 1. Potassium chloride (K-Dur) 20 mEq PO twice daily
 2. Potassium chloride (KCl) 40 mEq intramuscularly now
 3. Potassium chloride (KCl) 40 mEq intravenously over 4 hours
 4. Potassium chloride (K-Lor) 40 mEq powder dissolved in 4 oz of water
 5. Potassium chloride (KCl) 40 mEq subcutaneously

42. A nurse is caring for a child admitted with hypokalemia, hypophosphatemia, and metabolic acidosis secondary to starvation. Following treatment, a pediatrician orders a maintenance dose of potassium phosphate (Neutra-Phos) 2 mmol/kg/day in divided doses every 8 hours. The client weighs 24 lb. How many millimoles of potassium phosphate should the nurse administer every 8 hours? Record your answer using one decimal place.

____

43. A nurse is preparing to administer IV magnesium sulfate 50 mg/kg, as ordered, to a child who has been diagnosed with severe hypomagnesemia. The client weighs 84 lb. The dose on hand is 500 mg/mL. How many milliliters should the nurse administer? Record your answer using one decimal place.

____

44. Which electrocardiogram strips should a nurse associate with the development of a serum potassium imbalance? **Select all that apply.**

 1.

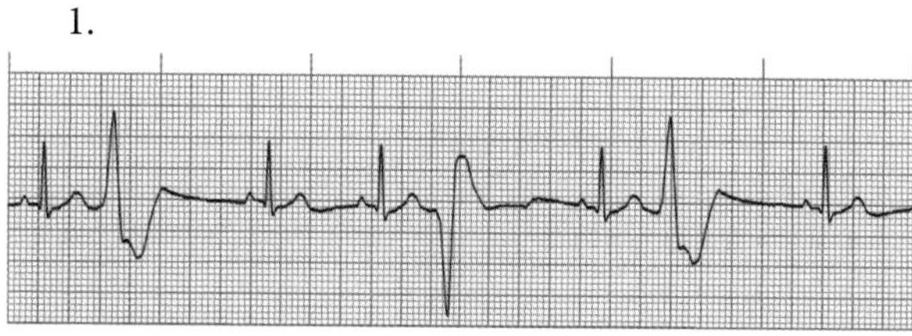

 2.

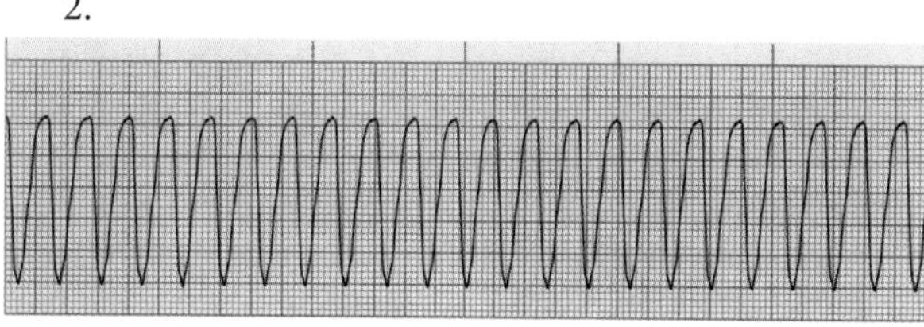

 3.

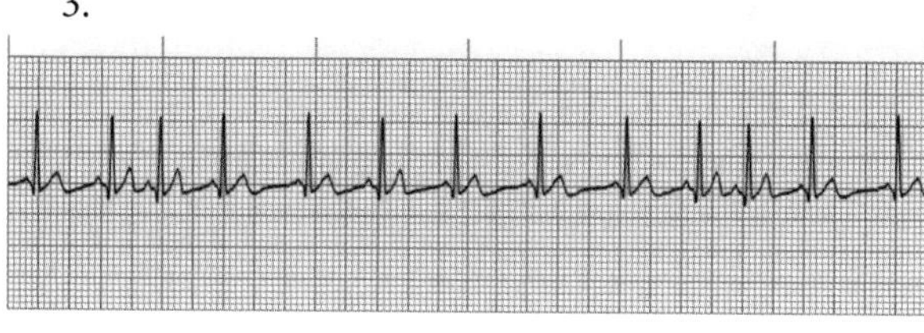

 4.

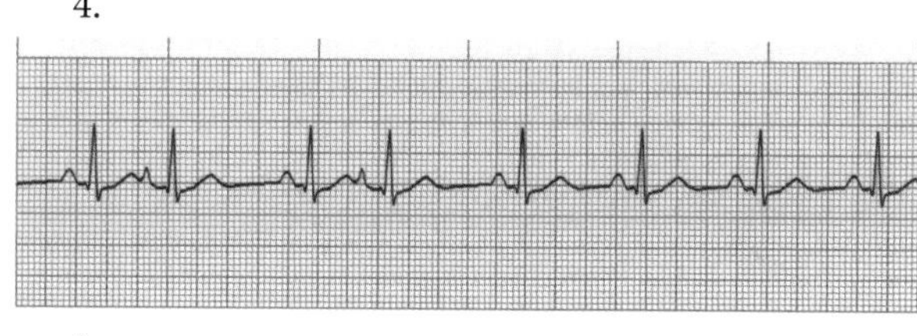

 5.

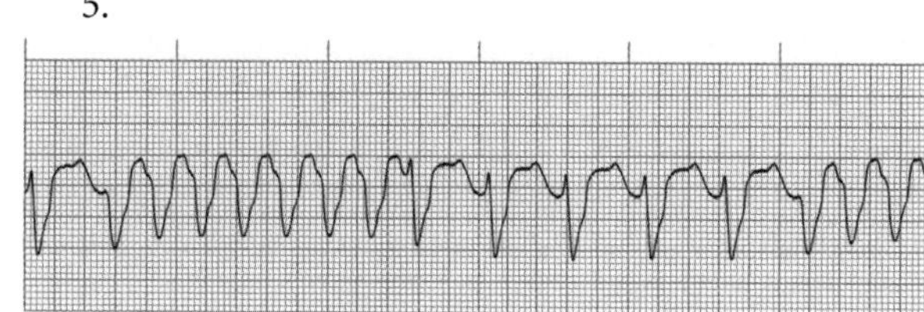

45. A nurse is caring for a client who has been diagnosed with uncompensated respiratory acidosis secondary to hypoxia. When reviewing this client's laboratory data, which value should the nurse anticipate?
 1. Increased pH
 2. Increased $PaCO_2$
 3. Decreased HCO_3^-
 4. Decreased serum calcium level

46. A nurse is providing discharge instructions to a client who has been diagnosed with hypophosphatemia. Which food should the nurse instruct the client to include as part of a high-phosphate diet?
 1. Fresh fruits
 2. Red meats
 3. Dairy products
 4. Green leafy vegetables

47. A health-care provider orders 0.9% saline solution at 125 mL/hr IV for a client with mild dehydration. In error, a nurse infuses the solution at a rate of 325 mL/hr throughout the night. Which type of fluid imbalance is this client most likely experiencing?
1. Hypotonic overhydration
2. Hypertonic dehydration
3. Isotonic overhydration
4. Hypotonic dehydration

48. A nurse is planning care for a client with hypokalemia secondary to prolonged gastric suctioning. Which outcome would be most appropriate to establish for the nursing diagnosis of Risk for Falls Related to Skeletal Muscle Weakness Secondary to Electrolyte Imbalance?
1. The client's oral fluid intake will equal urine output.
2. The client will remain free from injury throughout the hospital stay.
3. The client's serum electrolyte levels will return to the normal reference range.
4. The client will verbalize specific foods to ingest that increase dietary potassium intake.

49. A nurse is caring for a client diagnosed with a relative alkalosis. Which graphic should the nurse identify as the one that most accurately depicts the concept of *relative* alkalosis?

1.

ACID	BASE
ACID	BASE
ACID	BASE

2.

ACID	BASE
ACID	BASE
ACID	BASE
	BASE

3.

ACID	BASE
ACID	BASE
	BASE

4.

ACID	BASE
ACID	BASE
ACID	

50. A nurse is infusing 0.9% saline solution to a client diagnosed with fluid volume deficit. Which parameters are most important for the nurse to assess *during* IV rehydration of this client? **Select all that apply.**
1. Weight
2. Pulse rate and quality
3. Oxygen saturation
4. Urine output
5. Skin turgor

51. A nurse is caring for an older adult client who is at risk for seizures secondary to neuromuscular irritability associated with hypomagnesemia. Which actions should the nurse question in the implementation of seizure precautions for this client? **Select all that apply.**
1. Assess the functioning of suction equipment.
2. Place a tongue blade at the head of the client's bed.
3. Pad the side rails and headboard of the client's bed.
4. Maintain the bed in a low position with the wheels locked.
5. Ensure that the client's room is bright during daylight hours.

52. Which conditions, if noted when reviewing a client's laboratory data, should a nurse associate with the development of hypercalcemia? **Select all that apply.**
1. Hyperthyroidism
2. Hypophosphatemia
3. Hypermagnesemia
4. Metabolic alkalosis
5. Hyperparathyroidism

53. A nurse is caring for a client diagnosed with a relative acidosis. Which graphic should the nurse identify as the one that most accurately depicts the concept of *relative* acidosis?

1.

ACID	BASE
ACID	BASE
ACID	BASE

2.

ACID	BASE
ACID	BASE
ACID	BASE
	BASE

3.

ACID	BASE
ACID	BASE
	BASE

4.

ACID	BASE
ACID	BASE
ACID	

54. A weak and confused client presents to the emergency department reporting severe pain in the left calf muscle. A nurse assesses that the client has a heart rate of 48 bpm and circumoral cyanosis. Laboratory data reveal a serum calcium level of 11.6 mg/dL. Based on this information, which cardiac rhythm is the nurse most likely to observe on the electrocardiogram?

1.

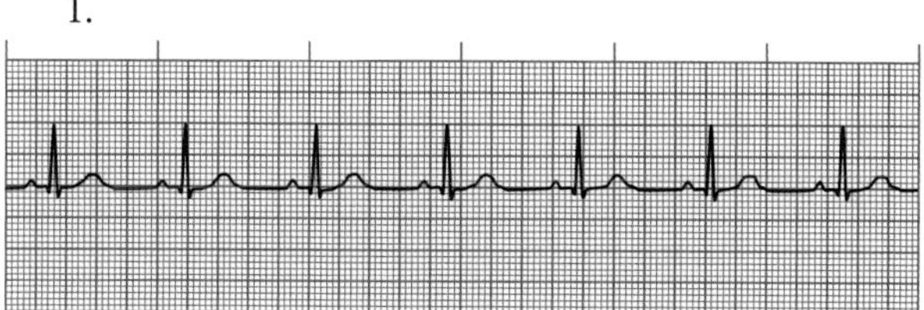

2.

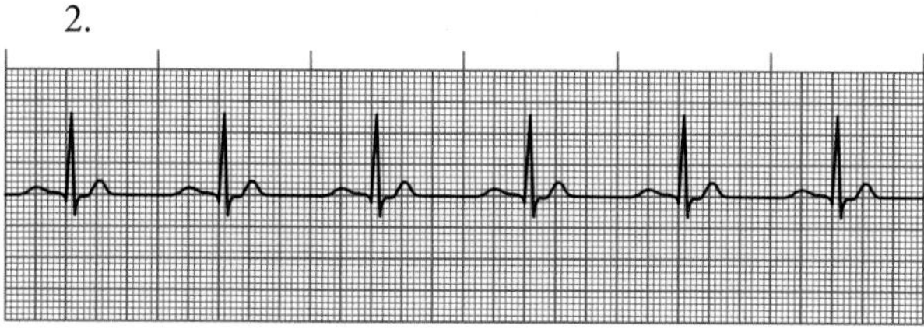

3.

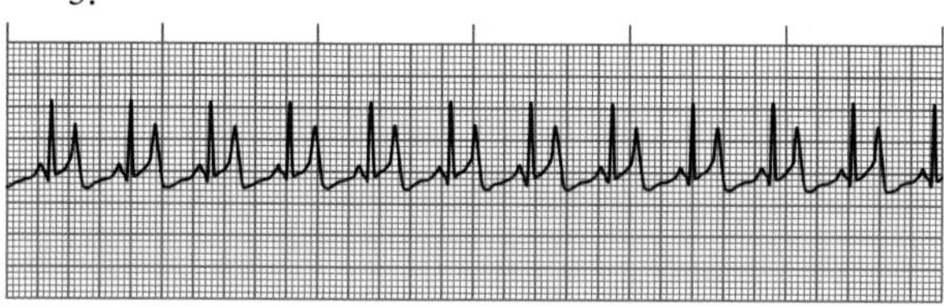

4.

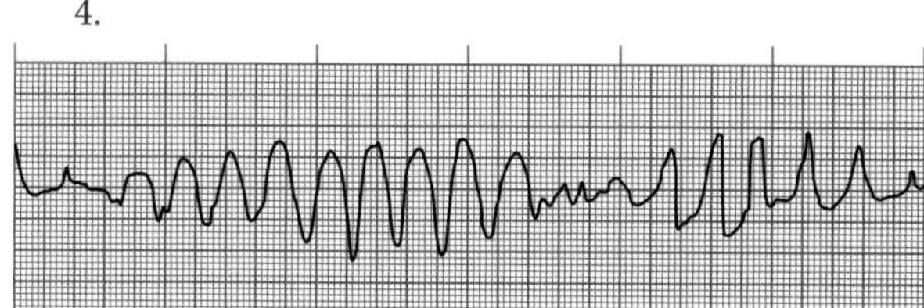

55. A nurse is caring for a postoperative client who is to receive IV lactated Ringer's solution 1,000 mL over 8 hours. At what rate should the nurse set the infusion pump? Record your answer as a whole number.

____

56. A nurse is preparing to administer 3% sodium chloride (NaCl) solution intravenously to a 75-lb child who has been diagnosed with acute hyponatremia. A health-care provider orders 0.5 mEq/kg/hr of 3% saline solution. The 3% saline solution contains 50 mEq of sodium per 100 mL. How many milliliters of this IV solution should the nurse administer hourly? Record your answer using a whole number.

____

57. A nurse is planning care for a client with a history of hypertension who is currently receiving treatment for breast cancer. The client is now diagnosed with metabolic alkalosis related to prolonged vomiting, secondary to chemotherapy and diuretic use. Which health-care provider order should the nurse question?
1. Administer IV furosemide (Lasix) 40 mg every 12 hours.
2. Administer IV 0.9% saline solution with 40 mEq/L KCl at 100 mL/hr.
3. Administer IV promethazine (Phenergan) 12.5 mg every 6 hours as needed for nausea.
4. Administer IV ondansetron (Zofran) 4 mg every 4 hours as needed for nausea.

58. A nurse identifies Risk for Falls Related to Skeletal Muscle Weakness as a diagnosis for an older adult client admitted with hypernatremia secondary to diabetes insipidus. Which nursing intervention would assist in maintaining this client's safety?
1. Position the client's wheelchair at the foot of the bed.
2. Ensure that the client's call bell is within reach at all times.
3. Assess the client's level of consciousness once every shift.
4. Weigh the client daily at the same time and using the same scale.

59. A nurse is counseling an older adult woman diagnosed with congestive heart failure. The client states, "I don't understand it. Both my husband and I are taking Lasix and he is fine. Why did this happen to me?" Which nursing response to the client's question is most accurate?
1. A woman has less fluid than a man and is at increased risk for imbalances.
2. A woman has more fluid than a man and is at increased risk for imbalances.
3. A woman has double the fluid of a man and is at increased risk for imbalances.
4. A woman has the same amount of fluid as a man and is at the same risk for imbalances.

60. A nurse is planning care for a client diagnosed with fluid volume deficit secondary to long-term chlorothiazide (Diuril) therapy. Which nursing diagnosis should the nurse assign to this client?
1. Risk for Decreased Cardiac Output
2. Chronic Urinary Retention
3. Risk for Deficient Fluid Volume
4. Deficient Fluid Volume: Isotonic

61. A nurse assesses a client diagnosed with hyperchloremia. Which findings would require immediate investigation by the nurse?
1. Respiratory rate 16 breaths per minute
2. Blood pressure 124/76 mm Hg
3. Kussmaul respirations
4. Decreased urinary output

62. A nurse is instructing a client who has been diagnosed with fluid volume excess and is being discharged on a non–potassium-sparing diuretic. Which foods should the nurse recommend to increase the amount of potassium in the client's diet? **Select all that apply.**
1. Baked potatoes
2. Apples
3. Yogurt
4. Bread
5. Clams

63. A mother brings her infant to the clinic with a fever of 103°F (39.4°C). The clinic nurse explains to the mother that a fever increases the infant's risk for dehydration. What are the reasons for this increased risk? **Select all that apply.**
1. Increased intake
2. Increased insensible loss
3. Decreased renal perfusion
4. Large surface area relative to volume

64. Which factor should a nurse identify as placing a client at risk for an acid-base imbalance?
1. Administration of PO ibuprofen
2. Administration of PO morphine sulfate
3. Administration of IV 0.9% saline solution
4. Administration of IV dextrose 5% in 0.45% saline solution

65. Which client should a nurse classify as having the greatest risk of fluid volume deficit (FVD)?
1. An older adult with congestive heart failure
2. An adolescent with ulcerative colitis
3. An infant with congenital heart disease
4. An older adult with hypertension

66. A nurse is caring for a client who has been diagnosed with metabolic alkalosis secondary to the excessive ingestion of baking soda for unrelieved chest pain. Which graphic should the nurse associate with metabolic alkalosis?

1.

Potassium (K^+)	Calcium (Ca^{2+})	Chloride (Cl^-)
↓	↓	↓

2.

Potassium (K^+)	Calcium (Ca^{2+})	Chloride (Cl^-)
↓	↓	↑

3.

Potassium (K^+)	Calcium (Ca^{2+})	Chloride (Cl^-)
↑	Normal	↑ or normal

4.

Potassium (K^+)	Calcium (Ca^{2+})	Chloride (Cl^-)
↑	Normal	↑↓

67. A nurse is preparing to administer a bolus of calcium gluconate 10% 7 mEq, as ordered, to a client who has been diagnosed with hypermagnesemia related to the administration of IV magnesium for the treatment of preterm labor. The concentration of the dose available is 0.45 mEq/mL. How many milliliters should the nurse administer? Record your answer using one decimal place.

____

68. A nurse calculates the pulse pressure of a client with fluid volume excess. The client's blood pressure is 152/105 mm Hg. What is the client's pulse pressure? Record your answer using a whole number.

____

69. A nurse is administering IV magnesium sulfate to a client who has been diagnosed with celiac disease. The client begins vomiting and sweating, exhibits facial flushing, and is becoming extremely lethargic. The nurse immediately notifies the client's healthcare provider and evaluates the client's electrocardiogram strip. Which cardiac rhythm is the nurse most likely to observe?

1.

2.

3.

4.

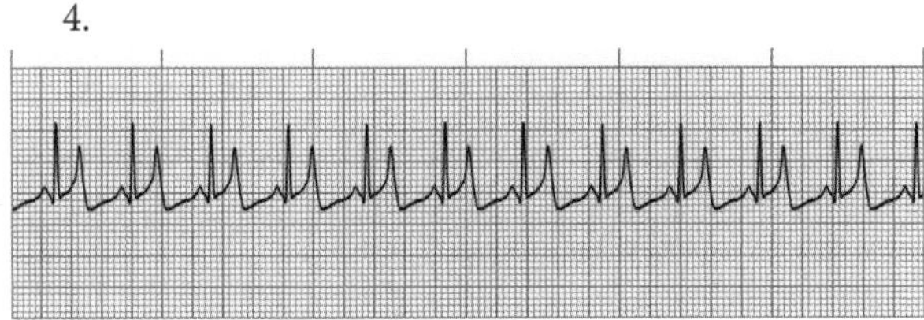

70. A client with type 1 diabetes mellitus has been experiencing nausea, vomiting, and anorexia for several days. The client has not been taking the prescribed insulin during this illness and currently has a blood glucose level of 435 mg/dL. Which arterial blood gas pH is the nurse most likely to find?
1. Less than 7.35
2. Greater than 7.35
3. Between 7.35 and 7.45
4. Greater than 7.45

71. A client with type 2 diabetes mellitus who is dehydrated presents to the emergency department. The client is diagnosed with hyperglycemic hyperosmolar state (HHS). Which laboratory findings should a nurse associate with HHS?
1. Serum blood glucose level 650 mg/dL
2. Urinalysis: blood positive
3. Serum pH less than 7.35
4. Urinalysis: ketones positive

72. A nurse is planning discharge education for a client diagnosed with syndrome of inappropriate antidiuretic hormone secretion (SIADH). Which instructions should the nurse include when teaching this client? **Select all that apply.**
1. Limit fluid intake.
2. Report muscle twitching.
3. Measure intake and output.
4. Perform mouth care once a day.
5. Report weight gain of 1 lb.

73. A 2-year-old child has had nausea, vomiting, and diarrhea for 3 days. Assessment by a nurse reveals dry oral mucosa, amber urine, and decreased skin turgor. Which measurements should a nurse obtain to best determine the child's current fluid status? **Select all that apply.**
1. Weight
2. Respiratory rate
3. Heart rate
4. Pulse oximetry
5. Blood pressure

74. A nurse assesses a client diagnosed with the syndrome of inappropriate antidiuretic hormone secretion (SIADH). Which factors, if assessed in a client with fluid volume excess, should the nurse associate with SIADH? **Select all that apply.**
1. Hyponatremia
2. Bradycardia
3. Polyuria
4. Headache
5. Recent pneumonia

75. A nurse admits an older adult client to the emergency department and notes that the client is cyanotic and has a respiratory rate of 6 breaths per minute. Which acid-base imbalance should the nurse associate with this finding?
1. Respiratory acidosis
2. Metabolic acidosis
3. Respiratory alkalosis
4. Metabolic alkalosis

76. Which serum chloride level should a nurse anticipate when evaluating the laboratory data of a client diagnosed with hypernatremia?
1. 85 mEq/L
2. 95 mEq/L
3. 105 mEq/L
4. 115 mEq/L

77. A community health nurse is teaching community members about nutrition. According to the recommendations of the National Institutes of Health, how much calcium should the nurse instruct women 19 to 50 years old to ingest daily?
1. 700 mg
2. 800 mg
3. 1,200 mg
4. 1,300 mg

78. A nurse is caring for a client who has developed acute respiratory acidosis. The nurse reviews the client's STAT laboratory values. Which electrolyte value should concern the nurse *most*?
1. Calcium
2. Sodium
3. Magnesium
4. Potassium

79. A nurse is planning care for a client who has been diagnosed with respiratory acidosis secondary to chronic obstructive pulmonary disease. Which intervention should be the nurse's *priority*?
1. Administering oxygen
2. Maintaining the client's airway
3. Teaching the client to perform deep breathing and coughing
4. Teaching the client pursed-lip breathing techniques

80. A nurse is evaluating the laboratory data of clients on a medical-surgical unit. Which laboratory result should the nurse report to a health-care provider?

Result A:	Result B:
Serum sodium: 136 mEq/L Serum potassium: 3.5 mEq/L Serum osmolality: 284 mOsm/kg	Serum sodium: 140 mEq/L Serum potassium: 3.7 mEq/L Serum osmolality: 286 mOsm/kg
Result C: Serum sodium: 128 mEq/L Serum potassium: 4.0 mEq/L Serum osmolality: 288 mOsm/kg	**Result D:** Serum sodium: 144 mEq/L Serum potassium: 4.5 mEq/L Serum osmolality: 290 mOsm/kg

1. Result A
2. Result B
3. Result C
4. Result D

81. A psychiatric nurse admits an anxious client who has experienced multiple panic attacks. The client is hyperventilating. After the client is calmed, laboratory studies are performed to identify any underlying illnesses. Based on this information, which laboratory values should the nurse anticipate? **Select all that apply.**
1. Serum pH less than 7.35
2. Serum pH greater than 7.45
3. Serum calcium level less than 8.2 mg/dL
4. Serum calcium level greater than 10.2 mg/dL
5. Serum phosphorus level less than 2.5 mg/dL
6. Serum phosphorus level greater than 4.5 mg/dL

82. A nurse is caring for a newly admitted client. Which factors, if noted, should the nurse associate with the development of hypochloremia? **Select all that apply.**
1. Metabolic alkalosis
2. Hyperparathyroidism
3. Diaphoresis
4. Excessive use of laxatives
5. Syndrome of inappropriate antidiuretic hormone secretion

83. A nurse analyzes a client's arterial blood gas (ABG) values. The client's serum pH is 7.42, $PaCO_2$ is 30 mm Hg, and HCO_3^- is 18 mEq/L. Which acid-base imbalance should the nurse associate with these ABG values?
1. Partially compensated metabolic acidosis
2. Fully compensated respiratory acidosis
3. Partially compensated metabolic alkalosis
4. Fully compensated respiratory alkalosis

84. A nurse admits a client diagnosed with malignant hypertension whose serum potassium level is 2.8 mEq/L. Based on this information, which health-care provider order should the nurse question?
1. Implement fall precautions.
2. Administer hydrochlorothiazide (Oretic) 12.5 mg PO daily.
3. Administer IV potassium chloride 10 mEq × 4.
4. Implement continuous cardiac telemetry.

85. A nurse is instructing a client on a low-sodium diet. Which foods should the nurse recommend the client avoid?
1. Pasta salad with mixed vegetables
2. Baked chicken and broccoli
3. Bologna and cheese sandwich
4. Dry cereal with skim milk and banana

86. A nurse is caring for a pregnant client who is in active labor. The client has a blood pressure of 126/72 mm Hg, heart rate of 90 bpm, and respiratory rate of 30 breaths per minute. Which acid-base imbalance should the nurse associate with these signs and symptoms?
1. Metabolic acidosis
2. Metabolic alkalosis
3. Respiratory acidosis
4. Respiratory alkalosis

87. A clinic nurse assesses an Asian client who reports having lactose intolerance. The client also reports having "charley horses" in the calf during sleep. Which nursing assessments should the nurse include? **Select all that apply.**
1. Assess the client for Chvostek's sign.
2. Ask the client about changes in height.
3. Assess for Trousseau's sign.
4. Measure the circumference of the client's calf.
5. Auscultate for hypoactive bowel sounds.

88. A nurse is caring for a client diagnosed with diabetes insipidus. The client's urinalysis reveals a low urine specific gravity, an elevated serum osmolality, and a serum sodium level of 160 mEq/L. Which IV solutions would be contraindicated for this client? **Select all that apply.**
1. 3% saline solution
2. 0.45% saline solution
3. 0.9% saline solution
4. Dextrose 2.5% in water

89. A nurse is assessing a client who has a history of multiple chronic illnesses. Which conditions should the nurse identify as placing the client at risk for fluid volume excess (FVE)? **Select all that apply.**
1. Diabetes insipidus
2. End-stage renal disease
3. Type 2 diabetes mellitus
4. Long-term corticosteroid therapy
5. Syndrome of inappropriate antidiuretic hormone secretion

90. A nurse evaluates the arterial blood gas values of a client who is being treated for diabetic ketoacidosis. Which finding should indicate to the nurse that the client is responding to the treatment plan?
1. pH 7.34
2. $PaCO_2$ 36 mm Hg
3. PaO_2 96 mm Hg
4. HCO_3^- 20 mEq

91. A nurse is instructing the parents of a 4-year-old child after a tonsillectomy. Which fluids should the nurse recommend that the parents administer during the immediate postoperative period to prevent dehydration?
1. Soft drinks
2. Ice cream
3. Popsicles
4. Beef broth

92. A health-care provider writes orders for a client diagnosed with hypervolemia. Which order should a nurse question?
1. Weigh the client daily.
2. Permit oral fluids as ordered.
3. Administer isotonic IV fluids as ordered.
4. Auscultate lung sounds every 4 hours and as needed.

93. A nurse reviews a client's arterial blood gas results. Which value should the nurse associate with long-term carbon dioxide retention?
1. pH 7.28
2. $PaCO_2$ 40 mm Hg
3. PaO_2 92 mm Hg
4. HCO_3^- 36 mEq

94. A nurse plans to administer calcium gluconate to an older adult client to treat hypocalcemia. Which routes of administration should the nurse identify as *contraindicated* when giving this medication? **Select all that apply.**
1. PO route
2. Subcutaneous route
3. Intramuscular route
4. IV route
5. Intradermal route
6. Rectal route

95. A nurse is reviewing a client's laboratory data. Which laboratory results should the nurse associate with the development of fluid volume excess (FVE)? **Select all that apply.**
1. Decreased blood urea nitrogen
2. Decreased hematocrit
3. Increased hemoglobin level
4. Decreased specific gravity of the urine
5. Increased urine osmolality

96. A nurse is assessing a client who reports numbness and tingling of the hands and face. The client's vital signs are temperature 99.0°F (37.2°C), blood pressure 142/86 mm Hg, heart rate 110 bpm, and respiratory rate 32 breaths per minute. Which blood pH value is the nurse most likely to find when evaluating this client's laboratory values?
1. 7.35
2. 7.40
3. 7.45
4. 7.50

97. A school nurse is teaching a high school football team about the dangers associated with dehydration. For which fluid imbalance would these clients be at highest risk?
1. Isotonic dehydration
2. Hypotonic dehydration
3. Hypertonic dehydration
4. Normotonic dehydration

98. A nurse is caring for a client diagnosed with hypercalcemia. Which health-care provider order should the nurse question?
1. Administer IV furosemide 20 mg.
2. Administer calcitonin 4 IU/kg intramuscularly every 12 hours.
3. Administer IV lactated Ringer's solution at 125 mL/hr.
4. Administer prednisolone 30 mg PO every 12 hours.

99. A nurse prepares to interpret the arterial blood gas values of a client suspected of having an acid-base imbalance. Which value should the nurse consider *first*?
1. pH
2. PaO_2
3. $PaCO_2$
4. HCO_3^-

100. A client diagnosed with renal failure experiences a 5% increase in total body weight over a 48-hour period. How should a nurse classify this increase in weight with regard to fluid volume excess (FVE)?
1. No FVE
2. Mild FVE
3. Moderate FVE
4. Severe FVE

REVIEW ANSWERS

1. ANSWER: 2.

Rationale:

1. Peripheral pulses may be bounding, but this finding would not be as important as assessing for signs of pulmonary edema.
2. **An assessment of the client's breath sounds is most important. This client is experiencing fluid volume excess, which can cause pulmonary edema and heart failure.**
3. Urine specific gravity may be increased, but this finding would not be as important as assessing for signs of pulmonary edema.
4. Blood urea nitrogen and creatinine levels may be increased, but these findings would not be as important as assessing for signs of pulmonary edema.

TEST-TAKING TIP: Recognize that the client's intake is much greater than the output, placing the client at risk for fluid volume excess. Use the "ABCs" to prioritize assessments and determine which should be performed first.

Content Area: *Adult Health*

Category of Health Alteration: *Fluid Volume Excess*

Integrated Processes: *Nursing Process: Assessment*

Client Need: *Physiological Integrity*

Cognitive Level: *Application*

Reference: *Ignatavicius, D., and Workman, M. (2012). Medical-Surgical Nursing: Patient-Centered Collaborative Care (7th ed.). St. Louis, MO: Saunders.*

2. ANSWER: 1.

Rationale:

1. **The nurse should associate these ABG values with uncompensated respiratory acidosis. The pH of 7.2 reflects *uncompensated* acidosis because it remains below the normal reference range of 7.35 to 7.45; the *increased* $PaCO_2$ of 48 mm Hg indicates that carbon dioxide is being retained, making the respiratory system responsible for the acidosis; and the *normal* HCO_3^- of 25 mEq/L indicates that the kidneys have not yet begun reabsorbing or producing bicarbonate to compensate for the increased $PaCO_2$ level.**
2. These values are not indicative of compensated respiratory acidosis.
3. These values are not indicative of uncompensated metabolic acidosis.
4. These values are not indicative of compensated metabolic acidosis.

TEST-TAKING TIP: Recall that in a compensated acid-base imbalance, the pH would be very near or within the normal reference range. Rule out all compensated acid-base imbalances because the pH is significantly low.

Content Area: *Adult Health*

Category of Health Alteration: *Acid-Base Imbalance*

Integrated Processes: *Nursing Process: Analysis*

Client Need: *Physiological Integrity*

Cognitive Level: *Analysis*

Reference: *Berman, A., Snyder, S., Kozier, B., and Erb, G. (2012). Kozier & Erb's Fundamentals of Nursing: Concepts, Process, and Practice (9th ed.). Upper Saddle River, NJ: Pearson.*

3. ANSWER: 2.

Rationale:

1. Grade 0 indicates no DTR response.
2. **When the client's DTRs are "less brisk than expected," the nurse should document that they are grade 1. Grade 1 indicates a weaker than normal (hypoactive) response. Monitoring DTRs in a client receiving magnesium sulfate therapy is extremely important to detect hypermagnesemia and prevent its complications.**
3. Grade 2 indicates a normal or expected response.
4. Grade 3 indicates a brisker than expected response.
5. Grade 4 indicates a brisk, hyperactive response with intermittent or transient clonus—a sudden, brief, jerking contraction of a muscle or muscle group that is often seen in seizures.

TEST-TAKING TIP: Review the grading scale for DTRs if you had difficulty answering this question correctly.

Content Area: *Maternal Health*

Category of Health Alteration: *Magnesium Imbalance*

Integrated Processes: *Nursing Process: Assessment*

Client Need: *Health Promotion and Maintenance*

Cognitive Level: *Comprehension*

Reference: *Ignatavicius, D., and Workman, M. (2012). Medical-Surgical Nursing: Patient-Centered Collaborative Care (7th ed.). St. Louis, MO: Saunders.*

4. ANSWER: 1.

Rationale:

1. **The nurse should associate a serum sodium level of 122 mEq/L with hyponatremia, which is defined as a serum sodium level less than 135 mEq/L.**
2. Hypernatremia is defined as a serum sodium level greater than 145 mEq/L.
3. Hypokalemia is defined as a serum potassium level less than 3.5 mEq/L.
4. Hyperkalemia is defined as a serum potassium level greater than 5.0 mEq/L.

TEST-TAKING TIP: Memorize the normal reference ranges for sodium and potassium because this information is tested on the NCLEX examination.

Content Area: *Adult Health*

Category of Health Alteration: *Sodium Imbalance*

Integrated Processes: *Nursing Process: Assessment*

Client Need: *Physiological Integrity*

Cognitive Level: *Comprehension*

Reference: *Williams, L., and Hopper, P. (2011). Understanding Medical-Surgical Nursing (4th ed.). Philadelphia, PA: F. A. Davis.*

5. ANSWER: 1, 4, 6.

Rationale:

1. **The client is most likely experiencing hyponatremia, metabolic alkalosis, and fluid volume deficit. Persistent vomiting can lead to dehydration and hyponatremia because both water and sodium are lost when vomiting.**
2. Hypernatremia may result when more water is lost than sodium; both water and sodium are lost when vomiting.
3. Respiratory acidosis occurs when hydrogen ions are retained because of inadequate gas exchange in the lungs.
4. **The client is most likely experiencing hyponatremia, metabolic alkalosis, and fluid volume deficit. Prolonged**

vomiting causes an acid deficit (loss of stomach acids) that may result in metabolic alkalosis.
5. Vomiting would cause a fluid volume *deficit*, not a fluid volume excess.
6. The client is most likely experiencing hyponatremia, metabolic alkalosis, and fluid volume deficit.
TEST-TAKING TIP: The key words are "intractable vomiting for 3 days." Consider how the client's serum sodium level, acid-base balance, and fluid volume status would be affected by prolonged vomiting.
Content Area: Older Adult Health
Category of Health Alteration: Fluid Volume Deficit, Sodium Imbalance, Acid-Base Imbalance
Integrated Processes: Nursing Process: Assessment
Client Need: Physiological Integrity
Cognitive Level: Application
***Reference:** Ignatavicius, D., and Workman, M. (2012). Medical-Surgical Nursing: Patient-Centered Collaborative Care (7th ed.). St. Louis, MO: Saunders.*

6. ANSWER: 1, 2.
Rationale:
1. When a client is taking Capoten (an angiotensin-converting enzyme [ACE] inhibitor), the nurse should assess the apical pulse for dysrhythmia secondary to hyperkalemia. Although ACE inhibitors usually have few side effects, they may cause hyperkalemia. Cardiovascular changes are the most severe problems associated with hyperkalemia.
2. The nurse should assess the client's breath sounds for the development of angioedema, which produces upper airway stridor. In rare cases, ACE inhibitors can cause angioedema, which is swelling (similar to hives) that occurs beneath the skin rather than on the surface. If angioedema occurs in the throat, that swelling can be life threatening.
3. Increased urine output would be associated with the use of diuretics, not ACE inhibitors.
4. Deep tendon hyporeflexia is seen in hypokalemia.
5. The client's short-term nutritional status would not be affected by the use of an ACE inhibitor, although reduced appetite is a potential adverse effect of long-term usage.
TEST-TAKING TIP: Recall that the adverse effects of all ACE inhibitors include hyperkalemia and, rarely, angioedema. Select the options that would address these potential problems.
Content Area: Adult Health
Category of Health Alteration: Potassium Imbalance
Integrated Processes: Nursing Process: Assessment
Client Need: Physiological Integrity
Cognitive Level: Application
***Reference:** Deglin, J. H., Vallerand, A. H., and Sanoski, C. A. (2013). Davis's Drug Guide for Nurses (13th ed.). Philadelphia, PA: F. A. Davis.*

7. ANSWER: 23.
Rationale:

250 lb÷ 2.2 lb/kg = 113.64 kg
113.64 kg × 0.1 unit of regular insulin = 11.36 units
11.36 units/X =50 units/100 mL = 50X = 1,136 units/mL
= 1,136 ÷ 50 = 22.73 = 23 mL/hr

TEST-TAKING TIP: Always double-check drug calculations. Recall that insulin is a high-alert drug. Ask another registered nurse to verify your calculation before administering an insulin infusion.
Content Area: Adult Health
Category of Health Alteration: Acid-Base Imbalance
Integrated Processes: Nursing Process: Analysis
Client Need: Physiological Integrity
Cognitive Level: Application
***Reference:** Deglin, J. H., Vallerand, A. H., and Sanoski, C. A.(2013). Davis's Drug Guide for Nurses (13th ed.). Philadelphia, PA: F. A. Davis.*

8. ANSWER: 1.3.
Rationale:

42 lb÷ 2.2 lb/kg = 19.09 kg
2 mg × 19.09 kg = 38.18 mg/day
38.18 mg (3 doses = 12.73 mg every 8 hours
10 mg/1 mL = 12.73/X(cross multiply) = 10X = 12.73
= 12.73÷ 10 = 1.27 mL = 1.3 mL every 8 hours

TEST-TAKING TIP: If rounding is necessary, perform the rounding at the end of the calculation.
Content Area: Child Health
Category of Health Alteration: Fluid Volume Excess
Integrated Processes: Nursing Process: Implementation
Client Need: Physiological Integrity
Cognitive Level: Application
***Reference:** Deglin, J. H., Vallerand, A. H., and Sanoski, C. A.(2013). Davis's Drug Guide for Nurses (13th ed.). Philadelphia, PA: F. A. Davis.*

9. ANSWER: 4.
Rationale:
1. Risk for Falls is an appropriate nursing diagnosis because severe hyponatremia causes muscle weakness, but it should not be the priority for this client.
2. Risk for Injury is an appropriate nursing diagnosis because severe hyponatremia causes muscle weakness, but it should not be the priority for this client.
3. Acute Confusion is an appropriate nursing diagnosis because severe hyponatremia causes lethargy and confusion, but it should not be the priority for this client.
4. The nurse should assign priority to the diagnosis Ineffective Breathing Pattern for a client with severe hyponatremia. This client is at increased risk for hypoventilation and respiratory distress or failure due to hyponatremia.
TEST-TAKING TIP: Remember the "ABCs." Protecting the client's airway and breathing should always be the first priority.
Content Area: Adult Health
Category of Health Alteration: Sodium Imbalance
Integrated Processes: Nursing Process: Planning
Client Need: Safe and Effective Care Environment
Cognitive Level: Analysis
***Reference:** Ignatavicius, D., and Workman, M. (2012). Medical-Surgical Nursing: Patient-Centered Collaborative Care (7th ed.). St. Louis, MO: Saunders.*

10. ANSWER: 2.
Rationale:
1. A 24-hour urine output of 1,000 mL is acceptable because it is greater than the obligatory urine output of 400

to 600 mL required to excrete toxic waste products, but it is not a reliable indicator of fluid volume status.

2. The best indicator of fluid volume status in a client with ulcerative colitis is a weight loss of 2 kg (equal to 4.4 lb) over 2 days. A weight loss of 1 lb corresponds with a fluid volume deficit of about 500 mL, or, in this case, about 2,200 mL.

3. Exact intake and output volumes are important in assessing fluid status, but they are not the most reliable measurements.

4. A stool count is not a reliable indicator of fluid volume status, even in the presence of liquid stools (diarrhea).

TEST-TAKING TIP: The key words are "best indicator of fluid volume status." Recall that weight is the most reliable indicator of fluid status.

Content Area: Adult Health
Category of Health Alteration: Fluid Volume Deficit
Integrated Processes: Nursing Process: Implementation
Client Need: Physiological Integrity
Cognitive Level: Application
***Reference:** Ignatavicius, D., and Workman, M. (2012). Medical-Surgical Nursing: Patient-Centered Collaborative Care (7th ed.). St. Louis, MO: Saunders.*

11. ANSWER: 4.

Rationale:

1. Hypokalemia results in hypoactive DTRs.
2. Hypercalcemia results in hypoactive DTRs.
3. Hypernatremia is not usually associated with abnormalities in DTRs.
4. **The nurse should suspect hypomagnesemia in a client with increased DTRs. Serum magnesium levels less than 1.6 mg/dL (hypomagnesemia) increase nerve cell membrane excitability, causing the cells to depolarize spontaneously, which results in hyperactive DTRs.**

TEST-TAKING TIP: Remember which electrolyte imbalances cause hyperactive DTRs (hypomagnesemia and hypocalcemia) and which cause hypoactive DTRs (hypermagnesemia and hypercalcemia).

Content Area: Adult Health
Category of Health Alteration: Magnesium Imbalance
Integrated Processes: Nursing Process: Assessment
Client Need: Physiological Integrity
Cognitive Level: Application
***Reference:** Ignatavicius, D., and Workman, M. (2012). Medical-Surgical Nursing: Patient-Centered Collaborative Care (7th ed.). St. Louis, MO: Saunders.*

12. ANSWER: 4.

Rationale:

1. A serum pH of 7.42 is within the normal range of 7.35 to 7.45, indicating full compensation. In partially compensated metabolic acidosis, the serum pH would still be below 7.35.
2. A serum pH of 7.42 is within the normal range of 7.35 to 7.45, indicating full compensation, but is closer to the upper (more alkalotic) end of the normal reference range. In fully compensated respiratory acidosis, the serum pH would be near or above 7.35 and both the carbon dioxide level ($PaCO_2$) and bicarbonate (HCO_3^-) levels would be increased to or beyond the upper levels of the normal range.
3. A serum pH of 7.42 is within the normal range of 7.35 to 7.45, indicating full compensation. In partially compensated metabolic alkalosis, the serum pH would still be above 7.45.
4. **The nurse should associate fully compensated respiratory alkalosis with these ABG values. The pH of 7.42 is within the normal reference range of 7.35 to 7.45, indicating full compensation. Note that the pH is on the upper (more alkalotic) end of the normal reference range and both carbon dioxide ($PaCO_2$) and bicarbonate (HCO_3^-) levels are decreased. Recall that a decreased carbon dioxide level would cause the blood to become alkalotic (pH above 7.45); however, the decreased bicarbonate level is pulling the pH down within the normal range, indicating that the kidneys are excreting bicarbonate to compensate for an imbalance that is respiratory in origin.**

TEST-TAKING TIP: First, look at the direction of the pH. Next, think about the other ABG values to determine the origin of the imbalance.

Content Area: Adult Health
Category of Health Alteration: Acid-Base Imbalance
Integrated Processes: Nursing Process: Analysis
Client Need: Physiological Integrity
Cognitive Level: Analysis
***Reference:** Berman, A., Snyder, S., Kozier, B., and Erb, G. (2012). Kozier & Erb's Fundamentals of Nursing: Concepts, Process, and Practice (9th ed.). Upper Saddle River, NJ: Pearson.*

13. ANSWER: 1, 3, 5.

Rationale:

1. **The nurse should observe a client with hyponatremia (serum sodium level less than 135 mEq/L) for confusion and headache, which are caused by cerebral edema.**
2. Constipation is not associated with sodium imbalance.
3. **Muscle spasms can occur in both hyponatremia and hypernatremia. Generalized weakness, nausea, vomiting, and diarrhea may also occur in hyponatremia.**
4. Tachypnea is not associated with sodium imbalance.
5. **The nurse should observe the client with hyponatremia (serum sodium level less than 135 mEq/L) for confusion and headache, which are caused by cerebral edema.**

TEST-TAKING TIP: Recognize that this client has a critically low serum sodium level. Recall the signs and symptoms of hyponatremia, and use the process of elimination to rule out incorrect options.

Content Area: Adult Health
Category of Health Alteration: Sodium Imbalance
Integrated Processes: Nursing Process: Assessment
Client Need: Physiological Integrity
Cognitive Level: Application
***Reference:** Ignatavicius, D., and Workman, M. (2012). Medical-Surgical Nursing: Patient-Centered Collaborative Care (7th ed.). St. Louis, MO: Saunders.*

14. ANSWER: 1, 4.

Rationale:

1. **The nurse should associate oliguria and the presence of crackles in lungs with fluid volume excess. Other signs of FVE include weight gain, bounding pulse, increased**

respiratory rate, increased blood pressure, and venous distention.
2. A weak pulse is associated with fluid volume deficit (FVD), not FVE.
3. Weight loss is associated with FVD, not FVE.
4. The nurse should associate the presence of crackles in lungs with FVE.
5. Decreased respirations are associated with FVD, not FVE.
TEST-TAKING TIP: Review the signs of FVE and FVD if you had difficulty answering this question.
Content Area: Adult Health
Category of Health Alteration: Fluid Volume Excess
Integrated Processes: Nursing Process: Assessment
Client Need: Physiological Integrity
Cognitive Level: Application
Reference: *Wilkinson, J., and Treas, L. (2011). Fundamentals of Nursing: Theory, Concepts & Applications (2nd ed.). Philadelphia, PA: F. A. Davis.*

15. ANSWER: 2, 4, 5.
Rationale:
1. Renal failure places the client at risk for *hyper*phosphatemia.
2. The nurse should identify acid-base imbalance as a risk factor for hypophosphatemia. Respiratory alkalosis can cause low serum phosphorus levels.
3. Chemotherapy place the client at risk for *hyper*phosphatemia.
4. The nurse should identify insulin administration as a risk factor for hypophosphatemia. Insulin administration can cause phosphate to shift into the cells from the extracellular fluid.
5. The nurse should identify total parenteral nutrition (TPN) administration as a risk factor for hypophosphatemia. TPN can cause phosphate to shift into the cells from the extracellular fluid. Phosphate imbalances are frequently related to therapeutic interventions for other disorders.
TEST-TAKING TIP: The key words are "risk for hypophosphatemia." Consider each option and rule out those that would cause the serum phosphorus level to increase.
Content Area: Adult Health
Category of Health Alteration: Phosphate Imbalance
Integrated Processes: Nursing Process: Analysis
Client Need: Physiological Integrity
Cognitive Level: Analysis
Reference: *Berman, A., Snyder, S., Kozier, B., and Erb, G. (2012). Kozier & Erb's Fundamentals of Nursing: Concepts, Process, and Practice (9th ed.). Upper Saddle River, NJ: Pearson.*

16. ANSWER: 2, 4.
Rationale:
1. A decrease in the serum albumin level may make the *total* serum calcium level *appear* to be decreased when it is actually within the normal reference range. Calcium binds with albumin, a carrier protein, in the blood. Because *free*, or *ionized*, calcium is actively regulated by the body and is not bound with albumin, this value (free, or ionized, calcium) is more clinically accurate in the presence of low serum albumin levels.
2. The nurse should associate an increased serum phosphorus level (hyperphosphatemia) with the development of hypocalcemia. Calcium and phosphorus have a balanced inverse relationship: when one value is increased, the other value is decreased.
3. Hypocalcemia is associated with alkalosis (pH greater than 7.45), not acidosis. As the hydrogen ion concentration in blood decreases, the freely ionized calcium concentration also decreases, thus decreasing the total serum calcium level.
4. The nurse should associate the presence of ethanol in the blood with the development of hypocalcemia. Alcoholism is a common cause of hypocalcemia and is related to inadequate nutrition.
5. A decrease, not an increase, in vitamin D would be associated with a decrease in calcium metabolism and absorption. Vitamin D is required for calcium metabolism and absorption.
TEST-TAKING TIP: Consider each option and rule out those that are not associated with a decreased serum calcium level.
Content Area: Adult Health
Category of Health Alteration: Calcium Imbalance
Integrated Processes: Nursing Process: Analysis
Client Need: Physiological Integrity
Cognitive Level: Application
Reference: *Van Leeuwen, A. M., Poelhuis-Leth, D., and Bladh, M. (2011). Davis's Comprehensive Handbook of Laboratory and Diagnostic Tests With Nursing Implications (4th ed.). Philadelphia, PA: F. A. Davis.*

17. ANSWER: 1,700.
Rationale: The nurse should administer 1,700 mL of rehydration fluid daily. For children weighing more than 20 kg (44 lb), the free liquid intake should be 1,500 mL + 20 mL/kg for each kilogram over 20.

$$66 \text{ lb} \div 2.2 \text{ lb/kg} = 30 \text{ kg}$$
$$1{,}500 \text{ mL} + 20 \text{ mL/kg for each kg over } 20 = 1{,}500 \text{ mL} + (20 \text{ mL} \times [30 \text{ kg} \_ 20 \text{ kg}]) = 1{,}500 \text{ mL} + (20 \text{ mL} \times 10 \text{ kg}) = 1{,}500 \text{ mL} + 200 \text{ mL} = 1{,}700 \text{ mL}$$

Oral rehydration solutions enhance and promote the reabsorption of sodium and water. The nurse should start by giving the child small sips to prevent vomiting. Water is not indicated for rehydration because it lacks sodium and glucose.
TEST-TAKING TIP: Review the Holliday-Segar method for calculating fluid requirements in Chapter 2 if you had difficulty answering this question.
Content Area: Child Health
Category of Health Alteration: Fluid Volume Deficit
Integrated Processes: Nursing Process: Implementation
Client Need: Physiological Integrity
Cognitive Level: Application
Reference: *Roberts, K. B. (2007). Dehydration. In The Merck Manuals Online Medical Library. http://www.merck.com/mmpe/sec19/ch276/ch276b.html.*

18. ANSWER: 122.7.
Rationale:

$$150 \text{ lb} \div 2.2 \text{ lb/kg} = 68.18 \text{ kg}$$
$$18 \text{ mEq/L} \_ 12 \text{ mEq/L} = 6 \text{ mEq/L}$$
$$0.3 \times 68.18 = 20.45 \times 6 = 122.7 \text{ mEq}$$

TEST-TAKING TIP: Always double-check your calculations before providing your answer on the NCLEX examination *and* before administering medication to a client.
Content Area: *Adult Health*
Category of Health Alteration: *Acid-Base Imbalance*
Integrated Processes: *Nursing Process: Implementation*
Client Need: *Physiological Integrity*
Cognitive Level: *Application*
Reference: *Deglin, J. H., Vallerand, A. H., and Sanoski, C. A.(2013). Davis's Drug Guide for Nurses (13th ed.). Philadelphia, PA: F. A. Davis.*

19. ANSWER: 5.7.
Rationale:

$$250 \text{ lb} \times 5\% = 12.5 \text{ lb}$$
$$12.5 \text{ lb} \div 2.2 \text{ lb/kg} = 5.68 \text{ kg} = 5.7 \text{ kg}$$

TEST-TAKING TIP: Remember that there are 2.2 lb in 1 kg.
Content Area: *Adult Health*
Category of Health Alteration: *Fluid Volume Excess*
Integrated Processes: *Nursing Process: Implementation*
Client Need: *Physiological Integrity*
Cognitive Level: *Application*
Reference: *Berman, A., Snyder, S., Kozier, B., and Erb, G. (2012). Kozier & Erb's Fundamentals of Nursing: Concepts, Process, and Practice (9th ed.). Upper Saddle River, NJ: Pearson.*

20. ANSWER: 4.
Rationale:
1. Furosemide may produce hypokalemia in a client with normal kidney function, but it is not used to decrease serum potassium, especially in a client with impaired renal function.
2. Sodium bicarbonate causes potassium to shift from the extracellular fluid to the intracellular fluid and may be used to quickly decrease serum potassium levels in the presence of severe hyperkalemia (greater than 7 mEq/L).
3. Regular insulin is not the first choice in lowering the client's serum potassium level because it does not eliminate potassium from the client's body, it just causes potassium to shift into the intracellular fluid temporarily.
4. The nurse should anticipate an order to administer sodium polystyrene sulfonate (Kayexalate), a cationic exchange resin that reduces serum potassium levels by exchanging sodium ions for potassium ions in the intestine and removes potassium via the gastrointestinal tract.
TEST-TAKING TIP: Remember that sodium polystyrene sulfonate is commonly used to lower serum potassium levels and can be administered by mouth or rectally as a retention enema.
Content Area: *Adult Health*
Category of Health Alteration: *Potassium Imbalance*
Integrated Processes: *Nursing Process: Planning*
Client Need: *Physiological Integrity*
Cognitive Level: *Knowledge*
Reference: *Deglin, J. H., Vallerand, A. H., and Sanoski, C. A. (2013). Davis's Drug Guide for Nurses (13th ed.). Philadelphia, PA: F. A. Davis.*

21. ANSWER: 1.
Rationale:
1. The nurse should anticipate a serum potassium level of 2.5 mEq/L (hypokalemia) because furosemide is a non–potassium-sparing loop diuretic. If the client's potassium level is less than 2.5 mEq/L, the nurse should notify the health-care provider immediately, because this is a critical value.
2. A serum potassium level of 4.0 mEq/L is within the normal reference range.
3. A serum potassium level of 5.0 mEq/L is within the normal reference range.
4. A serum potassium level of 6.5 mEq/L is higher than the normal reference range and would not be expected in a client taking furosemide (a non–potassium-sparing diuretic). If a client's potassium level is greater than 6.5 mEq/L, the nurse should notify the health-care provider immediately, because this is a critical value.
TEST-TAKING TIP: Recall that the normal serum potassium level in an adult is between 3.5 and 5.0 mEq/L. Knowledge of normal serum potassium levels is tested on the NCLEX examination.
Content Area: *Adult Health*
Category of Health Alteration: *Fluid Volume Excess*
Integrated Processes: *Nursing Process: Analysis*
Client Need: *Physiological Integrity*
Cognitive Level: *Application*
Reference: *Van Leeuwen, A. M., Poelhuis-Leth, D., and Bladh, M. (2011). Davis's Comprehensive Handbook of Laboratory and Diagnostic Tests With Nursing Implications (4th ed.). Philadelphia, PA: F. A. Davis.*

22. ANSWER: 1.
Rationale:
1. The nurse should determine that a regular cardiac rhythm (normal sinus rhythm) indicates that the client's hypomagnesemia is improving. Hypomagnesemia causes tachycardia and dysrhythmias. A regular heart rate is an indication of a resolving magnesium imbalance.
2. The presence of torsades de pointes and widened QRS complexes would indicate continued or worsened hypomagnesemia.
3. Prominent U waves are a sign of hypokalemia, not hypomagnesemia.
4. The presence of torsades de pointes and widened QRS complexes would indicate continued or worsened hypomagnesemia.
TEST-TAKING TIP: Recall the ECG signs of the different electrolyte imbalances.
Content Area: *Adult Health*
Category of Health Alteration: *Magnesium Imbalance*
Integrated Processes: *Nursing Process: Evaluation*
Client Need: *Physiological Integrity*
Cognitive Level: *Application*
Reference: *Berman, A., Snyder, S., Kozier, B., and Erb, G. (2012). Kozier & Erb's Fundamentals of Nursing: Concepts, Process, and Practice (9th ed.). Upper Saddle River, NJ: Pearson.*

23. ANSWER: 1.
Rationale:
1. The nurse should use adequate urine output to determine that fluid resuscitation has been effective. Normal urine output for children is 1 to 2 mL/kg/hr.
2. Blood pressure can remain normal, even in a state of hypovolemia.
3. Capillary refill time can remain normal, even in a state of hypovolemia.

4. Improvement in level of consciousness is not a reliable indicator of adequate fluid resuscitation because the child will be receiving medications for pain and anxiety control. Children with burns are usually treated with morphine sulfate (Duramorph) for pain and midazolam (Versed) for anxiety.
TEST-TAKING TIP: The key words are "adequacy of fluid resuscitation." Select the best indicator of fluid volume status among the options presented.
Content Area: Child Health
Category of Health Alteration: Fluid Volume Deficit
Integrated Processes: Nursing Process: Evaluation
Client Need: Physiological Integrity
Cognitive Level: Application
Reference: *Ward, S. L., and Hisley, S. M. (2011). Maternal-Child Nursing Care: Optimizing Outcomes for Mothers, Children and Families. Philadelphia, PA: F. A. Davis.*

24. ANSWER: 1.
Rationale:
1. The nurse should elicit Trousseau's sign by inflating a blood pressure cuff on the upper arm to a reading higher than the client's systolic blood pressure for 1 to 4 minutes and observing for carpopedal spasm, which indicates the presence of hypocalcemia.
2. Chvostek's sign is elicited by tapping the client's facial nerve anterior to the earlobe and observing for twitching of the mouth, nose, or cheek on the same side as the stimulus.
3. Hypocalcemia increases neuromuscular irritability and results in cells that depolarize more easily and at inappropriate times, increasing DTRs, but this does not constitute a positive Trousseau's sign.
4. Hyperventilation may elicit a positive Trousseau's sign, but one would not observe for muscle spasms in the hands and feet.
TEST-TAKING TIP: Know how to elicit Trousseau's sign and Chvostek's sign for the NCLEX examination.
Content Area: Adult Health
Category of Health Alteration: Calcium Imbalance
Integrated Processes: Nursing Process: Assessment
Client Need: Physiological Integrity
Cognitive Level: Comprehension
Reference: *Ignatavicius, D., and Workman, M. (2012). Medical-Surgical Nursing: Patient-Centered Collaborative Care (7th ed.). St. Louis, MO: Saunders.*

25. ANSWER: 2, 3, 4.
Rationale:
1. The nurse should instruct the client to wear lightweight, loose-fitting clothing, not constrictive clothing, when working in a hot environment.
2. The nurse should include instructions to gradually increase the amount of activity when working to prevent dehydration and possible heat exhaustion.
3. The nurse should include instructions to limit activity on hot or humid days to prevent dehydration and possible heat exhaustion.
4. The nurse should include instructions to drink plenty of fluids before, during, and after working to prevent dehydration and possible heat exhaustion.
5. Salt tablets should not be consumed because they can cause nausea, vomiting, and stomach irritation and can also increase the client's risk for hypernatremia and hypertonic dehydration.
TEST-TAKING TIP: The key words are "heat exhaustion." Select options that would decrease the client's risk for heat exhaustion.
Content Area: Adult Health
Category of Health Alteration: Fluid Volume Deficit
Integrated Processes: Nursing Process: Implementation
Client Need: Physiological Integrity
Cognitive Level: Application
Reference: *Ignatavicius, D., and Workman, M. (2012). Medical-Surgical Nursing: Patient-Centered Collaborative Care (7th ed.). St. Louis, MO: Saunders.*

26. ANSWER: 1, 2, 5.
Rationale:
1. The nurse should anticipate that the client will also have a decreased HCO_3^- level. Renal failure causes metabolic acidosis because the kidneys cannot make enough bicarbonate ions to balance the free hydrogen ions in the blood (decreased HCO_3^- level) and the kidney tubules cannot secrete hydrogen ions into the urine.
2. The client's serum potassium level is often increased in acidosis as the body attempts to buffer the blood pH by moving potassium out of the cells and into the bloodstream to counteract the hydrogen ions moving into the cells.
3. Acidosis may cause the client's serum calcium level to be decreased, not increased.
4. The client's PaO_2 would be either normal or increased.
5. The client's $PaCO_2$ level would be either normal or increased because the respiratory function is not impaired and the client may be "blowing off" carbon dioxide to compensate for the acidotic state.
TEST-TAKING TIP: Identify that renal failure results in metabolic acidosis. Rule out laboratory values that would not occur in the presence of metabolic acidosis.
Content Area: Adult Health
Category of Health Alteration: Acid-Base Imbalance
Integrated Processes: Nursing Process: Analysis
Client Need: Physiological Integrity
Cognitive Level: Application
Reference: *Ignatavicius, D., and Workman, M. (2012). Medical-Surgical Nursing: Patient-Centered Collaborative Care (7th ed.). St. Louis, MO: Saunders.*

27. ANSWER: 2.
Rationale:
1. Hypokalemia, not hyperkalemia, increases the cardiac muscle's sensitivity to digoxin and may result in digoxin toxicity, even when the digoxin level is within the therapeutic range.
2. The nurse should associate premature ventricular contractions (PVCs) and loss of the P wave on the ECG with the development of digoxin toxicity. A client taking a loop diuretic is at increased risk for digoxin toxicity because of the potassium-depleting effects of the diuretic.
3. Digoxin toxicity may be potentiated in clients with *hyper*calcemia.
4. Digoxin toxicity may be potentiated in clients with *hypo*magnesemia.
TEST-TAKING TIP: Associate the use of loop diuretics with potential potassium imbalances.
Content Area: Older Adult Health

Category of Health Alteration: Fluid Volume Excess
Integrated Processes: Nursing Process: Implementation
Client Need: Physiological Integrity
Cognitive Level: Application
Reference: Ignatavicius, D., and Workman, M. (2012). Medical-Surgical Nursing: Patient-Centered Collaborative Care (7th ed.). St. Louis, MO: Saunders.

28. ANSWER: 2.
Rationale:
1. These ABG values are not indicative of uncompensated respiratory acidosis. The normal $PaCO_2$ of 39 mm Hg indicates that the imbalance is not respiratory in origin.
2. The nurse should associate these ABG values with uncompensated metabolic acidosis. The pH of 7.31 reflects *uncompensated* acidosis because it remains less than the normal reference range of 7.35 to 7.45; the *decreased* HCO_3^- of 18 mEq/L indicates that there is not enough bicarbonate in the blood, making the imbalance metabolic in origin; and the *normal* $PaCO_2$ of 39 mm Hg indicates that the lungs have not yet begun to "blow off" carbon dioxide to compensate for the acidosis.
3. These ABG values are not indicative of compensated respiratory acidosis because the pH is below 7.35, indicating that the body has not yet compensated for the imbalance. The normal $PaCO_2$ of 39 mm Hg indicates that the imbalance is not respiratory in origin.
4. These ABG values are not indicative of compensated metabolic acidosis because the pH is below 7.35, indicating that the body has not yet compensated for the imbalance. The decreased HCO_3^- of 18 mEq/L means that there is not enough bicarbonate in the blood, indicating that the imbalance is metabolic in origin.
TEST-TAKING TIP: After first analyzing the blood pH to identify the presence of acidosis or alkalosis, look for abnormalities in the other ABG values to determine the underlying cause of the acid-base imbalance.
Content Area: Adult Health
Category of Health Alteration: Acid-Base Imbalance
Integrated Processes: Nursing Process: Analysis
Client Need: Physiological Integrity
Cognitive Level: Analysis
Reference: Berman, A., Snyder, S., Kozier, B., and Erb, G. (2012). Kozier & Erb's Fundamentals of Nursing: Concepts, Process, and Practice (9th ed.). Upper Saddle River, NJ: Pearson.

29. ANSWER: 3.
Rationale:
1. Oliguria would be a manifestation of fluid volume deficit, not hypokalemia.
2. Diarrhea is not a manifestation of the development of hypokalemia, although it is the cause of hypokalemia in this infant.
3. The nurse should suspect hypokalemia if the infant demonstrates muscle weakness. Infants require 2 to 3 mEq/kg/day of potassium to maintain growth, acid-base balance, cellular energy, and electrical charge balance. A potassium deficiency may result in myocardial damage, dysrhythmia, hypotension, and muscle weakness.
4. Hyperactive bowel sounds are associated with *hyper*kalemia.
TEST-TAKING TIP: Recognize that the signs of hypokalemia are similar in infants and adults. Review the signs of hypokalemia if you had difficulty with this question.
Content Area: Child Health
Category of Health Alteration: Potassium Imbalance
Integrated Processes: Nursing Process: Assessment
Client Need: Physiological Integrity
Cognitive Level: Application
Reference: Ward, S. L., and Hisley, S. M. (2011). Maternal-Child Nursing Care: Optimizing Outcomes for Mothers, Children and Families. Philadelphia, PA: F. A. Davis.

30. ANSWER: 4.
Rationale:
1. Placing the client on telemetry is appropriate but should not be the nurse's priority.
2. Oxygen administration, although appropriate, is not the first priority and requires an order.
3. Signs of hypokalemia are often vague, and there is no time to assess for this imbalance.
4. The nurse should notify the health-care provider first because this is a medical emergency that places the client at risk for life-threatening cardiac dysrhythmias.
TEST-TAKING TIP: Assessment, the first step in the nursing process, is usually a nurse's first action, *except* in the case of a life-threatening emergency.
Content Area: Adult Health
Category of Health Alteration: Fluid Volume Excess
Integrated Processes: Nursing Process: Implementation
Client Need: Physiological Integrity
Cognitive Level: Analysis
Reference: Dugdale, D. C. (2009). Digitalis toxicity. In Medline Plus Medical Encyclopedia. http://www.nlm.nih.gov/medlineplus/ency/article/000165.htm.

31. ANSWER: 205.
Rationale:

$$150 \text{ lb} \div 2.2 \text{ kg} = 68.18 \text{ kg}$$
$$68.18 \text{ kg} \times 3 \text{ mEq/kg} = 204.54 \text{ mEq} = 205 \text{ mEq}$$

TEST-TAKING TIP: Read the question carefully; in this scenario, the 4-hour administration period is irrelevant. Be sure to disregard extraneous information on the NCLEX examination.
Content Area: Adult Health
Category of Health Alteration: Acid-Base Imbalance
Integrated Processes: Nursing Process: Analysis
Client Need: Physiological Integrity
Cognitive Level: Application
Reference: Deglin, J. H., Vallerand, A. H., and Sanoski, C. A. (2013). Davis's Drug Guide for Nurses (13th ed.). Philadelphia, PA: F. A. Davis.

32. ANSWER: 1.
Rationale:

$$80 \text{ mEq} \div 4 \text{ doses} = 20 \text{ mEq/dose}$$
$$20 \text{ mEq} = 1 \text{ tablet}$$

TEST-TAKING TIP: Always double-check medication calculations, especially for high-alert drugs. Oral potassium may have to be given in divided doses because a single dose should not exceed 20 mEq.
Content Area: Adult Health
Category of Health Alteration: Potassium Imbalance

Integrated Processes: Nursing Process: Implementation
Client Need: Physiological Integrity
Cognitive Level: Application
***Reference:** Deglin, J. H., Vallerand, A. H., and Sanoski, C. A. (2013). Davis's Drug Guide for Nurses (13th ed.). Philadelphia, PA: F. A. Davis.*

33. ANSWER: 1.

Rationale:

1. The nurse should assess this client for metabolic acidosis and respiratory alkalosis because both occur with aspirin overdose. Aspirin, also known as acetylsalicylic acid, is a salicylate drug. A severe metabolic acidosis with compensatory respiratory alkalosis may develop with severe salicylate intoxication.

2. Metabolic alkalosis is not associated with aspirin overdose.

3. Respiratory acidosis is not associated with aspirin overdose.

4. Respiratory acidosis and metabolic alkalosis are not associated with aspirin overdose.

TEST-TAKING TIP: The key words are "ingesting a bottle of baby aspirin." Recall that aspirin is acetylsalicylic acid; excess ingestion would increase the amount of acid in the body.

Content Area: Child Health
Category of Health Alteration: Acid-Base Imbalance
Integrated Processes: Nursing Process: Assessment
Client Need: Physiological Integrity
Cognitive Level: Application
***Reference:** Perry, S., Hockenberry, M., Lowdermilk, D., and Wilson, D. (2010). Maternal Child Nursing Care (4th ed.). St. Louis, MO: Mosby.*

34. ANSWER: 1.

Rationale:

1. The nurse should associate anorexia, nausea, vomiting, muscle cramps, paresthesias, and confusion with the development of digoxin toxicity. Digoxin is frequently prescribed to improve the symptoms associated with fluid volume excess.

2. Increased appetite, muscle weakness, and tinnitus are not signs of digoxin toxicity.

3. Hemoptysis is not a manifestation of digoxin toxicity.

4. Euphoria and productive cough are not signs of digoxin toxicity.

TEST-TAKING TIP: The key words are "digoxin toxicity." Select the option that best describes its manifestations.

Content Area: Older Adult Health
Category of Health Alteration: Fluid Volume Excess
Integrated Processes: Nursing Process: Assessment
Client Need: Physiological Integrity
Cognitive Level: Application
***Reference:** Deglin, J. H., Vallerand, A. H., and Sanoski, C. A. (2013). Davis's Drug Guide for Nurses (13th ed.). Philadelphia, PA: F. A. Davis.*

35. ANSWER: 4.

Rationale:

1. Each day, 300 to 500 mL of fluid may be lost through perspiration.

2. Fluid lost through the gastrointestinal tract accounts for approximately 100 to 200 mL/day.

3. Insensible fluid loss, through the skin and lungs, accounts for 350 to 400 mL/day.

4. The client is most likely losing weight despite fluid replacement because total fluid loss, other than urine, can exceed 1,000 mL/day (1 L equals 2.2 lb). Each day, 300 to 500 mL of fluid may be lost through perspiration, 100 to 200 mL through the gastrointestinal tract, and 350 to 400 mL through the skin and lungs (insensible fluid loss).

TEST-TAKING TIP: The key words are "the client is losing weight." Recognize that the client continues to experience FVD despite fluid replacement, and rule out the incorrect statements related to fluid loss.

Content Area: Adult Health
Category of Health Alteration: Fluid Volume Deficit
Integrated Processes: Nursing Process: Analysis
Client Need: Physiological Integrity
Cognitive Level: Knowledge
***Reference:** Wilkinson, J., and Treas, L. (2011). Fundamentals of Nursing: Theory, Concepts & Applications (2nd ed.). Philadelphia, PA: F. A. Davis.*

36. ANSWER: 1.

Rationale:

1. The nurse should interpret an anion gap of 19 mEq/L as confirmation of metabolic acidosis. The normal range for the anion gap is 8 to 16 mEq/L, and an anion gap greater than 16 mEq/L indicates the presence of metabolic acidosis. The anion gap [(Na^+ – (Cl^- + HCO_3^-)] is nonspecific. It is calculated to identify the presence of metabolic acidosis but does not indicate the underlying cause of the imbalance.

2. An anion gap less than 8 mEq/L would indicate the presence of metabolic alkalosis.

3. The anion gap is calculated to identify only metabolic imbalances, not respiratory imbalances.

4. The anion gap is calculated to identify only metabolic imbalances, not respiratory imbalances.

TEST-TAKING TIP: Recall that the anion gap is a measurement with a normal reference range of 8 to 16 mEq/L, and it is used to determine the presence of metabolic acidosis.

Content Area: Adult Health
Category of Health Alteration: Acid-Base Imbalance
Integrated Processes: Nursing Process: Planning
Client Need: Physiological Integrity
Cognitive Level: Application
***Reference:** Van Leeuwen, A. M., Poelhuis-Leth, D., and Bladh, M. (2011). Davis's Comprehensive Handbook of Laboratory and Diagnostic Tests With Nursing Implications (4th ed.). Philadelphia, PA: F. A. Davis.*

37. ANSWER: 2.

Rationale:

1. Decreased milk and vitamin D intake would worsen hypocalcemia.

2. The nurse should include monitoring for tingling and numbness around the mouth (circumoral paresthesia) when teaching a client diagnosed with hypoparathyroidism because this is a sign of hypocalcemia. Decreased serum calcium levels occur due to the lack of parathyroid hormone, which, with vitamin D and calcitonin, regulates serum calcium levels.

3. The client should consume foods that are low in phosphorus because of the inverse relationship between calcium and phosphorus.

4. Anorexia, nausea, vomiting, and constipation are signs of *hyper*calcemia.
TEST-TAKING TIP: Recall that hypoparathyroidism results in hypocalcemia. Review the signs of hypocalcemia.
Content Area: Adult Health
Category of Health Alteration: Calcium Imbalance
Integrated Processes: Teaching/Learning
Client Need: Physiological Integrity
Cognitive Level: Application
Reference: *Ignatavicius, D., and Workman, M. (2012). Medical-Surgical Nursing: Patient-Centered Collaborative Care (7th ed.). St. Louis, MO: Saunders.*

38. ANSWER: 4.
Rationale:
1. ECG strip 1 is normal sinus rhythm.
2. ECG strip 2 shows sinus bradycardia to sinus rhythm with a wandering atrial pacemaker, a rhythm associated with sinoatrial node dysfunction, not hypokalemia.
3. ECG strip 3 illustrates sinus tachycardia (heart rate greater than 100 bpm).
4. The nurse should identify ECG strip 4 as indicative of hypokalemia because it displays a normal sinus rhythm with prominent U waves, which are classic ECG changes associated with serum potassium levels less than 3.5 mEq/L.
TEST-TAKING TIP: Select the option that reflects the effects of hypokalemia on the electrical conduction of the heart. Review the effects of hypokalemia and hyperkalemia observed on an ECG rhythm strip if you had difficulty with this question.
Content Area: Adult Health
Category of Health Alteration: Potassium Imbalance
Integrated Processes: Nursing Process: Evaluation
Client Need: Physiological Integrity
Cognitive Level: Analysis
Reference: *Jones, S. (2010). ECG Notes: Interpretation and Management Guide (2nd ed.). Philadelphia, PA: F. A. Davis.*

39. ANSWER: 1, 3, 5.
Rationale:
1. 0.9% saline would not be administered at 50 mL/hr because the first goal of fluid therapy in diabetic ketoacidosis (DKA) is to restore volume in a severely volume-depleted client; thus, 50 mL/hr would be an inappropriate rate.
2. 0.9% saline solution should be infused at a rate of 1,000 mL/hr × 2, up to a total of 10 L in the first 24 hours of treatment.
3. 3% saline solution would be contraindicated in this client because it is a hypertonic solution that would worsen the client's dehydration.
4. Administration of a dextrose-containing solution is recommended, beginning when the client's blood glucose reaches 250 mg/dL.
5. Dextrose 5% in lactated Ringer's solution when the blood glucose reaches 500 mg/dL is inappropriate because the blood sugar is still too high for the infusion of a dextrose-containing solution.
TEST-TAKING TIP: The key words are "which health-care provider orders should a nurse question." Recognize that fluid volume deficit is a hallmark of DKA. Select the options that are *incorrect* orders.
Content Area: Adult Health
Category of Health Alteration: Fluid Volume Deficit
Integrated Processes: Nursing Process: Analysis
Client Need: Physiological Integrity
Cognitive Level: Analysis
Reference: *Ignatavicius, D., and Workman, M. (2012). Medical-Surgical Nursing: Patient-Centered Collaborative Care (7th ed.). St. Louis, MO: Saunders.*

40. ANSWER: 1, 3.
Rationale:
1. The nurse should anticipate that this client will experience metabolic acidosis and possibly respiratory acidosis because the client has ingested excessive amounts of alcohol, which is an acid. Substances that cause acidosis when ingested include ethanol, methyl alcohol, and acetylsalicylic acid (aspirin).
2. Excessive acid intake would not cause alkalosis.
3. Ethanol toxicity can cause muscle weakness that results in respiratory depression, placing the client at risk for respiratory acidosis as well as metabolic acidosis.
4. Excessive acid intake would not cause alkalosis.
TEST-TAKING TIP: The key words are "ethanol intoxication." Recall that ethanol (alcohol) intoxication causes acidosis. Use the process of elimination to rule out incorrect options.
Content Area: Adult Health
Category of Health Alteration: Acid-Base Imbalance
Integrated Processes: Nursing Process: Planning
Client Need: Physiological Integrity
Cognitive Level: Application
Reference: *Ignatavicius, D., and Workman, M. (2012). Medical-Surgical Nursing: Patient-Centered Collaborative Care (7th ed.). St. Louis, MO: Saunders.*

41. ANSWER: 1, 2, 4, 5.
Rationale:
1. The nurse should question oral (PO), intramuscular (IM), and subcutaneous (sub-cu) potassium replacement therapy in this client. A serum potassium level less than 3.0 mEq/L is considered severe, necessitating rapid intravenous (IV) replacement.
2. Potassium is never given intramuscularly because it is a severe tissue irritant.
3. A client with severe hypokalemia would receive IV potassium replacement. KCl 40 mEq/L over 4 hours is an appropriate dosage.
4. A serum potassium level less than 3.0 mEq/L is considered severe, necessitating rapid IV replacement.
5. Potassium is never given subcutaneously because it is a severe tissue irritant.
TEST-TAKING TIP: First, recall the routes of administration for medications that cause tissue irritation; second, evaluate the seriousness of the electrolyte deficiency, and use the process of elimination to find the correct answer.
Content Area: Adult Health
Category of Health Alteration: Potassium Imbalance

Integrated Processes: Nursing Process: Implementation
Client Need: Physiological Integrity
Cognitive Level: Application
Reference: *Ignatavicius, D., and Workman, M. (2012). Medical-Surgical Nursing: Patient-Centered Collaborative Care (7th ed.). St. Louis, MO: Saunders.*

42. ANSWER: 7.3.
Rationale:

24 lb÷ 2.2 lb/kg = 10.91 kg
10.91 kg × 2 mmol/kg/day = 21.82 mmol/day
21.82 mmol/day ÷ 3 doses per day = 7.27 = 7.3 mmol every 8 hours

TEST-TAKING TIP: Read the question carefully. Recall that there are three 8-hour periods in each day.
Content Area: Child Health
Category of Health Alteration: Acid-Base Imbalance
Integrated Processes: Nursing Process: Implementation
Client Need: Physiological Integrity
Cognitive Level: Application
Reference: *Deglin, J. H., Vallerand, A. H., and Sanoski, C. A. (2013). Davis's Drug Guide for Nurses (13th ed.). Philadelphia, PA: F. A. Davis.*

43. ANSWER: 3.8.
Rationale:

84 lb÷ 2.2 lb/kg = 38.18 kg
38.18 kg × 50 mg/kg = 1,909 mg
1,909 mg/*X*× 500 mg/1 mL= 500*X* = 1,909 = 1,909 ÷ 500= 3.81 mL = 3.8 mL

TEST-TAKING TIP: Always double-check your calculations before providing your answer on the NCLEX examination *and* before administering medication to a client.
Content Area: Child Health
Category of Health Alteration: Magnesium Imbalance
Integrated Processes: Nursing Process: Implementation
Client Need: Physiological Integrity
Cognitive Level: Application
Reference: *Deglin, J. H., Vallerand, A. H., and Sanoski, C. A. (2013). Davis's Drug Guide for Nurses (13th ed.). Philadelphia, PA: F. A. Davis.*

44. ANSWER: 1, 2, 5.
Rationale:
1. ECG strip 1 is a sinus rhythm with premature ventricular contractions, which may be indicative of potassium imbalance.
2. ECG strips 2 and 5 illustrate different types of ventricular tachycardia. Both hypokalemia and hyperkalemia can cause ventricular dysrhythmias.
3. ECG strip 3 depicts atrial tachycardia, an abnormal sinus rhythm.
4. ECG strip 4 is a sinus rhythm with premature atrial contractions. Atrial dysrhythmias are not usually associated with potassium imbalances.
5. ECG strips 2 and 5 illustrate different types of ventricular tachycardia. Both hypokalemia and hyperkalemia can cause ventricular dysrhythmias.
TEST-TAKING TIP: Associate potassium imbalances with potentially life-threatening ventricular dysrhythmias. Review the differences between atrial and ventricular dysrhythmias.
Content Area: Adult Health
Category of Health Alteration: Potassium Imbalance
Integrated Processes: Nursing Process: Evaluation
Client Need: Physiological Integrity
Cognitive Level: Analysis
Reference: *Jones, S. (2010). ECG Notes: Interpretation and Management Guide (2nd ed.). Philadelphia, PA: F. A. Davis.*

45. ANSWER: 2.
Rationale:
1. Respiratory acidosis would cause the serum pH to decrease.
2. The nurse should anticipate that this client's laboratory values will show a decreased pH (acidosis), increased $PaCO_2$ (respiratory origin of pH alteration), and normal HCO_3^- (no metabolic compensation yet). Hypoventilation causes carbon dioxide retention, resulting in respiratory acidosis.
3. If the client's renal system had begun to compensate, the client's HCO_3^- would be increased in an attempt to increase the pH to the normal reference range.
4. In the presence of acidosis, the client's serum calcium level would be increased.
TEST-TAKING TIP: Recall that in a respiratory acid-base imbalance, $PaCO_2$ is abnormal; increased carbon dioxide equals increased acid, and decreased carbon dioxide equals decreased acid.
Content Area: Adult Health
Category of Health Alteration: Acid-Base Imbalance
Integrated Processes: Nursing Process: Evaluation
Client Need: Physiological Integrity
Cognitive Level: Application
Reference: *Williams, L. ,and Hopper, P. (2011). Understanding Medical-Surgical Nursing (4th ed.). Philadelphia, PA: F. A. Davis.*

46. ANSWER: 2.
Rationale:
1. Fresh fruits, although healthy, are low in phosphorus.
2. The nurse should instruct the client to include red meats, eggs, nuts, whole grain breads, and cereal in the diet to increase phosphorus intake.
3. Dairy products should be avoided because they are rich in calcium. The higher the serum calcium level is, the lower the serum phosphorus level will become.
4. Green leafy vegetables, although healthy, are low in phosphorus.
TEST-TAKING TIP: The key word is "hypophosphatemia." Consider the amount of phosphorus in each item, and select the option with the highest phosphorus content.
Content Area: Adult Health
Category of Health Alteration: Phosphate Imbalance
Integrated Processes: Nursing Process: Implementation
Client Need: Physiological Integrity
Cognitive Level: Application
Reference: *Berman, A., Snyder, S., Kozier, B., and Erb, G. (2012). Kozier & Erb's Fundamentals of Nursing: Concepts, Process, and Practice (9th ed.). Upper Saddle River, NJ: Pearson.*

47. ANSWER: 3.
Rationale:
1. Hypotonic overhydration (water intoxication) results from the excessive intake or retention of salt-free solutions, such as water.

2. Hypertonic dehydration is a fictitious term.

3. The client is most likely experiencing isotonic overhydration because 0.9% saline solution (normal saline) is an isotonic solution that increases vascular fluid volume but does not cause a shift in fluids. Isotonic overhydration is the most common type of fluid volume excess and may result from the excessive administration, ingestion, or retention of isotonic fluids.

4. Hypotonic dehydration is a fictitious term.

TEST-TAKING TIP: Rule out dehydration because the nurse has administered excess IV fluids. Recall that 0.9% saline solution is an isotonic solution.

Content Area: Adult Health
Category of Health Alteration: Fluid Volume Excess
Integrated Processes: Nursing Process: Implementation
Client Need: Physiological Integrity
Cognitive Level: Application
Reference: Ignatavicius, D., and Workman, M. (2012). Medical-Surgical Nursing: Patient-Centered Collaborative Care (7th ed.). St. Louis, MO: Saunders.

48. ANSWER: 2.

Rationale:

1. The goal "The client's oral fluid intake will equal urine output" does not pertain to the nursing diagnosis Risk for Falls Related to Skeletal Muscle Weakness Secondary to Electrolyte Imbalance.

2. The most appropriate outcome for a client with a nursing diagnosis of Risk for Falls Related to Skeletal Muscle Weakness Secondary to Electrolyte Imbalance is to remain free from injury throughout the hospital stay.

3. The statement regarding the client's serum electrolyte levels would be an appropriate outcome for the nursing diagnosis Electrolyte Imbalance.

4. The goal "The client will verbalize specific foods to ingest that increase dietary potassium intake" does not pertain to the nursing diagnosis Risk for Falls Related to Skeletal Muscle Weakness Secondary to Electrolyte Imbalance.

TEST-TAKING TIP: Rule out options that do not specifically apply to the nursing diagnosis in the question.

Content Area: Adult Health
Category of Health Alteration: Potassium Imbalance
Integrated Processes: Nursing Process: Planning
Client Need: Safe and Effective Care Environment
Cognitive Level: Application
Reference: Ignatavicius, D., and Workman, M. (2012). Medical-Surgical Nursing: Patient-Centered Collaborative Care (7th ed.). St. Louis, MO: Saunders.

49. ANSWER: 3.

Rationale:

1. Graphic 1 depicts normal acid-base balance.

2. Graphic 2 depicts an *actual* alkalosis because there is an increased number of bases (base excess), usually bicarbonate.

3. The nurse should identify Graphic 3 as the most accurate depiction of *relative* alkalosis because it displays a decrease in acid, not an increase in base (acid deficit).

4. Graphic 4 displays a relative acidosis because there is a decreased number of bases, not an increased number of acids.

TEST-TAKING TIP: The key words are "relative alkalosis." Recognize that in relative alkalosis, the number of bases exceeds the number of acids because the acid is decreased.

Content Area: Adult Health
Category of Health Alteration: Acid-Base Imbalance
Integrated Processes: Nursing Process: Analysis
Client Need: Physiological Integrity
Cognitive Level: Comprehension
Reference: Ignatavicius, D., and Workman, M. (2012). Medical-Surgical Nursing: Patient-Centered Collaborative Care (7th ed.). St. Louis, MO: Saunders.

50. ANSWER: 2, 4.

Rationale:

1. Although weight is an indicator of fluid volume status, it should be assessed daily, not *during* the infusion.

2. The most important parameters for the nurse to monitor *during* rehydration are pulse rate and quality and urine output. An excessive increase in pulse rate and quality may indicate fluid overload.

3. Oxygen saturation is not directly affected by fluid volume status.

4. Urine output should be closely monitored during IV infusions to ensure that the client is voiding at least 30 mL/hr (obligatory urine output) to prevent fluid overload.

5. Skin turgor is not a parameter that would determine the adequacy of fluid replacement therapy *during* the infusion.

TEST-TAKING TIP: The key words are "*during* IV rehydration." Rule out the parameters that would not be important to monitor *during* an infusion.

Content Area: Adult Health
Category of Health Alteration: Fluid Volume Deficit
Integrated Processes: Nursing Process: Assessment
Client Need: Physiological Integrity
Cognitive Level: Application
Reference: Ignatavicius, D., and Workman, M. (2012). Medical-Surgical Nursing: Patient-Centered Collaborative Care (7th ed.). St. Louis, MO: Saunders.

51. ANSWER: 2, 5.

Rationale:

1. Assessing the functioning of suction equipment is an appropriate action when implementing seizure precautions.

2. When implementing seizure precautions for this client, the nurse should question placing a tongue blade at the head of the client's bed. This is inappropriate because a client who is having a seizure should never have anything placed in the mouth.

3. Padding the side rails and headboard of the client's bed is an appropriate action when implementing seizure precautions.

4. Maintaining the bed in a low position with the wheels locked is an appropriate action when implementing seizure precautions.

5. When implementing seizure precautions for this client, the nurse should question ensuring that the client's room is bright. The nurse should decrease environmental stimuli by darkening the room for a client who is at risk for seizures.

TEST-TAKING TIP: Read the question carefully; the *correct* options are the *incorrect* nursing actions.
Content Area: Older Adult Health
Category of Health Alteration: Magnesium Imbalance
Integrated Processes: Nursing Process: Implementation
Client Need: Safe and Effective Care Environment
Cognitive Level: Application
Reference: *Ignatavicius, D., and Workman, M. (2012). Medical-Surgical Nursing: Patient-Centered Collaborative Care (7th ed.). St. Louis, MO: Saunders.*

52. ANSWER: 1, 2, 3, 5.
Rationale:
1. **The nurse should identify hyperthyroidism as a factor that contributes to the development of hypercalcemia. An overactive thyroid causes increased serum calcium levels related to increased bone turnover and release of calcium into the blood.**
2. **The nurse should identify hypophosphatemia as a factor that contributes to the development of hypercalcemia. The presence of hypophosphatemia is related to hypercalcemia because phosphorus and calcium have an inverse relationship.**
3. **The nurse should identify hypermagnesemia as a factor that contributes to the development of hypercalcemia. Hypermagnesemia increases parathyroid hormone (PTH), thereby increasing calcium levels.**
4. Alkalosis (increased blood pH) causes ionized calcium to bind with proteins, resulting in *hypo*calcemia.
5. **The nurse should identify hyperparathyroidism as a factor that contributes to the development of hypercalcemia. Hyperparathyroidism (an excess of PTH) increases circulating calcium levels.**
TEST-TAKING TIP: Think about how the calcium level is affected by each condition. Use the process of elimination to rule out options that are *not* signs of hypercalcemia.
Content Area: Adult Health
Category of Health Alteration: Calcium Imbalance
Integrated Processes: Nursing Process: Analysis
Client Need: Physiological Integrity
Cognitive Level: Analysis
Reference: *Van Leeuwen, A. M., Poelhuis-Leth, D.,and Bladh, M. (2011). Davis's Comprehensive Handbook of Laboratory and Diagnostic Tests With Nursing Implications (4th ed.). Philadelphia, PA: F. A. Davis.*

53. ANSWER: 4.
Rationale:
1. Graphic 1 depicts normal acid-base balance.
2. Graphic 2 depicts an actual alkalosis because there is an increased number of bases (base excess), usually bicarbonate.
3. Graphic 3 displays a relative alkalosis because there is a decreased number of acids, not an increased number of bases.
4. **The nurse should identify Graphic 4 as the most accurate depiction of *relative* acidosis because it displays a decrease in base, not an increase in acid (base deficit).**
TEST-TAKING TIP: The key words are "relative acidosis." Recognize that in relative acidosis, the number of acids exceeds the number of bases because the base is decreased.
Content Area: Adult Health
Category of Health Alteration: Acid-Base Imbalance
Integrated Processes: Nursing Process: Analysis
Client Need: Physiological Integrity
Cognitive Level: Comprehension
Reference: *Ignatavicius, D., and Workman, M. (2012). Medical-Surgical Nursing: Patient-Centered Collaborative Care (7th ed.). St. Louis, MO: Saunders.*

54. ANSWER: 2.
Rationale:
1. ECG strip 1 is a normal sinus rhythm.
2. **The nurse is most likely to observe the cardiac rhythm in ECG strip 2 because the client is exhibiting signs and symptoms of hypercalcemia. This rhythm strip shows shortened Q-T intervals, which is a classic ECG change associated with serum calcium levels greater than 10.2 mg/dL.**
3. ECG strip 3 illustrates the peaked T waves associated with hyperkalemia.
4. ECG strip 4 shows torsades de pointes, which is a dysrhythmia associated with hypomagnesemia.
TEST-TAKING TIP: Select the option that best illustrates the effect of hypercalcemia on the electrical conduction of the heart.
Content Area: Adult Health
Category of Health Alteration: Calcium Imbalance
Integrated Processes: Nursing Process: Assessment
Client Need: Physiological Integrity
Cognitive Level: Analysis
References: *Jones, S. (2010). ECG Notes: Interpretation and Management Guide (2nd ed.). Philadelphia, PA: F. A. Davis; Ignatavicius, D., and Workman, M. (2012). Medical-Surgical Nursing: Patient-Centered Collaborative Care (7th ed.). St. Louis, MO: Saunders.*

55. ANSWER: 125.
Rationale:

$$1{,}000 \text{ mL} \div 8 \text{ hours} = 125 \text{ mL/hr}$$

TEST-TAKING TIP: Always double-check your calculations. An incorrect fluid calculation could result in fluid deficit or fluid overload.
Content Area: Adult Health
Category of Health Alteration: Fluid Volume Deficit
Integrated Processes: Nursing Process: Implementation
Client Need: Physiological Integrity
Cognitive Level: Application
Reference: *Deglin, J. H., Vallerand, A. H., and Sanoski, C. A.(2013). Davis's Drug Guide for Nurses (13th ed.). Philadelphia, PA: F. A. Davis.*

56. ANSWER: 34.
Rationale:

$$75 \text{ lb} \div 2.2 \text{ lb/kg} = 34.09 \text{ kg}$$
$$34.09 \text{ kg} \times 0.5 \text{ mEq/kg} = 17.05 \text{ mEq/hr}$$
$$50 \text{ mEq/100 mL} = 0.5 \text{ mEq/mL}$$
$$17.05 \text{ mEq} \div 0.5 \text{ mEq/mL} = 34.09 \text{ mL} = 34 \text{ mL/hr}$$

TEST-TAKING TIP: Always double-check medication calculations. Accidental administration of hypertonic saline solution can result in life-threatening electrolyte imbalances.
Content Area: Child Health
Category of Health Alteration: Sodium Imbalance
Integrated Processes: Nursing Process: Analysis
Client Need: Physiological Integrity
Cognitive Level: Application

Reference: Deglin, J. H., Vallerand, A. H., and Sanoski, C. A.(2013). Davis's Drug Guide for Nurses (13th ed.). Philadelphia, PA: F. A. Davis.

57. ANSWER: 1.

Rationale:

1. The nurse should question the order for furosemide because it is a loop diuretic and may exacerbate the client's fluid volume deficit and metabolic alkalosis.

2. Administering 0.9% saline solution with 40 mEq/L KCl IV at 100 mL/hr would be an appropriate order for this client.

3. Administering promethazine (Phenergan) 12.5 mg IV every 6 hours as needed for nausea would be an appropriate order for this client.

4. Administering ondansetron (Zofran) 4 mg IV every 4 hours as needed for nausea would be an appropriate order for this client.

TEST-TAKING TIP: The key words are "diuretic use." Be familiar with drug classifications. Use the process of elimination to rule out options that would be appropriate in the plan of care.

Content Area: Adult Health
Category of Health Alteration: Acid-Base Imbalance
Integrated Processes: Nursing Process: Analysis
Client Need: Physiological Integrity
Cognitive Level: Analysis
Reference: Ignatavicius, D., and Workman, M. (2012). Medical-Surgical Nursing: Patient-Centered Collaborative Care (7th ed.). St. Louis, MO: Saunders.

58. ANSWER: 2.

Rationale:

1. The client's wheelchair should be placed beside the client's bed, not at the foot of the bed.

2. Ensuring that the client's call bell is within reach at all times is the appropriate choice. This is an important intervention for maintaining the safety of a client with a diagnosis of Risk for Falls Related to Skeletal Muscle Weakness because it ensures that the client can call for assistance when getting out of bed.

3. Neurological checks should be performed every 4 hours.

4. Weighing the client is an important intervention for determining fluid volume status, but it is not applicable to injury prevention.

TEST-TAKING TIP: The key words are "Risk for Falls." Identify the option that correctly addresses client safety.

Content Area: Older Adult Health
Category of Health Alteration: Sodium Imbalance
Integrated Processes: Nursing Process: Analysis
Client Need: Safe and Effective Care Environment
Cognitive Level: Application
Reference: Ignatavicius, D., and Workman, M. (2012). Medical-Surgical Nursing: Patient-Centered Collaborative Care (7th ed.). St. Louis, MO: Saunders.

59. ANSWER: 1.

Rationale:

1. The nurse should teach the client that a woman of any age has less total body water than a man of similar size and age because men have more muscle mass and less body fat than women. Muscle cells contain mostly water, whereas fat cells contain very little water. This difference in water distribution may be responsible for the different ways women and men respond to drugs.

2. A woman has less body fluid than a man.

3. A woman has less body fluid than a man.

4. A woman has less body fluid than a man.

TEST-TAKING TIP: Select the statement that is true. Recall that older adults, infants, children, and obese clients are at risk for fluid and electrolyte imbalances.

Content Area: Older Adult Health
Category of Health Alteration: Fluid Volume Excess
Integrated Processes: Teaching/Learning
Client Need: Physiological Integrity
Cognitive Level: Application
Reference: Ignatavicius, D., and Workman, M. (2012). Medical-Surgical Nursing: Patient-Centered Collaborative Care (7th ed.). St. Louis, MO: Saunders.

60. ANSWER: 1.

Rationale:

1. The nurse should assign the nursing diagnosis Risk for Decreased Cardiac Output to this client because circulating blood volume is decreased in fluid volume deficit (FVD).

2. Although this client would have a decreased urinary output, the nursing diagnosis Chronic Urinary Retention is not appropriate because it is used for a client who has difficulty voiding or is unable to void.

3. Risk for Deficient Fluid Volume is incorrect because the client is already experiencing FVD.

4. Deficient Fluid Volume: Isotonic is incorrect because chronic thiazide therapy results in *hypotonic* dehydration because the urine is concentrated and more sodium than water is lost.

TEST-TAKING TIP: The key words are "long-term chlorothiazide (Diuril) therapy." Thiazide diuretics increase the excretion of both sodium and water; however, more sodium than water is lost, potentially creating a state of hypotonic dehydration.

Content Area: Adult Health
Category of Health Alteration: Fluid Volume Deficit
Integrated Processes: Nursing Process: Analysis
Client Need: Physiological Integrity
Cognitive Level: Application
Reference: Deglin, J. H., Vallerand, A. H., and Sanoski, C. A. (2013). Davis's Drug Guide for Nurses (13th ed.). Philadelphia, PA: F. A. Davis.

61. ANSWER: 3.

Rationale:

1. A respiratory rate of 16 breaths per minute is within normal limits.

2. Blood pressure of 124/76 mm Hg is within normal limits.

3. The nurse caring for a client with hyperchloremia should intervene immediately if the client displays Kussmaul respirations, an ineffective breathing pattern. Kussmaul respirations are a classic sign of metabolic acidosis, a potential life-threatening complication of hyperchloremia.

4. Decreased urinary output is an expected finding in hyperchloremia and would not necessitate intervention by the nurse.

TEST-TAKING TIP: Review the signs and symptoms of hyperchloremia. Rule out options that are within normal limits.

Content Area: Adult Health
Category of Health Alteration: Chloride Imbalance
Integrated Processes: Nursing Process: Analysis

Client Need: *Physiological Integrity*
Cognitive Level: *Analysis*
Reference: *Ignatavicius, D., and Workman, M. (2012). Medical-Surgical Nursing: Patient-Centered Collaborative Care (7th ed.). St. Louis, MO: Saunders.*

62. **ANSWER: 1, 3, 5.**
Rationale:
1. The nurse should recommend that the client increase the consumption of baked potatoes because they are an excellent source of potassium.
2. Apples would be appropriate for a low-potassium diet.
3. The nurse should recommend that the client increase the consumption of yogurt because it is an excellent source of potassium.
4. Bread would be appropriate for a low-potassium diet.
5. The nurse should recommend that the client increase the consumption of clams because they are an excellent source of potassium.
TEST-TAKING TIP: The key words are "increase the amount of potassium." Select the options that contain the *most* potassium.
Content Area: *Adult Health*
Category of Health Alteration: *Potassium Imbalance*
Integrated Processes: *Teaching/Learning*
Client Need: *Physiological Integrity*
Cognitive Level: *Application*
Reference: *U.S. Department of Agriculture, Agricultural Research Service. (2009). USDA National Nutrient Database for Standard Reference. Release 22. Nutrient Data Laboratory Home Page. Retrieved from http://www.ars.usda.gov/ba/bhnrc/ndl.*

63. **ANSWER: 2, 4.**
Rationale:
1. An increase in intake would decrease the infant's risk for dehydration.
2. The nurse should explain to the mother that a fever increases the infant's risk for dehydration because of insensible water loss. Fever increases insensible water loss by approximately 7 mL/kg/24 hours for each degree above 99°F.
3. Renal perfusion is not affected until dehydration is present.
4. The nurse should explain to the mother that a fever increases the infant's risk for dehydration because a child has a larger surface area relative to volume compared with an adult, which also contributes to insensible loss.
TEST-TAKING TIP: The key words are "increases the infant's risk for dehydration." Select options that would contribute to dehydration.
Content Area: *Child Health*
Category of Health Alteration: *Fluid Volume Deficit*
Integrated Processes: *Nursing Process: Implementation*
Client Need: *Physiological Integrity*
Cognitive Level: *Application*
Reference: *Ward, S. L., and Hisley, S. M. (2011). Maternal-Child Nursing Care: Optimizing Outcomes for Mothers, Children and Families. Philadelphia, PA: F. A. Davis.*

64. **ANSWER: 2.**
Rationale:
1. Ibuprofen, an NSAID, should not directly affect acid-base balance.
2. The nurse should identify the administration of morphine sulfate as a factor that increases the client's risk for an acid-base imbalance. Opioid administration can cause respiratory depression and increase the client's risk of respiratory acidosis.
3. 0.9% saline solution should not cause a fluid shift in electrolytes and would not directly affect acid-base balance.
4. Dextrose 5% in 0.45% saline solution should not cause a fluid shift in electrolytes and would not directly affect acid-base balance.
TEST-TAKING TIP: The key words are "at risk for an acid-base imbalance." Consider the effect of each option on acid-base balance, and rule out options that would have no significant effect.
Content Area: *Adult Health*
Category of Health Alteration: *Acid-Base Imbalance*
Integrated Processes: *Nursing Process: Implementation*
Client Need: *Physiological Integrity*
Cognitive Level: *Application*
Reference: *Ignatavicius, D., and Workman, M. (2012). Medical-Surgical Nursing: Patient-Centered Collaborative Care (7th ed.). St. Louis, MO: Saunders.*

65. **ANSWER: 2.**
Rationale:
1. Although an older adult is at increased risk for FVD in general, this client would not be at *greatest* risk for FVD.
2. The nurse should identify the client with ulcerative colitis as being at greatest risk for FVD. Ulcerative colitis is an inflammatory bowel disease characterized by frequent bloody diarrhea and fecal incontinence. Clients with ulcerative colitis can experience more than 10 bloody stools per day (depending on severity), losing fluid, electrolytes, and blood with each stool.
3. Although an infant is at increased risk for FVD in general, this client would not be at *greatest* risk for FVD.
4. Although an older adult is at increased risk for FVD in general, this client would not be at *greatest* risk for FVD.
TEST-TAKING TIP: To choose which client has the greatest risk for FVD, determine which client has an actual rather than potential risk. In most instances, children and older adult adults have the greatest risk of FVD. In this case, however, a client with ulcerative colitis would have the greatest risk.
Content Area: *Adult Health*
Category of Health Alteration: *Fluid Volume Deficit*
Integrated Processes: *Nursing Process: Analysis*
Client Need: *Physiological Integrity*
Cognitive Level: *Application*
Reference: *Ignatavicius, D., and Workman, M. (2012). Medical-Surgical Nursing: Patient-Centered Collaborative Care (7th ed.). St. Louis, MO: Saunders.*

66. **ANSWER: 1.**
Rationale:
1. The nurse should associate Graphic 1 with metabolic alkalosis. In the presence of alkalosis, the body attempts to decrease the blood pH. Thus, the serum potassium level is decreased because potassium moves into the cells in response to the release of hydrogen ions from the cells. The serum calcium level is decreased because an increase in

blood pH causes an increase in the intracellular uptake of calcium. The serum chloride level is also decreased because intracellular chloride levels increase in an effort to reduce the alkalinity of the extracellular fluid.
2. Graphic 2 displays the movement of electrolytes in the presence of *respiratory* alkalosis.
3. Graphic 3 displays the movement of electrolytes in the presence of metabolic *acidosis.*
4. Graphic 4 displays the movement of electrolytes in the presence of *respiratory acidosis.*
TEST-TAKING TIP: The key words are "metabolic alkalosis." Consider the effect of metabolic alkalosis on each electrolyte.
Content Area: Adult Health
Category of Health Alteration: Acid-Base Imbalance
Integrated Processes: Nursing Process: Analysis
Client Need: Physiological Integrity
Cognitive Level: Application
Reference: *Van Leeuwen, A. M., Poelhuis-Leth, D., and Bladh, M. (2011). Davis's Comprehensive Handbook of Laboratory and Diagnostic Tests With Nursing Implications (4th ed.). Philadelphia, PA: F. A. Davis.*

67. ANSWER: 15.6.
Rationale:

$$7 \text{ mEq}/X = 0.45 \text{ mEq}/1 \text{ mL} = 0.45X = 7 = 7 \div 0.45 = 15.55 \text{ mL} = 15.6 \text{ mL}$$

TEST-TAKING TIP: Read the question carefully. It is asking you to calculate how *many milliliters (not milliequivalents) to administer.*
Content Area: Maternal Health
Category of Health Alteration: Magnesium Imbalance
Integrated Processes: Nursing Process: Implementation
Client Need: Physiological Integrity
Cognitive Level: Application
Reference: *Deglin, J. H., Vallerand, A. H., and Sanoski, C. A.(2013). Davis's Drug Guide for Nurses (13th ed.). Philadelphia, PA: F. A. Davis.*

68. ANSWER: 47.
Rationale: The pulse pressure is the difference between the systolic blood pressure and the diastolic blood pressure.

$$152 \text{ mm Hg} - 105 \text{ mm Hg} = 47 \text{ mm Hg}$$

The pulse pressure represents the force the heart generates each time it contracts. In adults, the normal resting pulse pressure is 30 to 50 mm Hg, so this client's pulse pressure is within normal limits. A pulse pressure less than 30 mm Hg (narrow pulse pressure) could indicate a low cardiac stroke volume, which occurs with congestive heart failure or stroke. An elevated pulse pressure (widening pulse pressure) could indicate atherosclerosis, heart block, or increased intracranial pressure.
TEST-TAKING TIP: This nursing calculation requires only subtraction, but you must memorize the formula to calculate the value correctly.
Content Area: Adult Health
Category of Health Alteration: Fluid Volume Excess
Integrated Processes: Nursing Process: Implementation
Client Need: Physiological Integrity
Cognitive Level: Application
Reference: *Ignatavicius, D., and Workman, M. (2012). Medical-Surgical Nursing: Patient-Centered Collaborative Care (7th ed.). St. Louis, MO: Saunders.*

69. ANSWER: 3.
Rationale:
1. ECG strip 1 shows sinus tachycardia, which is associated with hypomagnesemia.
2. ECG strip 2 is a normal sinus rhythm.
3. The nurse is most likely to observe sinus bradycardia, which is illustrated by ECG strip 3, because the client is exhibiting signs of hypermagnesemia.
4. ECG strip 4 illustrates the peaked T waves associated with hyperkalemia.
TEST-TAKING TIP: Select the answer that illustrates the effects of hypermagnesemia on the electrical conduction of the heart.
Content Area: Adult Health
Category of Health Alteration: Magnesium Imbalance
Integrated Processes: Nursing Process: Analysis
Client Need: Physiological Integrity
Cognitive Level: Analysis
References: *Jones, S. (2010). ECG Notes: Interpretation and Management Guide (2nd ed.). Philadelphia, PA: F. A. Davis; Williams, L., and Hopper, P. (2011). Understanding Medical-Surgical Nursing (4th ed.). Philadelphia, PA: F. A. Davis.*

70. ANSWER: 1.
Rationale:
1. The nurse should expect the arterial blood gas pH to be less than 7.35 because this client is experiencing diabetic ketoacidosis (DKA), a life-threatening complication caused by insulin deficiency. DKA may be precipitated by an acute illness or infection, or it may occur in a client who is noncompliant with insulin therapy.
2. The normal pH reference range is 7.35 to 7.45.
3. The normal pH reference range is 7.35 to 7.45.
4. A serum pH greater than 7.45 indicates a state of alkalosis.
TEST-TAKING TIP: Associate diabetes mellitus with an increased risk for metabolic acidosis; choose the pH value that reflects acidosis.
Content Area: Adult Health
Category of Health Alteration: Acid-Base Imbalance
Integrated Processes: Nursing Process: Analysis
Client Need: Physiological Integrity
Cognitive Level: Application
Reference: *Ignatavicius, D., and Workman, M. (2012). Medical-Surgical Nursing: Patient-Centered Collaborative Care (7th ed.). St. Louis, MO: Saunders.*

71. ANSWER: 1.
Rationale:
1. The nurse should associate a serum blood glucose level of 650 mg/dL with hyperglycemic hyperosmolar state (HHS). Although both diabetic ketoacidosis (DKA) and HHS are caused by hyperglycemia and dehydration, blood glucose levels in HHS may exceed 600 mg/dL, a much higher level than that seen in DKA.
2. A urinalysis positive for blood is usually not associated with either HHS or DKA.

3. A serum pH less than 7.35 is diagnostic for DKA, not HHS.
4. Urinalysis positive for ketones is diagnostic for DKA, not HHS.

TEST-TAKING TIP: The key words are "hyperglycemic hyperosmolar state (HHS)." Recall that HHS is characterized by extremely high blood glucose levels and the absence of ketone formation.

Content Area: *Adult Health*
Category of Health Alteration: *Fluid Volume Deficit*
Integrated Processes: *Nursing Process: Analysis*
Client Need: *Physiological Integrity*
Cognitive Level: *Application*
Reference: *Ignatavicius, D., and Workman, M. (2012). Medical-Surgical Nursing: Patient-Centered Collaborative Care (7th ed.). St. Louis, MO: Saunders.*

72. ANSWER: 1, 2, 3.

Rationale:

1. The nurse should advise the client diagnosed with SIADH to limit fluid intake. In SIADH, excessive amounts of water are reabsorbed by the kidneys, creating potentially disastrous dilutional hyponatremia. Water must be restricted to prevent water intoxication.
2. The nurse should advise the client diagnosed with SIADH to report muscle twitching to the health-care provider immediately because it could indicate hyponatremia, which can lead to seizures or coma.
3. The nurse should advise the client diagnosed with SIADH to measure intake and output. Intake and output should be monitored carefully to assess the amount of fluid restriction needed.
4. The nurse should teach the client to rinse the mouth frequently—not just once a day—to keep mucous membranes moist during fluid restriction.
5. Weight gain of 2 lb or more should be reported to the health-care provider because this is an indication of fluid retention and increases the client's risk for fluid volume excess.

TEST-TAKING TIP: Recall that SIADH causes water retention and dilutional hyponatremia. Select the instructions that address these manifestations.

Content Area: *Adult Health*
Category of Health Alteration: *Sodium Imbalance*
Integrated Processes: *Teaching/Learning*
Client Need: *Physiological Integrity*
Cognitive Level: *Application*
Reference: *Ignatavicius, D., and Workman, M. (2012). Medical-Surgical Nursing: Patient-Centered Collaborative Care (7th ed.). St. Louis, MO: Saunders.*

73. ANSWER: 1, 5.

Rationale:

1. To best determine the client's fluid status, the nurse should obtain the client's weight. This client has signs and symptoms of fluid volume deficit (FVD), and weight is the most accurate indicator of fluid status in children.
2. Although respiratory rate may be affected by FVD, it would not reveal the client's fluid status as precisely as weight and blood pressure.
3. Although heart rate may be affected by FVD, it would not reveal the client's fluid status as precisely as weight and blood pressure.
4. Pulse oximetry should not be affected by the client's fluid status.
5. To best determine the client's fluid status, the nurse should obtain the client's blood pressure. A decrease in blood pressure is an indicator of FVD related to a lack of circulating vascular volume.

TEST-TAKING TIP: The key words are "to best determine the child's current fluid status." Consider each option, and select the most sensitive indicators of fluid status.

Content Area: *Child Health*
Category of Health Alteration: *Fluid Volume Deficit*
Integrated Processes: *Nursing Process: Assessment*
Client Need: *Physiological Integrity*
Cognitive Level: *Application*
Reference: *Ward, S. L., and Hisley, S. M. (2011). Maternal-Child Nursing Care: Optimizing Outcomes for Mothers, Children and Families. Philadelphia, PA: F. A. Davis.*

74. ANSWER: 1, 4, 5.

Rationale:

1. The nurse should associate hyponatremia with SIADH. SIADH is a disorder of the posterior pituitary gland in which antidiuretic hormone (ADH) continues to be released even though plasma osmolarity is normal or near normal. The excess ADH, also called *vasopressin*, leads to water retention by interfering with the renal excretion of water, producing concentrated urine and hyponatremia. ADH decreases urine production by causing the renal tubules to reabsorb water from the urine and return it to the intravascular compartment.
2. SIADH may cause tachycardia, not bradycardia.
3. SIADH causes fluid retention, not polyuria.
4. The nurse should associate headache with SIADH. The drop in the serum sodium level may cause headaches and changes in level of consciousness.
5. The nurse should associate recent pneumonia with SIADH. Current or recent viral or bacterial pneumonia may cause SIADH to occur.

TEST-TAKING TIP: Recall that SIADH causes fluid retention, resulting in dilutional hyponatremia. Review the possible causes and signs and symptoms of SIADH if you had difficulty with this question.

Content Area: *Adult Health*
Category of Health Alteration: *Fluid Volume Excess*
Integrated Processes: *Nursing Process: Assessment*
Client Need: *Physiological Integrity*
Cognitive Level: *Application*
Reference: *Ignatavicius, D., and Workman, M. (2012). Medical-Surgical Nursing: Patient-Centered Collaborative Care (7th ed.). St. Louis, MO: Saunders.*

75. ANSWER: 1.

Rationale:

1. The nurse should associate hypoventilation (respiratory rate of 6 breaths per minute) with an increased risk for respiratory acidosis because hypoventilation leads to the retention of carbon dioxide, causing an increase in the production of free hydrogen ions.
2. The client's respiratory status would not produce metabolic acidosis.
3. An elevated (not reduced) respiratory rate would increase the client's risk for respiratory alkalosis.

4. The client's respiratory status would not produce metabolic alkalosis.

TEST-TAKING TIP: Recall that in adults, the normal respiratory rate is 12 to 20 breaths per minute. Associate hypoventilation with respiratory acidosis and hyperventilation with respiratory alkalosis.

Content Area: Older Adult Health
Category of Health Alteration: Acid-Base Imbalance
Integrated Processes: Nursing Process: Analysis
Client Need: Physiological Integrity
Cognitive Level: Application
***Reference:** Ignatavicius, D., and Workman, M. (2012). Medical-Surgical Nursing: Patient-Centered Collaborative Care (7th ed.). St. Louis, MO: Saunders.*

76. ANSWER: 4.

Rationale:

1. A serum chloride level of 85 mEq/L is below normal limits.
2. A serum chloride level of 95 mEq/L is within normal limits.
3. A serum chloride level of 105 mEq/L is within normal limits.
4. The nurse should expect a client with hypernatremia to exhibit hyperchloremia because imbalances in chloride usually occur as a result of other electrolyte imbalances, most frequently sodium. A serum chloride level of 115 mEq/L is higher than normal and should be interpreted as hyperchloremia.

TEST-TAKING TIP: Remember that chloride follows sodium. Review the normal ranges for both sodium and chloride.

Content Area: Adult Health
Category of Health Alteration: Chloride Imbalance
Integrated Processes: Nursing Process: Analysis
Client Need: Physiological Integrity
Cognitive Level: Application
***Reference:** Ignatavicius, D., and Workman, M. (2012). Medical-Surgical Nursing: Patient-Centered Collaborative Care (7th ed.). St. Louis, MO: Saunders.*

77. ANSWER: 3.

Rationale:

1. Toddlers 1 to 3 years old need approximately 700 mg/day.
2. School-aged children, from 4 to 8 years old, also require approximately 1,000 mg per day, not 800 mg.
3. According to the recommendations of the National Institutes of Health, the nurse should instruct women 19 to 50 years old to ingest 1,200 mg of calcium per day.
4. Women older than age 50 need 1,300 mg/day.

TEST-TAKING TIP: Refer to Table 5.5, Recommended Daily Intake of Calcium.

Content Area: Adult Health
Category of Health Alteration: Calcium Imbalance
Integrated Processes: Teaching/Learning
Client Need: Physiological Integrity
Cognitive Level: Knowledge
***Reference:** National Institutes of Health, Office of Dietary Supplements. (Reviewed 2012). Dietary supplement fact sheet: calcium. http://ods.od.nih.gov/factsheets/Calcium-HealthProfessional/.*

78. ANSWER: 4.

Rationale:

1. Calcium levels are not directly affected by uncompensated acidosis.
2. Sodium levels are not directly affected by uncompensated acidosis.
3. Magnesium levels are not directly affected by uncompensated acidosis.
4. Although the nurse should review all the laboratory values, the nurse should be most concerned with the client's serum potassium level. The serum potassium level is often high in the presence of acidosis, as the body attempts to maintain neutrality during buffering. In acidosis, hydrogen ions increase and move into the intracellular fluid (ICF). To keep the ICF neutral, an equal number of potassium ions moves out of the ICF and into the extracellular fluid, causing relative hyperkalemia.

TEST-TAKING TIP: The key words are "acute respiratory acidosis." The term "acute" indicates a recent or rapid onset, so compensation would not have occurred yet. Select the electrolyte that would most likely be affected by this condition.

Content Area: Adult Health
Category of Health Alteration: Potassium Imbalance
Integrated Processes: Nursing Process: Assessment
Client Need: Physiological Integrity
Cognitive Level: Application
***Reference:** Ignatavicius, D., and Workman, M. (2012). Medical-Surgical Nursing: Patient-Centered Collaborative Care (7th ed.). St. Louis, MO: Saunders.*

79. ANSWER: 2.

Rationale:

1. Oxygen therapy is ineffective if the client's airway is not patent.
2. The nurse's priority intervention should always be airway maintenance to improve gas exchange. The nurse should keep the client's head, neck, and chest in alignment and should assist the client in liquefying and clearing airway secretions.
3. Adequate gas exchange is the priority, not client education.
4. Adequate gas exchange is the priority, not client education.

TEST-TAKING TIP: Each of the interventions is appropriate for a client with chronic obstructive pulmonary disease, but maintaining a patent airway is the priority intervention.

Content Area: Adult Health
Category of Health Alteration: Acid-Base Imbalance
Integrated Processes: Nursing Process: Planning
Client Need: Physiological Integrity
Cognitive Level: Analysis
***Reference:** Ignatavicius, D., and Workman, M. (2012). Medical-Surgical Nursing: Patient-Centered Collaborative Care (7th ed.). St. Louis, MO: Saunders.*

80. ANSWER: 3.

Rationale:

1. The normal reference range for serum sodium is 135 to 145 mEq/L.
2. The normal reference range for serum sodium is 135 to 145 mEq/L.
3. The nurse should report Result C to the health-care provider because it reflects hyponatremia (serum sodium level less than 135 mEq/L).

4. Result D is within normal limits.

TEST-TAKING TIP: Memorize the normal reference range for serum sodium because this information is tested on the NCLEX examination.

Content Area: Adult Health
Category of Health Alteration: Sodium Imbalance
Integrated Processes: Nursing Process: Evaluation
Client Need: Physiological Integrity
Cognitive Level: Application
Reference: *Ignatavicius, D., and Workman, M. (2012). Medical-Surgical Nursing: Patient-Centered Collaborative Care (7th ed.). St. Louis, MO: Saunders.*

81. ANSWER: 2, 3, 6.

Rationale:
1. Hyperventilation results in respiratory alkalosis.
2. The nurse should anticipate a serum pH greater than 7.45 because the client is in a state of respiratory alkalosis secondary to hyperventilation.
3. The nurse should anticipate hypocalcemia (serum calcium level less than 8.2 mg/dL). In the presence of alkalosis, calcium ions shift into the cells in an attempt to buffer the high pH, decreasing the circulating serum calcium level (hypocalcemia).
4. The serum calcium level would be decreased, not increased.
5. The serum phosphorus level would be increased, not decreased.
6. The nurse should anticipate hyperphosphatemia (serum phosphorus level greater than 4.5 mg/dL). The client's serum phosphorus level would be above normal (hyperphosphatemia) because of phosphorus's inverse relationship with calcium.

TEST-TAKING TIP: The key word is "hyperventilating." Hyperventilation is the primary cause of respiratory alkalosis. Consider how a state of alkalosis would affect pH and calcium and phosphorus levels.

Content Area: Adult Health
Category of Health Alteration: Calcium Imbalance
Integrated Processes: Nursing Process: Analysis
Client Need: Physiological Integrity
Cognitive Level: Application
Reference: *Van Leeuwen, A. M., Poelhuis-Leth, D., and Bladh, M. (2011). Davis's Comprehensive Handbook of Laboratory and Diagnostic Tests With Nursing Implications (4th ed.). Philadelphia, PA: F. A. Davis.*

82. ANSWER: 1, 3, 4, 5.

Rationale:
1. The nurse should associate metabolic alkalosis with the development of hypochloremia. Chloride depletion produces metabolic alkalosis.
2. Hyperparathyroidism is associated with the development of *hyper*chloremia.
3. The nurse should associate diaphoresis (excessive sweating) with the development of hypochloremia. Diaphoresis results in excessive loss of sodium and chloride, increasing the client's risk for hyponatremia and hypochloremia.
4. The nurse should associate the excessive use of laxatives with the development of hypochloremia. Excessive laxative use results in excessive loss of sodium and chloride, increasing the client's risk for hyponatremia and hypochloremia.
5. The nurse should associate the syndrome of inappropriate antidiuretic hormone secretion (SIADH) with the development of hypochloremia. SIADH causes hypochloremia because retained fluid dilutes sodium and chloride levels.

TEST-TAKING TIP: Remember that chloride follows sodium. Select options associated with decreased sodium levels.

Content Area: Adult Health
Category of Health Alteration: Chloride Imbalance
Integrated Processes: Nursing Process: Analysis
Client Need: Physiological Integrity
Cognitive Level: Application
Reference: *Ignatavicius, D., and Workman, M. (2012). Medical-Surgical Nursing: Patient-Centered Collaborative Care (7th ed.). St. Louis, MO: Saunders.*

83. ANSWER: 4.

Rationale:
1. These ABG values are not associated with partially compensated metabolic acidosis.
2. These ABG values are not associated with fully compensated respiratory acidosis.
3. These ABG values are not associated with partially compensated metabolic alkalosis.
4. The nurse should associate fully compensated respiratory alkalosis with these ABG values. The pH of 7.42 is within the normal reference range of 7.35 to 7.45, indicating full compensation. However, the pH is still on the upper (more alkalotic) end of the normal reference range, and both carbon dioxide ($PaCO_2$) and bicarbonate (HCO_3^-) levels are decreased. A decreased carbon dioxide level would cause the blood to become alkalotic (pH greater than 7.45), but the decreased bicarbonate level is pulling the pH down within the normal range, indicating that the kidneys are excreting bicarbonate to compensate for an imbalance that is respiratory in origin.

TEST-TAKING TIP: First, look at the direction of the pH. Next, think about the other ABG values to determine the origin of the imbalance.

Content Area: Adult Health
Category of Health Alteration: Acid-Base Imbalance
Integrated Processes: Nursing Process: Analysis
Client Need: Physiological Integrity
Cognitive Level: Analysis
Reference: *Berman, A., Snyder, S., Kozier, B., and Erb, G. (2012). Kozier & Erb's Fundamentals of Nursing: Concepts, Process, and Practice (9th ed.). Upper Saddle River, NJ: Pearson.*

84. ANSWER: 2.

Rationale:
1. Fall precautions should be implemented because hypokalemia causes muscle weakness, increasing the client's risk of falls.
2. The nurse should question the order to administer hydrochlorothiazide, which would further deplete the already low serum potassium level. Use of any non–potassium-sparing diuretic would be contraindicated for this client.
3. Intravenous potassium replacement is required to correct severe hypokalemia.
4. Cardiac monitoring is important with potassium imbalances because of the potential for dysrhythmias resulting from hypokalemia and during replacement therapy.

TEST-TAKING TIP: Recall the signs, symptoms, and treatment of hypokalemia. Select the option that would not correct hypokalemia or the problems associated with it.
Content Area: Adult Health
Category of Health Alteration: Potassium Imbalance
Integrated Processes: Nursing Process: Analysis
Client Need: Physiological Integrity
Cognitive Level: Application
Reference: *Ignatavicius, D., and Workman, M. (2012). Medical-Surgical Nursing: Patient-Centered Collaborative Care (7th ed.). St. Louis, MO: Saunders.*

85. ANSWER: 3.
Rationale:
1. Pasta salad with mixed vegetables would be appropriate for a low-sodium diet.
2. Baked chicken and broccoli would be appropriate for a low-sodium diet.
3. The nurse should recommend that the client avoid the bologna and cheese sandwich as part of a low-sodium diet. Sandwich meat and processed cheese are high in sodium.
4. Dry cereal with skim milk and banana would be appropriate for a low-sodium diet.
TEST-TAKING TIP: The key words are "low-sodium." Select the option that contains the *most* sodium.
Content Area: Adult Health
Category of Health Alteration: Sodium Imbalance
Integrated Processes: Teaching/Learning
Client Need: Physiological Integrity
Cognitive Level: Application
Reference: *U.S. Department of Agriculture, Agricultural Research Service. (2009). USDA National Nutrient Database for Standard Reference. Release 22. Nutrient Data Laboratory Home Page. http://www.ars.usda.gov/ba/bhnrc/ndl.*

86. ANSWER: 4.
Rationale:
1. Hyperventilation results in respiratory alkalosis, not metabolic acidosis.
2. Hyperventilation results in respiratory alkalosis, not metabolic alkalosis.
3. Hyperventilation results in respiratory alkalosis, not respiratory acidosis.
4. The nurse should associate respiratory alkalosis with these signs and symptoms. Hyperventilation (respiratory rate of 30 breaths per minute) is the cause of the imbalance.
TEST-TAKING TIP: Recall that hyperventilation (mechanical or spontaneous) is the *only* cause of respiratory alkalosis.
Content Area: Maternal Health
Category of Health Alteration: Acid-Base Imbalance
Integrated Processes: Nursing Process: Evaluation
Client Need: Physiological Integrity
Cognitive Level: Application
Reference: *Perry, S., Hockenberry, M., Lowdermilk, D., and Wilson, D. (2010). Maternal Child Nursing Care (4th ed.). St. Louis, MO: Mosby.*

87. ANSWER: 1, 2, 3.
Rationale:
1. The nurse should include an assessment for Chvostek's sign. Because of a deficiency in the enzyme lactase, 75% to 90% of all Asians, African Americans, and American Indians have lactose intolerance, preventing them from consuming calcium-rich dairy products and placing them at risk for hypocalcemia. A positive Chvostek's sign is indicative of hypocalcemia.
2. The nurse should ask the client about changes in height because the client is exhibiting signs of hypocalcemia.
3. The nurse should assess for Trousseau's sign. A positive Trousseau's sign is indicative of hypocalcemia.
4. Measuring the circumference of the client's calf is an assessment for *hypercalcemia.*
5. Auscultating for hypoactive bowel sounds is an assessment for *hypercalcemia.*
TEST-TAKING TIP: The key words are "lactose intolerance" and "charley horses." These factors are related to calcium deficiency. Select the options that are appropriate when assessing for hypocalcemia.
Content Area: Adult Health
Category of Health Alteration: Calcium Imbalance
Integrated Processes: Nursing Process: Assessment
Client Need: Physiological Integrity
Cognitive Level: Application
Reference: *Ignatavicius, D., and Workman, M. (2012). Medical-Surgical Nursing: Patient-Centered Collaborative Care (7th ed.). St. Louis, MO: Saunders.*

88. ANSWER: 1, 4.
Rationale:
1. The nurse should recognize that hypertonic IV solutions, such as 3% saline solution, would be contraindicated because this client is dehydrated and hypernatremic.
2. Isotonic solutions, such as 0.45% saline solution, are more appropriate for a dehydrated client with hypernatremia because they increase circulating blood volume without causing a fluid shift.
3. Isotonic solutions, such as 0.9% saline solution (normal saline), are more appropriate for a dehydrated client with hypernatremia because they increase circulating blood volume without causing a fluid shift.
4. The nurse should recognize that hypertonic IV solutions, such as dextrose 2.5% in water, would be contraindicated because this client is dehydrated and hypernatremic.
TEST-TAKING TIP: The key word is "contraindicated." Understand what happens in the body when each type of IV solution is administered. Rule out hypertonic solutions because they would worsen the client's dehydration and hypernatremia.
Content Area: Adult Health
Category of Health Alteration: Fluid Volume Deficit
Integrated Processes: Nursing Process: Implementation
Client Need: Physiological Integrity
Cognitive Level: Application
Reference: *Ignatavicius, D., and Workman, M. (2012). Medical-Surgical Nursing: Patient-Centered Collaborative Care (7th ed.). St. Louis, MO: Saunders.*

89. ANSWER: 2, 4, 5.
Rationale:
1. Diabetes insipidus would result in polyuria and dehydration.
2. The nurse should identify end-stage renal disease as placing this client at risk for the development of FVE, which occurs when fluid intake or retention is greater than the body's fluid needs.

3. Although type 2 diabetes increases the client's risk for renal failure, early-phase renal failure would result in dehydration, not FVE.
4. The nurse should identify long-term corticosteroid therapy as placing this client at risk for the development of FVE. The conditions most commonly associated with FVE are those related to excessive intake or inadequate excretion of fluid.
5. The nurse should identify syndrome of inappropriate antidiuretic hormone secretion (SIADH) as placing this client at risk for the development of FVE. Causes of FVE include excessive fluid replacement, renal failure, heart failure, long-term corticosteroid therapy, SIADH, psychiatric disorders with polydipsia, and water intoxication.
TEST-TAKING TIP: Select the conditions that would cause the client to retain fluid or prevent the elimination of excess fluid.
Content Area: Adult Health
Category of Health Alteration: Fluid Volume Excess
Integrated Processes: Nursing Process: Assessment
Client Need: Physiological Integrity
Cognitive Level: Application
Reference: Ignatavicius, D., and Workman, M. (2012). Medical-Surgical Nursing: Patient-Centered Collaborative Care (7th ed.). St. Louis, MO: Saunders.

90. ANSWER: 1.
Rationale:
1. The nurse should determine that a normal or near-normal serum pH indicates that the client is responding to the treatment plan because the desired outcome for the treatment of diabetic ketoacidosis is resolution of acidosis. The serum pH is the primary determinant of the success of the treatment plan.
2. $PaCO_2$ 36 mm Hg is within the normal reference range and is not the value that determines whether the client is responding to the treatment plan.
3. PaO_2 96 mm Hg is within normal reference range and is not the value that determines whether the client is responding to the treatment plan.
4. HCO_3^- 20 mEq is within the normal reference range and is not the value that determines whether the client is responding to the treatment plan.
TEST-TAKING TIP: Recognize that pH is the primary indicator of acid-base imbalance.
Content Area: Adult Health
Category of Health Alteration: Acid-Base Imbalance
Integrated Processes: Nursing Process: Evaluation
Client Need: Physiological Integrity
Cognitive Level: Application
Reference: Wilkinson, J., and Treas, L. (2011). Fundamentals of Nursing: Theory, Concepts & Applications (2nd ed.). Philadelphia, PA: F. A. Davis.

91. ANSWER: 3.
Rationale:
1. Soft drinks can be irritating and are often not well tolerated.
2. Milk products leave a residue and should be avoided.
3. The nurse should recommend cold or frozen fluids, such as popsicles, in the immediate postoperative period because they provide comfort as well as fluid intake.
4. Beef broth and other brown- or red-colored fluids should be avoided to allow recognition of the presence of fresh or old blood.
TEST-TAKING TIP: Select the noncarbonated fluid that would provide comfort, hydrate the client, and not mask bleeding.
Content Area: Child Health
Category of Health Alteration: Fluid Volume Deficit
Integrated Processes: Nursing Process: Implementation
Client Need: Physiological Integrity
Cognitive Level: Application
Reference: Ward, S. L., and Hisley, S. M. (2011). Maternal-Child Nursing Care: Optimizing Outcomes for Mothers, Children and Families. Philadelphia, PA: F. A. Davis.

92. ANSWER: 3.
Rationale:
1. Daily weighing is recommended because weight is one of the most important indicators of fluid balance.
2. Cautious administration of oral fluids is advised, while adhering to any prescribed fluid restrictions.
3. The nurse should question the order to administer isotonic IV fluids because the administration of such fluids would increase the client's vascular volume, worsening the fluid volume excess (FVE).
4. Auscultating the lungs to detect the presence or worsening of crackles and wheezes should be performed on an ongoing basis.
TEST-TAKING TIP: Recall that the administration of oral or IV fluids increases FVE. Read the question carefully, and recognize that the correct answer is the incorrect order for this client.
Content Area: Adult Health
Category of Health Alteration: Fluid Volume Excess
Integrated Processes: Nursing Process: Analysis
Client Need: Physiological Integrity
Cognitive Level: Analysis
Reference: Lemone, P., and Burke, K. (2010). Medical-Surgical Nursing: Critical Thinking in Client Care (5th ed.). Upper Saddle River, NJ: Pearson Prentice Hall.

93. ANSWER: 4.
Rationale:
1. The client's pH should be in the low-normal to normal range in this situation.
2. The client's $PaCO_2$ value should be elevated.
3. The client's PaO_2 should not be affected.
4. The nurse should associate an elevated bicarbonate (HCO_3^-) level with long-term carbon dioxide retention because the kidneys compensate for the chronically elevated carbon dioxide levels to correct the respiratory acidosis.
TEST-TAKING TIP: Visualize the process of long-term carbon dioxide retention and what happens during compensation.
Content Area: Adult Health
Category of Health Alteration: Acid-Base Imbalance
Integrated Processes: Nursing Process: Planning
Client Need: Physiological Integrity
Cognitive Level: Analysis
Reference: Wilkinson, J., and Treas, L. (2011). Fundamentals of Nursing: Theory, Concepts & Applications (2nd ed.).Philadelphia, PA: F. A. Davis.

94. ANSWER: 2, 3, 5, 6.
Rationale:
1. Oral (PO) administration is appropriate for calcium gluconate. Calcium is usually administered orally to prevent the development of hypocalcemia and osteoporosis or to treat mild hypocalcemia.
2. The nurse should identify the subcutaneous route as contraindicated when administering calcium gluconate because this medication is highly irritating and may cause cellulitis, necrosis, and tissue sloughing.
3. The nurse should identify the intramuscular (IM) route as contraindicated when administering calcium gluconate because this medication is highly irritating and may cause cellulitis, necrosis, and tissue sloughing.
4. IV administration is appropriate for calcium gluconate. The IV route is used to treat acute hypocalcemia.
5. The nurse should identify the intradermal route as contraindicated when administering calcium gluconate because this medication is highly irritating and may cause cellulitis, necrosis, and tissue sloughing.
6. The nurse should identify the rectal route as contraindicated when administering calcium gluconate because this medication is highly irritating and may cause cellulitis, necrosis, and tissue sloughing.
TEST-TAKING TIP: Recall that calcium gluconate should be administered orally or by the IV route, using great care to prevent extravasation.
Content Area: Older Adult Health
Category of Health Alteration: Calcium Imbalance
Integrated Processes: Nursing Process: Planning
Client Need: Physiological Integrity
Cognitive Level: Application
Reference: *Deglin, J. H., Vallerand, A. H., and Sanoski, C. A. (2013). Davis's Drug Guide for Nurses (13th ed.). Philadelphia, PA: F. A. Davis.*

95. ANSWER: 1, 2, 4.
Rationale:
1. The nurse should associate decreased blood urea nitrogen (BUN) with the development of FVE, which involves the excessive retention of sodium and water in the extracellular fluid. The increase in fluid volume results in hemodilution and causes the BUN, hematocrit, and urine specific gravity to decrease.
2. The nurse should associate decreased hematocrit with the development of FVE, which involves the excessive retention of sodium and water in the extracellular fluid.
3. The hemoglobin (the oxygen-carrying protein on red blood cells) level is not affected.
4. The nurse should associate decreased urine specific gravity with the development of FVE, which involves the excessive retention of sodium and water in the extracellular fluid.
5. Urine osmolality is a measure of urine concentration. Excess fluid would cause a decrease in urine concentration.
TEST-TAKING TIP: Recall that water retention causes hemodilution. Think about which laboratory values would decrease as vascular volume increased.
Content Area: Adult Health
Category of Health Alteration: Fluid Volume Excess
Integrated Processes: Nursing Process: Implementation
Client Need: Physiological Integrity
Cognitive Level: Application
Reference: *Wilkinson, J., and Treas, L. (2011). Fundamentals of Nursing: Theory, Concepts & Applications (2nd ed.). Philadelphia, PA: F. A. Davis.*

96. ANSWER: 4.
Rationale:
1. The normal serum pH reference range is 7.35 to 7.45.
2. The normal serum pH reference range is 7.35 to 7.45.
3. The normal serum pH reference range is 7.35 to 7.45.
4. The nurse is most likely to find that this client has a blood pH value greater than 7.50 because the client is experiencing respiratory alkalosis secondary to hyperventilation.
TEST-TAKING TIP: The client's respiratory rate is 32 breaths per minute, indicating hyperventilation. Recall that hyperventilation causes the blood pH to increase, resulting in respiratory alkalosis.
Content Area: Adult Health
Category of Health Alteration: Acid-Base Imbalance
Integrated Processes: Nursing Process: Analysis
Client Need: Physiological Integrity
Cognitive Level: Application
Reference: *Ignatavicius, D., and Workman, M. (2012). Medical-Surgical Nursing: Patient-Centered Collaborative Care (7th ed.). St. Louis, MO: Saunders.*

97. ANSWER: 1.
Rationale:
1. These clients would be at highest risk for isotonic dehydration because they lose water and sodium in equal amounts through perspiration and other insensible routes. Isotonic dehydration occurs when sodium and water deficits are present in balanced proportions. This is the most common type of dehydration, which, if untreated, may lead to hypovolemic shock.
2. In hypotonic dehydration, electrolyte loss exceeds water loss.
3. In hypertonic dehydration, the most dangerous type of dehydration, water loss exceeds electrolyte loss.
4. Normotonic is not a classification for dehydration.
TEST-TAKING TIP: The key words are "football team." These athletes experience both fluid and electrolyte losses.
Content Area: Child Health
Category of Health Alteration: Fluid Volume Deficit
Integrated Processes: Nursing Process: Implementation
Client Need: Physiological Integrity
Cognitive Level: Comprehension
Reference: *Ward, S. L., and Hisley, S. M. (2011). Maternal-Child Nursing Care: Optimizing Outcomes for Mothers, Children and Families. Philadelphia, PA: F. A. Davis.*

98. ANSWER: 3.
Rationale:
1. Furosemide (Lasix) is a thiazide diuretic that would increase the excretion of calcium by the kidneys.
2. Calcitonin (Calcimar) inhibits calcium resorption from bone.
3. The nurse should question the health-care provider's order for lactated Ringer's solution. This IV solution contains calcium, which would worsen the client's hypercalcemia.
4. Prednisolone is a corticosteroid that counteracts the effect of vitamin D to prevent calcium absorption.

TEST-TAKING TIP: Recall that lactated Ringer's solution contains sodium, chloride, lactate, potassium, and *calcium*.
Content Area: Adult Health
Category of Health Alteration: Calcium Imbalance
Integrated Processes: Nursing Process: Analysis
Client Need: Physiological Integrity
Cognitive Level: Analysis
Reference: Ignatavicius, D., and Workman, M. (2012). Medical-Surgical Nursing: Patient-Centered Collaborative Care (7th ed.). St. Louis, MO: Saunders.

99. ANSWER: 1.
Rationale:
1. When interpreting a client's arterial blood gas (ABG) values, it is most important for the nurse to consider the client's blood pH first. If the client's blood pH is less than 7.35 or greater than 7.45, the nurse should interpret that the client has an acid-base imbalance of some type.
2. PaO_2 is not useful in determining the etiology of acid-base imbalances.
3. Reviewing the client's $PaCO_2$ level may aid in determining the origin of the imbalance, but it should not be considered first.
4. Reviewing the client's HCO_3^- level may aid in determining the origin of the imbalance, but it should not be considered first.
TEST-TAKING TIP: The key word is "first." The nurse should always assess the client's blood pH before looking at any other ABG values.
Content Area: Adult Health
Category of Health Alteration: Acid-Base Imbalance
Integrated Processes: Nursing Process: Planning
Client Need: Physiological Integrity
Cognitive Level: Comprehension
Reference: Berman, A., Snyder, S., Kozier, B., and Erb, G. (2012). Kozier & Erb's Fundamentals of Nursing: Concepts, Process, and Practice (9th ed.). Upper Saddle River, NJ: Pearson.

100. ANSWER: 3.
Rationale:
1. Weight gain is the most reliable indicator of FVE.
2. Mild FVE is characterized by a 2% increase in total body weight.
3. The nurse should classify a sudden 5% increase in total body weight as moderate FVE.
4. Severe FVE is characterized by an 8% increase in total body weight.
TEST-TAKING TIP: Calculate that a 5% increase in total body weight in a 100-lb client would be about 5 lb, suggesting moderate FVE.
Content Area: Adult Health
Category of Health Alteration: Fluid Volume Excess
Integrated Processes: Nursing Process: Analysis
Client Need: Physiological Integrity
Cognitive Level: Application
Reference: Berman, A., Snyder, S., Kozier, B., and Erb, G. (2012). Kozier & Erb's Fundamentals of Nursing: Concepts, Process, and Practice (9th ed.). Upper Saddle River, NJ: Pearson.

Chapter 10

Comprehensive Test II

REVIEW QUESTIONS

1. A registered nurse (RN) is planning care for several clients. Which client would be most appropriate for the RN to delegate to a licensed practical nurse?
   1. An older adult postoperative client who has uncontrolled pain
   2. A child who has a temperature of 103.5°F (39.7°C)
   3. A client who is receiving IV fluids for dehydration
   4. A client who is receiving an IV insulin drip for diabetic ketoacidosis

2. Which laboratory result should a nurse anticipate when assessing a child who has persistent projectile vomiting secondary to gastroenteritis?
   1. Serum chloride 85 mEq/L
   2. Serum chloride 95 mEq/L
   3. Serum chloride 105 mEq/L
   4. Serum chloride 110 mEq/L

3. A nurse admits an older adult client with a history of chronic bronchitis and emphysema who is currently experiencing confusion, severe headache, and lethargy. The client's skin is flushed, with a slight bluish tinge to the mucous membranes; respirations are rapid and shallow; blood pressure is 80/40 mm Hg; and heart rate is 138 bpm. Which acid-base imbalance should the nurse identify in this client?
   1. Respiratory acidosis
   2. Metabolic acidosis
   3. Respiratory alkalosis
   4. Metabolic alkalosis

4. Which manifestation should a nurse associate with a serum calcium level of 11.2 mg/dL if it is noted during the assessment of a client diagnosed with hyperparathyroidism?
   1. Paresthesias
   2. Painful muscle cramps
   3. Positive Chvostek's sign
   4. Decreased deep tendon reflexes

5. Which nursing diagnoses should a nurse assign to an adult client diagnosed with respiratory alkalosis related to hyperventilation secondary to excessive mechanical ventilation effects? **Select all that apply.**
   1. Risk for Injury Related to Confusion
   2. Risk for Falls Related to Skeletal Muscle Weakness
   3. Impaired Gas Exchange Related to Mechanical Ventilation
   4. Decreased Cardiac Output Related to Increased Respiratory Rate
   5. Ineffective Breathing Pattern Related to Inability to Sustain Spontaneous Ventilation

6. Which findings should a nurse associate with a nursing diagnosis of Deficient Fluid Volume Secondary to Dehydration, if noted when assessing an adult client? **Select all that apply.**
   1. Thready pulse
   2. Increased pulse rate
   3. Jugular venous distention
   4. Decreased blood pressure
   5. Decreased hemoglobin level and hematocrit

7. A nurse is preparing to administer a loading dose of aminophylline 6 mg/kg (as ordered) to a client who has been diagnosed with respiratory acidosis related to an acute exacerbation of emphysema. The client weighs 240 lb. The dose on hand is 25 mg/mL. How many milliliters should the nurse administer? Record your answer using one decimal place.

   ____

8. A nurse is recording intake and output of an adult client. The client reports consuming a 240-mL cup of coffee, a 350-mL canned soft drink, and two 8-oz cartons of milk; the client has received 100 mL/hr of IV fluids for a total of 8 hours and has voided 1,200 mL of urine. Determine the client's intake in milliliters. Record your answer as a whole number.

   ____

9. A nurse assesses the edematous extremities of a 6-month-old client. Based on the exhibit provided, which grade of edema should the nurse document?

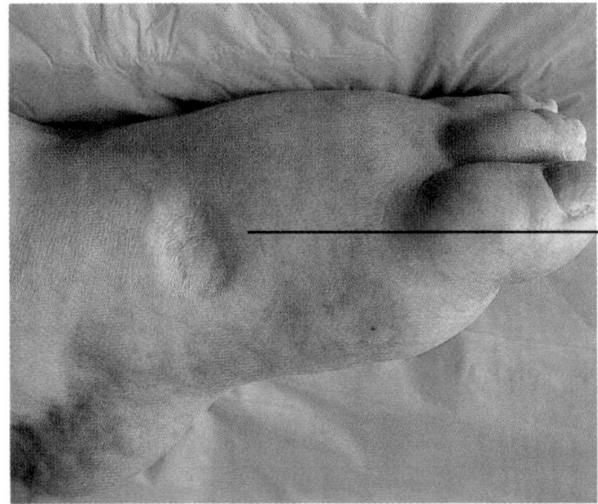

1. Grade 1+
2. Grade 2+
3. Grade 3+
4. Grade 4+

10. A nurse is managing the care of a client who was just admitted with a diagnosis of diabetic ketoacidosis. Which health-care provider order should the nurse question?
    1. Monitor blood sugar every hour.
    2. Assess vital signs every 15 minutes until stable.
    3. Administer regular insulin subcutaneously per sliding scale.
    4. Administer 0.9% saline solution IV at 1,000 mL/hr × 2 L.

11. In error, a nurse administers 3% saline solution intravenously to a preoperative client with a normal fluid and electrolyte balance. Which physiological reaction should the nurse anticipate as a result of this error?
    1. The client would experience only an increase in plasma volume.
    2. The client would experience only an increase in interstitial volume.
    3. The client would experience an increase in plasma volume and a decrease in interstitial volume.
    4. The client would experience an increase in plasma volume and an increase in interstitial volume.

12. A nurse is preparing discharge teaching for a client recently diagnosed with end-stage renal disease and started on hemodialysis. Which food should the nurse teach the client to avoid to decrease the client's daily intake of phosphorus and potassium?
    1. Milk
    2. Broth
    3. Pretzels
    4. Fresh fruits

13. A nurse is caring for a critically ill client who begins exhibiting deep, rapid respirations and has developed a fruity breath odor. Which acid-base imbalance should the nurse associate with these manifestations?
    1. Metabolic acidosis
    2. Metabolic alkalosis
    3. Respiratory acidosis
    4. Respiratory alkalosis

14. A nurse assesses a 6-year-old postoperative client who has returned to the pediatric unit after undergoing a tonsillectomy and adenoidectomy 2 hours ago. The client is lethargic, irritable, and confused and is vomiting small amounts of clear, blood-tinged fluid. Based on the assessment findings in the following chart, which intervention should the nurse identify as most appropriate for this client?

Temperature: 99°F (37.2°C) axillary	Serum Na^+: 125 mEq/L
Blood pressure: 90/48 mm Hg	Serum Cl^-: 90 mEq/L
Heart rate: 114 bpm, regular	Serum K^+: 3.7 mEq/L
Respiratory rate: 12 breaths/min	Blood glucose: 76 mg/dL
Oxygen saturation: 98%	Serum creatinine: 0.6 mg/dL

    1. Provide water and ice chips by mouth.
    2. Perform neurological checks daily.
    3. Administer 0.9% saline solution at 250 mL/hr IV.
    4. Administer ondansetron (Zofran) 0.15 mg/kg IV every 6 hours as needed for nausea.

15. Which laboratory values should a nurse expect when evaluating the arterial blood gas (ABG) values of a client diagnosed with partially compensated respiratory alkalosis? **Select all that apply.**
    1. Decrease in $PaCO_2$
    2. Increase in $PaCO_2$
    3. Decrease in HCO_3^-
    4. Increase in HCO_3^-
    5. pH increasing toward 7.35
    6. pH decreasing toward 7.45

16. For which potential complications should a nurse monitor in an older adult client receiving an IV isotonic saline solution for the treatment of dehydration? **Select all that apply.**
    1. Lung crackles
    2. Decreased pulse rate
    3. Weight gain
    4. Dependent edema
    5. Bounding pulse quality

17. A nurse analyzes the laboratory data of a client admitted to the emergency department after choking on a piece of steak. Which laboratory results should the nurse expect to be abnormal? **Select all that apply.**
 1. pH
 2. HCO_3^- level
 3. PaO_2 level
 4. $PaCO_2$ level
 5. Sodium level

18. A nurse assesses a 6-day-old infant who has just been diagnosed with formula intolerance. Worrying that her baby is not getting enough to drink, the mother has been giving the infant water from a bottle. Other than an increased intake of water, which factor should the nurse identify as predisposing this infant to fluid imbalances?
 1. Decreased cardiac output
 2. Decreased kidney function
 3. Decreased body surface area
 4. Decreased extracellular fluid

19. A nurse analyzes a client's arterial blood gas (ABG) values. The client's serum pH is 7.55, $PaCO_2$ is 33 mm Hg, and HCO_3^- is 27 mEq/L. Which acid-base imbalance should the nurse associate with these ABG values?
 1. Uncompensated metabolic alkalosis
 2. Compensated metabolic alkalosis
 3. Uncompensated respiratory alkalosis
 4. Compensated respiratory alkalosis

20. A nursing instructor prepares a student to administer potassium chloride intravenously. Which statement by the student indicates the need for additional instruction?
 1. "I am going to use an infusion pump to administer this medication."
 2. "I plan to monitor the client's urine output during and after the administration of this medication."
 3. "I have drawn up this medication for IV push administration."
 4. "I plan to monitor the client's electrocardiogram during the administration of this medication."

21. A nurse admits a client diagnosed with fluid volume deficit secondary to diabetic ketoacidosis. Which IV solution should the nurse identify as *initially* appropriate for this client?
 1. 0.45% saline solution
 2. Dextrose 5% in 0.9% saline solution
 3. Lactated Ringer's solution
 4. 3% sodium chloride solution

22. A nurse is preparing to administer a 14 mEq IV bolus of calcium gluconate 10% to a postpartum client diagnosed with magnesium toxicity. Calcium gluconate 10% contains 0.45 mEq/mL. How many milliliters should the nurse administer to this client? Record your answer using one decimal place.

____

23. A hospitalized infant who weighs 16 lb has voided 240 mL at the end of a 12-hour shift. How many mL/kg/hr of urine has this infant voided? Record your answer using one decimal point.

____

24. A nurse is preparing to administer an insulin drip to a client diagnosed with diabetic ketoacidosis. A health-care provider orders an initial infusion of 23 units/hr of regular insulin IV. The pharmacy supplies 100 units of regular insulin in 500 mL of 0.9% (normal) saline solution. How many milliliters of solution should the nurse infuse hourly? Record your answer as a whole number.

____

25. A nurse performing an assessment suspects that a client has fluid volume excess related to right-sided heart failure. Which finding, if identified in this client, should the nurse associate with the development of right-sided heart failure? **Select all that apply.**
 1. Peripheral edema
 2. Bilateral crackles in lung fields
 3. Hypotension
 4. S_4 heart sound
 5. Jugular venous distention

26. When caring for a client with an acid-base imbalance, which serum electrolytes are essential for a nurse to monitor? **Select all that apply.**
 1. Calcium (Ca^{2+})
 2. Sodium (Na^+)
 3. Potassium (K^+)
 4. Phosphate (PO_4^-)
 5. Magnesium (Mg^{2+})

27. A nurse is teaching the parents of a toddler diagnosed with hyponatremia secondary to syndrome of inappropriate antidiuretic hormone secretion (SIADH). Which instructions should the nurse include in the teaching? **Select all that apply.**
 1. Weigh the child daily.
 2. Provide frequent mouth care.
 3. Give the child water to drink.
 4. Feed the child a high-sodium diet.
 5. Measure the urine output accurately.
 6. Allow the child to suck on hard candy if thirsty.

28. Which clinical manifestations should a nurse associate with chronic hypophosphatemia if assessed in a newly admitted client? **Select all that apply.**
   1. Lethargy
   2. Muscle and joint aches
   3. Weak peripheral pulses
   4. Positive Chvostek's sign
   5. Hypoactive bowel sounds

29. Which actions should a nurse take to assess a child for Chvostek's sign? Place each nursing action in the correct sequence (1 to 5).
   ________ Report and document the findings.
   ________ Monitor twitching of the mouth, nose, or cheek.
   ________ Tap the client's face just below the zygomatic arch.
   ________ Explain the procedure to the client's parents.
   ________ Observe for the appearance of facial twitching on the ipsilateral side.

30. A school nurse is teaching 12-year-old middle school students about the importance of including calcium-rich foods in the diet. According to the National Institutes of Health, how many milligrams of calcium should the nurse advise the students to consume daily?
   1. 700 mg
   2. 1,000 mg
   3. 1,100 mg
   4. 1,300 mg

31. A nurse analyzes a client's arterial blood gas (ABG) values. The client's serum pH is 7.48, $PaCO_2$ is 44 mm Hg, and HCO_3^- is 30 mEq/L. Which acid-base imbalance should the nurse associate with these ABG values?
   1. Uncompensated metabolic alkalosis
   2. Compensated metabolic alkalosis
   3. Uncompensated respiratory alkalosis
   4. Compensated respiratory alkalosis

32. A nurse is evaluating education for a client with fluid volume excess. Which statement by the client should indicate to the nurse that the client understands the education?
   1. "I do not need to worry about my diet because I am taking a fluid pill."
   2. "I plan to avoid luncheon meats and canned vegetables."
   3. "I will notify my health-care provider if I lose weight."
   4. "I should restrict the amount of fresh vegetables in my diet."

33. Which laboratory value should a nurse anticipate when caring for a client diagnosed with hypophosphatemia?
   1. Serum calcium level 9.5 mg/dL
   2. Serum calcium level 12 mg/dL
   3. Serum phosphorus level 3.5 mg/dL
   4. Serum phosphorus level 4.7 mg/dL

34. A nurse is preparing to administer a sodium bicarbonate infusion to a client diagnosed with moderate metabolic acidosis. A health-care provider orders 3 mEq/kg of sodium bicarbonate 5% solution to be infused intravenously over 8 hours. The dose on hand is 0.6 mEq/mL in 500 mL of 0.9% (normal) saline solution. The client weighs 145 lb. How many milliliters of sodium bicarbonate 5% solution should the nurse administer? Record your answer as a whole number.

   ____

35. A nurse is preparing to administer 20 mEq of potassium chloride intravenously, diluted in 500 mL of normal (0.9%) saline solution. The nurse plans to infuse the solution via peripheral IV access, using tubing with a drop factor of 30 gtt/mL, over 2 hours. How many mL/hr should the nurse program the IV pump to deliver? Record your answer as a whole number.

   ____

36. A neonate who weighs 7.5 lb is to receive a transfusion of 10 mL/kg packed red blood cells (PRBCs) to replace a fluid volume deficit resulting from a torn umbilical cord at delivery. How many milliliters of PRBCs should a nurse administer to this client? Record your answer as a whole number.

   ____

37. A nurse on a neurosurgical care unit notes that a client recovering from laminectomy surgery is lethargic and difficult to arouse. The client's respiratory rate is 12 breaths per minute, with a shallow pattern. The client has been receiving controlled-release oxycodone hydrochloride (OxyContin) 15 mg orally twice daily and IV morphine sulfate via patient-controlled analgesia as needed for pain. Which arterial blood gas values should the nurse associate with this client's manifestations?

Lab Report A		Lab Report B		Lab Report C		Lab Report D	
pH	7.21	pH	7.31	pH	7.43	pH	7.50
$PaCO_2$	66 mm Hg	$PaCO_2$	42 mm Hg	$PaCO_2$	40 mm Hg	$PaCO_2$	29 mm Hg
HCO_3^-	22 mEq/L	HCO_3^-	15 mEq/L	HCO_3^-	24 mEq/L	HCO_3^-	23 mEq/L

1. Lab Report A
2. Lab Report B
3. Lab Report C
4. Lab Report D

38. Which assessment should be performed by a nurse to identify whether a client is developing a potentially dangerous side effect of the medication magnesium oxide (Mag-Ox 400)?
1. Assess for constipation.
2. Assess for tachycardia.
3. Assess for hypertension.
4. Assess for deep tendon hyporeflexia.

39. A nurse is providing IV fluids to a dehydrated infant who weighs 4 kg. The nurse calculates that the infant has voided 170 mL of urine over a 24-hour period. How should the nurse interpret this measurement?
1. Urine output is low, and the infant is still dehydrated.
2. Urine output is within normal limits.
3. Urine output is high, and the infant is at risk for fluid overload.
4. It is the responsibility of the health-care provider to interpret intake and output values.

40. A nurse is caring for an older adult client who has been transferred from a long-term care facility after experiencing vomiting and diarrhea for several days. The client is now lethargic and hypotensive. A health-care provider writes orders for the client. Which order should the nurse question?
1. Monitor and record intake and output.
2. Administer 3% sodium chloride solution IV at 150 mL/hr.
3. Administer 0.9% saline solution IV at 150 mL/hr.
4. Weigh the client daily.

41. A nurse assesses a client who has been vomiting for several days. The client is diagnosed with seasonal flu. The nurse should correctly identify that the client is experiencing which fluid and acid-base imbalance?
1. Fluid volume deficit and metabolic acidosis
2. Fluid volume deficit and metabolic alkalosis
3. Fluid volume excess and respiratory acidosis
4. Fluid volume excess and respiratory alkalosis

42. When calculating a client's intake and output, how should a nurse address the irrigation fluid of the client's percutaneous endoscopic gastrostomy tube?
1. Add the amount to total output.
2. Add the amount to total intake.
3. Deduct the amount from total output.
4. Deduct the amount from total intake.

43. A nurse is caring for an older adult client who is experiencing a fluid imbalance. Which age-related change should a nurse associate with fluid imbalance in an older adult?
1. Efficient temperature regulation
2. Increased glomerular filtration rate
3. Decreased perception of thirst, interfering with the thirst mechanism
4. Higher percentage of total body water than younger or middle-aged adults

44. A nurse is admitting a client diagnosed with chronic kidney disease who is receiving calcium acetate (PhosLo) 2 tablets with each meal three times per day as ordered. Each tablet contains 667 mg of calcium acetate. How many milligrams of calcium acetate should the nurse record that the client receives daily? Record your answer as a whole number.

____

45. A nurse calculates the anion gap of a client suspected of having metabolic acidosis. The client's serum sodium level is 146 mEq/L, serum chloride level is 104 mEq/L, and serum bicarbonate level is 18 mEq/L. What is the value of this client's anion gap in mEq/L? Record your answer as a whole number.

____

46. A health-care provider orders eplerenone (Inspra) 100 mg/day in two divided doses PO for a client diagnosed with fluid volume excess and hypertension secondary to primary hyperaldosteronism. The dose of eplerenone on hand is 50 mg/tablet. How many tablets should a nurse administer to the client every 12 hours? Record your answer as a whole number.

____

47. A nurse obtains the recent medical history of a newly admitted client. Which factors in this client's history should the nurse identify as placing the client at risk for respiratory acidosis? **Select all that apply.**
   1. Emphysema
   2. Multiple sclerosis
   3. Coronary artery disease
   4. Type 2 diabetes mellitus
   5. Current methadone (Dolophine) use

48. A nurse is assessing the lungs of an older adult client admitted with chemotherapy-induced anemia who is receiving 1 unit of blood. The nurse auscultates bilateral crackles in the lower bases. The previous nurse had reported clear lung sounds in this client. Which actions should the nurse take *immediately*? **Select all that apply.**
   1. Discontinue the transfusion.
   2. Slow the rate of the transfusion.
   3. Assess the client's blood pressure.
   4. Notify the primary health-care provider.
   5. Continue the transfusion at the current rate.

49. Which clinical manifestations should a nurse associate with the development of hyperkalemia if it is observed in a newly admitted client? **Select all that apply.**
   1. Bradycardia
   2. Hypotension
   3. Paresthesias
   4. Peaked T waves
   5. Prominent U waves

50. Which safety interventions should a nurse include when planning care for a client diagnosed with severe hypernatremia? **Select all that apply.**
   1. Fall precautions
   2. Seizure precautions
   3. Contact precautions
   4. Isolation precautions
   5. Aspiration precautions

51. A nurse is reviewing the electrocardiogram strip of a client diagnosed with a fluid and electrolyte imbalance. Based on the exhibit provided, which imbalance should the nurse suspect?

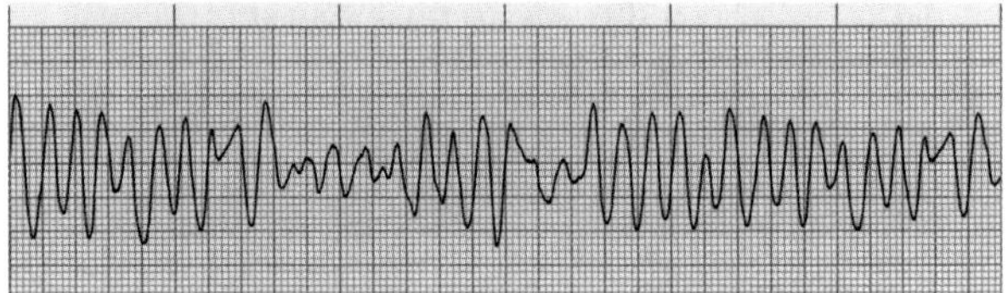

   1. Hypocalcemia
   2. Hyponatremia
   3. Hypochloremia
   4. Hypomagnesemia

52. A nurse administers digoxin to a client to treat atrial fibrillation and systolic heart failure. For which other reason should the nurse administer digoxin to this client?
   1. To increase the client's cardiac output
   2. To decrease the client's potassium loss
   3. To increase the client's heart rate
   4. To decrease the client's urinary output

53. A nurse is caring for a client diagnosed with hypovolemic hyponatremia. Which IV solution order should the nurse anticipate?
   1. 0.45% saline solution
   2. 0.9% saline solution
   3. 3% saline solution
   4. Dextrose 5% in water

54. A nurse is preparing to administer a continuous IV insulin infusion to a client diagnosed with diabetic ketoacidosis. Which agent should the nurse identify as the insulin of choice for this client?
   1. Novolin N
   2. Humulin N
   3. Humulin R
   4. Novolin 70/30

55. Which vital sign reading should a nurse associate with the development of fluid volume deficit (FVD)?
   1. Blood pressure (BP) 82/58 mm Hg, pulse 115 bpm, respirations 24 breaths per minute
   2. BP 100/70 mm Hg, pulse 86 bpm, respirations 20 breaths per minute
   3. BP 110/80 mm Hg, pulse 72 bpm, respirations 18 breaths per minute
   4. BP 140/70 mm Hg, pulse 68 bpm, respirations 16 breaths per minute

56. Which factor in a client's medical history should a nurse associate with the development of hypercalcemia?
1. Hypoparathyroidism
2. Hyperparathyroidism
3. Hypothyroidism
4. Hyperphosphatemia

57. A nurse is assessing a client who may be experiencing metabolic alkalosis. Which sign or symptom, if noted during the assessment, should the nurse associate with this particular acid-base imbalance?
1. Tetany
2. Lethargy
3. Hyporeflexia
4. Deep respirations

58. A nurse is caring for a client diagnosed with fluid volume excess (FVE) secondary to end-stage renal failure. Which manifestations, if exhibited by the client, should the nurse associate with FVE? **Select all that apply.**
1. Increased blood pressure
2. Decreased urinary output
3. Decreased fluid intake
4. Increased weight
5. Decreased weight

59. A nurse is reviewing the electrocardiogram (ECG) strip of a client who has been diagnosed with a fluid and electrolyte imbalance. Based on the exhibit provided, which imbalance should the nurse suspect?

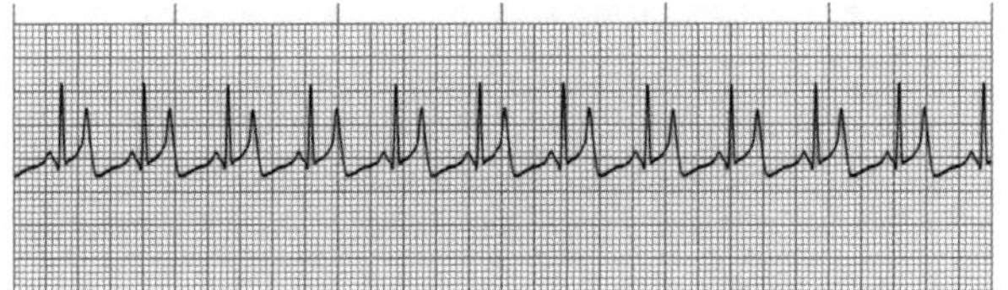

1. Hyperkalemia
2. Hypercalcemia
3. Hypophosphatemia
4. Hypomagnesemia

60. A nurse assesses a 6-year-old postoperative client recovering from a tonsillectomy and adenoidectomy 2 hours ago. The client is lethargic, irritable, and confused and is vomiting small amounts of clear, blood-tinged fluid. How should the nurse interpret the client's assessment data in the following chart?

Temperature: 99°F (37.2°C) axillary	Serum Na^+: 125 mEq/L
Blood pressure: 90/48 mm Hg	Serum Cl^-: 90 mEq/L
Heart rate: 114 bpm, regular	Serum K^+: 3.7 mEq/L
Respiratory rate: 12 breaths/min	Blood glucose: 76 mg/dL
Oxygen saturation: 98%	Serum creatinine: 0.6 mg/dL

1. The serum potassium level is decreased, suggesting hypokalemia.
2. The serum sodium level is decreased, suggesting hyponatremia.
3. The serum glucose level is increased, suggesting hyperglycemia.
4. The temperature is increased, suggesting the presence of infection.

61. A nurse is caring for a postoperative client who has a nasogastric tube. The nurse notes that the nasogastric tube is draining a large amount of secretions and that the client is now confused, has shallow respirations, and exhibits hand flexion during blood pressure measurement. Which acid-base imbalance should the nurse associate with this client's manifestations?
1. Metabolic acidosis
2. Metabolic alkalosis
3. Respiratory acidosis
4. Respiratory alkalosis

62. Which urine output value should a nurse associate with the development of fluid volume deficit (FVD) in an unstressed adult client?
1. 20 mL/hr
2. 30 mL/hr
3. 40 mL/hr
4. 50 mL/hr

63. A nurse is caring for a client admitted with respiratory acidosis secondary to accidental oxycodone (OxyContin) overdose. Which IV medication should the nurse determine to be the *priority* intervention for this client?
1. Potassium chloride
2. Regular insulin
3. Sodium bicarbonate
4. Naloxone hydrochloride

64. Which manifestation should a nurse identify as the most serious complication associated with hypernatremia?
 1. Hypertension
 2. Seizure activity
 3. Muscle cramps and twitching
 4. Decreased level of consciousness

65. Which clinical manifestation, if noted, should a nurse associate with *ineffective* IV fluid replacement therapy for a client diagnosed with fluid volume deficit (FVD)?
 1. Jugular venous distention
 2. Urine output of 40 mL/hr
 3. Blood pressure of 89/58 mm Hg
 4. Temperature of 99.8°F (37.7°C)

66. A home health nurse is preparing to administer calcitonin 4 IU/kg every 12 hours intramuscularly to an older adult client diagnosed with severe hypercalcemia. The client weighs 110 lb. The dose on hand is 200 IU/mL. How many milliliters of calcitonin should the nurse administer to this client every 12 hours? Record your answer as a whole number.

____

67. A health-care provider orders hydrochlorothiazide 3 mg/kg/day in two divided doses PO for an 85-lb child with edema secondary to congestive heart failure. How many milligrams of hydrochlorothiazide should a nurse administer to this child every 12 hours (twice daily)? Record your answer as a whole number.

____

68. A nurse is caring for a client who has recently been diagnosed with type 1 diabetes mellitus and is now recovering from diabetic ketoacidosis. The client's prescribed insulin dose per sliding scale to correct high blood sugar is the actual blood sugar level minus 120 (the desired blood sugar), divided by 50 (the correction factor) before each meal and at bedtime. If the client's before-meal blood sugar is 256 mg/dL, how many units of rapid-acting insulin does the client require to cover this level? Record your answer as a whole number.

____

69. Which steps should a nurse take to correctly assess a client diagnosed with fluid volume deficit for postural hypotension? Place each action in the correct sequence (1–5).
 ______ Document the results of the assessments.
 ______ Compare the client's blood pressures and pulse rates.
 ______ Check the client's blood pressure and pulse rate in the standing position.
 ______ Check the client's blood pressure and pulse rate in the supine position.
 ______ Check the client's blood pressure and pulse rate in the sitting position.

70. Which clinical manifestation should a nurse associate with the development of hypomagnesemia if observed in a newly admitted client?
 1. Tetany
 2. Diarrhea
 3. Lethargy
 4. Bradycardia

71. A nurse interprets that a client has an arterial blood pH of 7.49 that is metabolic in origin. Which other abnormal laboratory finding should the nurse associate with this pH imbalance?
 1. Increased serum chloride level
 2. Decreased serum calcium level
 3. Increased serum potassium level
 4. Decreased serum bicarbonate level

72. A nurse is evaluating a client's education regarding bumetanide (Bumex). The nurse should determine that which statement by the client indicates the need for further education regarding the medication?
 1. "I will continue taking this medication as directed even when I lose 3 lb in a week."
 2. "I will notify my health-care provider if I urinate more frequently."
 3. "I will notify my health-care provider if I notice any loss of hearing."
 4. "I will take my daily dose of this medication when I wake up in the morning."

73. A client's arterial blood gas report reveals a pH of 6.82. How should a nurse interpret this value?
 1. The pH is slightly decreased.
 2. The pH is extremely increased.
 3. The pH is incompatible with life.
 4. The pH is within the normal reference range.

74. A nurse is reviewing the electrocardiogram (ECG) strip of a client who has been diagnosed with a fluid and electrolyte imbalance. Based on the exhibit provided, which imbalance should the nurse suspect?

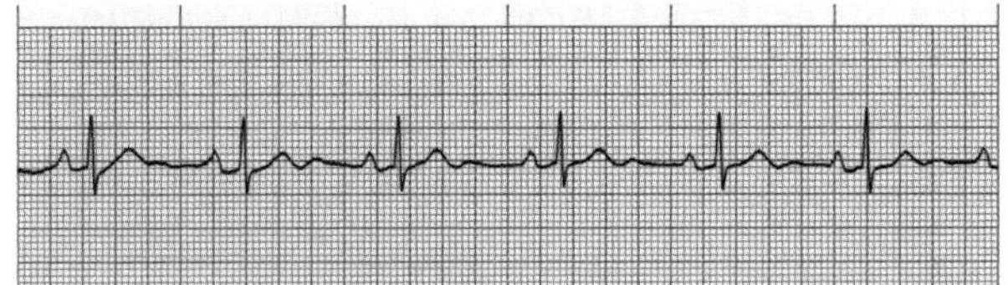

1. Hypernatremia
2. Hypokalemia
3. Hypercalcemia
4. Hypomagnesemia

75. A nurse reviews the laboratory values of multiple clients on a medical-surgical unit. Which arterial blood gas (ABG) values should the nurse associate with a client reporting surgical pain who has a blood pressure of 142/86 mm Hg, a heart rate of 104 bpm, and a respiratory rate of 34 breaths per minute?

1.

pH	7.33
$PaCO_2$	36 mm Hg
HCO_3^-	15 mEq/L

2.

pH	7.49
$PaCO_2$	45 mm Hg
HCO_3^-	33 mEq/L

3.

pH	7.31
$PaCO_2$	51 mm Hg
HCO_3^-	23mEq/L

4.

pH	7.51
$PaCO_2$	29 mm Hg
HCO_3^-	24 mEq/L

76. A nurse is educating a client regarding a prescribed loop diuretic. Which instruction should the nurse include in the client's education?

1. Follow a low-potassium diet.
2. Take a double dose if one dose is missed to avoid edema.
3. Change positions slowly to avoid orthostatic hypotension.
4. Notify the health-care provider of weight gain of more than 2 lb in 1 day.

77. An emergency department nurse admits an unconscious client who is diagnosed with possible ingestion of gamma-hydroxybutyric acid. For which acid-base imbalance should the nurse assess this client?

1. Metabolic acidosis
2. Metabolic alkalosis
3. Respiratory acidosis
4. Respiratory alkalosis

78. A nurse draws blood from a client diagnosed with Graves' disease for laboratory tests. The client reports recent weight loss, nausea, and constipation. The nurse notes that the client's heart rate is 122 bpm and that the client has a widening pulse pressure and decreased deep tendon reflexes (DTRs). Which serum calcium level should the nurse anticipate?

1. 7.5 mg/dL
2. 8.5 mg/dL
3. 9.5 mg/dL
4. 10.5 mg/dL

79. While a nurse is assessing a client who has been admitted after a motor vehicle collision, the client has a panic attack and begins to hyperventilate. Which intervention should the nurse initiate *first* when caring for this client?

1. Obtain vital signs.
2. Place the client in a supine position.
3. Administer oxygen via nasal cannula.
4. Assist the client to breathe more slowly.

80. A nurse evaluates a client who has received diuretic therapy for fluid volume excess (FVE). Which finding should indicate to the nurse that the therapy has been effective?

1. Decrease in hematocrit
2. Decrease in urine output
3. Decrease in body weight
4. Decrease in blood urea nitrogen

81. A nurse prepares to administer calcium chloride 10% 12 mEq IV push to a client diagnosed with hypocalcemia. The dose on hand is 1.36 mEq/mL. How many milliliters of calcium chloride 10% should the nurse administer to this client? Record your answer as a whole number.

____

82. A nurse is preparing to administer 40 mEq of potassium gluconate (Kaylixir) PO to a client diagnosed with hypokalemia. To ensure that the medication is diluted properly, how many milliliters of solution would be required to obtain a concentration of 20 mEq/15 mL? Record your answer as a whole number.

____

83. Which assessment findings should a nurse associate with left-sided heart failure when caring for a client diagnosed with fluid volume excess (FVE)? **Select all that apply.**
   1. Peripheral edema
   2. Hepatic enlargement
   3. Crackles in all lung fields
   4. Jugular venous distention
   5. Persistent nonproductive cough

84. A nurse in an emergency department admits a client who experienced a near drowning in a freshwater pond. Which sodium imbalance should the nurse associate with this incident?
   1. Hypernatremia related to an actual increase in sodium
   2. Hypernatremia related to a relative increase in sodium
   3. Hyponatremia related to an actual decrease in sodium
   4. Hyponatremia related to a relative decrease in sodium

85. A client's IV solution of 0.9% saline is infusing at 150 mL/hr, as ordered. After 4 hours of infusion, the client reports difficulty breathing and develops a bounding pulse volume. Which intervention should be the nurse's *priority*?
   1. Elevate the client's legs.
   2. Monitor the client's weight.
   3. Notify the health-care provider.
   4. Assess the client's lung sounds.

86. A nurse analyzes a client's arterial blood gas (ABG) values. The client's serum pH is 7.36, $PaCO_2$ is 48 mm Hg, and HCO_3^- is 30 mEq/L. Which acid-base imbalance should the nurse associate with these ABG values?
   1. Partially compensated metabolic acidosis
   2. Fully compensated respiratory acidosis
   3. Partially compensated metabolic alkalosis
   4. Fully compensated respiratory alkalosis

87. A client has been vomiting for 3 days. A nurse understands that this client is at increased risk for developing fluid volume deficit and hyponatremia and prepares to infuse 0.9% saline solution 1,000 mL intravenously at 125 mL/hr, as ordered by a health-care provider. The nurse selects IV tubing that has a drop factor of 30 gtt/mL. How many drops per minute should the nurse infuse to administer the prescribed 125 mL/hr? Record your answer using a whole number.

____

88. A nurse on a medical-surgical unit notes that a client recently diagnosed with diverticulitis is now reporting dizziness, weakness, and numbness and tingling of the face and hands. The client's respiratory rate is 36 breaths per minute, with a shallow pattern. Which arterial blood gas values should the nurse associate with this client's manifestations?

Lab Report A		**Lab Report B**		**Lab Report C**		**Lab Report D**	
pH	7.29	pH	7.31	pH	7.45	pH	7.49
$PaCO_2$	62 mm Hg	$PaCO_2$	41 mm Hg	$PaCO_2$	43 mm Hg	$PaCO_2$	29 mm Hg
HCO_3^-	24 mEq/L	HCO_3^-	17 mEq/L	HCO_3^-	25 mEq/L	HCO_3^-	25 mEq/L

   1. Lab Report A
   2. Lab Report B
   3. Lab Report C
   4. Lab Report D

89. A nurse is preparing to transfuse packed red blood cells to a client with a history of right-sided heart failure. Which infusion rate should the nurse use when performing this infusion?
1. 50 mL/hr
2. 100 mL/hr
3. 150 mL/hr
4. 200 mL/hr

90. Which manifestation, if identified during the assessment of a client, should a nurse associate with the development of hypernatremia?
1. Polyuria
2. Paresthesia
3. Increased thirst
4. Muscle weakness

91. A nurse is caring for a client diagnosed with uncompensated metabolic alkalosis secondary to prolonged vomiting. When reviewing this client's laboratory data, which value should the nurse anticipate?
1. Decreased pH
2. Increased $PaCO_2$
3. Decreased $PaCO_2$
4. Increased HCO_3^-

92. A nurse is instructing a client who is at risk for hypocalcemia. Which food should the nurse advise the client to choose to prevent the development of this imbalance?
1. Apple
2. Pizza
3. Popcorn
4. Chicken noodle soup

93. Which nursing diagnosis should a nurse assign to a client who has a serum potassium level of 3.0 mEq/L and is exhibiting muscle weakness, smooth muscle atony, and cardiac dysrhythmias?
1. Diarrhea Related to Spastic Colonic Activity
2. Decreased Cardiac Output Related to Dysrhythmia
3. Risk for Falls Related to Orthostatic Hypotension
4. Risk for Acute Confusion Related to Electrolyte Imbalance

94. A client diagnosed with hyperparathyroidism presents to an emergency department reporting severe generalized weakness. The client is diagnosed with hypophosphatemia and hypercalcemia. Which electrocardiogram (ECG) finding should a nurse identify as indicative of these electrolyte imbalances?
1.

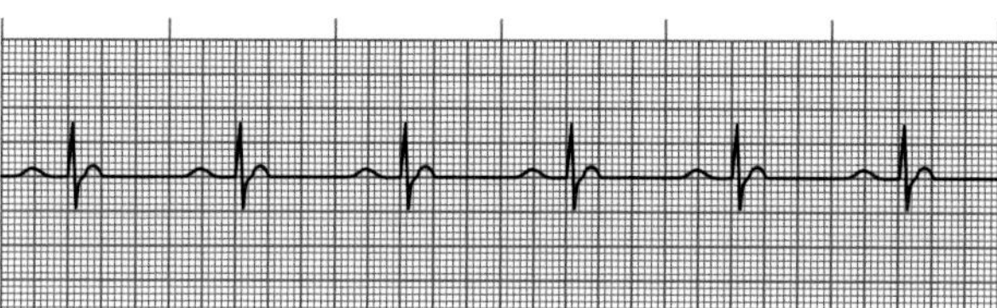

2.

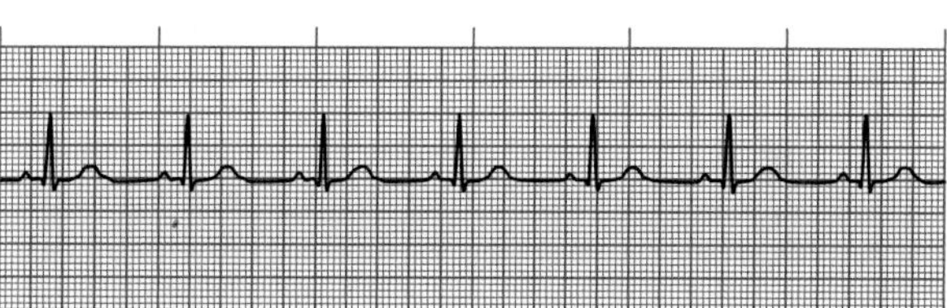

3.

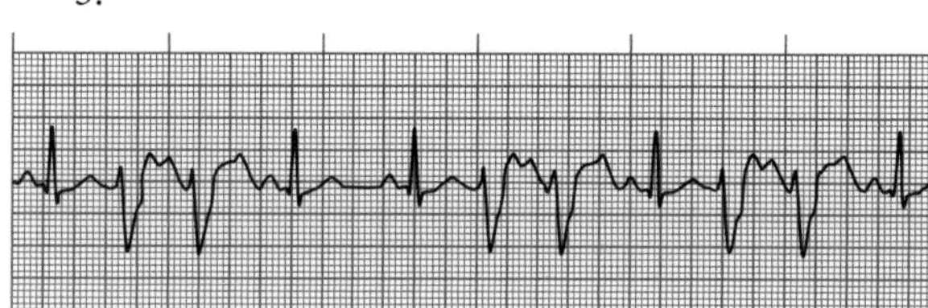

4.

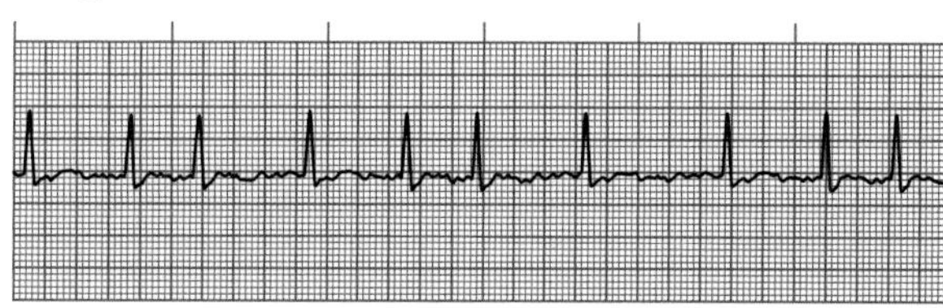

95. A nurse is caring for a hospitalized client who has been diagnosed with hyperemesis gravidarum and has a serum potassium level of 3.0 mEq/L. Which intervention is most appropriate for this client?
1. Administer potassium chloride (K-Dur) 20 mEq PO twice daily, as ordered by the health-care provider.
2. Administer furosemide (Lasix) 40 mg intravenously, as ordered by the health-care provider.
3. Infuse the potassium at a rate of 40 mEq/hr IV, as ordered by the health-care provider.
4. Use a controlled infusion device to administer an IV potassium solution.

96. A nurse who is instructing a client on a low-sodium diet should advise the client that which food is naturally low in sodium?
    1. Shrimp
    2. Spinach
    3. Carrots
    4. Oranges

97. A postoperative client with a history of anxiety begins to hyperventilate for an extended period. Metabolic causes of hyperventilation are ruled out. A unit nurse is unable to calm the client, who continues to hyperventilate despite efforts to slow the rate of breathing. Which medication should the nurse anticipate an order to administer?
    1. alprazolam (Xanax) PO
    2. lorazepam (Ativan) by IV push
    3. sodium bicarbonate (Neut) PO
    4. naloxone hydrochloride (Narcan) by IV push

98. A nurse is assessing a newly admitted client who reports frequent charley horses, diarrhea, and irritability for the past week. Which condition should the nurse suspect?
    1. Hyperkalemia
    2. Hypocalcemia
    3. Hypermagnesemia
    4. Hypophosphatemia

99. Which manifestation should a nurse investigate *first* when assessing a client admitted with severe preeclampsia that is being treated with a continuous infusion of IV magnesium sulfate?
    1. Oral temperature 100.6°F (38°C)
    2. Pulse 110 bpm
    3. Blood pressure 170/110 mm Hg
    4. Respiratory rate 10 breaths per minute

100. A nurse is caring for an adult client with a serum potassium level of 2.3 mEq/L. Which order for potassium chloride should the nurse identify as being most appropriate for this client?
    1. Administer potassium chloride 40 mEq/L intramuscularly now.
    2. Administer potassium chloride 40 mEq/L by IV push now.
    3. Administer potassium chloride 40 mEq/L by IV infusion over 4 hours.
    4. Administer potassium chloride 40 mEq/L PO three times daily.

REVIEW ANSWERS

1. ANSWER: 3.

Rationale:

1. An older adult postoperative client who has uncontrolled pain requires frequent assessment by the RN, and care of this client cannot be delegated to a licensed practical nurse.
2. A child who has a temperature of 103.5°F (39.7°C) requires frequent assessment by the RN, and care of this client cannot be delegated to a licensed practical nurse.
3. **It is most appropriate for the RN to delegate care of a client with dehydration to a licensed practical nurse because this client is the most stable and does not require frequent monitoring, evaluation, and planning of care.**
4. A client who is receiving an IV insulin drip for diabetic ketoacidosis requires frequent assessment by the RN, and care of this client cannot be delegated to a licensed practical nurse. IV insulin is a high-alert drug that can be administered only by licensed health-care providers (health-care providers, nurse practitioners, and health-care provider assistants) and RNs.

TEST-TAKING TIP: Rule out clients who require ongoing assessment. Recognize that the age of the client is not always relevant when deciding which one requires the most frequent monitoring, evaluation, and care.

Content Area: Adult Health
Category of Health Alteration: Fluid Volume Deficit
Integrated Processes: Nursing Process: Planning
Client Need: Safe and Effective Care Environment
Cognitive Level: Analysis
Reference: Ignatavicius, D., and Workman, M. (2012). Medical-Surgical Nursing: Patient-Centered Collaborative Care (7th ed.). St. Louis, MO: Saunders.

2. ANSWER: 1.

Rationale:

1. **The nurse should expect a child with persistent projectile vomiting secondary to gastroenteritis to exhibit hypochloremia. Severe gastroenteritis may cause projectile vomiting, dehydration, and metabolic alkalosis. Specifically, excessive vomiting causes the client to lose chloride in the form of hydrochloric acid. A serum chloride level of 85 mEq/L reflects hypochloremia.**
2. The nurse should expect a child with persistent projectile vomiting secondary to gastroenteritis to exhibit hypochloremia, not a normal serum chloride level. A serum chloride level of 95 mEq/L is within the normal reference range.
3. The nurse should expect a child with persistent projectile vomiting secondary to gastroenteritis to exhibit hypochloremia, not a normal serum chloride level. A serum chloride level of 105 mEq/L is within the normal reference range.
4. The nurse should expect a child with persistent projectile vomiting secondary to gastroenteritis to exhibit hypochloremia, not an elevated serum chloride level. A serum chloride level of 110 mEq/L is elevated (hyperchloremia).

TEST-TAKING TIP: Recall that the normal reference range for serum chloride is 95 to 108 mEq/L (varies by laboratory).

Content Area: Child Health
Category of Health Alteration: Chloride Imbalance
Integrated Processes: Nursing Process: Assessment
Client Need: Physiological Integrity
Cognitive Level: Application
Reference: Ignatavicius, D., and Workman, M. (2012). Medical-Surgical Nursing: Patient-Centered Collaborative Care (7th ed.). St. Louis, MO: Saunders.

3. ANSWER: 1.

Rationale:

1. **The nurse should identify that the client is experiencing respiratory acidosis, based on the client's medical history and signs and symptoms. Confusion, headache, lethargy, flushed skin, cyanotic mucous membranes, hypotension, and tachycardia are classic signs of respiratory acidosis. This client is most likely experiencing carbon dioxide narcosis as well. Arterial blood gas values would need to be obtained to evaluate this possibility and the client's status.**
2. The nurse should identify that the client is experiencing respiratory acidosis, not metabolic acidosis. Metabolic acidosis is caused by the excessive breakdown of fatty acids, lactic acid production, or excessive intake of acids.
3. The nurse should identify that the client is experiencing respiratory acidosis, not respiratory alkalosis. Alkalosis is a decrease in the number of free hydrogen ions circulating in the blood, which results in an increase in blood pH.
4. The nurse should identify that the client is experiencing respiratory acidosis, not metabolic alkalosis. Alkalosis is a decrease in the number of free hydrogen ions circulating in the blood, which results in an increase in blood pH.

TEST-TAKING TIP: The key words are "chronic bronchitis and emphysema." Respiratory acidosis may result whenever respiratory function is impaired.

Content Area: Older Adult Health
Category of Health Alteration: Acid-Base Imbalance
Integrated Processes: Nursing Process: Analysis
Client Need: Physiological Integrity
Cognitive Level: Application
Reference: Ignatavicius, D., and Workman, M. (2012). Medical-Surgical Nursing: Patient-Centered Collaborative Care (7th ed.). St. Louis, MO: Saunders.

4. ANSWER: 4.

Rationale:

1. Paresthesias are associated with hypocalcemia, not hypercalcemia. A serum calcium (total) level of 11.2 mg/dL is above the normal reference range of 8.2 to 10.2 mg/dL (adults).
2. Painful muscle cramps are associated with hypocalcemia, not hypercalcemia. A serum calcium (total) level of 11.2 mg/dL is above the normal reference range of 8.2 to 10.2 mg/dL (adults).
3. A positive Chvostek's sign is associated with hypocalcemia, not hypercalcemia. A serum calcium (total) level of 11.2 mg/dL is above the normal reference range of 8.2 to 10.2 mg/dL (adults).
4. **The nurse should associate decreased deep tendon reflexes (DTRs) with a serum calcium level of 11.2 mg/dL (hypercalcemia). The normal total serum calcium level is 8.2 to 10.2 mg/dL (adults). Calcium is an excitable membrane stabilizer that causes severe weakness, decreased reflexes, and altered mental status when levels are elevated. Hyperparathyroidism is the most common cause of hypercalcemia.**

TEST-TAKING TIP: Recall that calcium is an excitable membrane stabilizer. Excess calcium "slows down" physiological processes. Memorize the normal reference range for this electrolyte.
Content Area: Adult Health
Category of Health Alteration: Calcium Imbalance
Integrated Processes: Nursing Process: Assessment
Client Need: Physiological Integrity
Cognitive Level: Application
***Reference:** Ignatavicius, D., and Workman, M. (2012). Medical-Surgical Nursing: Patient-Centered Collaborative Care (7th ed.). St. Louis, MO: Saunders.*

5. ANSWER: 1, 2, 3, 5.
Rationale:
1. **The nurse should assign the diagnosis Risk for Injury Related to Confusion to this client experiencing respiratory alkalosis caused by mechanical hyperventilation. Respiratory alkalosis results in confusion, skeletal muscle weakness, further impairment of gas exchange, and inadequate tissue oxygenation.**
2. **The nurse should assign the diagnosis Risk for Falls Related to Skeletal Muscle Weakness to this client experiencing respiratory alkalosis caused by mechanical hyperventilation. Respiratory alkalosis results in confusion, skeletal muscle weakness, further impairment of gas exchange, and inadequate tissue oxygenation.**
3. **The nurse should assign the diagnosis Impaired Gas Exchange Related to Mechanical Ventilation to this client experiencing respiratory alkalosis caused by mechanical hyperventilation. Respiratory alkalosis results in confusion, skeletal muscle weakness, further impairment of gas exchange, and inadequate tissue oxygenation.**
4. The diagnosis Decreased Cardiac Output Related to Increased Respiratory Rate is inaccurate because decreased cardiac output usually is not related to an increased respiratory rate.
5. **The nurse should assign the diagnosis Ineffective Breathing Pattern Related to Inability to Sustain Spontaneous Ventilation to this client experiencing respiratory alkalosis caused by mechanical hyperventilation. Respiratory alkalosis results in confusion, skeletal muscle weakness, further impairment of gas exchange, and inadequate tissue oxygenation.**

TEST-TAKING TIP: The key words are "respiratory alkalosis related to hyperventilation." Choose the options that are related to hyperventilation.
Content Area: Adult Health
Category of Health Alteration: Acid-Base Imbalance
Integrated Processes: Nursing Process: Analysis
Client Need: Physiological Integrity
Cognitive Level: Analysis
***Reference:** Ignatavicius, D., and Workman, M. (2012). Medical-Surgical Nursing: Patient-Centered Collaborative Care (7th ed.). St. Louis, MO: Saunders.*

6. ANSWER: 1, 2, 4.
Rationale:
1. **The nurse should associate a thready pulse with a nursing diagnosis of Deficient Fluid Volume Secondary to Dehydration. Thready pulse is a sign of fluid volume deficit (FVD).**
2. **The nurse should associate an increased pulse rate with a nursing diagnosis of Deficient Fluid Volume Secondary to Dehydration. An increased pulse rate is a sign of FVD.**
3. Jugular venous distention would be present with excess fluid volume, not with a nursing diagnosis of Deficient Fluid Volume.
4. **The nurse should associate decreased blood pressure with a nursing diagnosis of Deficient Fluid Volume Secondary to Dehydration. Decreased blood pressure is a sign of FVD.**
5. Isotonic and hypotonic dehydration with plasma volume deficits would cause hemoconcentration, resulting in *increased*, not decreased, hemoglobin and hematocrit levels. Decreased hemoglobin and hematocrit values may be indicative of hemorrhage.

TEST-TAKING TIP: The key words are "Deficient Fluid Volume" and "Dehydration." Rule out options that are signs of fluid volume excess.
Content Area: Adult Health
Category of Health Alteration: Fluid Volume Deficit
Integrated Processes: Nursing Process: Assessment
Client Need: Physiological Integrity
Cognitive Level: Application
***Reference:** Ignatavicius, D., and Workman, M. (2012). Medical-Surgical Nursing: Patient-Centered Collaborative Care (7th ed.). St. Louis, MO: Saunders.*

7. ANSWER: 26.4.
Rationale:

240 lb ÷ 2.2 lb/kg = 109.09 kg
109.09 kg × 6 mg/kg = 659.4 mg
659.4 mg/*X* × 25 mg/1 mL = 25*X* = 659.4 = 659.4 ÷ 25 =
26.38 mL = 26.4 mL

TEST-TAKING TIP: Always double-check your calculations before providing your answer on the NCLEX-RN examination *and* before administering medication to a client.
Content Area: Adult Health
Category of Health Alteration: Acid-Base Imbalance
Integrated Processes: Nursing Process: Implementation
Client Need: Physiological Integrity
Cognitive Level: Application
***References:** Deglin, J. H., Vallerand, A. H., and Sanoski, C. A. (2013). Davis's Drug Guide for Nurses (13th ed.). Philadelphia, PA: F. A. Davis; Beaman, N. (2008). Pharmacology Clear and Simple: A Drug Classifications and Dosage Calculations Approach. Philadelphia, PA: F. A. Davis.*

8. ANSWER: 1,870.
Rationale:

(240 mL + 350 mL + 16 oz [480 mL] oral intake) + 800 mL parenteral intake = 1,870 mL total intake
The 1,200 mL voided is output, not intake.

TEST-TAKING TIP: If a client reports oral intake in ounces, 1 oz = 30 mL.
Content Area: Adult Health
Category of Health Alteration: Fluid Volume Excess
Integrated Processes: Nursing Process: Implementation
Client Need: Physiological Integrity
Cognitive Level: Application
***Reference:** Berman, A., Snyder, S., Kozier, B., and Erb, G. (2012). Kozier & Erb's Fundamentals of Nursing: Concepts, Process, and Practice (9th ed.). Upper Saddle River, NJ: Pearson.*

9. ANSWER: 2.

Rationale:

1. On the scale for grading edema, a 2-mm indentation = 1+, 4-mm indentation = 2+, 6-mm indentation = 3+, and 8-mm indentation = 4+.

2. The nurse should document that the client has grade 2+ edema. On the scale for grading edema, a 4-mm indentation = 2+. Edema is the presence of excess interstitial fluid. An area of edema appears shiny, swollen, and taut and tends to blanch; if edema is accompanied by inflammation, it may appear reddened. Pitting refers to the degree to which the skin remains indented or pitted after pressure is applied, usually by a finger.

3. On the scale for grading edema, a 2-mm indentation = 1+, 4-mm indentation = 2+, 6-mm indentation = 3+, and 8-mm indentation = 4+.

4. On the scale for grading edema, a 2-mm indentation = 1+, 4-mm indentation = 2+, 6-mm indentation = 3+, and 8-mm indentation = 4+.

TEST-TAKING TIP: Review Figure 1.3 on page 8 if you were unable to answer this question correctly.

Content Area: Child Health

Category of Health Alteration: Fluid Volume Excess

Integrated Processes: Nursing Process: Assessment

Client Need: Physiological Integrity

Cognitive Level: Comprehension

Reference: *Berman, A., Snyder, S., Kozier, B., and Erb, G. (2012). Kozier & Erb's Fundamentals of Nursing: Concepts, Process, and Practice (9th ed.). Upper Saddle River, NJ: Pearson.*

10. ANSWER: 3.

Rationale:

1. "Monitor blood sugar every hour" (or more frequently, if necessary) is an appropriate intervention for diabetic ketoacidosis and does not need to be questioned by the nurse.

2. "Assess vital signs every 15 minutes until stable" is an appropriate intervention for diabetic ketoacidosis and does not need to be questioned by the nurse.

3. The nurse should question the order to administer regular insulin subcutaneously per sliding scale. Regular insulin should be administered initially by IV bolus, followed by a continuous IV infusion to decrease the client's serum glucose level quickly. Subcutaneous insulin therapy is started when the client can take oral fluids and the ketosis has stopped.

4. "Administer 0.9% saline solution IV at 1,000 mL/hr × 2 L" is an appropriate intervention for diabetic ketoacidosis and does not need to be questioned by the nurse.

TEST-TAKING TIP: Read the question carefully. Recognize that the *correct* answer is the *wrong* treatment.

Content Area: Adult Health

Category of Health Alteration: Acid-Base Imbalance

Integrated Processes: Nursing Process: Implementation

Client Need: Physiological Integrity

Cognitive Level: Analysis

Reference: *Ignatavicius, D., and Workman, M. (2012). Medical-Surgical Nursing: Patient-Centered Collaborative Care (7th ed.). St. Louis, MO: Saunders.*

11. ANSWER: 3.

Rationale:

1. The nurse should anticipate that this client would experience an increase in plasma volume and a decrease in interstitial volume, not just an increase in plasma volume.

2. The nurse should anticipate that this client would experience an increase in plasma volume and a decrease, not an increase, in interstitial volume.

3. The nurse should anticipate that a client with a normal fluid and electrolyte balance who mistakenly received a 3% saline IV solution would experience an increase in plasma volume and a decrease in interstitial volume. If a hypertonic IV solution is infused into a client with normal extracellular fluid osmolarity, the infusing fluid will make the client's intravascular compartment hyperosmotic (or hypertonic). In an attempt to balance this, the client's interstitial fluid will be pulled into the intravascular compartment to dilute the blood osmolarity back to normal, resulting in an increase in plasma volume and a decrease in the interstitial volume. Isotonic solutions, such as 0.9% saline solution, would increase plasma volume without causing a fluid shift between compartments. Hypotonic solutions, such as 0.45% saline solution, would cause an increase in both plasma volume and interstitial volume because fluid is pulled out of the intravascular compartment and into the interstitial fluid and cells.

4. The nurse should anticipate that this client would experience an increase in plasma volume and a decrease in interstitial volume, not an increase in both plasma and interstitial volume.

TEST-TAKING TIP: Read each option carefully. Be familiar with the fluid shifts caused by different types of IV solutions.

Content Area: Adult Health

Category of Health Alteration: Fluid Volume Excess

Integrated Processes: Nursing Process: Implementation

Client Need: Physiological Integrity

Cognitive Level: Comprehension

Reference: *Ignatavicius, D., and Workman, M. (2012). Medical-Surgical Nursing: Patient-Centered Collaborative Care (7th ed.). St. Louis, MO: Saunders.*

12. ANSWER: 1.

Rationale:

1. The nurse should teach the client to avoid milk because it is high in both phosphorus and potassium.

2. Broth does not contain significant amounts of phosphorus or potassium and would be a good source of dietary sodium and chloride. A client attempting to decrease the daily intake of phosphorus and potassium would not need to avoid this food.

3. Pretzels do not contain significant amounts of phosphorus or potassium and would be a good source of dietary sodium and chloride. A client attempting to decrease the daily intake of phosphorus and potassium would not need to avoid this food.

4. Fresh fruits are a source of potassium but do not contain significant amounts of phosphorus. A client attempting to decrease the daily intake of *both* phosphorus and potassium would not need to avoid this food. A client attempting to decrease the daily intake of potassium alone would need to avoid fresh fruits.

TEST-TAKING TIP: Read the question carefully and select the option that is high in *both* electrolytes.
Content Area: Adult Health
Category of Health Alteration: Phosphate Imbalance
Integrated Processes: Teaching/Learning
Client Need: Health Promotion and Maintenance
Cognitive Level: Application
Reference: *Ignatavicius, D., and Workman, M. (2012). Medical-Surgical Nursing: Patient-Centered Collaborative Care (7th ed.). St. Louis, MO: Saunders.*

13. ANSWER: 1.
Rationale:
1. The nurse should associate the development of deep, rapid respirations (Kussmaul respirations) and a fruity breath odor with metabolic acidosis, most likely diabetic ketoacidosis (DKA). Kussmaul respirations are very deep, rapid respirations that are not under the client's voluntary control. This type of breathing occurs when excess acids, caused by the absence of insulin, increase hydrogen and carbon dioxide levels in the blood, triggering the body to excrete more carbon dioxide by increasing the rate and depth of breathing (respiratory compensation). A fruity breath odor is characteristic of diabetic ketoacidosis.
2. The nurse should associate the development of deep, rapid respirations (Kussmaul respirations) and a fruity breath odor with metabolic acidosis, most likely diabetic ketoacidosis, not with metabolic alkalosis.
3. The nurse should associate the development of deep, rapid respirations (Kussmaul respirations) and a fruity breath odor with metabolic acidosis, most likely diabetic ketoacidosis, not with respiratory acidosis.
4. The nurse should associate the development of deep, rapid respirations (Kussmaul respirations) and a fruity breath odor with metabolic acidosis, most likely diabetic ketoacidosis, not with respiratory alkalosis.
TEST-TAKING TIP: Recall that Kussmaul respirations and a fruity breath odor are associated with metabolic acidosis and are most often caused by diabetic ketoacidosis. Review the signs and symptoms of acid-base imbalances if you had difficulty with this question.
Content Area: Adult Health
Category of Health Alteration: Acid-Base Imbalance
Integrated Processes: Nursing Process: Implementation
Client Need: Physiological Integrity
Cognitive Level: Application
Reference: *Ignatavicius, D., and Workman, M. (2012). Medical-Surgical Nursing: Patient-Centered Collaborative Care (7th ed.). St. Louis, MO: Saunders.*

14. ANSWER: 4.
Rationale:
1. The nurse should provide fluids that contain electrolytes (such as Gatorade), not just water and ice chips, when the client can tolerate oral fluids. Water would exacerbate the client's nausea and vomiting and worsen the client's dilutional hyponatremia.
2. Neurological checks should be performed at least every 6 hours, not just daily.
3. Although 0.9% saline solution would be appropriate for this client, the rate (250 mL/hr) is too high and would place the child at risk for fluid overload.
4. The nurse should identify the administration of IV ondansetron 0.15 mg/kg every 6 hours as appropriate to effectively control this client's nausea and vomiting.
TEST-TAKING TIP: Review the chart carefully, and identify the abnormal findings. Then think about how these findings relate to the possible interventions. Select the option that is most appropriate for a child with hyponatremia, mental status changes, and vomiting.
Content Area: Child Health
Category of Health Alteration: Sodium Imbalance
Integrated Processes: Nursing Process: Assessment
Client Need: Physiological Integrity
Cognitive Level: Analysis
Reference: *Ward, S. L., and Hisley, S. M. (2011). Maternal-Child Nursing Care: Optimizing Outcomes for Mothers, Children and Families. Philadelphia, PA: F. A. Davis.*

15. ANSWER: 1, 3, 6.
Rationale:
1. A nurse evaluating the ABG values of a client diagnosed with partially compensated respiratory alkalosis should expect the pH to decrease toward 7.45, with a decrease in HCO_3^- and a decreased $PaCO_2$. The kidneys excrete additional HCO_3^- to decrease the amount of base and increase available hydrogen ions in an attempt to lower the client's pH.
2. A nurse evaluating the ABG values of a client diagnosed with partially compensated respiratory alkalosis should expect the pH to decrease toward 7.45, with a decrease in HCO_3^- and a decreased, not increased, $PaCO_2$.
3. A nurse evaluating the ABG values of a client diagnosed with partially compensated respiratory alkalosis should expect the pH to decrease toward 7.45, with a decrease in HCO_3^- and a decreased $PaCO_2$. The kidneys excrete additional HCO_3^- to decrease the amount of base and increase available hydrogen ions in an attempt to lower the client's pH.
4. A nurse evaluating the ABG values of a client diagnosed with partially compensated respiratory alkalosis should expect the pH to decrease toward 7.45, with a decrease, not an increase, in HCO_3^- and a decreased $PaCO_2$.
5. A nurse evaluating the ABG values of a client diagnosed with partially compensated respiratory alkalosis should expect the pH to decrease toward 7.45, not increase toward 7.35, with a decrease in HCO_3^- and a decreased $PaCO_2$. The kidneys excrete additional HCO_3^- to decrease the amount of base and increase available hydrogen ions in an attempt to lower, not raise, the client's pH.
6. A nurse evaluating the ABG values of a client diagnosed with partially compensated respiratory alkalosis should expect the pH to decrease toward 7.45, with a decrease in HCO_3^- and a decreased $PaCO_2$. The kidneys excrete additional HCO_3^- to decrease the amount of base and increase available hydrogen ions in an attempt to lower the client's pH.
TEST-TAKING TIP: Associate respiratory alkalosis with an increase in pH, a decrease in $PaCO_2$, and a decrease in HCO_3^- because of the kidneys' attempt to compensate.

Content Area: Adult Health
Category of Health Alteration: Acid-Base Imbalance
Integrated Processes: Nursing Process: Analysis
Client Need: Physiological Integrity
Cognitive Level: Application
Reference: *Williams, L., and Hopper, P. (2011). Understanding Medical-Surgical Nursing (4th ed.). Philadelphia, PA: F. A. Davis.*

16. ANSWER: 1, 3, 4, 5.
Rationale:
1. The nurse should monitor any client receiving an isotonic IV solution, regardless of age, for moist crackles in the lungs. Lung crackles, increased pulse rate, weight gain, dependent edema, and bounding pulse quality indicate the development of hypervolemia. Although any client receiving isotonic IV solutions is at risk for developing hypervolemia, older adult clients are at increased risk because of age-related decreases in the glomerular filtration rate and other comorbidities.
2. The nurse should monitor any client receiving an isotonic IV solution, regardless of age, for an increased, not decreased, pulse rate. An increased pulse rate, lung crackles, weight gain, dependent edema, and bounding pulse quality indicate the development of hypervolemia.
3. The nurse should monitor any client receiving an isotonic IV solution, regardless of age, for weight gain. Lung crackles, increased pulse rate, weight gain, dependent edema, and bounding pulse quality indicate the development of hypervolemia.
4. The nurse should monitor any client receiving an isotonic IV solution, regardless of age, for dependent edema. Lung crackles, increased pulse rate, weight gain, dependent edema, and bounding pulse quality indicate the development of hypervolemia.
5. The nurse should monitor any client receiving an isotonic IV solution, regardless of age, for bounding pulse quality. Lung crackles, increased pulse rate, weight gain, dependent edema, and bounding pulse quality indicate the development of hypervolemia.
TEST-TAKING TIP: The key words are "isotonic saline solution." Recognize that excessive administration of isotonic IV solutions may result in fluid volume overload.
Content Area: Older Adult Health
Category of Health Alteration: Fluid Volume Excess
Integrated Processes: Nursing Process: Assessment
Client Need: Physiological Integrity
Cognitive Level: Application
Reference: *Ignatavicius, D., and Workman, M. (2012). Medical-Surgical Nursing: Patient-Centered Collaborative Care (7th ed.). St. Louis, MO: Saunders.*

17. ANSWER: 1, 3, 4.
Rationale:
1. The nurse should expect the client's serum pH to be abnormal. Obstruction of the airway impairs gas exchange, resulting in respiratory acidosis. The serum pH would be decreased because carbon dioxide is being retained in the lungs.
2. The nurse should not expect the client's serum HCO_3^- level to be abnormal. A client with rapid-onset respiratory acidosis usually has a normal HCO_3^- level because compensation by the kidneys has not started.
3. The nurse should expect the client's serum PaO_2 level to be abnormal. Obstruction of the airway impairs gas exchange, resulting in respiratory acidosis. The PaO_2 level would be decreased because gas exchange is impaired.
4. The nurse should expect the client's serum $PaCO_2$ level to be abnormal. Obstruction of the airway impairs gas exchange, resulting in respiratory acidosis. The $PaCO_2$ level would be increased because gas exchange is impaired.
5. The nurse should not expect the client's serum sodium level to be abnormal. Serum sodium levels are not usually affected in acidosis.
TEST-TAKING TIP: Recognize that the client's situation would produce respiratory acidosis, and select the options that reflect that imbalance.
Content Area: Adult Health
Category of Health Alteration: Acid-Base Imbalance
Integrated Processes: Nursing Process: Analysis
Client Need: Physiological Integrity
Cognitive Level: Application
Reference: *Ignatavicius, D., and Workman, M. (2012). Medical-Surgical Nursing: Patient-Centered Collaborative Care (7th ed.). St. Louis, MO: Saunders.*

18. ANSWER: 2.
Rationale:
1. An infant has a higher (not lower) cardiac output per kilogram of body weight.
2. The nurse should identify that the infant is predisposed to fluid and electrolyte imbalances because of decreased kidney function. The kidneys are functionally immature at birth and are inefficient in excreting waste. The kidneys of an infant are also unable to concentrate or dilute urine efficiently, conserve or excrete sodium, and acidify urine. This infant is less able to handle large quantities of solute-free water than an older child and is more likely to become dehydrated when given concentrated formulas or to become overhydrated when given excessive water or dilute formula.
3. An infant has greater (not less) body surface area proportionally.
4. An infant has an increased (not decreased) amount of extracellular fluid.
TEST-TAKING TIP: Recall that clients with immature or decreased kidney function are at greater risk for fluid and electrolyte imbalances.
Content Area: Child Health
Category of Health Alteration: Fluid Volume Excess
Integrated Processes: Nursing Process: Assessment
Client Need: Physiological Integrity
Cognitive Level: Application
Reference: *Ward, S. L., and Hisley, S. M. (2011). Maternal-Child Nursing Care: Optimizing Outcomes for Mothers, Children and Families. Philadelphia, PA: F. A. Davis.*

19. ANSWER: 3.
Rationale:
1. The client's serum pH of 7.55, $PaCO_2$ of 33 mm Hg, and HCO_3^- of 27 mEq/L are not indicative of uncompensated metabolic alkalosis.
2. The client's serum pH of 7.55, $PaCO_2$ of 33 mm Hg, and HCO_3^- of 27 mEq/L are not indicative of compensated metabolic alkalosis.

3. The nurse should associate the client's serum pH of 7.55, $PaCO_2$ of 33 mm Hg, and HCO_3^- of 27 mEq/L with uncompensated respiratory alkalosis. The pH of 7.55 reflects *uncompensated* alkalosis because it remains greater than the normal reference range of 7.35 to 7.45; the *decreased* $PaCO_2$ of 33 mm Hg indicates that the client's lungs are exhaling excessive amounts of carbon dioxide, making the respiratory system the source of the alkalosis; and the *normal* HCO_3^- of 27 mEq/L indicates that the kidneys have not yet begun to compensate.
4. The client's serum pH of 7.55, $PaCO_2$ of 33 mm Hg, and HCO_3^- of 27 mEq/L are not indicative of compensated respiratory alkalosis.
TEST-TAKING TIP: Review normal arterial blood gas levels and which imbalances are indicated by abnormal values if you had difficulty answering this question correctly.
Content Area: Adult Health
Category of Health Alteration: Acid-Base Imbalance
Integrated Processes: Nursing Process: Analysis
Client Need: Physiological Integrity
Cognitive Level: Analysis
Reference: *Berman, A., Snyder, S., Kozier, B., and Erb, G. (2012). Kozier & Erb's Fundamentals of Nursing: Concepts, Process, and Practice (9th ed.). Upper Saddle River, NJ: Pearson.*

20. ANSWER: 3.
Rationale:
1. The nursing student's statement "I am going to use an infusion pump to administer this medication" is correct when preparing to administer IV potassium chloride and does not indicate the need for additional instruction.
2. The nursing student's statement "I plan to monitor the client's urine output during and after the administration of this medication" is correct when preparing to administer IV potassium chloride and does not indicate the need for additional instruction.
3. The nursing instructor should identify that the nursing student needs additional instruction if, when preparing to administer IV potassium chloride, the student states, "I have drawn up this medication for IV push administration." Rapid infusion of potassium may cause cardiac arrest. Potassium should *never* be administered by IV push.
4. The nursing student's statement "I plan to monitor the client's electrocardiogram during the administration of this medication" is correct when preparing to administer IV potassium chloride and does not indicate the need for additional instruction.
TEST-TAKING TIP: Select the statement that is incorrect.
Content Area: Adult Health
Category of Health Alteration: Potassium Imbalance
Integrated Processes: Nursing Process: Evaluation
Client Need: Physiological Integrity
Cognitive Level: Analysis
Reference: *Ignatavicius, D., and Workman, M. (2012). Medical-Surgical Nursing: Patient-Centered Collaborative Care (7th ed.). St. Louis, MO: Saunders.*

21. ANSWER: 1.
Rationale:
1. The nurse should identify 0.45% saline solution, a hypotonic solution, as the appropriate initial IV solution for a client diagnosed with fluid volume deficit (FVD) secondary to diabetic ketoacidosis. Clients with diabetic ketoacidosis are hyperglycemic. The high serum glucose pulls fluid out of the cells and into the vascular and interstitial compartments. Hypotonic solutions, such as 0.45% saline solution, pull fluid from the intravascular and interstitial compartments and into the cells, correcting the imbalance. Hypotonic fluids must be administered slowly to prevent a sudden fluid shift from the intravascular space into the cells.
2. The nurse should identify a hypotonic solution as the appropriate initial IV solution for a client diagnosed with FVD secondary to diabetic ketoacidosis. Dextrose 5% in 0.9% saline solution is an isotonic, not a hypotonic, solution.
3. The nurse should identify a hypotonic solution as the appropriate initial IV solution for a client diagnosed with FVD secondary to diabetic ketoacidosis. Lactated Ringer's solution is an isotonic, not a hypotonic, solution.
4. The nurse should identify a hypotonic solution as the appropriate initial IV solution for a client diagnosed with FVD secondary to diabetic ketoacidosis. The 3% sodium chloride solution is a hypertonic, not a hypotonic, solution.
TEST-TAKING TIP: The key words are "diabetic ketoacidosis." Consider each type of IV fluid, identify the type of solution, and visualize how each solution affects the movement of fluids and electrolytes into and out of the cells.
Content Area: Adult Health
Category of Health Alteration: Fluid Volume Deficit
Integrated Processes: Nursing Process: Implementation
Client Need: Physiological Integrity
Cognitive Level: Application
Reference: *Wilkinson, J., and Treas, L. (2011). Fundamentals of Nursing: Theory, Concepts & Applications (2nd ed.). Philadelphia, PA: F. A. Davis.*

22. ANSWER: 31.1.
Rationale:

$$0.45 \text{ mEq}/1 \text{ mL} = 14 \text{ mEq}/X = 0.45X = 14 = 14 \div 0.45 = 31.11 \text{ mL} = 31.1 \text{ mL}$$

TEST-TAKING TIP: Always double-check your calculations before providing your answer on the NCLEX-RN examination *and* before administering medication to a client.
Content Area: Maternal Health
Category of Health Alteration: Magnesium Imbalance
Integrated Processes: Nursing Process: Implementation
Client Need: Physiological Integrity
Cognitive Level: Application
Reference: *Beaman, N. (2008). Pharmacology Clear and Simple: A Drug Classifications and Dosage Calculations Approach. Philadelphia, PA: F. A. Davis.*

23. ANSWER: 2.8.
Rationale:

$$16 \text{ lb} \div 2.2 \text{ lb/kg} = 7.27 \text{ kg}$$
$$[240 \text{ mL (volume excreted)} \div 7.27 \text{ kg (current weight)}] \div 12 \text{ hours} = 2.8 \text{ mL/kg/hr}$$

TEST-TAKING TIP: Be sure to convert the infant's weight to kilograms before performing the calculation.
Content Area: Child Health
Category of Health Alteration: Fluid Volume Deficit

Integrated Processes: Nursing Process: Implementation
Client Need: Physiological Integrity
Cognitive Level: Application
Reference: *Beaman, N. (2008). Pharmacology Clear and Simple: A Drug Classifications and Dosage Calculations Approach. Philadelphia, PA: F. A. Davis.*

24. ANSWER: 115.
Rationale:

$$23 \text{ units}/X = 100 \text{ units}/500 \text{ mL} = 100X = 11{,}500 = 11{,}500 \div 100 = 115 \text{ mL/hr}$$

TEST-TAKING TIP: Review your calculations before providing your answer on the NCLEX examination, *and* always have another nurse double-check your calculations before administering high-alert drugs.
Content Area: Adult Health
Category of Health Alteration: Acid-Base Imbalance
Integrated Processes: Nursing Process: Analysis
Client Need: Physiological Integrity
Cognitive Level: Application
Reference: *Beaman, N. (2008). Pharmacology Clear and Simple: A Drug Classifications and Dosage Calculations Approach. Philadelphia, PA: F. A. Davis.*

25. ANSWER: 1, 5.
Rationale:
1. The nurse should associate peripheral edema with the development of right-sided heart failure. Edema develops with changes in normal hydrostatic pressure, such as occur in right-sided heart failure. Right-sided heart failure may be caused by left ventricular failure, right ventricular myocardial infarction, or pulmonary hypertension. In this type of heart failure, the right ventricle cannot empty completely, which causes increased volume and pressure in the venous system and results in jugular venous distention, hepatic enlargement, and peripheral edema.
2. Bilateral crackles are signs of left-sided, not right-sided, heart failure.
3. Hypotension is more often a sign of fluid volume deficit, not fluid volume excess related to right-sided heart failure.
4. An S_4 heart sound is a sign of left-sided, not right-sided, heart failure.
5. The nurse should associate jugular venous distention with the development of right-sided heart failure. Edema develops with changes in normal hydrostatic pressure, such as occur in right-sided heart failure. Right-sided heart failure may be caused by left ventricular failure, right ventricular myocardial infarction, or pulmonary hypertension. In this type of heart failure, the right ventricle cannot empty completely, which causes increased volume and pressure in the venous system and results in jugular venous distention, hepatic enlargement, and peripheral edema.
TEST-TAKING TIP: Review the signs of left-sided and right-sided heart failure if you were unable to answer this question correctly.
Content Area: Adult Health
Category of Health Alteration: Fluid Volume Excess
Integrated Processes: Nursing Process: Assessment
Client Need: Physiological Integrity
Cognitive Level: Analysis
Reference: *Ignatavicius, D., and Workman, M. (2012). Medical-Surgical Nursing: Patient-Centered Collaborative Care (7th ed.). St. Louis, MO: Saunders.*

26. ANSWER: 1, 3.
Rationale:
1. When caring for a client with an acid-base imbalance, the nurse should monitor the client for related electrolyte imbalances, including calcium, potassium, and chloride imbalances. Serum calcium levels usually decrease in both respiratory alkalosis and respiratory acidosis, with a variable response in metabolic acidosis.
2. Sodium levels are not directly affected by acid-base imbalances.
3. When caring for a client with an acid-base imbalance, the nurse should monitor the client for related electrolyte imbalances, including calcium, potassium, and chloride imbalances. Serum potassium levels are elevated in the presence of acidosis, as the body attempts to buffer the decrease in blood pH; conversely, serum potassium levels decrease in alkalosis.
4. Phosphate levels are not directly affected by acid-base imbalances.
5. Magnesium levels are not directly affected by acid-base imbalances.
TEST-TAKING TIP: Recall which electrolytes are directly affected by acid-base imbalances.
Content Area: Adult Health
Category of Health Alteration: Acid-Base Imbalance
Integrated Processes: Nursing Process: Implementation
Client Need: Physiological Integrity
Cognitive Level: Knowledge
Reference: *Ignatavicius, D., and Workman, M. (2012). Medical-Surgical Nursing: Patient-Centered Collaborative Care (7th ed.). St. Louis, MO: Saunders.*

27. ANSWER: 1, 2, 4, 5.
Rationale:
1. The nurse should instruct the parents of a toddler diagnosed with SIADH to weigh the child daily. Weight gain is the primary sign of fluid retention. SIADH is a disorder of the posterior pituitary that causes the excessive production of antidiuretic hormone, resulting in fluid retention and hyponatremia.
2. The nurse should instruct the parents of a toddler diagnosed with SIADH to provide frequent mouth care to keep the mucous membranes moist.
3. The nurse should not instruct the parents of a child diagnosed with SIADH to give the child water to drink. Restriction of free water is necessary to help the body hemoconcentrate sodium and correct dilutional hyponatremia.
4. The nurse should instruct the parents of a toddler diagnosed with SIADH to feed the child a diet that is high in sodium and protein to replace the nutrients commonly lost as a result of SIADH. SIADH is a disorder of the posterior pituitary that causes the excessive production of antidiuretic hormone, resulting in fluid retention and hyponatremia.

5. The nurse should instruct the parents of a toddler diagnosed with SIADH to measure the child's urine output accurately to detect hypervolemia.
6. The nurse should not instruct the parents of a toddler diagnosed with SIADH to allow the child to suck on hard candy if thirsty. Although sucking on hard candy to diminish thirst is appropriate for older children and adults, this is not an appropriate instruction when caring for a toddler.
TEST-TAKING TIP: Recall that SIADH results in fluid retention and hyponatremia. Clients with hyponatremia should always be instructed to restrict their free water intake.
Content Area: Child Health
Category of Health Alteration: Sodium Imbalance
Integrated Processes: Teaching/Learning
Client Need: Physiological Integrity
Cognitive Level: Application
***Reference:** Ward, S. L., and Hisley, S. M. (2011). Maternal-Child Nursing Care: Optimizing Outcomes for Mothers, Children and Families. Philadelphia, PA: F. A. Davis.*

28. ANSWER: 1, 2, 3, 5.
Rationale:
1. The nurse should associate lethargy with hypophosphatemia and hypercalcemia, which accompanies chronic hypophosphatemia.
2. The nurse should associate muscle and joint aches with hypophosphatemia and hypercalcemia, which accompanies chronic hypophosphatemia.
3. The nurse should associate weak peripheral pulses with hypophosphatemia and hypercalcemia, which accompanies chronic hypophosphatemia.
4. A positive Chvostek's sign is indicative of hypocalcemia, which would be related to hyperphosphatemia, not hypophosphatemia.
5. The nurse should associate hypoactive bowel sounds with hypophosphatemia and hypercalcemia, which accompanies chronic hypophosphatemia.
TEST-TAKING TIP: Recall that *hypo*phosphatemia occurs with *hyper*calcemia. Select the options that are signs of hypercalcemia.
Content Area: Adult Health
Category of Health Alteration: Phosphate Imbalance
Integrated Processes: Nursing Process: Assessment
Client Need: Physiological Integrity
Cognitive Level: Application
***Reference:** Berman, A., Snyder, S., Kozier, B., and Erb, G. (2012). Kozier & Erb's Fundamentals of Nursing: Concepts, Process, and Practice (9th ed.). Upper Saddle River, NJ: Pearson.*

29. ANSWER: 5, 3, 2, 1, 4.
Rationale: The nurse who is assessing a child for Chvostek's sign first should explain the procedure to the client's parents. Next, the nurse places a finger just below and in front of the client's ear and taps the client's face just below the zygomatic arch. The nurse should then monitor for twitching of the mouth, nose, or cheek and observe for the appearance of facial twitching on the ipsilateral side. Finally, the nurse should report and document the findings.
TEST-TAKING TIP: First, envision the procedure in your mind's eye. Next, number the actions from first to last.
Content Area: Child Health
Category of Health Alteration: Calcium Imbalance
Integrated Processes: Nursing Process: Assessment
Client Need: Physiological Integrity
Cognitive Level: Application
***Reference:** Ignatavicius, D., and Workman, M. (2012). Medical-Surgical Nursing: Patient-Centered Collaborative Care (7th ed.). St. Louis, MO: Saunders.*

30. ANSWER: 4.
Rationale:
1. According to the National Institutes of Health, children 1 to 3 years old require 700 mg of calcium daily. Students 9 to 18 years old should consume 1,300 mg of calcium per day.
2. According to the National Institutes of Health, children 4 to 8 years old require 1,000 mg of calcium per day. Students 9 to 18 years old should consume 1,300 mg of calcium per day.
3. According to the National Institutes of Health, adults 19 to 50 years old require 1,000 mg of calcium per day. Students 9 to 18 years old should consume 1,300 mg of calcium per day.
4. According to the National Institutes of Health, the nurse should advise students 9 to 18 years old to consume 1,300 mg of calcium per day.
TEST-TAKING TIP: Recall that the most important period for bone formation is age 9 to 18 years.
Content Area: Child Health
Category of Health Alteration: Calcium Imbalance
Integrated Processes: Teaching/Learning
Client Need: Physiological Integrity
Cognitive Level: Knowledge
***Reference:** National Institutes of Health, Office of Dietary Supplements. (Reviewed 2012). Dietary supplement fact sheet: calcium. http://ods.od.nih.gov/factsheets/Calcium-HealthProfessional/.*

31. ANSWER: 1.
Rationale:
1. The nurse should associate these ABG values with uncompensated metabolic alkalosis. The pH of 7.48 reflects *uncompensated* alkalosis because it remains greater than the normal reference range of 7.35 to 7.45; the *increased* HCO_3^- of 30 mEq/L shows that there is too much bicarbonate in the blood, indicating that the imbalance is metabolic in origin; and the high-normal $PaCO_2$ of 44 mm Hg indicates that the lungs have begun to compensate for the alkalotic state by retaining excess carbon dioxide but have not fully compensated for the imbalance.
2. The nurse should associate these ABG values with uncompensated, not compensated, metabolic alkalosis.
3. The nurse should associate these ABG values with uncompensated metabolic alkalosis, not uncompensated respiratory alkalosis.
4. The nurse should associate these ABG values with uncompensated metabolic alkalosis, not compensated respiratory alkalosis.
TEST-TAKING TIP: Recall that the normal reference range for $PaCO_2$ is 35 to 45 mm Hg. Note that a $PaCO_2$ level of 44 mm Hg is in the high-normal range, indicating that respiratory compensation is beginning, whereas the completely abnormal HCO_3^- level indicates that the imbalance is metabolic in origin.
Content Area: Adult Health
Category of Health Alteration: Acid-Base Imbalance

Integrated Processes: Nursing Process: Analysis
Client Need: Physiological Integrity
Cognitive Level: Analysis
Reference: Berman, A., Snyder, S., Kozier, B., and Erb, G. (2012). Kozier & Erb's Fundamentals of Nursing: Concepts, Process, and Practice (9th ed.). Upper Saddle River, NJ: Pearson.

32. ANSWER: 2.
Rationale:
1. The statement "I do not need to worry about my diet because I am taking a fluid pill" is incorrect because a client with fluid volume excess who is taking a diuretic ("fluid pill") must also monitor dietary intake, especially sodium and potassium.
2. The statement "I plan to avoid luncheon meats and canned vegetables" should indicate to the nurse that the client with fluid volume excess understands the education. This client must also verbalize an understanding of how to incorporate a low-sodium diet into his or her lifestyle. Teaching clients about diet therapy is essential to prevent fluid and electrolyte imbalances.
3. The statement "I will notify my health-care provider if I lose weight" is incorrect because weight loss is a desired effect in a client with fluid volume excess; weight *gain* should be reported to the health-care provider.
4. The statement "I should restrict the amount of fresh vegetables in my diet" is incorrect; this client with fluid volume excess should not restrict fresh vegetables and should choose fresh, instead of canned, vegetables.
TEST-TAKING TIP: Review the goals for a client with fluid volume excess, and rule out options that do not correspond with these goals.
Content Area: Adult Health
Category of Health Alteration: Fluid Volume Excess
Integrated Processes: Teaching/Learning
Client Need: Physiological Integrity
Cognitive Level: Analysis
Reference: Williams, L., and Hopper, P. (2011). Understanding Medical-Surgical Nursing (4th ed.). Philadelphia, PA: F. A. Davis.

33. ANSWER: 2.
Rationale:
1. When caring for a client diagnosed with hypophosphatemia, the nurse should anticipate a decreased serum phosphorus level and an elevated serum calcium level (hypercalcemia). A serum calcium level of 9.5 mg/dL is within the normal reference range.
2. When caring for a client diagnosed with hypophosphatemia, the nurse should anticipate a decreased serum phosphorus level and an elevated serum calcium level (hypercalcemia), as reflected by the serum calcium level of 12 mg/dL. Because of the inverse relationship between phosphate and calcium, a *decrease* in serum phosphorus results in an *increase* in serum calcium. The normal total serum calcium level is 8.2 to 10.2 mg/dL (adults). (Reference ranges vary by laboratory.) The normal serum phosphorus level in adults is 2.5 to 4.5 mg/dL (3.0 to 4.5 mEq/L).
3. When caring for a client diagnosed with hypophosphatemia, the nurse should anticipate a decreased serum phosphorus level and an elevated serum calcium level (hypercalcemia). A serum phosphorus level of 3.5 mg/dL is within the normal reference range.
4. When caring for a client diagnosed with hypophosphatemia, the nurse should anticipate a decreased serum phosphorus level and an elevated serum calcium level (hypercalcemia). A serum phosphorus level of 4.7 mg/dL is elevated (hyperphosphatemia).
TEST-TAKING TIP: Memorize the normal reference ranges for electrolytes. Recall that serum phosphorus and serum calcium levels are inversely proportionate.
Content Area: Adult Health
Category of Health Alteration: Phosphate Imbalance
Integrated Processes: Nursing Process: Analysis
Client Need: Physiological Integrity
Cognitive Level: Application
Reference: Ignatavicius, D., and Workman, M. (2012). Medical-Surgical Nursing: Patient-Centered Collaborative Care (7th ed.). St. Louis, MO: Saunders.

34. ANSWER: 119.
Rationale:

$$145 \text{ lb} \div 2.2 \text{ kg} = 65.9 \text{ kg}$$
$$65.9 \text{ kg} \times 3 \text{ mEq/kg} = 197.7 \text{ mEq}$$
$$197.7 \text{ mEq} \times 0.6 \text{ mEq/mL} = 118.62 \text{ mL} = 119 \text{ mL}$$

TEST-TAKING TIP: Read the question carefully. Disregard information that does not pertain to the calculation.
Content Area: Adult Health
Category of Health Alteration: Acid-Base Imbalance
Integrated Processes: Nursing Process: Analysis
Client Need: Physiological Integrity
Cognitive Level: Application
Reference: Deglin, J. H., Vallerand, A. H., and Sanoski, C. A. (2013). Davis's Drug Guide for Nurses (13th ed.). Philadelphia, PA: F. A. Davis.

35. ANSWER: 125.
Rationale: Use the following formula to calculate the dose:

$$\text{Volume} \times \text{Drop factor/Time} = \text{Rate}$$
$$500 \text{ mL} \times 30 \text{ gtt/60 min} = 15{,}000/60 = 250 \text{ mL/hr} \div 2 \text{ hours} = 125 \text{ mL/hr}$$

TEST-TAKING TIP: Read the question carefully; note that the solution is to be infused over 2 hours.
Content Area: Adult Health
Category of Health Alteration: Potassium Imbalance
Integrated Processes: Nursing Process: Implementation
Client Need: Physiological Integrity
Cognitive Level: Application
Reference: Deglin, J. H., Vallerand, A. H., and Sanoski, C. A. (2013). Davis's Drug Guide for Nurses (13th ed.). Philadelphia, PA: F. A. Davis.

36. ANSWER: 34.
Rationale:

$$7.5 \text{ lb} \div 2.2 \text{ lb/kg} = 3.41 \text{ kg}$$
$$3.41 \text{ kg} \times 10 \text{ mL} = 34.1 = 34 \text{ mL}$$

TEST-TAKING TIP: Recall that there are 2.2 lb in each kilogram.
Content Area: Child Health
Category of Health Alteration: Fluid Volume Deficit
Integrated Processes: Nursing Process: Implementation
Client Need: Physiological Integrity
Cognitive Level: Application
Reference: Beaman, N. (2008). Pharmacology Clear and Simple: A Drug Classifications and Dosage Calculations Approach. Philadelphia, PA: F. A. Davis.

37. ANSWER: 1.

Rationale:

1. **The nurse should associate the client's manifestations and current medication regimen with Lab Report A, indicating respiratory acidosis resulting from hypoventilation (respiratory rate of 12 breaths per minute) secondary to respiratory depression caused by narcotic administration. The client's pH (7.21) is less than 7.35 and the $PaCO_2$ level (66 mm Hg) is increased, indicating that the client is retaining carbon dioxide. The normal HCO_3^- value (22 mEq/L) indicates that the kidneys have not yet begun to compensate for the respiratory origin of the acidosis.**
2. Lab Report B indicates metabolic acidosis.
3. Lab Report C is within the normal reference range.
4. Lab Report D indicates respiratory alkalosis.

TEST-TAKING TIP: Recognize that the administration of narcotics can cause respiratory depression, potentially leading to respiratory acidosis.

Content Area: Adult Health
Category of Health Alteration: Acid-Base Imbalance
Integrated Processes: Nursing Process: Analysis
Client Need: Physiological Integrity
Cognitive Level: Analysis
Reference: *Ignatavicius, D., and Workman, M. (2012). Medical-Surgical Nursing: Patient-Centered Collaborative Care (7th ed.). St. Louis, MO: Saunders.*

38. ANSWER: 4.

Rationale:

1. Hypermagnesemia is a potentially dangerous side effect of magnesium oxide (Mag-Ox 400). Constipation is associated with hypomagnesemia, not hypermagnesemia.
2. Hypermagnesemia is a potentially dangerous side effect of magnesium oxide (Mag-Ox 400). Tachycardia is associated with hypomagnesemia, not hypermagnesemia.
3. Hypermagnesemia is a potentially dangerous side effect of magnesium oxide (Mag-Ox 400). Hypertension is associated with hypomagnesemia, not hypermagnesemia.
4. **Hypermagnesemia is a potentially dangerous side effect of magnesium oxide (Mag-Ox 400). The nurse should assess the client for deep tendon hyporeflexia because it is a sign of hypermagnesemia.**

TEST-TAKING TIP: Recall that supplementation of any electrolyte increases the client's risk for excessive intake of that substance. Choose the option that is a manifestation of the opposite imbalance being treated (treatment for hypomagnesemia may result in hypermagnesemia).

Content Area: Adult Health
Category of Health Alteration: Magnesium Imbalance
Integrated Processes: Nursing Process: Assessment
Client Need: Physiological Integrity
Cognitive Level: Application
Reference: *Deglin, J. H., Vallerand, A. H., and Sanoski, C. A. (2013). Davis's Drug Guide for Nurses (13th ed.). Philadelphia, PA: F. A. Davis.*

39. ANSWER: 2.

Rationale:

1. The nurse should interpret that the infant's urine output is within normal limits, not that the output is low and the infant is still dehydrated.
2. **The nurse should interpret that the infant's urine output is within normal limits. The normal urine output for children is 1 to 2 mL/kg/hr, so a normal output for an infant who weighs 4 kg would be 4 to 8 mL/hr. This 4-kg infant has voided 170 mL over 24 hours, which equals 7.08 mL/hr (170 mL/24 hours).**
3. The nurse should interpret that the infant's urine output is within normal limits, not that the output is high and the infant is at risk for fluid overload.
4. It is essential that the nurse interpret these data and report abnormal findings to the health-care provider as necessary.

TEST-TAKING TIP: Recall that normal urine output for children is 1 to 2 mL/kg/hr. Assessment of intake and output is a nursing responsibility.

Content Area: Child Health
Category of Health Alteration: Fluid Volume Deficit
Integrated Processes: Nursing Process: Implementation
Client Need: Physiological Integrity
Cognitive Level: Application
Reference: *Ward, S. L., and Hisley, S. M. (2011). Maternal-Child Nursing Care: Optimizing Outcomes for Mothers, Children and Families. Philadelphia, PA: F. A. Davis.*

40. ANSWER: 2.

Rationale:

1. This client, who has been experiencing vomiting and diarrhea for several days and is now lethargic and hypotensive, is showing signs of fluid volume deficit (FVD) and hyponatremia. Monitoring and recording intake and output are necessary to evaluate the client's fluid volume status. This order should not be questioned.
2. **This client, who has been experiencing vomiting and diarrhea for several days and is now lethargic and hypotensive, is showing signs of FVD and hyponatremia. The nurse should question the health-care provider's order to administer IV 3% sodium chloride solution (a hypertonic solution), which would worsen the client's FVD and potentially correct the client's hyponatremia too rapidly, causing cellular lysis and destruction.**
3. This client, who has been experiencing vomiting and diarrhea for several days and is now lethargic and hypotensive, is showing signs of FVD and hyponatremia. Normal saline solution (0.9% saline) is an appropriate intervention because it would correct the client's FVD and hyponatremia. This order should not be questioned.
4. This client, who has been experiencing vomiting and diarrhea for several days and is now lethargic and hypotensive, is showing signs of FVD and hyponatremia. Weighing the client daily is necessary to evaluate the client's fluid volume status. This order should not be questioned.

TEST-TAKING TIP: The key words are "Which order should the nurse question?" Select the option that is an incorrect order.

Content Area: Older Adult Health
Category of Health Alteration: Sodium Imbalance
Integrated Processes: Nursing Process: Analysis
Client Need: Physiological Integrity
Cognitive Level: Analysis
Reference: *Williams, L., and Hopper, P. (2011). Understanding Medical-Surgical Nursing (4th ed.). Philadelphia, PA: F. A. Davis.*

41. ANSWER: 2.

Rationale:

1. The nurse should correctly identify that a client with seasonal flu who has been vomiting for several days is experiencing fluid volume deficit (FVD) and metabolic alkalosis, not metabolic acidosis.

2. The nurse should correctly identify that a client with seasonal flu who has been vomiting for several days is experiencing FVD and metabolic alkalosis. The client has lost a significant amount of body fluid and gastric acid through vomiting, causing a decrease in hydrogen ions in the body and resulting in an increase in serum pH (alkalosis) that is metabolic in origin.

3. The nurse should correctly identify that a client with seasonal flu who has been vomiting for several days is experiencing FVD and metabolic alkalosis, not fluid volume excess and respiratory acidosis.

4. The nurse should correctly identify that a client with seasonal flu who has been vomiting for several days is experiencing FVD and metabolic alkalosis, not fluid volume excess and respiratory alkalosis.

TEST-TAKING TIP: Use the process of elimination: rule out options that include fluid volume excess, because vomiting causes dehydration, and exclude options that include respiratory-related imbalances, because there is no indication of impaired respiratory function.

Content Area: Adult Health

Category of Health Alteration: Acid-Base Imbalance, Fluid Volume Deficit

Integrated Processes: Nursing Process: Assessment

Client Need: Physiological Integrity

Cognitive Level: Application

Reference: *Berman, A., Snyder, S., Kozier, B., and Erb, G. (2012). Kozier & Erb's Fundamentals of Nursing: Concepts, Process, and Practice (9th ed.). Upper Saddle River, NJ: Pearson.*

42. ANSWER: 2.

Rationale:

1. When calculating a client's intake and output, the nurse should add irrigation fluid for a percutaneous endoscopic gastrostomy tube to the client's total intake, not total output.

2. When calculating a client's intake and output, the nurse should add irrigation fluid for a percutaneous endoscopic gastrostomy tube to the client's total intake. To measure fluid intake, the nurse should record each fluid item *taken in* by the client, including oral fluids, ice chips, foods that are liquid or tend to become a liquid at room temperature, tube feedings, parenteral fluids, IV medications, and catheter or tube irrigation fluids. To measure fluid output, the nurse should record urine output, vomitus, and liquid feces, and tube drainage, such as gastric or intestinal drainage, wound drainage, or draining fistulas.

3. When calculating a client's intake and output, the nurse should add irrigation fluid for a percutaneous endoscopic gastrostomy tube to the client's total intake, not deduct it from total output.

4. When calculating a client's intake and output, the nurse should add irrigation fluid for a percutaneous endoscopic gastrostomy tube to the client's total intake, not deduct it from total intake.

TEST-TAKING TIP: Read each option carefully. Use the process of elimination to rule out incorrect options.

Content Area: Adult Health

Category of Health Alteration: Fluid Volume Deficit

Integrated Processes: Nursing Process: Implementation

Client Need: Physiological Integrity

Cognitive Level: Comprehension

Reference: *Berman, A., Snyder, S., Kozier, B., and Erb, G. (2012). Kozier & Erb's Fundamentals of Nursing: Concepts, Process, and Practice (9th ed.). Upper Saddle River, NJ: Pearson.*

43. ANSWER: 3.

Rationale:

1. Older adults have *less* efficient temperature regulation, increasing their risk for fluid imbalance.

2. Older adults have a *decreased* glomerular filtration rate, increasing their risk for fluid imbalance.

3. The nurse should associate a decreased perception of thirst with fluid imbalance in an older adult client. Older adults also have less efficient temperature regulation, a decreased glomerular filtration rate, and a lower percentage of total body water than younger adults, increasing their risk for fluid imbalance.

4. Older adults have a *lower* percentage of total body water than younger adults, increasing their risk for fluid imbalance.

TEST-TAKING TIP: *Recall that older adults experience a "slowing down" or "decrease" in functioning and have less body water than younger adults or children.*

Content Area: Older Adult Health

Category of Health Alteration: Fluid Volume Excess

Integrated Processes: Nursing Process: Implementation

Client Need: Physiological Integrity

Cognitive Level: Application

Reference: *Lemone, P., and Burke, K. (2010). Medical-Surgical Nursing: Critical Thinking in Client Care (5th ed.). Upper Saddle River, NJ: Pearson Prentice Hall.*

44. ANSWER: 4,002.

Rationale:

2 tablets × 3 times per day = 6 tablets per day
667 mg × 6 = 4,002 mg

TEST-TAKING TIP: *The key words are "three times per day." Read the question carefully to answer correctly.*

Content Area: Adult Health

Category of Health Alteration: Phosphate Imbalance

Integrated Processes: Nursing Process: Implementation

Client Need: Physiological Integrity

Cognitive Level: Application

Reference: *Beaman, N. (2008). Pharmacology Clear and Simple: A Drug Classifications and Dosage Calculations Approach. Philadelphia, PA: F. A. Davis.*

45. ANSWER: 24.

Rationale:

Anion gap = Serum sodium - (Serum chloride + Serum bicarbonate)
Anion gap = 146 - (104 + 18) = 146 - 122 = 24 mEq/L

TEST-TAKING TIP: *When doing mathematical calculations, perform them in the correct order. Add the values in parentheses before subtracting in this calculation.*

Content Area: Adult Health
Category of Health Alteration: Acid-Base Imbalance
Integrated Processes: Nursing Process: Planning
Client Need: Physiological Integrity
Cognitive Level: Comprehension
Reference: Van Leeuwen, A. M., Poelhuis-Leth, D., and Bladh, M. (2011). Davis's Comprehensive Handbook of Laboratory and Diagnostic Tests With Nursing Implications (4th ed.). Philadelphia, PA: F. A. Davis.

46. ANSWER: 1.
Rationale:

100 mg ÷ 50 mg/tablet = 2 tablets per day
2 tablets ÷ 2 doses = 1 tablet every 12 hours (twice daily)

TEST-TAKING TIP: Calculate the total number of tablets daily and divide by 2. The key words are "two divided doses" and "every 12 hours."
Content Area: Adult Health
Category of Health Alteration: Fluid Volume Excess
Integrated Processes: Nursing Process: Implementation
Client Need: Physiological Integrity
Cognitive Level: Application
Reference: Beaman, N. (2008). Pharmacology Clear and Simple: A Drug Classifications and Dosage Calculations Approach. Philadelphia, PA: F. A. Davis.

47. ANSWER: 1, 5.
Rationale:
1. The nurse should identify that a history of emphysema places the client at risk for respiratory acidosis. Emphysema results in decreased alveolar-capillary diffusion, leading to poor gas exchange and carbon dioxide retention.
2. Multiple sclerosis alone would not cause respiratory acidosis.
3. Coronary artery disease alone would not cause respiratory acidosis.
4. Type 2 diabetes mellitus is a risk factor for metabolic acidosis, not respiratory acidosis.
5. The nurse should identify that the use of methadone (a synthetic narcotic similar to morphine sulfate) places the client at risk for respiratory acidosis. Opioids cause respiratory depression by decreasing the function of the brainstem neurons that trigger breathing movements.
TEST-TAKING TIP: Read the question carefully. Select the options that would affect the client's respiratory function because the question is asking about respiratory acidosis.
Content Area: Adult Health
Category of Health Alteration: Acid-Base Imbalance
Integrated Processes: Nursing Process: Assessment
Client Need: Physiological Integrity
Cognitive Level: Application
Reference: Ignatavicius, D., and Workman, M. (2012). Medical-Surgical Nursing: Patient-Centered Collaborative Care (7th ed.). St. Louis, MO: Saunders.

48. ANSWER: 2, 3, 4.
Rationale:
1. The nurse should not stop the transfusion because signs of a transfusion reaction are not noted.
2. The nurse should immediately slow the transfusion. The development of bilateral lung crackles is a sign of fluid volume excess (FVE) and must be treated appropriately.
3. The nurse should immediately assess the client's blood pressure and other vital signs. The development of bilateral lung crackles is a sign of FVE and must be treated appropriately.
4. The nurse should notify the primary health-care provider. The development of bilateral lung crackles is a sign of FVE and must be treated appropriately.
5. Continuing the transfusion at the current rate would worsen the client's developing FVE.
TEST-TAKING TIP: Remember that client safety is always a priority. Select the actions the nurse should take to maintain client safety in this situation.
Content Area: Older Adult Health
Category of Health Alteration: Fluid Volume Excess
Integrated Processes: Nursing Process: Implementation
Client Need: Physiological Integrity
Cognitive Level: Application
Reference: Ignatavicius, D., and Workman, M. (2012). Medical-Surgical Nursing: Patient-Centered Collaborative Care (7th ed.). St. Louis, MO: Saunders.

49. ANSWER: 1, 2, 3, 4.
Rationale:
1. The nurse should associate bradycardia with the development of hyperkalemia.
2. The nurse should associate hypotension with the development of hyperkalemia.
3. The nurse should associate paresthesias with the development of hyperkalemia.
4. The nurse should associate peaked T waves with the development of hyperkalemia.
5. Prominent U waves are a classic sign of hypokalemia, not hyperkalemia.
TEST-TAKING TIP: Recall that cardiovascular changes are the most common effects of hyperkalemia.
Content Area: Adult Health
Category of Health Alteration: Potassium Imbalance
Integrated Processes: Nursing Process: Assessment
Client Need: Physiological Integrity
Cognitive Level: Application
Reference: Ignatavicius, D., and Workman, M. (2012). Medical-Surgical Nursing: Patient-Centered Collaborative Care (7th ed.). St. Louis, MO: Saunders.

50. ANSWER: 1. 2, 5.
Rationale:
1. The nurse should include fall precautions when planning care for a client with severe hypernatremia. Fall precautions should be implemented because muscles, which twitch in mild hypernatremia, become progressively weaker as serum sodium levels increase.
2. The nurse should include seizure precautions when planning care for a client with severe hypernatremia. Seizures are the most serious complication and can lead to traumatic injury, asphyxiation, and death.
3. Contact precautions are unnecessary for clients with hypernatremia but should be used for clients with specific infectious processes.
4. Isolation precautions are unnecessary for clients with hypernatremia but should be used for clients with specific infectious processes.

5. The nurse should include aspiration precautions when planning care for a client with severe hypernatremia. Aspiration precautions should be implemented because seizure activity and muscle weakness both increase the client's risk for aspiration.

TEST-TAKING TIP: The key words are "severe hypernatremia." Recall that neuromuscular irritability is associated with increased serum sodium levels, and muscles lose the ability to respond to stimuli as sodium levels increase.

Content Area: *Adult Health*

Category of Health Alteration: *Sodium Imbalance*

Integrated Processes: *Nursing Process: Planning*

Client Need: *Safe and Effective Care Environment*

Cognitive Level: *Analysis*

Reference: *Ignatavicius, D., and Workman, M. (2012). Medical-Surgical Nursing: Patient-Centered Collaborative Care (7th ed.). St. Louis, MO: Saunders.*

51. ANSWER: 4.

Rationale:

1. The electrocardiogram strip shows torsades de pointes, an unusual variant of ventricular tachycardia. Although calcium abnormalities may cause cardiac dysrhythmias such as ventricular tachycardia and ventricular fibrillation, hypomagnesemia is usually the cause of torsades de pointes.

2. The electrocardiogram strip shows torsades de pointes, an unusual variant of ventricular tachycardia. Hyponatremia is not usually associated with ventricular dysrhythmias.

3. The electrocardiogram strip shows torsades de pointes, an unusual variant of ventricular tachycardia. Hypochloremia is not usually associated with ventricular dysrhythmias.

4. The nurse should suspect that the client is experiencing hypomagnesemia because the electrocardiogram strip shows torsades de pointes, an unusual variant of ventricular tachycardia. Although potassium, calcium, and magnesium abnormalities may cause cardiac dysrhythmias such as ventricular tachycardia and ventricular fibrillation, hypomagnesemia is usually the cause of torsades de pointes.

TEST-TAKING TIP: Associate hypomagnesemia with ventricular dysrhythmias and, in particular, with torsades de pointes.

Content Area: *Adult Health*

Category of Health Alteration: *Magnesium Imbalance*

Integrated Processes: *Nursing Process: Evaluation*

Client Need: *Physiological Integrity*

Cognitive Level: *Application*

Reference: *Jones, S. (2010). ECG Notes: Interpretation and Management Guide (2nd ed.). Philadelphia, PA: F. A. Davis.*

52. ANSWER: 1.

Rationale:

1. The nurse should administer digoxin to treat the client's atrial fibrillation and to treat the client's heart failure by increasing cardiac output. An increase in cardiac output promotes diuresis, reducing fluid volume excess. The therapeutic effects of digoxin include increased cardiac output (positive inotropic effect) and slowing of the heart rate (negative chronotropic effect).

2. Digoxin does not increase potassium.

3. The therapeutic effects of digoxin include slowing, not increasing, the heart rate.

4. Digoxin does not decrease urinary output.

TEST-TAKING TIP: Recall that the need to prevent fluid volume excess by increasing cardiac output is associated with a condition such as systolic heart failure.

Content Area: *Adult Health*

Category of Health Alteration: *Fluid Volume Excess*

Integrated Processes: *Nursing Process: Implementation*

Client Need: *Physiological Integrity*

Cognitive Level: *Application*

Reference: *Deglin, J. H., Vallerand, A. H., and Sanoski, C. A. (2013). Davis's Drug Guide for Nurses (13th ed.). Philadelphia, PA: F. A. Davis.*

53. ANSWER: 2.

Rationale:

1. A 0.45% saline solution would replace minimal sodium, increasing the risk of exacerbating the client's hyponatremia.

2. The nurse should anticipate an order for 0.9% saline solution. A client with hypovolemic hyponatremia requires the replacement of sodium and fluid. The best choice in this case is 0.9% (normal) saline solution because it replaces both.

3. A 3% saline solution replaces primarily sodium, leaving the client at risk for hypernatremia because the fluid deficit still exists.

4. Dextrose 5% in water would replace no sodium at all, increasing the risk of exacerbating the client's hyponatremia.

TEST-TAKING TIP: Select an isotonic IV solution when replacing both fluid volume and sodium.

Content Area: *Adult Health*

Category of Health Alteration: *Sodium Imbalance*

Integrated Processes: *Nursing Process: Implementation*

Client Need: *Physiological Integrity*

Cognitive Level: *Application*

Reference: *Williams, L., and Hopper, P. (2011). Understanding Medical-Surgical Nursing (4th ed.). Philadelphia, PA: F. A. Davis.*

54. ANSWER: 3.

Rationale:

1. Novolin N, also known as NPH insulin, is an intermediate-acting insulin that is administered subcutaneously and has a duration of 18 to 24 hours.

2. Humulin N, also known as NPH insulin, is an intermediate-acting insulin that is administered subcutaneously and has a duration of 18 to 24 hours.

3. The nurse should identify Humulin R as the insulin of choice for this client because this is regular insulin, which is the only type of insulin that can be administered intravenously via continuous infusion to quickly correct the hyperglycemia associated with diabetic ketoacidosis.

4. Novolin 70/30, also known as NPH/regular insulin, is a combination of intermediate-acting and short-acting insulin that is administered subcutaneously and provides a rapid onset and constant concentration over a 24-hour period.

TEST-TAKING TIP: Become familiar with the various insulin preparations and the onset, peak, and duration of each to help you select the correct insulin for a specific indication.

Content Area: *Adult Health*

Category of Health Alteration: *Acid-Base Imbalance*

Integrated Processes: *Nursing Process: Implementation*

Client Need: *Physiological Integrity*

Cognitive Level: *Application*

Reference: *Ignatavicius, D., and Workman, M. (2012). Medical-Surgical Nursing: Patient-Centered Collaborative Care (7th ed.). St. Louis, MO: Saunders.*

55. ANSWER: 1.

Rationale:

1. The nurse should recognize a decrease in blood pressure (82/58 mm Hg) and an increase in pulse rate (115 bpm) as indicative of FVD. The normal accepted adult range is 100 to 120 mm Hg for systolic blood pressure and 60 to 80 mm Hg for diastolic blood pressure. The normal resting adult heart rate ranges from 60 to 100 bpm. The normal adult respiratory rate is 12 to 20 breaths per minute.

2. These vital signs are all within normal limits.

3. These vital signs are all within normal limits.

4. A blood pressure of 140/70 mm Hg would be associated with fluid volume excess, not FVD. The pulse and respiratory rates are within normal limits.

TEST-TAKING TIP: Recall that the signs of FVD include a decrease in blood pressure, an increase in heart and respiratory rates, and a decrease in urine output.

Content Area: Adult Health
Category of Health Alteration: Fluid Volume Deficit
Integrated Processes: Nursing Process: Assessment
Client Need: Physiological Integrity
Cognitive Level: Application

Reference: *Wilkinson, J., and Treas, L. (2011). Fundamentals of Nursing: Theory, Concepts & Applications (2nd ed.). Philadelphia, PA: F. A. Davis.*

56. ANSWER: 2.

Rationale:

1. *Hypo*parathyroidism is associated with *hypo*calcemia, not *hyper*calcemia.

2. The nurse should associate the development of *hyper*calcemia with *hyper*parathyroidism. Hyperparathyroidism is the most common cause of hypercalcemia. Excess parathyroid hormone (PTH) causes serum calcium levels to increase because PTH releases free calcium from bone storage sites and decreases the kidneys' excretion of calcium.

3. *Hyper*thyroidism, not *hypo*thyroidism, causes elevated serum calcium levels. Excess circulating thyroid hormone stimulates bone resorption and bone demineralization, resulting in hypercalcemia.

4. *Hypo*phosphatemia, not *hyper*phosphatemia, causes *hyper*calcemia. A decrease in serum phosphorus levels results in an increase in serum calcium levels (an inverse relationship).

TEST-TAKING TIP: The key word is "hypercalcemia." Think about how each condition would affect a client's serum calcium level.

Content Area: Adult Health
Category of Health Alteration: Calcium Imbalance
Integrated Processes: Nursing Process: Analysis
Client Need: Physiological Integrity
Cognitive Level: Application

Reference: *Ignatavicius, D., and Workman, M. (2012). Medical-Surgical Nursing: Patient-Centered Collaborative Care (7th ed.). St. Louis, MO: Saunders.*

57. ANSWER: 1.

Rationale:

1. The nurse should associate tetany with metabolic alkalosis. Many symptoms of alkalosis are a result of the hypocalcemia and hypokalemia that usually accompany this imbalance. Metabolic alkalosis is also characterized by a decreased respiratory effort secondary to skeletal muscle weakness, whereas respiratory alkalosis is characterized by an increased rate and depth of respirations.

2. Lethargy is associated with acidosis, not alkalosis.

3. Hyporeflexia is associated with acidosis, not alkalosis.

4. Metabolic alkalosis is characterized by a *decreased* respiratory effort secondary to skeletal muscle weakness, whereas respiratory alkalosis is characterized by an increased rate and depth of respirations.

TEST-TAKING TIP: Recall that hypocalcemia and hypokalemia accompany metabolic alkalosis. Select options that are signs or symptoms of hypocalcemia and hypokalemia.

Content Area: Adult Health
Category of Health Alteration: Acid-Base Imbalance
Integrated Processes: Nursing Process: Assessment
Client Need: Physiological Integrity
Cognitive Level: Application

Reference: *Ignatavicius, D., and Workman, M. (2012). Medical-Surgical Nursing: Patient-Centered Collaborative Care (7th ed.). St. Louis, MO: Saunders.*

58. ANSWER: 1, 2, 4.

Rationale:

1. The nurse should recognize increased blood pressure as a manifestation of FVE. The client's end-stage renal failure causes decreased urinary output, which results in fluid retention. FVE is characterized by changes in vital signs, such as increased blood pressure, and by increased weight.

2. The nurse should recognize decreased urinary output as a manifestation of FVE. The client's end-stage renal failure causes decreased urinary output, which results in fluid retention.

3. Decreased fluid intake is usually related to fluid volume deficit (FVD), not FVE.

4. The nurse should recognize increased weight as a manifestation of FVE. The client's end-stage renal failure causes decreased urinary output, which results in fluid retention. FVE is characterized by changes in vital signs, such as increased blood pressure, and by increased weight.

5. Decreased weight is often related to FVD, not FVE.

TEST-TAKING TIP: Use the process of elimination by ruling out options associated with FVD rather than FVE.

Content Area: Adult Health
Category of Health Alteration: Fluid Volume Excess
Integrated Processes: Nursing Process: Implementation
Client Need: Physiological Integrity
Cognitive Level: Application

Reference: *Wilkinson, J., and Treas, L. (2011). Fundamentals of Nursing: Theory, Concepts & Applications (2nd ed.). Philadelphia, PA: F. A. Davis.*

59. ANSWER: 1.

Rationale:

1. The nurse should suspect that the client is experiencing hyperkalemia because this rhythm strip shows peaked, tented T waves, which are a classic ECG change associated with serum potassium levels greater than 5.0 mEq/L.

2. Hypercalcemia results in shortened Q-T intervals, not peaked, tented T waves.

3. Hypophosphatemia results in shortened Q-T intervals, not peaked, tented T waves.

4. Hypomagnesemia results in torsades de pointes and premature ventricular contractions, not peaked, tented T waves.

TEST-TAKING TIP: Recall that peaked T waves, caused by excitable tissues that are more sensitive to stimuli, are a classic sign of hyperkalemia.

Content Area: Adult Health
Category of Health Alteration: Potassium Imbalance
Integrated Processes: Nursing Process: Analysis
Client Need: Physiological Integrity
Cognitive Level: Application
***Reference:** Ignatavicius, D., and Workman, M. (2012). Medical-Surgical Nursing: Patient-Centered Collaborative Care (7th ed.). St. Louis, MO: Saunders.*

60. ANSWER: 2.

Rationale:

1. The client's serum potassium level is within normal limits. It does not suggest hypokalemia.
2. **The nurse should interpret that the client's serum sodium level is decreased, suggesting hyponatremia. Lethargy, irritability, confusion, and vomiting are all signs of hyponatremia.**
3. The client's serum glucose level is within normal limits. It does not reflect hyperglycemia.
4. The client's low-grade temperature is most likely related to nothing-by-mouth status before the surgical procedure and general anesthesia. An oral temperature of 100.5°F (38°C) or greater would indicate infection.

TEST-TAKING TIP: Review the chart carefully, and identify abnormal findings. Think about how these findings would relate to the clinical scenario provided. You must memorize the normal ranges for sodium, potassium, and glucose for the NCLEX-RN examination.

Content Area: Child Health
Category of Health Alteration: Sodium Imbalance
Integrated Processes: Nursing Process: Assessment
Client Need: Physiological Integrity
Cognitive Level: Analysis
***Reference:** Ward, S. L., and Hisley, S. M. (2011). Maternal-Child Nursing Care: Optimizing Outcomes for Mothers, Children and Families. Philadelphia, PA: F. A. Davis.*

61. ANSWER: 2.

Rationale:

1. The nurse should associate the client's manifestations with the development of metabolic alkalosis, not metabolic acidosis.
2. **The nurse should associate the client's manifestations with the development of metabolic alkalosis. Risk factors for metabolic alkalosis include excessive nasogastric tube drainage, which this client is experiencing. Many symptoms of alkalosis, including confusion, respiratory weakness, and positive Trousseau's sign, are a result of the electrolyte imbalances that accompany this acid-base imbalance.**
3. The nurse should associate the client's manifestations with the development of metabolic alkalosis, not respiratory acidosis.
4. The nurse should associate the client's manifestations with the development of metabolic alkalosis, not respiratory alkalosis. The client is not exhibiting hyperventilation, the only cause of respiratory alkalosis.

TEST-TAKING TIP: Review the risk factors for acid-base imbalances to determine which imbalance a specific client is at increased risk for. Rule out options that do not cause the manifestations the client is experiencing.

Content Area: Adult Health
Category of Health Alteration: Acid-Base Imbalance
Integrated Processes: Nursing Process: Assessment
Client Need: Physiological Integrity
Cognitive Level: Application
***Reference:** Ignatavicius, D., and Workman, M. (2012). Medical-Surgical Nursing: Patient-Centered Collaborative Care (7th ed.). St. Louis, MO: Saunders.*

62. ANSWER: 1.

Rationale:

1. **The nurse should identify a urine output of 20 mL/hr as indicative of FVD. The obligatory urine output (minimal amount required to excrete waste products from the body) for an unstressed adult is 30 mL/hr; this rate may be higher in clients who are physically stressed. The average adult urine output is 35 to 40 mL/hr. Dehydration should be considered in any adult with a urine output of less than 30 mL/hr.**
2. A client with a urine output of 30 mL/hr would warrant close monitoring for the potential development of FVD but is not manifesting FVD at present.
3. Urine output of 40 mL/hr is average and does not indicate FVD. The average adult urine output is 35 to 40 mL/hr.
4. Urine output of 50 mL/hr is above average and does not indicate FVD. The average adult urine output is 35 to 40 mL/hr.

TEST-TAKING TIP: Recall that the signs of FVD include a decrease in blood pressure, an increase in heart and respiratory rates, and a *decrease* in urine output.

Content Area: Adult Health
Category of Health Alteration: Fluid Volume Deficit
Integrated Processes: Nursing Process: Assessment
Client Need: Physiological Integrity
Cognitive Level: Application
***Reference:** Williams, L., and Hopper, P. (2011). Understanding Medical-Surgical Nursing (4th ed.). Philadelphia, PA: F. A. Davis.*

63. ANSWER: 4.

Rationale:

1. Potassium chloride may or may not be indicated for this client, depending on the serum potassium level; it is not the priority intervention.
2. Regular insulin would be used to treat diabetic ketoacidosis, not respiratory acidosis.
3. Sodium bicarbonate therapy would be indicated only in severe *metabolic* acidosis.
4. **The nurse caring for a client admitted with respiratory acidosis secondary to accidental oxycodone (OxyContin) overdose should determine that the administration of naloxone hydrochloride is the priority intervention for this client. Naloxone hydrochloride is an opioid antagonist indicated for the complete or partial reversal of opioid depression, including respiratory depression severe enough to cause respiratory acidosis.**

TEST-TAKING TIP: Select the option that would treat the underlying cause of the acid-base imbalance.

Content Area: Adult Health
Category of Health Alteration: Acid-Base Imbalance
Integrated Processes: Nursing Process: Assessment
Client Need: Physiological Integrity
Cognitive Level: Application
Reference: Berman, A., Snyder, S., Kozier, B., and Erb, G. (2012). Kozier & Erb's Fundamentals of Nursing: Concepts, Process, and Practice (9th ed.). Upper Saddle River, NJ: Pearson.

64. ANSWER: 2.
Rationale:
1. Hypertension is a sign of hypernatremia, but it is not as serious as seizures.
2. The nurse should identify seizure activity as the most serious complication associated with hypernatremia. Seizure activity is related to neuromuscular irritability caused by elevated serum sodium levels. Seizures may lead to aspiration, asphyxiation, coma, and death. The other options are signs of hypernatremia but are not as serious as seizures.
3. Muscle cramps and twitching are signs of hypernatremia, but they are not as serious as seizures.
4. A decreased level of consciousness is a sign of hypernatremia, but it is not as serious as seizures.
TEST-TAKING TIP: The key words are "most serious." Select the most life-threatening manifestation by asking yourself, "Which is going to cause my client the most harm the quickest?"
Content Area: Adult Health
Category of Health Alteration: Sodium Imbalance
Integrated Processes: Nursing Process: Assessment
Client Need: Physiological Integrity
Cognitive Level: Application
Reference: Ignatavicius, D., and Workman, M. (2012). Medical-Surgical Nursing: Patient-Centered Collaborative Care (7th ed.). St. Louis, MO: Saunders.

65. ANSWER: 3.
Rationale:
1. Jugular venous distention indicates that fluid resuscitation has been too aggressive and the client is now experiencing fluid volume excess.
2. A urine output of 40 mL/hr indicates effective IV fluid replacement therapy.
3. The nurse should associate blood pressure of 89/58 mm Hg with ineffective IV fluid replacement therapy for FVD. Low blood pressure indicates that the circulating volume is still decreased. Average blood pressure in a healthy adult is 120/80 mm Hg.
4. A low-grade fever is not indicative of ineffective IV therapy.
TEST-TAKING TIP: The key word is "*ineffective*." Select the option that describes the abnormal assessment finding related to FVD.
Content Area: Adult Health
Category of Health Alteration: Fluid Volume Deficit
Integrated Processes: Nursing Process: Evaluation
Client Need: Physiological Integrity
Cognitive Level: Analysis
Reference: Williams, L., and Hopper, P. (2011). Understanding Medical-Surgical Nursing (4th ed.). Philadelphia, PA: F. A. Davis.

66. ANSWER: 1.
Rationale:

$$110 \text{ lb} \div 2.2 \text{ lb/kg} = 50 \text{ kg}$$
$$50 \text{ kg} \times 4 \text{ IU/kg} = 200 \text{ IU} = 1 \text{ mL}$$

TEST-TAKING TIP: Always double-check medication calculations, especially if they seem too simple.
Content Area: Older Adult Health
Category of Health Alteration: Calcium Imbalance
Integrated Processes: Nursing Process: Analysis
Client Need: Physiological Integrity
Cognitive Level: Application
Reference: Beaman, N. (2008). Pharmacology Clear and Simple: A Drug Classifications and Dosage Calculations Approach. Philadelphia, PA: F. A. Davis.

67. ANSWER: 58.
Rationale:

$$85 \text{ lb} \div 2.2 \text{ lb/kg} = 38.64 \text{ kg}$$
$$3 \text{ mg} \times 38.64 \text{ kg} = 115.92 \text{ mg/day}$$
$$115.9 \text{ mg} \div 2 \text{ doses} = 57.95 \text{ mg} = 58 \text{ mg}$$

TEST-TAKING TIP: The key words are "every 12 hours"; be sure to divide the total daily dosage by 2.
Content Area: Child Health
Category of Health Alteration: Fluid Volume Excess
Integrated Processes: Nursing Process: Implementation
Client Need: Physiological Integrity
Cognitive Level: Application
Reference: Beaman, N. (2008). Pharmacology Clear and Simple: A Drug Classifications and Dosage Calculations Approach. Philadelphia, PA: F. A. Davis.

68. ANSWER: 3.
Rationale:

Difference between actual and target blood glucose (120 mg/dL) ÷ Correction factor (50) = Number of units of rapid-acting insulin

$$(256 - 120) \div 50 = 2.72 = 3$$

TEST-TAKING TIP: Double-check all medication calculations. Remember that insulin is a high-alert drug and should be administered in whole units, using only an insulin syringe for proper measurement.
Content Area: Adult Health
Category of Health Alteration: Acid-Base Imbalance
Integrated Processes: Teaching/Learning
Client Need: Physiological Integrity
Cognitive Level: Application
Reference: Diabetes Education Online, Diabetes Teaching Center at the University of California, San Francisco. (2010). Type 1 diabetes: diabetes treatment: calculating insulin dose. http://www.deo.ucsf.edu/type1/diabetes-treatment/medications-and-therapies/type-1-insulin-rx/calculating-insuliin-dose.html.

69. ANSWER: 5, 4, 3, 1, 2.
Rationale: Orthostatic, or postural, hypotension is assessed by measuring the blood pressure and pulse rate with the client in the supine position, then in the sitting position, and finally in the standing position. A significant change in both blood pressure and pulse rate signifies hypovolemia

or dehydration. A positive result occurs if the client becomes dizzy or loses consciousness or if the pulse rate increases by 20 bpm or more and the systolic blood pressure decreases by 20 mm Hg within 3 minutes of changing from supine to sitting or from sitting to standing. Always remember to document the findings.

TEST-TAKING TIP: Envision this assessment in your mind's eye, and determine the proper order to perform the steps.

Content Area: Adult Health
Category of Health Alteration: Fluid Volume Deficit
Integrated Processes: Nursing Process: Implementation
Client Need: Physiological Integrity
Cognitive Level: Application
Reference: *Wilkinson, J., and Treas, L. (2011). Fundamentals of Nursing: Theory, Concepts & Applications (2nd ed.). Philadelphia, PA: F. A. Davis.*

70. ANSWER: 1.

Rationale:

1. The nurse should associate tetany with hypomagnesemia because a lack of magnesium causes increased cellular irritability and hyperexcitability.
2. Constipation, not diarrhea, is associated with hypomagnesemia.
3. Lethargy is a manifestation of hypermagnesemia, not hypomagnesemia.
4. Bradycardia is a cardiac dysrhythmia associated with hypermagnesemia; ventricular dysrhythmias are usually associated with hypomagnesemia.

TEST-TAKING TIP: Recall that hypomagnesemia is often associated with hypocalcemia and has similar signs and symptoms.

Content Area: Adult Health
Category of Health Alteration: Magnesium Imbalance
Integrated Processes: Nursing Process: Assessment
Client Need: Physiological Integrity
Cognitive Level: Application
Reference: *Ignatavicius, D., and Workman, M. (2012). Medical-Surgical Nursing: Patient-Centered Collaborative Care (7th ed.). St. Louis, MO: Saunders.*

71. ANSWER: 2.

Rationale:

1. The nurse should *not* associate a serum pH of 7.49 that is metabolic in origin (metabolic alkalosis) with an increased serum chloride level. Alkalosis is associated with decreased, not increased, serum chloride levels.
2. The nurse should associate a serum pH of 7.49 that is metabolic in origin (metabolic alkalosis) with a decreased serum calcium level. Alkalosis is also associated with decreased serum chloride and potassium levels and an increased bicarbonate level.
3. The nurse should *not* associate a serum pH of 7.49 that is metabolic in origin (metabolic alkalosis) with an increased serum potassium level. Alkalosis is associated with decreased, not increased, serum potassium levels.
4. The nurse should *not* associate a serum pH of 7.49 that is metabolic in origin (metabolic alkalosis) with a decreased serum bicarbonate level. Alkalosis is associated with an increased bicarbonate level.

TEST-TAKING TIP: Recognize that a serum pH of 7.49 indicates alkalosis. Recall that hypokalemia, hypochloremia, and hypocalcemia are often associated with alkalosis.

Content Area: Adult Health
Category of Health Alteration: Acid-Base Imbalance
Integrated Processes: Nursing Process: Implementation
Client Need: Physiological Integrity
Cognitive Level: Application
Reference: *Ignatavicius, D., and Workman, M. (2012). Medical-Surgical Nursing: Patient-Centered Collaborative Care (7th ed.). St. Louis, MO: Saunders.*

72. ANSWER: 2.

Rationale:

1. The statement "I will continue taking this medication as directed even when I lose 3 lb in a week" is correct and shows an adequate understanding of the indications for use of the medication.
2. The nurse should determine that the client requires further education regarding loop diuretics if the client states that he or she will report more frequent urination. Increased frequency of urination is a desired and expected effect of loop diuretics and would not need to be reported to the health-care provider.
3. The statement "I will notify my health-care provider if I notice any loss of hearing" is correct because loop diuretics may cause tinnitus or hearing loss, and the development of this adverse effect should be reported to the health-care provider.
4. The statement "I will take my daily dose of this medication when I wake up in the morning" is correct because clients who receive a daily diuretic are advised to take the dose at breakfast to avoid nocturnal diuresis.

TEST-TAKING TIP: Read the question carefully. Realize that you should choose the statement by the client that is *incorrect.*

Content Area: Adult Health
Category of Health Alteration: Fluid Volume Excess
Integrated Processes: Nursing Process: Evaluation
Client Need: Physiological Integrity
Cognitive Level: Analysis
Reference: *Deglin, J. H., Vallerand, A. H., and Sanoski, C. A. (2013). Davis's Drug Guide for Nurses (13th ed.). Philadelphia, PA: F. A. Davis.*

73. ANSWER: 3.

Rationale:

1. The nurse should interpret a blood pH of 6.82 as being incompatible with life, not just slightly decreased.
2. The nurse should interpret a blood pH of 6.82 as being severely decreased and incompatible with life, not extremely increased.
3. The nurse should interpret a blood pH of 6.82 as being incompatible with life. The body's pH range is normally 7.35 to 7.45. Values less than 6.9 or greater than 7.8 are generally considered incompatible with life. If the nurse assesses that this client is physiologically more stable than the results indicate, the possibility of a laboratory error should be considered.
4. The nurse should interpret a blood pH of 6.82 as being incompatible with life and well outside the normal reference range.

TEST-TAKING TIP: Recall that the body must maintain pH within a narrow range to sustain life.

Content Area: Adult Health
Category of Health Alteration: Acid-Base Imbalance

Integrated Processes: Nursing Process: Evaluation
Client Need: Physiological Integrity
Cognitive Level: Application
Reference: *Williams, L., and Hopper, P. (2011). Understanding Medical-Surgical Nursing (4th ed.). Philadelphia, PA: F. A. Davis.*

74. ANSWER: 2.

Rationale:

1. The nurse should suspect that the client is experiencing hypokalemia, not hypernatremia, because this rhythm strip shows a normal sinus rhythm with prominent U waves. Although both hyponatremia and hypernatremia result in cardiovascular changes, they are not associated with ECG changes.

2. The nurse should suspect that the client is experiencing hypokalemia because this rhythm strip shows a normal sinus rhythm with prominent U waves, which is a classic ECG change associated with serum potassium levels less than 3.5 mEq/L.

3. The nurse should suspect that the client is experiencing hypokalemia, not hypercalcemia, because this rhythm strip shows a normal sinus rhythm with prominent U waves. Hypercalcemia results in shortened Q-T intervals.

4. The nurse should suspect that the client is experiencing hypokalemia, not hypomagnesemia, because this rhythm strip shows a normal sinus rhythm with prominent U waves. Hypomagnesemia results in torsades de pointes and premature ventricular contractions.

TEST-TAKING TIP: Recall that in hypokalemia, the body's electrical activity slows down, resulting in depressed ST segments, flat T waves, and increased U waves visible on an ECG.

Content Area: Adult Health
Category of Health Alteration: Potassium Imbalance
Integrated Processes: Nursing Process: Analysis
Client Need: Physiological Integrity
Cognitive Level: Application
Reference: *Ignatavicius, D., and Workman, M. (2012). Medical-Surgical Nursing: Patient-Centered Collaborative Care (7th ed.). St. Louis, MO: Saunders.*

75. ANSWER: 4.

Rationale:

1. The nurse should recognize that this client's ABG values would indicate respiratory alkalosis. ABG values of pH 7.33, $PaCO_2$ 36 mm Hg, and HCO_3^- 15 mEq/L indicate metabolic acidosis, not respiratory alkalosis.

2. The nurse should recognize that this client's ABG values would indicate respiratory alkalosis. ABG values of pH 7.49, $PaCO_2$ 45 mm Hg, and HCO_3^- 33 mEq/L indicate metabolic alkalosis, not respiratory alkalosis.

3. The nurse should recognize that this client's ABG values would indicate respiratory alkalosis. ABG values of pH 7.31, $PaCO_2$ 51 mm Hg, and HCO_3^- 23 mEq/L indicate respiratory acidosis, not respiratory alkalosis.

4. The nurse should recognize that this client's ABG values would indicate respiratory alkalosis. In this situation, respiratory alkalosis is shown by ABG values of pH 7.51, $PaCO_2$ 29 mm Hg, and HCO_3^- 24 mEq/L. The client's hyperventilation (respiratory rate of 34 breaths per minute) causes the pH to become alkalotic (greater than 7.45) because carbon dioxide is being lost rapidly. Thus, a client with an increased respiratory rate of 34 breaths per minute would not have a normal or elevated $PaCO_2$ level. The client's elevated blood pressure and heart rate are physiological signs of pain.

TEST-TAKING TIP: Recognize that an abnormal respiratory rate would have a significant effect on the client's $PaCO_2$ level. Rule out options that include normal $PaCO_2$ levels.

Content Area: Adult Health
Category of Health Alteration: Acid-Base Imbalance
Integrated Processes: Nursing Process: Evaluation
Client Need: Physiological Integrity
Cognitive Level: Analysis
Reference: *Williams, L., and Hopper, P. (2011). Understanding Medical-Surgical Nursing (4th ed.). Philadelphia, PA: F. A. Davis.*

76. ANSWER: 3.

Rationale:

1. The nurse should instruct the client to consume foods that are high in potassium, not follow a low-potassium diet, because loop diuretics increase potassium excretion by the kidneys.

2. The nurse should instruct the client to take missed doses as soon as possible, but the client should not take a double dose.

3. The nurse should instruct the client to change positions slowly to minimize orthostatic hypotension. The fluid loss caused by diuretic therapy increases this client's risk for the occurrence of orthostatic hypotension.

4. The nurse should instruct the client to notify a health-care professional of weight gain more than 3 lb, not 2 lb, in 1 day.

TEST-TAKING TIP: The key words are "loop diuretic." Recognize that these medications cause potassium loss. Recall that weight gain of 1 kg (2.2 lb) equals approximately 1 L of fluid retained.

Content Area: Adult Health
Category of Health Alteration: Fluid Volume Excess
Integrated Processes: Teaching/Learning
Client Need: Physiological Integrity
Cognitive Level: Application
Reference: *Deglin, J. H., Vallerand, A. H., and Sanoski, C. A. (2013). Davis's Drug Guide for Nurses (13th ed.). Philadelphia, PA: F. A. Davis.*

77. ANSWER: 3.

Rationale:

1. The nurse should assess an unconscious client diagnosed with possible ingestion of gamma-hydroxybutyric acid for respiratory acidosis, not metabolic acidosis.

2. The nurse should assess an unconscious client diagnosed with possible ingestion of gamma-hydroxybutyric acid for respiratory acidosis, not metabolic alkalosis.

3. The nurse should assess an unconscious client diagnosed with possible ingestion of gamma-hydroxybutyric acid for respiratory acidosis because gamma-hydroxybutyric acid, also known as GHB, Ecstasy, or the date rape drug, may cause respiratory depression or coma. Increased carbon dioxide retention leads to a decrease in blood pH (acidosis).

4. The nurse should assess an unconscious client diagnosed with possible ingestion of gamma-hydroxybutyric acid for respiratory acidosis, not respiratory alkalosis.

TEST-TAKING TIP: Recall that the effects of many illicit substances can result in respiratory depression. Associate respiratory depression with respiratory acidosis.
Content Area: Adult Health
Category of Health Alteration: Acid-Base Imbalance
Integrated Processes: Nursing Process: Assessment
Client Need: Physiological Integrity
Cognitive Level: Application
Reference: Berman, A., Snyder, S., Kozier, B., and Erb, G. (2012). Kozier & Erb's Fundamentals of Nursing: Concepts, Process, and Practice (9th ed.). Upper Saddle River, NJ: Pearson.

78. ANSWER: 4.
Rationale:
1. The nurse should anticipate a total serum calcium level of 10.5 mg/dL or greater, indicating hypercalcemia. A serum calcium level of 7.5 mg/dL indicates hypocalcemia. The normal reference range for total serum calcium is 8.2 to 10.2 mg/dL.
2. The nurse should anticipate a total serum calcium level of 10.5 mg/dL or greater, indicating hypercalcemia. A total serum calcium level of 8.5 mg/dL is within the normal reference range of 8.2 to 10.2 mg/dL.
3. The nurse should anticipate a total serum calcium level of 10.5 mg/dL or greater, indicating hypercalcemia. A total serum calcium level of 9.5 mg/dL is within the normal reference range of 8.2 to 10.2 mg/dL.
4. The nurse should anticipate a total serum calcium level of 10.5 mg/dL or greater. Clients with hyperthyroidism (Graves' disease) are at increased risk for developing hypercalcemia. Tachycardia, nausea, constipation, widening pulse pressure, and decreased DTRs are all manifestations of hypercalcemia. The normal reference range for total serum calcium is 8.2 to 10.2 mg/dL.
TEST-TAKING TIP: Recall that hyperthyroidism may cause elevated serum calcium levels.
Content Area: Adult Health
Category of Health Alteration: Calcium Imbalance
Integrated Processes: Nursing Process: Implementation
Client Need: Physiological Integrity
Cognitive Level: Application
Reference: Ignatavicius, D., and Workman, M. (2012). Medical-Surgical Nursing: Patient-Centered Collaborative Care (7th ed.). St. Louis, MO: Saunders.

79. ANSWER: 4.
Rationale:
1. Obtaining vital signs is a necessary part of the client's assessment, but it is not the priority at this time.
2. Positioning the client in a supine position is inappropriate because this would decrease oxygenation and most likely worsen the client's hyperventilation.
3. Administration of supplemental oxygen may be indicated if the client's oxygenation is compromised, but this is not the priority in this situation.
4. The nurse's first intervention for a client who is having a panic attack and begins to hyperventilate should be to assist the client to breathe more slowly. This client is exhaling too much carbon dioxide, potentially resulting in respiratory alkalosis. Breathing through pursed lips or cupped hands would slow the client's rate of breathing.

TEST-TAKING TIP: Recall that hyperventilation causes respiratory alkalosis. Choose the option that would decrease the effects of hyperventilation.
Content Area: Adult Health
Category of Health Alteration: Acid-Base Imbalance
Integrated Processes: Nursing Process: Implementation
Client Need: Physiological Integrity
Cognitive Level: Application
Reference: Berman, A., Snyder, S., Kozier, B., and Erb, G. (2012). Kozier & Erb's Fundamentals of Nursing: Concepts, Process, and Practice (9th ed.). Upper Saddle River, NJ: Pearson.

80. ANSWER: 3.
Rationale:
1. A decrease in hematocrit is a potential sign of FVE, not of improvement in FVE.
2. A decrease in urine output is a potential sign of FVE, not of improvement in FVE.
3. A decrease in body weight should indicate to the nurse that therapy for FVE has been effective. A decrease in body weight corresponds with a decrease in excess fluid, the goal of diuretic therapy. Decreases in hematocrit, urine output, and blood urea nitrogen are all potential signs of FVE.
4. A decrease in blood urea nitrogen is a potential sign of FVE, not of improvement in FVE.
TEST-TAKING TIP: Use the process of elimination to rule out options 1, 2, and 4 because these are signs of FVE.
Content Area: Adult Health
Category of Health Alteration: Fluid Volume Excess
Integrated Processes: Nursing Process: Evaluation
Client Need: Physiological Integrity
Cognitive Level: Application
Reference: Ignatavicius, D., and Workman, M. (2012). Medical-Surgical Nursing: Patient-Centered Collaborative Care (7th ed.). St. Louis, MO: Saunders.

81. ANSWER: 9.
Rationale:

12 mEq/X = 1.36 mEq/1 mL (cross multiply) =
1.36X = 12 = 8.82 mL = 9 mL

TEST-TAKING TIP: Always double-check medication calculations, especially if they seem too simple.
Content Area: Adult Health
Category of Health Alteration: Calcium Imbalance
Integrated Processes: Nursing Process: Analysis
Client Need: Physiological Integrity
Cognitive Level: Application
Reference: Beaman, N. (2008). Pharmacology Clear and Simple: A Drug Classifications and Dosage Calculations Approach. Philadelphia, PA: F. A. Davis.

82. ANSWER: 30.
Rationale: Use the following formula to calculate the dose:

Dose on hand/Dose unit = Desired dose/Dose given
20 mEq/15 mL = 40 mEq/X mL (cross multiply) =
20X = 600 = 30 mL

TEST-TAKING TIP: Always double-check medication calculations. Because potassium is a high-alert drug, confirm the concentration of all potassium-containing solutions with another registered nurse before administration.

Content Area: Adult Health
Category of Health Alteration: Potassium Imbalance
Integrated Processes: Nursing Process: Implementation
Client Need: Physiological Integrity
Cognitive Level: Application
Reference: *Deglin, J. H., Vallerand, A. H., and Sanoski, C. A. (2013). Davis's Drug Guide for Nurses (13th ed.). Philadelphia, PA: F. A. Davis.*

83. ANSWER: 3, 5.

Rationale:

1. Peripheral edema is a sign of right-sided, not left-sided, heart failure. In right-sided heart failure, the right ventricle cannot empty completely, causing increased volume and pressure in the venous system and resulting in peripheral edema.
2. Hepatic enlargement is a sign of right-sided, not left-sided, heart failure. In right-sided heart failure, the right ventricle cannot empty completely, causing increased volume and pressure in the venous system and resulting in hepatic enlargement.
3. **The nurse should suspect FVE related to left-sided heart failure if the client develops crackles in all lung fields. In left-sided heart failure, as the amount of blood ejected from the left ventricle diminishes, hydrostatic pressure builds in the pulmonary venous system and results in fluid-filled alveoli and pulmonary congestion. Cough is often an early manifestation of heart failure, and crackles are auscultated as the problem progresses.**
4. Jugular venous distention is a sign of right-sided, not left-sided, heart failure. In right-sided heart failure, the right ventricle cannot empty completely, causing increased volume and pressure in the venous system and resulting in jugular venous distention.
5. **The nurse should suspect FVE related to left-sided heart failure if the client develops a persistent, nonproductive cough. In left-sided heart failure, as the amount of blood ejected from the left ventricle diminishes, hydrostatic pressure builds in the pulmonary venous system and results in fluid-filled alveoli and pulmonary congestion. Cough is often an early manifestation of heart failure, and crackles are auscultated as the problem progresses. A client in early heart failure describes the cough as irritating, frequently nocturnal, and usually nonproductive.**

TEST-TAKING TIP: Review the signs of left-sided and right-sided heart failure if you were unable to answer this question correctly.

Content Area: Adult Health
Category of Health Alteration: Fluid Volume Excess
Integrated Processes: Nursing Process: Assessment
Client Need: Physiological Integrity
Cognitive Level: Application
Reference: *Ignatavicius, D., and Workman, M. (2012). Medical-Surgical Nursing: Patient-Centered Collaborative Care (7th ed.). St. Louis, MO: Saunders.*

84. ANSWER: 4.

Rationale:

1. The nurse should associate a near drowning in fresh water with hyponatremia related to a relative decrease in sodium, not hypernatremia related to an actual increase in sodium. The client likely ingested excessive amounts of water alone and is experiencing a relative decrease in sodium secondary to hypervolemia, causing a dilution of the serum sodium.
2. The nurse should associate a near drowning in fresh water with hyponatremia related to a relative decrease in sodium, not hypernatremia related to a relative increase in sodium. The client likely ingested excessive amounts of water alone and is experiencing a relative decrease in sodium secondary to hypervolemia, causing a dilution of the serum sodium.
3. The nurse should associate a near drowning in fresh water with hyponatremia related to a relative decrease in sodium, not hyponatremia related to an actual decrease in sodium. The client likely ingested excessive amounts of water alone and is experiencing a relative decrease in sodium secondary to hypervolemia, causing a dilution of the serum sodium.
4. **The nurse should associate a near drowning in fresh water with hyponatremia related to a relative decrease in sodium. The client likely ingested excessive amounts of water alone and is experiencing a relative decrease in sodium secondary to hypervolemia, causing a dilution of the serum sodium.**

TEST-TAKING TIP: Differentiate between actual and relative decreases or increases in electrolytes. Recognize that relative decreases and increases are always due to alterations in fluid volume.

Content Area: Adult Health
Category of Health Alteration: Sodium Imbalance
Integrated Processes: Nursing Process: Implementation
Client Need: Physiological Integrity
Cognitive Level: Application
Reference: *Williams, L., and Hopper, P. (2011). Understanding Medical-Surgical Nursing (4th ed.). Philadelphia, PA: F. A. Davis.*

85. ANSWER: 4.

Rationale:

1. Elevation of the client's legs could worsen the client's respiratory status because vascular volume is increased by gravity.
2. Simply continuing to monitor the client's weight may result in serious consequences as the fluid volume excess (FVE) increases.
3. The health-care provider should be notified following the assessment.
4. **The nurse's priority intervention should be to assess the client's lung sounds. Assessments of vital signs, heart sounds, and lung sounds are critical when monitoring for FVE. Gas exchange may be impaired by edema of the pulmonary interstitial tissues. Acute pulmonary edema is a serious and potentially life-threatening complication of pulmonary congestion, and auscultation of the lungs for the presence or worsening of crackles and wheezes should be performed routinely and with any change in the client's status.**

TEST-TAKING TIP: Follow the nursing process: Assess *first*, then implement.

Content Area: Adult Health
Category of Health Alteration: Fluid Volume Excess
Integrated Processes: Nursing Process: Implementation
Client Need: Physiological Integrity
Cognitive Level: Analysis
Reference: *Lemone, P., and Burke, K. (2010). Medical-Surgical Nursing: Critical Thinking in Client Care (5th ed.). Upper Saddle River, NJ: Pearson Prentice Hall.*

86. ANSWER: 2.

Rationale:

1. The nurse should associate these ABG values with fully compensated respiratory acidosis, not partially compensated metabolic acidosis.

2. The nurse should associate these ABG values with fully compensated respiratory acidosis. The pH of 7.36 is within the normal reference range of 7.35 to 7.45, indicating full compensation. The pH is still on the lower (more acidotic) end of the normal reference range, and both the $PaCO_2$ (48 mm Hg) and HCO_3^- (30 mEq/L) levels are elevated. An elevated $PaCO_2$ would cause the blood to become acidotic (pH less than 7.35), but the elevated HCO_3^- level is pulling the pH up within the normal range, indicating that the kidneys are compensating for an imbalance that is respiratory in origin.

3. The nurse should associate these ABG values with fully compensated respiratory acidosis, not partially compensated metabolic alkalosis.

4. The nurse should associate these ABG values with fully compensated respiratory acidosis, not fully compensated respiratory alkalosis.

TEST-TAKING TIP: First, look at the direction of the pH. Next, think about the other ABG values to determine the origin of the imbalance.

Content Area: Adult Health

Category of Health Alteration: Acid-Base Imbalance

Integrated Processes: Nursing Process: Analysis

Client Need: Physiological Integrity

Cognitive Level: Analysis

Reference: Berman, A., Snyder, S., Kozier, B., and Erb, G. (2012). Kozier & Erb's Fundamentals of Nursing: Concepts, Process, and Practice (9th ed.). Upper Saddle River, NJ: Pearson.

87. ANSWER: 63.

Rationale:

Volume × Drop factor/Time = Rate
125 mL/hr × 30 gtt/mL/60 min = 3,750/60 = 62.5 = 63 gtt/min

TEST-TAKING TIP: Read the question carefully. The question is asking you to calculate a manual drip rate to infuse a solution at 125 mL/hr using tubing with a drop factor of 30 gtt/mL. When performing this particular calculation, the total amount of solution to be infused is irrelevant.

Content Area: Adult Health

Category of Health Alteration: Sodium Imbalance

Integrated Processes: Nursing Process: Analysis

Client Need: Physiological Integrity

Cognitive Level: Application

Reference: Beaman, N. (2008). Pharmacology Clear and Simple: A Drug Classifications and Dosage Calculations Approach. Philadelphia, PA: F. A. Davis.

88. ANSWER: 4.

Rationale:

1. The nurse should associate the client's manifestations with the development of respiratory alkalosis. Lab Report A indicates respiratory acidosis.

2. The nurse should associate the client's manifestations with the development of respiratory alkalosis. Lab Report B indicates metabolic acidosis.

3. The nurse should associate the client's manifestations with the development of respiratory alkalosis. Lab Report C is within the normal reference ranges.

4. The nurse should associate the client's manifestations with the development of respiratory alkalosis secondary to hyperventilation (respiratory rate of 36 breaths per minute). The client's arterial blood gas pH (7.49) is greater than 7.45, and the $PaCO_2$ (29 mm Hg) is decreased, indicating that the client is losing carbon dioxide. The normal HCO_3^- (25 mEq/L) indicates that the kidneys have not yet begun to compensate for the respiratory origin of the acidosis.

TEST-TAKING TIP: Recognize that hyperventilation results in respiratory alkalosis, indicated by a pH greater than 7.45, decreased $PaCO_2$, and normal (if uncompensated) HCO_3^-.

Content Area: Adult Health

Category of Health Alteration: Acid-Base Imbalance

Integrated Processes: Nursing Process: Analysis

Client Need: Physiological Integrity

Cognitive Level: Analysis

Reference: Ignatavicius, D., and Workman, M. (2012). Medical-Surgical Nursing: Patient-Centered Collaborative Care (7th ed.). St. Louis, MO: Saunders.

89. ANSWER: 2.

Rationale:

1. An infusion rate of 50 mL/hr would not deliver the unit within the 4-hour time limit.

2. The nurse should use an infusion rate of 100 mL/hr when administering packed red blood cells to a client diagnosed with right-sided heart failure. Circulatory overload can occur when a blood product is infused too quickly. Older adults are at increased risk for this complication.

3. An infusion rate of 150 mL/hr is not recommended for this client because it is too rapid and increases the client's risk of fluid volume excess.

4. An infusion rate of 200 mL/hr is not recommended for this client because it is too rapid and increases the client's risk of fluid volume excess.

TEST-TAKING TIP: Review the administration of IV fluid therapy or blood products in clients with compromised heart function if you had difficulty with this question.

Content Area: Adult Health

Category of Health Alteration: Fluid Volume Excess

Integrated Processes: Nursing Process: Planning

Client Need: Physiological Integrity

Cognitive Level: Application

Reference: Ignatavicius, D., and Workman, M. (2012). Medical-Surgical Nursing: Patient-Centered Collaborative Care (7th ed.). St. Louis, MO: Saunders.

90. ANSWER: 3.

Rationale:

1. Polyuria, or increased urinary output, would not be seen in hypernatremia because the body would be trying to dilute the elevated serum sodium by conserving, rather than excreting, water.

2. Paresthesia is associated with hyperkalemia, hypocalcemia, and hyperphosphatemia, not hypernatremia.

3. The nurse should associate increased thirst with the development of hypernatremia. Thirst is usually one of

the first symptoms to appear. Other signs and symptoms of hypernatremia include alterations in mental status, such as agitation, restlessness, and confusion.
4. Muscle weakness is associated with hyponatremia, not hypernatremia.
TEST-TAKING TIP: Recall the signs and symptoms of hypernatremia, and use the process of elimination to rule out incorrect options.
Content Area: Adult Health
Category of Health Alteration: Sodium Imbalance
Integrated Processes: Nursing Process: Assessment
Client Need: Physiological Integrity
Cognitive Level: Application
Reference: *Williams, L., and Hopper, P. (2011). Understanding Medical-Surgical Nursing (4th ed.). Philadelphia, PA: F. A. Davis.*

91. ANSWER: 4.
Rationale:
1. A decreased pH would be indicative of acidosis, not alkalosis.
2. An increased $PaCO_2$ would be seen only if the imbalance was compensated.
3. If the client's respiratory system had begun to compensate, the $PaCO_2$ would be increased, not decreased, in an attempt to lower pH to the normal reference range.
4. The nurse caring for a client diagnosed with uncompensated metabolic alkalosis should anticipate an increased HCO_3^- because the pH alteration is metabolic in origin. Prolonged vomiting causes excessive loss of hydrochloric acid from the stomach, resulting in metabolic alkalosis. The nurse should also expect to see increased pH (alkalosis) and normal $PaCO_2$ (no respiratory compensation) in uncompensated metabolic alkalosis. If the client's respiratory system had begun to compensate, the $PaCO_2$ would be increased in an attempt to decrease pH to the normal reference range.
TEST-TAKING TIP: The key words are "metabolic alkalosis." Rule out decreased pH (acidosis) and increased and decreased $PaCO_2$ (respiratory origin).
Content Area: Adult Health
Category of Health Alteration: Acid-Base Imbalance
Integrated Processes: Nursing Process: Evaluation
Client Need: Physiological Integrity
Cognitive Level: Application
Reference: *Williams, L., and Hopper, P. (2011). Understanding Medical-Surgical Nursing (4th ed.). Philadelphia, PA: F. A. Davis.*

92. ANSWER: 2.
Rationale:
1. An apple is low in calcium (3 mg) and should not be recommended.
2. The nurse should advise the client to choose pizza, which is the option that provides the greatest amount of calcium (240 mg).
3. Popcorn is low in calcium (5 mg) and should not be recommended.
4. Chicken noodle soup is low in calcium (3 mg) and should not be recommended.
TEST-TAKING TIP: Recognize that pizza is topped with cheese—a good source of calcium.
Content Area: Adult Health
Category of Health Alteration: Calcium Imbalance
Integrated Processes: Nursing Process: Analysis
Client Need: Physiological Integrity
Cognitive Level: Comprehension
Reference: *National Institutes of Health, Office of Dietary Supplements. (Reviewed 2012). Dietary supplement fact sheet: calcium. http://ods.od.nih.gov/factsheets/Calcium-HealthProfessional/.*

93. ANSWER: 2.
Rationale:
1. The nursing diagnosis Diarrhea Related to Spastic Colonic Activity would be appropriate for a client experiencing hyperkalemia, not hypokalemia.
2. The nurse should assign the nursing diagnosis Decreased Cardiac Output Related to Dysrhythmia because the client is experiencing hypokalemia, which results in muscle weakness, smooth muscle atony, and cardiac dysrhythmias.
3. The nursing diagnosis Risk for Falls Related to Orthostatic Hypotension would be appropriate for a client experiencing hyperkalemia, not hypokalemia.
4. The nursing diagnosis Risk for Acute Confusion Related to Electrolyte Imbalance would not be appropriate because confusion is usually not associated with potassium imbalances. Confusion is associated with sodium imbalances.
TEST-TAKING TIP: Become familiar with the similarities and differences in the signs and symptoms of hypokalemia and hyperkalemia.
Content Area: Adult Health
Category of Health Alteration: Potassium Imbalance
Integrated Processes: Nursing Process: Analysis
Client Need: Physiological Integrity
Cognitive Level: Application
Reference: *Ignatavicius, D., and Workman, M. (2012). Medical-Surgical Nursing: Patient-Centered Collaborative Care (7th ed.). St. Louis, MO: Saunders.*

94. ANSWER: 1.
Rationale:
1. The nurse should identify ECG strip 1 as indicative of hypophosphatemia and, more specifically, hypercalcemia because it shows a shortened Q-T interval. This is a classic ECG change associated with hypercalcemia (which is often associated with hypophosphatemia).
2. ECG strip 2 is a normal sinus rhythm.
3. ECG strip 3 illustrates sinus rhythm with premature ventricular contractions (in couplets), which might be associated with potassium or magnesium imbalances.
4. ECG strip 4 shows atrial fibrillation, which is not related to electrolyte imbalances.
TEST-TAKING TIP: Review the effects of hypercalcemia on the electrical conduction of the heart, and select the answer that illustrates those effects.
Content Area: Adult Health
Category of Health Alteration: Phosphate Imbalance
Integrated Processes: Nursing Process: Evaluation
Client Need: Physiological Integrity
Cognitive Level: Analysis
References: *Jones, S. (2010). ECG Notes: Interpretation and Management Guide (2nd ed.). Philadelphia, PA: F. A. Davis; Ignatavicius, D., and Workman, M. (2012). Medical-Surgical Nursing: Patient-Centered Collaborative Care (7th ed.). St. Louis, MO: Saunders.*

95. ANSWER: 4.

Rationale:

1. Oral potassium supplements would be contraindicated for this client because she is vomiting.

2. The nurse should not administer furosemide because it is a non–potassium-sparing diuretic, which would worsen the client's fluid volume deficit and hypokalemia.

3. The nurse should question an order to infuse potassium at a rate of 40 mEq/hr. Potassium should *never* be administered at a rate greater than 20 mEq/hr.

4. The nurse should use a controlled infusion device to administer an IV potassium solution to ensure that the medication is infused slowly at *no more than 20 mEq/hr.*

TEST-TAKING TIP: Read each option carefully, and rule out those that would be contraindicated for this client.

Content Area: Maternal Health

Category of Health Alteration: Potassium Imbalance

Integrated Processes: Nursing Process: Implementation

Client Need: Physiological Integrity

Cognitive Level: Application

***Reference:** Deglin, J. H., Vallerand, A. H., and Sanoski, C. A. (2013). Davis's Drug Guide for Nurses (13th ed.). Philadelphia, PA: F. A. Davis.*

96. ANSWER: 4.

Rationale:

1. Shrimp are naturally high in sodium (1,590 mg).

2. Spinach is naturally high in sodium (120 mg).

3. Carrots are naturally high in sodium (100 mg).

4. The nurse should advise the client that oranges are low in sodium and are an excellent source of potassium. A whole orange contains approximately 2 mg of sodium per 100 gm.

TEST-TAKING TIP: Consider each option and eliminate foods known to be high in sodium.

Content Area: Adult Health

Category of Health Alteration: Sodium Imbalance

Integrated Processes: Teaching/Learning

Client Need: Physiological Integrity

Cognitive Level: Application

***Reference:** Lemone, P., and Burke, K. (2010). Medical-Surgical Nursing: Critical Thinking in Client Care (5th ed.). Upper Saddle River, NJ: Pearson Prentice Hall.*

97. ANSWER: 2.

Rationale:

1. Administration of alprazolam is not contraindicated, but it would be less effective than IV lorazepam because with oral (PO) administration, it would take longer to obtain the desired effect.

2. The nurse should anticipate an order to administer lorazepam, a sedative, at this time. Sedation and attempts to help the client breathe more slowly are the appropriate treatments. The IV route would provide sedation more quickly than the PO route.

3. Administration of sodium bicarbonate is contraindicated because the client's hyperventilation increases the risk for respiratory alkalosis; sodium bicarbonate would worsen alkalosis.

4. Administration of naloxone would not have any effect on the client's respiratory rate; this medication is used to treat respiratory depression secondary to narcotic effects.

TEST-TAKING TIP: Recall that the primary treatment of respiratory alkalosis is reversal of hyperventilation.

Content Area: Adult Health

Category of Health Alteration: Acid-Base Imbalance

Integrated Processes: Nursing Process: Implementation

Client Need: Physiological Integrity

Cognitive Level: Application

***Reference:** Berman, A., Snyder, S., Kozier, B., and Erb, G. (2012). Kozier & Erb's Fundamentals of Nursing: Concepts, Process, and Practice (9th ed.). Upper Saddle River, NJ: Pearson.*

98. ANSWER: 2.

Rationale:

1. The nurse should suspect that the client is experiencing hypocalcemia, not hyperkalemia. Hyperkalemia may also cause diarrhea, but it is characterized by bradycardia, hypotension, paresthesias, and cardiac dysrhythmias (primarily cardiovascular effects).

2. The nurse should suspect that the client is experiencing hypocalcemia. Low serum calcium levels increase cell membrane irritability (speed things up), causing muscle spasms, increased bowel motility, hyperreflexia, and irritability.

3. The nurse should suspect that the client is experiencing hypocalcemia, not hypermagnesemia. Hypermagnesemia causes bradycardia, hypotension, and possible respiratory depression related to muscle weakness (slows things down).

4. The nurse should suspect that the client is experiencing hypocalcemia, not hypophosphatemia. Hypophosphatemia is associated with hypercalcemia, not hypocalcemia.

TEST-TAKING TIP: When thinking about calcium imbalances, think opposites: *decreased* calcium levels cause an *increase* in bowel motility (diarrhea), muscle spasms, twitching, hyperreflexia, and irritability; *increased* calcium levels cause a *decrease* in bowel motility (constipation), severe muscle weakness, and fatigue.

Content Area: Adult Health

Category of Health Alteration: Calcium Imbalance

Integrated Processes: Nursing Process: Analysis

Client Need: Physiological Integrity

Cognitive Level: Application

***Reference:** Ignatavicius, D., and Workman, M. (2012). Medical-Surgical Nursing: Patient-Centered Collaborative Care (7th ed.). St. Louis, MO: Saunders.*

99. ANSWER: 4.

Rationale:

1. Although alterations in temperature are important to assess, respiratory alterations should be the priority.

2. Although alterations in pulse rate are important to assess, respiratory alterations should be the priority.

3. Although alterations in blood pressure are important to assess, respiratory alterations should be the priority.

4. The nurse should first investigate the client's respiratory rate of 10 breaths per minute because she may be experiencing profound respiratory depression related to hypermagnesemia. Administration of IV magnesium sulfate places the client at increased risk for hypermagnesemia and magnesium toxicity. Loss of patellar reflexes, respiratory and neuromuscular depression, oliguria, and decreased level of consciousness are signs of magnesium toxicity.

TEST-TAKING TIP: Remember that alterations in the client's airway or breathing require priority assessment.
Content Area: *Maternal Health*
Category of Health Alteration: *Magnesium Imbalance*
Integrated Processes: *Nursing Process: Implementation*
Client Need: *Safe and Effective Care Environment*
Cognitive Level: *Analysis*
Reference: *Perry, S., Hockenberry, M., Lowdermilk, D., and Wilson, D. (2010). Maternal Child Nursing Care (4th ed.). St. Louis, MO: Mosby.*

100. ANSWER: 3.

Rationale:

1. Potassium should not be administered intramuscularly because it is a severe tissue irritant.
2. Potassium should *never* be given by IV push or bolus because rapid infusions of potassium chloride can cause death.
3. **The nurse should identify an order for IV potassium chloride 40 mEq/L over 4 hours as the most appropriate order to treat hypokalemia in this client. A serum potassium level of 2.3 mEq/L is considered critical and requires an IV infusion of potassium for replacement.**
4. Oral potassium supplements are given once or twice daily to treat mild to moderate hypokalemia, not severe hypokalemia.

TEST-TAKING TIP: Recall that potassium is a high-alert drug. IV infusions of potassium should not exceed a rate of 10 mEq/hr via peripheral site or 20 mEq/hr via central venous access (with cardiac monitoring) for adults.
Content Area: *Adult Health*
Category of Health Alteration: *Potassium Imbalance*
Integrated Processes: *Nursing Process: Planning*
Client Need: *Physiological Integrity*
Cognitive Level: *Application*
Reference: *Deglin, J. H., Vallerand, A. H., and Sanoski, C. A. (2013). Davis's Drug Guide for Nurses (13th ed.). Philadelphia, PA: F. A. Davis.*

Case Study Answers

Chapter 1

A. The following *subjective* assessment findings indicate that the client is experiencing a health alteration:

1. **Shortness of breath and dyspnea on exertion:** Pulmonary edema results from excessive shifting of fluid from the vascular space to the pulmonary interstitial space and alveoli. Pulmonary edema can interfere with oxygen–carbon dioxide exchange, resulting in dyspnea and orthopnea.
2. **Swelling of feet and ankles:** Peripheral edema is caused by fluid retention, which is seen most often in the lower extremities. Dependent edema is a primary defining characteristic of fluid volume excess (FVE).
3. **Weight gain of 10 lb over the past week:** Weight gain is the most reliable indicator of FVE.
4. **History of myocardial infarction:** Damage to the heart muscle (myocardium) places the client at risk for congestive heart failure. In 40% to 50% of clients, acute myocardial infarction results in either transient or persistent congestive heart failure. According to the American Heart Association, heart failure affects the kidneys' ability to dispose of sodium and water.
5. **30–pack year smoking history:** Severe chronic lung disease, which is caused by smoking in the majority of cases, causes fluid retention and edema because of increased capillary pressure from the heart to the lungs, which may result in congestive heart failure.
6. **Obesity:** Congestive heart failure is a well-established comorbidity of obesity. Severe obesity can result in fluid retention, which can easily be overlooked until large volumes of fluid have accumulated.
7. **Aspirin 81 mg daily:** NSAIDs, such as aspirin, naproxen, and ibuprofen, cause fluid retention and swelling, increasing the risk for congestive heart failure in some clients.

B. The following *objective* clinical findings indicate that the client is experiencing a health alteration:

1. **Shallow, rapid respirations and decreased pulse oximetry:** An increase in respiratory rate and shallow respirations may be signs of pulmonary edema caused by FVE. Low oxygen saturation in the blood is often indicative of a preexisting respiratory illness or the retention of excess fluid in the body.
2. **Presence of moist crackles in anterior and posterior bilateral lower lobes:** The presence of moist crackles (rales) bilaterally on auscultation is a classic sign of pulmonary edema.
3. **Occasional moist, nonproductive cough:** A moist, productive cough and frothy sputum are signs of pulmonary edema.
4. **3+ pedal and ankle edema present bilaterally:** In 3+ deep, pitting edema, the indentation remains for a short time, and the leg looks swollen. This indicates a significant amount of fluid retention in the lower extremities.
5. **Pedal and radial pulses regular, 4+, and bounding bilaterally:** Bounding pulses on both sides of the body indicate increased blood volume resulting from FVE.
6. **Skin of lower extremities is pale and taut bilaterally:** Fluid retention causes the skin of edematous extremities to become pale due to decreased perfusion to the capillaries. Swelling makes the skin appear tight.
7. **Current weight 256 lb:** The client currently weighs 256 lb (116 kg) and reports a 10-lb (4.5-kg) weight gain over the past week. Divide the weight gain (10 lb) by the client's pre-illness weight (256 − 10 = 246 lb) and multiply by 100 to determine that this represents an increase of about 4% of the client's body weight, which is indicative of mild FVE. Weight gain is the most reliable indicator of FVE. Recall that fluid retention in obese clients can easily be overlooked until large volumes of fluid have accumulated.
8. **Increased blood pressure:** The client's blood pressure of 188/96 mm Hg, despite taking an antihypertensive medication (metoprolol), indicates hypertension secondary to FVE.
9. **Heart rate of 126 bpm:** As fluid retention increases, the heart must pump faster to maintain adequate tissue perfusion; the normal resting heart rate in a healthy adult client is 60 to 100 bpm.
10. **Increased respiratory rate:** The client's respiratory rate has increased to 24 breaths per minute because air exchange in the lungs is decreased, secondary to pulmonary edema. The normal respiratory rate in an adult client is 12 to 20 breaths per minute.

11. Elevated laboratory values: Decreased serum sodium and decreased serum potassium are caused by dilution of electrolytes by excess circulating fluid (relative hyponatremia and hypokalemia). The brain natriuretic peptide (BNP) is a cardiac biomarker that helps diagnose heart failure. A BNP greater than 100 pg/mL indicates that the client is experiencing heart failure.

C. After analyzing the client's data, the nurse should assign a **primary** nursing diagnosis of **Excess Fluid Volume Secondary to Fluid Retention**. Other appropriate nursing diagnoses include, but are not limited to, Activity Intolerance, Decreased Cardiac Output, Risk for Electrolyte Imbalance, Impaired Gas Exchange, Imbalanced Nutrition: More than Body Requirements, Risk for Impaired Skin Integrity, Risk for Decreased Cardiac Tissue Perfusion, and Risk for Falls.

D. The nurse should plan to implement the following interventions to meet the client's needs:

1. **Administer oxygen at a rate of 6 L/min via mask until O_2 saturation is greater than 95%:** This increases perfusion to the tissues and organs. The head of the bed should be elevated 45 degrees (semi-Fowler's position) to ease the client's respiratory effort.
2. **Administer furosemide (Lasix) 40 mg IV × 1 now:** This drug promotes diuresis and reduces the heart's workload.
3. **Administer labetalol HCl 20 mg IV bolus over 2 minutes, then 20 mg IV bolus every 10 minutes until systolic blood pressure is less than 140 mm Hg. Do not exceed 300 mg:** The goal is to lower blood pressure until the systolic reading is less than 140 mm Hg.
4. **Insert a Foley catheter; monitor intake and output:** The catheter promotes client comfort while the kidneys eliminate excess fluid. Intake and output are monitored to determine the client's fluid status; adult clients should produce a minimum of 30 mL/hr of urine, but this client should void large volumes of fluid.
5. **Provide only ice chips PO; no fluids:** Limiting fluids prevents worsening of FVE; educate the client regarding the need for fluid restriction, and advise family members not to provide fluids to the client.
6. **Obtain vital signs every 15 minutes × 1 hour, then every 30 minutes × 1 hour:** Establish a baseline before administering medications, and closely monitor the client's status during diuresis.
7. **Reevaluate after 2 hours:** If the client is not eliminating excess fluid via urine or if the client's blood pressure cannot be adequately controlled, hospital admission may be required.
8. **Educate the client:** Inform the client about the current treatment regimen; teach the client the signs and symptoms of FVE and related electrolyte imbalances; and instruct the client to eat foods high in potassium if she will be receiving loop diuretic therapy after discharge.
9. **Document interventions:** Accurately record all assessment findings, nursing interventions, and the client's response to interventions.

E. The following outcomes should indicate to the nurse that the client's FVE has resolved:

1. **Increase in O_2 saturation levels:** Oxygen saturation as measured by pulse oximetry should be 95% or greater.
2. **Increase in urinary output:** The minimum urinary output for an adult client is 30 mL/hr.
3. **Decrease in blood pressure:** The client's blood pressure should decrease to 140/90 mm Hg or less; the ideal blood pressure for a healthy adult is less than 120/80 mm Hg.
4. **Decrease in heart and respiratory rates:** The client's heart rate should decrease below 100 bpm, and the respiratory rate should decrease to 12 to 20 breaths per minute; the depth of respirations should be within normal limits, and breathing should be unlabored.
5. **Lungs clear on auscultation:** There should be no audible crackles bilaterally on auscultation; lung bases should be clear; there should be no moist, productive cough.
6. **No peripheral edema noted:** There should be no indentation when the lower extremities are pressed; the dependent edema score should be no more than 1+.
7. **Laboratory values:** All laboratory values should be within the normal reference ranges: serum sodium, 135 to 145 mEq/L; serum potassium, 3.5 to 5.0 mEq/L; BNP, less than 100 pg/mL.

Chapter 2

A. The following *subjective* assessment findings indicate that the client is experiencing a health alteration:

1. **Fatigue and malaise:** These symptoms are commonly associated with fluid and electrolyte imbalances, as well as many other disorders.
2. **Dizziness when standing:** Orthostatic hypotension (sudden decrease in blood pressure when moving from a lying to a sitting position or from a sitting to a standing position) is associated with a decrease in blood volume (hypovolemia).
3. **Intermittent confusion:** Confusion, or altered mental status, is a symptom commonly associated with fluid and electrolyte imbalances, as well as many other disorders.
4. **3-day history of nausea, vomiting, and diarrhea:** The client has been losing fluid and electrolytes for 3 days and has most likely been unable to tolerate food or liquids.

5. **Reported weight loss of 6 lb (2.7 kg) in 3 days:** Because a weight loss of 1 kg equals the loss of about 1 L of fluid, the client has lost almost 3 L of fluid over the past 3 days—or about a liter of body fluid per day.
6. **Recent fluid volume excess (FVE) necessitating acute treatment with IV furosemide (Lasix):** The client has recently been treated for congestive heart failure related to FVE. The client's 3-day history of vomiting and diarrhea, inability to tolerate oral intake, and treatment with a loop diuretic for FVE increases the client's risk for fluid volume deficit (FVD).
7. **Metoprolol (Toprol-XL):** This medication is a beta blocker used to treat hypertension. The use of an antihypertensive agent in the presence of significant body fluid loss could cause the client to become hypotensive. Note that the client's dosage of metoprolol was increased following treatment for FVE.
8. **Furosemide and potassium by mouth:** The client is currently taking furosemide, a loop diuretic that increases the excretion of water via urine, increasing the client's risk for FVD. Oral potassium replacement in the presence of FVD can result in an increased serum potassium level (actual or relative hyperkalemia).

B. The following *objective* clinical findings indicate that the client is experiencing a health alteration:

1. **Shallow, rapid respirations and a decreased pulse oximetry.**
2. **Dry oral mucous membranes:** Dryness of the lips, mouth, and throat are early signs of dehydration.
3. **Pale, cool skin:** Dehydrated skin becomes pale and cool as fluid moves out of the cells and into the vascular system in an attempt to maintain circulating blood volume.
4. **Poor skin turgor:** The tenting of skin for longer than 3 seconds is indicative of dehydration.
5. **Weak bilateral radial and pedal pulses:** Pulses are weak when palpated because of a decrease in blood pressure related to a decrease in circulating blood volume.
6. **Current weight 135 lb:** The client currently weighs 135 lb (61 kg) and reports a 6-lb (2.7-kg) weight loss over 3 days. Divide the weight loss (6 lb) by the client's pre-illness weight (135 + 6 = 141 lb) and multiply by 100 to determine that this weight loss represents about 4% of the client's body weight, which is indicative of mild FVD. Weight loss is the most reliable indicator of FVD.
7. **Temperature 99.8°F (37.7°C) orally:** Although this would be considered a low-grade fever in an adult client, it may represent a significant fever in an older adult. Older adults normally have lower core body temperatures due to a decreased metabolic rate and inefficient thermoregulatory mechanisms. FVD increases the core body temperature due to a decrease in perspiration; this also contributes to insensible fluid loss.
8. **Heart rate of 124 bpm:** As the blood volume decreases, the heart pumps faster in an attempt to maintain adequate tissue perfusion; the normal resting heart rate in a healthy adult client is 60 to 100 bpm.
9. **Decreased blood pressure:** A decrease in blood pressure is a late and often unreliable sign of dehydration because many conditions can cause hypotension. Normal blood pressure for an adult is about 120/80 mm Hg; 90/60 mm Hg is considered borderline low blood pressure.
10. **Elevated laboratory values:** Increased serum Na^+, K^+, BUN, and creatinine levels are due to hemoconcentration secondary to dehydration; potassium supplementation may also increase serum K^+ levels.

C. After analyzing the client's data, the nurse should assign a **primary** nursing diagnosis of **Deficient Fluid Volume Secondary to Vomiting and Diarrhea.** Other appropriate nursing diagnoses include, but are not limited to, Acute Confusion, Hyperthermia, Nausea, Imbalanced Nutrition: Less than Body Requirements, Impaired Oral Mucous Membrane, Ineffective Self Health Management, Risk for Impaired Skin Integrity, and Risk for Falls.

D. The nurse should plan to implement the following interventions to meet the client's needs:

1. **Administer oxygen at a rate of 2 L/min via nasal cannula:** This increases perfusion to the tissues and organs. The head of the bed should be elevated 45 degrees (semi-Fowler's position) to ease the client's respiratory effort.
2. **Keep the client NPO:** The goal is to decrease vomiting until the health-care provider prescribes clear liquids, progressing to full liquids and then a regular diet.
3. **Administer IV normal saline solution at a rate of 200 mL over 1 hour, then decrease to 100 mL/hr:** This slowly corrects FVD and prevents rebound hyponatremia as the blood volume expands. Rapid administration of IV fluids may cause serious electrolyte imbalances and result in overcorrection of FVD.
4. **Repeat the basic metabolic panel:** This will determine the client's fluid volume status and response to interventions.
5. **Obtain vital signs every 15 minutes × 1 hour, then every 30 minutes × 1 hour:** Establish a baseline before administering medications, and closely monitor the client's status during rehydration.
6. **Administer 12.5 mg promethazine (Phenergan) intravenously now:** This drug prevents nausea and vomiting.

7. **Monitor intake and output, skin turgor, and level of consciousness:** These interventions are intended to evaluate the client's fluid volume status; also auscultate lung sounds, listening for crackles, which are a sign of potential fluid overload.
8. **Hold Lasix, K-Dur, and Toprol-XL:** Do not administer furosemide (Lasix) to prevent further diuresis; do not administer potassium chloride (K-Lor) because the client's serum potassium level is elevated; do not administer metoprolol (Toprol-XL) because the client is hypotensive.
9. **Educate the client:** Inform the client about the current treatment regimen; teach the client the signs and symptoms of FVD and related electrolyte imbalances; and instruct the client to eat foods high in potassium if she will be receiving loop diuretic therapy after discharge.
10. **Document interventions:** Accurately record all assessment findings, nursing interventions, and the client's response to interventions.

E. The following outcomes should indicate to the nurse that the client's FVD has resolved:

1. **Increase in O_2 saturation levels:** Oxygen saturation as measured by pulse oximetry should be 95% or greater.
2. **Increase in oral intake and urinary output:** The client should be able to tolerate oral fluids and a regular, low-sodium diet. The minimum urinary output for an adult client is 30 mL/hr.
3. **Increase in blood pressure:** The client's blood pressure should increase to greater than 90/60 mm Hg; no sign of orthostatic hypotension should be present.
4. **Decrease in heart and respiratory rates:** The client's heart rate should decrease below 100 bpm, and the respiratory rate should decrease to 12 to 20 breaths per minute.
5. **Laboratory values:** All laboratory values should be within the normal reference ranges.
6. **Client should be alert and oriented to person, time, and place:** The client should no longer be confused.

Chapter 3

A. The following *subjective* assessment findings indicate that the client is experiencing a health alteration:

1. **Postoperative for tonsillectomy and adenoidectomy (T&A):** The client is at increased risk for fluid and electrolyte imbalances secondary to surgical stress, administration of IV fluids and multiple anesthetic agents, and blood loss.
2. **Administration of 500 mL IV D_5W intraoperatively:** D_5W is a hypotonic IV solution that does not contain sodium; postoperatively, children are at high risk for acute hyponatremia secondary to free water retention (water intoxication), and many fatalities have resulted from this disorder. When the serum sodium concentration rapidly falls below 120 mEq/L, the body's compensatory mechanism is often overwhelmed; severe cerebral edema ensues, resulting in brainstem herniation, compression of vital midbrain structures, and death.
3. **Sore throat:** It is common for the throat to be extremely sore following T&A.
4. **Nausea:** Many clients, especially children, experience postoperative nausea, which is a side effect of many general anesthetic agents. In addition, the child may have swallowed blood during or immediately after the procedure, resulting in nausea and vomiting.

B. The following *objective* clinical findings indicate that the client is experiencing a health alteration:

1. **Lethargy and confusion:** Low serum sodium levels, resulting from decreased sodium intake or excess body water, can affect the nervous system, producing symptoms such as lethargy and confusion. Note that high serum sodium levels (which commonly result from dehydration or a decrease in body water) can produce similar symptoms, including confusion, muscle twitches, seizures, and death.
2. **Vomiting frequent small amounts of clear, blood-tinged fluid:** This would be an expected finding following T&A under general anesthesia.
3. **Tachycardia; weak, thready pulse; and decreased blood pressure:** The heart rate of 154 bpm and blood pressure of 90/48 mm Hg are secondary to hyponatremia, NPO status, and postoperative intake of hypotonic IV fluids (D_5W). A decrease in blood volume may cause the heart to pump faster but less powerfully, causing a rapid, weak, thready pulse.
4. **Shallow, slow respirations and decreased oxygen saturation:** Signs of hyponatremia include slow breathing (respiratory rate less than 12 to 20 breaths per minute); shallow breathing may also be a side effect of anesthesia. An oxygen saturation of 94% is low for a child with healthy lungs (normal would be 99% or 100%).
5. **Cool, pale skin:** Skin becomes pale and cool as fluid moves out of the cells and into the vascular system in an attempt to maintain circulating blood volume.
6. **Pedal and radial pulses regular, 1+, and weak bilaterally:** Pulses are weak when palpated because of a decrease in blood pressure related to decreased circulating blood volume.
7. **Temperature 100°F (37.8°C) axillary:** Temperatures ranging from 100°F to 101°F (37.8°C to 38.3°C)

must be interpreted in the light of the child's overall condition; reassess the child's temperature using a temporal artery thermometer, which reads a core temperature analogous to the rectal temperature. The normal temperature range is 97°F to 100° F (36°C to 37.8°C); fever is defined as a temperature greater than 101°F (38.3°C).

8. **Decreased serum Na^+:** A serum sodium level of 125 mEq/L is a definitive sign of hyponatremia; the normal range is 135 to 145 mEq/L.
9. **Decreased serum Cl^-:** A serum chloride level of 90 mEq/L is a definitive sign of hypochloremia, which often accompanies hyponatremia (remember that chloride follows sodium). The normal range for serum chloride is 95 to 108 mEq/L.

C. After analyzing the client's data, other than Acute Pain, the nurse should assign a **primary** nursing diagnosis of **Deficient Fluid Volume [Hypotonic] Secondary to NPO Status and Intake of Postoperative IV Hypotonic Fluids (D_5W).** Other appropriate nursing diagnoses include, but are not limited to, Risk for Electrolyte Imbalance, Risk for Imbalanced Body Temperature, Acute Confusion, Impaired Gas Exchange, Nausea, Acute Pain, Impaired Swallowing, Risk for Bleeding, and Risk for Infection.

D. The nurse should plan to implement the following interventions to meet the client's needs:

1. **Administer oxygen at a rate of 2 L/min via nasal cannula:** This increases perfusion to the tissues and organs. The head of the bed should be elevated 45 degrees (semi-Fowler's position) to ease the client's respiratory effort.
2. **Measure vital signs every 15 minutes × 2 hours, then every 30 minutes:** Establish a baseline before administering medication, and monitor the client's status.
3. **Discontinue D_5W:** Intravenous infusion of a hypotonic solution, such as D_5W, will worsen the client's hyponatremia and hypochloremia and could potentiate additional electrolyte imbalances.
4. **Administer IV normal saline solution: 100 mL over 1 hour, then 50 mL/hr × 1 L; correct serum sodium over 24 hours, no faster than 1 to 2 mEq/hr:** This corrects serum sodium and chloride deficits and increases blood volume. Electrolytes should be replaced slowly to avoid overcorrection and unwanted electrolyte shifts.
5. **Administer IV ondansetron (Zofran) 0.15 mg/kg every 6 hours as necessary for nausea:** This drug relieves nausea and prevents vomiting; vomiting may cause bleeding and pain at the surgical site.
6. **Repeat the basic metabolic panel every 4 hours × 2 after normal saline IV fluid is started:** This determines the client's fluid volume status, electrolyte levels, and overall response to interventions.
7. **Monitor intake and output:** This ensures that the client is receiving enough fluids either intravenously or orally and that the client's urinary output is within normal limits based on age and weight; in a healthy client, intake is generally equivalent to output.
8. **Assess neurological status every hour × 8:** This assessment identifies changes in neurological status, including alertness and orientation to time, place, and person.
9. **Implement seizure precautions:** Sodium imbalance places the client at risk for seizure activity; client safety is always a priority.
10. **Provide a clear liquid diet when the client is awake; avoid free water; use electrolyte supplemental fluids (Pedialyte, Gatorade) as tolerated:** This helps rehydrate the client, provides supplemental electrolytes, and decreases nausea and vomiting.

E. The following outcomes should indicate to the nurse that the client's FVD and electrolyte imbalances have resolved:

1. **Increase in O_2 saturation levels:** Oxygen saturation as measured by pulse oximetry should be 95% or greater.
2. **Gradual increase in serum sodium and chloride levels to the normal reference range:** The client's laboratory results should reflect a serum sodium level of 135 to 145 mEq/L and a serum chloride level of 95 to 108 mEq/L.
3. **Increase in respiratory rate and blood pressure:** The client's respiratory rate should increase to 12 to 20 breaths per minute; children aged 6 to 9 should have a systolic blood pressure of 108 to 121 mm Hg and a diastolic blood pressure of 71 to 81 mm Hg, depending on height and gender.
4. **Decrease in heart rate:** The client's heart rate should decrease below 100 bpm; the heart rate should decrease as the fluid volume deficit is corrected.
5. **Decrease in nausea and vomiting; toleration of a normal diet:** The client should be able to tolerate clear liquids without the sensation of nausea or vomiting.
6. **Resolution of abnormal neurological findings:** The client should no longer be lethargic or confused and should be oriented to time, place, and person.

Chapter 4

A. The following *subjective* assessment findings indicate that the client is experiencing a health alteration:

1. **Fatigue, muscle aches, weakness, and muscle cramping:** Weakness and fatigue are the most common complaints in clients with hypokalemia;

with severe hypokalemia, muscle cramps and pain can occur with rhabdomyolysis. Other symptoms of hypokalemia include increased urination, irregular heartbeat (arrhythmia), orthostatic hypotension, muscle pain, and tetany.

2. **Recent nausea, vomiting, and diarrhea:** Diarrhea is a common cause of hypokalemia. Vomiting is also a common cause, but gastric fluid contains little potassium; vomiting produces volume depletion and metabolic alkalosis, which result in sodium retention and potassium loss via the urine.
3. **History of congestive heart failure:** Clients with heart failure usually take several medications to lessen their symptoms and prevent worsening of the underlying disease; medications such as furosemide (Lasix) cause the body to lose potassium.
4. **Metoprolol (Toprol-XL) 100 mg PO daily:** This long-acting beta blocker slows the heart rate, lowers the blood pressure, and lessens the heart's workload by blocking the action of norepinephrine to improve the systolic function of the left ventricle. Beta blockers do not *cause* potassium loss.
5. **Lisinopril (Zestril) 5 mg PO daily:** This angiotensin-converting enzyme (ACE) inhibitor enlarges the small arteries, which relieves the systolic workload of the left ventricle and lowers the blood pressure. ACE inhibitors block the production of angiotensin II, which is elevated in congestive heart failure, causes vasoconstriction, and increases the left ventricle's workload; it is toxic to the left ventricle at excessive levels.
6. **Digoxin (Lanoxin) 0.25 mg PO daily:** This inotrope causes the heart to pump more forcefully, but it is now used only as an add-on therapy with ACE inhibitors and beta blockers. *Excessive digoxin can build up in the blood and cause potentially dangerous abnormal heart rhythms (arrhythmias)*; the risk of developing arrhythmias increases if the dose is excessive, the kidneys do not excrete digoxin from the body properly, or the potassium level is too low (diuretics may cause low potassium levels).
7. **Potassium chloride (K-Lor) 20 mEq PO daily:** To prevent hypokalemia, clients are usually prescribed 10 to 20 mEq of potassium chloride daily; to treat mild to moderate hypokalemia, clients are prescribed 40 to 100 mEq daily. Under normal circumstances, this client's daily dose of 20 mEq would prevent hypokalemia, but not in the presence of diarrhea and vomiting coupled with diuretic therapy.
8. **Furosemide (Lasix) 40 mg PO daily:** This loop diuretic causes the kidneys to remove excess salt and water from the bloodstream, thereby reducing the amount of blood volume in circulation and decreasing the heart's workload. Loop diuretics (non–potassium-sparing) also cause potassium to be lost via the urine.

B. The following *objective* assessment findings indicate that the client is experiencing a health alteration:

1. **Weakness and severe cramping × 2 days after nausea, vomiting, and diarrhea:** These abnormal findings are signs and symptoms of hypokalemia related to nausea, vomiting, diarrhea, and diuretic use.
2. **Decreased blood pressure and orthostatic hypotension:** The client has a fluid volume deficit (FVD) secondary to diarrhea and vomiting; the decrease in circulating blood volume results in a decrease in blood pressure. The client's blood pressure drops to 92/54 mm Hg when he stands, indicating orthostatic hypotension. Low blood pressure is also a sign of hypokalemia.
3. **Increased heart rate and weak, irregular peripheral pulses:** Hypokalemia, in the absence of FVD, would normally cause a slow heart rate (sinus bradycardia) progressing to life-threatening ventricular fibrillation, depending on the severity of the potassium imbalance. This client's elevated heart rate of 112 bpm and irregular peripheral pulses are most likely a result of FVD.
4. **Hypoactive deep tendon reflexes and bowel sounds:** Hypoactive deep tendon reflexes and decreased bowel motility are associated with potassium deficit and calcium excess.
5. **Increased serum digoxin level:** The client is at increased risk for cardiac dysrhythmias because of an elevated digoxin level in the presence of hypokalemia and long-term use of furosemide (a potassium-depleting diuretic) for the treatment of CHF.
6. **Moderately decreased serum potassium level:** The client is taking a subtherapeutic dose of oral potassium, as evidenced by his decreased serum potassium level.
7. **Increased BUN:** The client's BUN is most likely increased because of a fluid volume deficit, but the normal creatinine level indicates adequate renal function.
8. **Abnormal ECG showing sinus tachycardia with intraventricular conduction defect (left anterior fascicular block), occasional to frequent PVCs, and a prominent U wave:** An ECG shows the electrical activity of the heart; an extra "bump" on the ECG tracing, called a U wave, is indicative of hypokalemia.

C. After analyzing the client's data, the nurse should assign a **primary** nursing diagnosis of **Deficient Fluid Volume [Hypotonic] Secondary to Vomiting,**

Diarrhea, and Loop Diuretic Therapy. Other appropriate nursing diagnoses include, but are not limited to, Risk for Electrolyte Imbalance, Decreased Cardiac Output, Diarrhea, Fatigue, Nausea, Risk for Falls, and Risk for Unstable Blood Glucose Level.

D. The nurse should plan to implement the following interventions to meet the client's needs:
1. **Place on telemetry:** It is especially important to monitor the cardiac rhythm for dysrhythmias when administering IV potassium supplements.
2. **Institute fall precautions:** The client is at increased risk for falls secondary to muscle weakness caused by hypokalemia.
3. **Vital signs every 15 minutes × 1 hour and every 30 minutes × 1 hour, then every 4 hours if stable:** This monitors the client's overall status until he is stabilized; it is especially important to do so when administering IV potassium supplements.
4. **Monitor intake and output:** This assesses the client's fluid volume status and kidney function.
5. **Administer IV solution now: 40 mEq potassium diluted in 500 mL normal saline solution at 10 mEq/hr:** IV potassium in saline resolves the client's FVD and corrects hypokalemia. It is important to note that most institutions do not allow nursing staff to dilute potassium chloride on the unit; it is most often administered piggyback via an infusing IV solution. For peripheral IV infusion, the usual concentration is 20 to 40 mEq/L infused at a maximum rate of 10 mEq/hr.
6. **Hold digoxin, metoprolol, and lisinopril:** Withholding these drugs prevents a worsening of digoxin toxicity and any further decrease in blood pressure.
7. **Administer IV ondansetron (Zofran) 4 mg every 6 hours as needed for nausea:** Ondansetron works by blocking the action of serotonin, a natural substance that may cause nausea and vomiting.
8. **Clear liquid diet:** A clear liquid diet is recommended for clients with nausea and vomiting. It consists of only clear fluids and clear foods that become fluid at room temperature, such as clear broth, tea, cranberry juice, Jell-O, and popsicles.
9. **Repeat the ECG, serum potassium, glucose, and electrolytes in 4 to 6 hours, and notify the health-care provider of the results:** This monitors the client's response to interventions.
10. **Refer to the primary health-care provider to restart digoxin and adjust potassium chloride, furosemide, metoprolol, and lisinopril dosages:** Because the client is presenting to an emergency department, he would be referred to a primary care provider for further monitoring and to reestablish a medication regimen.

E. The following outcomes should indicate to the nurse that the client's FVD has resolved:
1. Decrease in the heart rate to below 100 bpm.
2. Decrease in cardiac dysrhythmias and U wave formation.
3. Increase in serum potassium to the normal reference range; the normal range for an adult client is 3.5 to 5.0 mEq/L.
4. Increase in pulse volume, deep tendon reflexes, and bowel sounds.
5. Increase in blood pressure to the normal reference range; no orthostatic hypotension.
6. Decrease in BUN.
7. Absence of nausea and vomiting; tolerance of a normal diet.
8. Client's intention to schedule an appointment with his primary health-care provider for a repeat assessment of the digoxin level.

Chapter 5

A. The following *subjective* assessment findings indicate that the client is experiencing a health alteration:
1. **Thyroidectomy 2 days ago:** Hypocalcemia develops in only 1% to 2% of clients following total thyroidectomy. If hypocalcemia occurs, accidental damage to the parathyroid glands (located near the thyroid gland) during surgery should be suspected. Hypoparathyroidism is the most common cause of hypocalcemia.
2. **Fatigue and anxiety:** These symptoms may be due to surgical stress and hospitalization, but they are also symptoms of hypocalcemia.
3. **"My hands are asleep and I feel prickly pins around my mouth":** The sensation of tingling or "pins and needles" in and around the mouth and lips and in the hands and feet is called oral, perioral, and acral (pertaining to a limb or extremity) paresthesia, respectively. This is often the earliest symptom of hypocalcemia.
4. **History of goiter:** Goiter is an abnormal enlargement of the thyroid gland, which most likely necessitated the thyroidectomy. Goiter is associated with both hypocalcemia and hypercalcemia, depending on the underlying etiology.

B. The following *objective* assessment findings indicate that the client is experiencing a health alteration:
1. **Alert; irritable; anxious; oriented to person, place, and time:** Confusion, irritability, anxiety, lethargy, and altered mental status are signs of hypocalcemia.
2. **Heart sounds S_1 and S_2 regular, heart rate 58 bpm:** The client has been taking atenolol (Tenormin) 50 mg PO daily; this is a beta blocker that works by relaxing the blood vessels and slowing the heart rate to improve blood flow and decrease blood pressure.

Hypocalcemia may be associated with bradycardia or tachycardia, depending on the etiology.

3. **Blood pressure 90/60 mm Hg (hypotension):** The client has been taking hydrochlorothiazide/triamterene (Dyazide) 1 capsule daily for hypertension. Prolonged NPO status prior to surgery and fluid volume deficit may have increased the blood level of the drug, resulting in low blood pressure. Low serum calcium levels (hypocalcemia) are associated with hypertension in some individuals.
4. **Trousseau's sign and Chvostek's sign present:** Positive Chvostek's and Trousseau's signs are indicative of hypocalcemia.
5. **Deep tendon reflexes 3+ bilaterally:** Calcium is a membrane stabilizer. When calcium levels are low, neuromuscular irritability occurs, making the deep tendon reflexes hyperactive.
6. **Pedal and radial pulses regular, 1+, and weak bilaterally:** Weak bilateral pulses are caused by a decrease in blood pressure.
7. **Bowel sounds hyperactive in all four quadrants:** Hyperactive bowel sounds, abdominal cramping, and diarrhea are signs of hypocalcemia caused by the neuromuscular irritability that results when serum calcium levels are low.
8. **Serum calcium of 7.4 mg/dL and ionized calcium of 3.2 mg/dL:** For adults, the normal total serum calcium level is 8.2 to 10.2 mg/dL, and the normal ionized serum calcium level is 4.6 to 5.3 mg/dL. Because calcium binds with albumin in the blood, a lack of serum albumin results in a lack of circulating calcium. Therefore, when a client's serum albumin level is abnormal, it is essential to analyze the *ionized* calcium level; ionized, or unbound, calcium is not attached to albumin, thus providing more accurate information about the client's calcium status. These laboratory values confirm that the client is experiencing true hypocalcemia.
9. **Serum albumin of 2.5 gm/dL:** A low serum albumin level (hypoalbuminemia) is the most common cause of hypocalcemia. The normal reference range for serum albumin is 3.4 to 4.8 gm/dL.
10. **Serum phosphorus of 4.9 mg/dL:** Serum phosphorus and serum calcium levels have an inverse relationship. When serum phosphorus levels are high, serum calcium levels are low because phosphorus binds with calcium, decreasing the amount of calcium available in the bloodstream. The normal serum phosphorus level in adults is 2.5 to 4.5 mg/dL (3.0 to 4.5 mEq/L).
11. **Serum magnesium of 1.3 mEq/L:** Serum magnesium and serum calcium levels usually move in the same direction because they are both cations, so hypomagnesemia often accompanies hypocalcemia. The normal serum magnesium level is 1.6 to 2.6 mg/dL (1.3 to 2.1 mEq/L).
12. **Vitamin D level of 8 pg/mL:** Vitamin D is required for calcium metabolism and absorption. Thus, low vitamin D levels can cause hypocalcemia. The normal vitamin D reference range is 15 to 60 pg/mL.
13. **ECG showing sinus bradycardia with prolonged Q-T intervals:** If serum calcium levels become too low, the heart will not contract as it should. Acute hypocalcemia is characterized by prolongation of the Q-T interval and a prolonged ST segment.

C. After analyzing the client's data, the nurse should assign a **primary** nursing diagnosis of **Delayed Surgical Recovery Secondary to Hypocalcemia.** Other appropriate nursing diagnoses include, but are not limited to, Deficient Fluid Volume, Risk for Electrolyte Imbalance, Decreased Cardiac Output, Anxiety, Fatigue, Risk for Falls, and Risk for Seizures.

D. The nurse should plan to implement the following interventions to meet the client's needs:

1. **Oxygen 2 L/min via nasal cannula:** This increases perfusion to the tissues and organs. The head of the bed should be elevated 45 degrees (semi-Fowler's position) to ease the client's respiratory effort.
2. **0.9% saline solution IV 1,000 mL at 125 mL/hr:** IV saline corrects the fluid deficiency and increases the client's blood pressure.
3. **Start telemetry and monitor closely during calcium administration:** Close monitoring during calcium administration checks for improvement in the cardiac rhythm and signs of hypercalcemia resulting from overcorrection of hypocalcemia.
4. **Vital signs every 15 minutes × 1 hour and every 30 minutes × 1 hour, then every 4 hours if stable:** When administering IV calcium supplements, it is especially important to monitor the client's overall status until the client is stabilized.
5. **Administer 10% calcium gluconate IV 30 mL over no less than 15 minutes now and every 6 hours × 2 doses:** Calcium gluconate is recommended in cases of symptomatic or severe hypocalcemia; it should be administered IV piggyback in 50 to 100 mL 0.9% saline solution (normal saline) or 5% dextrose in water (D_5W) over 15 to 30 minutes to safely raise the ionized (unbound) calcium level.
6. **Hold atenolol (Tenormin) and hydrochlorothiazide/triamterene (Dyazide):** Withholding these drugs prevents a further decrease in blood pressure.
7. **Implement seizure precautions and fall precautions:** This client is at increased risk for falls and seizure activity related to neuromuscular irritability secondary to hypocalcemia.
8. **Monitor intake and output:** This assesses the client's fluid volume status and kidney function.

9. **Reevaluate clinical signs and symptoms; repeat ECG, serum calcium, ionized calcium, magnesium, phosphorus, and potassium in 6 hours, and notify the health-care provider of the results:** These assessments monitor the client's response to interventions; serum calcium should be measured every 4 to 6 hours to maintain levels at 8 to 9 mg/dL. If low albumin is present, ionized calcium should also be monitored.

E. The following outcomes should indicate to the nurse that the client's hypocalcemia has resolved:
1. **Increased O_2 saturation levels:** Oxygen saturation as measured by pulse oximetry should be 95% or greater.
2. **Laboratory values returned to the normal reference ranges:** Increased total calcium, ionized calcium, serum albumin, serum phosphorus, serum magnesium, and vitamin D levels should return to the normal reference ranges.
3. **Increased heart rate, blood pressure, and peripheral pulses:** The client's heart rate should increase to 60 to 100 bpm. The client's blood pressure should increase to greater than 90/60 mm Hg, and the peripheral pulses should be palpable.
4. **Improvement in ECG rhythms:** The client should achieve a normal sinus rhythm.
5. **Normal deep tendon reflexes and bowel sounds:** The client's deep tendon reflexes should be within normal limits, and bowel sounds should be intermittently audible on auscultation.
6. **Decrease in the client's report of circumoral paresthesia and numbness of the fingertips:** The absence of these signs indicates that the client's hypocalcemia is being corrected.
7. **Negative Chvostek's and Trousseau's signs:** The absence of these classic signs of hypocalcemia indicates a reduction in neuromuscular irritability secondary to an increased ionized calcium level.

Chapter 6

A. The following *subjective* assessment findings indicate that the client is experiencing a health alteration:
1. **Dizziness and nausea:** The symptoms may be attributed to fluid volume deficit and alcohol intoxication in a client with a history of chronic alcohol abuse.
2. **Generalized weakness and leg twitching bilaterally:** Early manifestations of hypomagnesemia, such as weakness and leg twitching, are caused by neuromuscular excitability.
3. **History of chronic alcohol abuse:** Alcoholism is the most common cause of hypomagnesemia.
4. **Hypertension:** Magnesium lowers blood pressure and alters peripheral vascular resistance. Thus, low serum magnesium levels may result in increased peripheral vascular resistance and hypertension.
5. **Metoprolol (Lopressor) 25 mg PO twice a day:** Metoprolol is a beta-adrenergic receptor blocking agent that reduces the heart rate and cardiac output, thus reducing the systolic blood pressure when taken as prescribed.

B. The following *objective* assessment findings indicate that the client is experiencing a health alteration:
1. **Oriented to person but not to place or time:** Alcohol intoxication may cause alterations in mental status.
2. **Lethargy, generalized weakness, and muscle twitching:** Signs of hypomagnesemia include tremor, lethargy, muscle cramps, depression, generalized weakness, anorexia, and vomiting.
3. **Heart sounds S_1 and S_2 irregular, rapid:** The client is tachycardic with a heart rate of 134 bpm. In this client, tachycardia may be due to fluid volume deficit (FVD) secondary to decreased water intake, diarrhea, or hypomagnesemia.
4. **Cardiac monitor reveals a 30-beat run of ventricular tachycardia with a torsades de pointes configuration:** Torsades de pointes is a life-threatening type of ventricular tachycardia that can be caused by hypomagnesemia. The American Heart Association recommends that magnesium sulfate be added to the regimen used to manage torsades de pointes and other types of ventricular fibrillation.
5. **Pedal and radial pulses irregular, 1+, and weak bilaterally:** Weak peripheral pulses and tachycardia are suggestive of FVD.
6. **DTRs 3+ bilaterally:** Hyperactive deep tendon reflexes are associated with hypomagnesemia and accompanying hypocalcemia. These electrolyte imbalances cause neuromuscular irritability.
7. **Bowel sounds hyperactive in all four quadrants:** Hyperactive bowel sounds are associated with hypomagnesemia, hypocalcemia, and hyperkalemia.
8. **Incontinent of moderate amount of liquid brown stool:** The client's incontinence is most likely related to bowel hypermotility and alcohol intoxication.
9. **Blood pressure 168/94 mm Hg:** This client's hypertension may be related to hypomagnesemia, dehydration secondary to alcohol intake, or failure to take prescribed antihypertensive medications.
10. **O_2 saturation 93% on room air:** Muscle weakness caused by hypomagnesemia, hypocalcemia, and hypokalemia may affect the diaphragm, resulting in shallow respirations and a decreased respiratory rate, decreasing the oxygen saturation of the blood.
11. **Serum magnesium of 1 mEq/L:** This laboratory value confirms that the client is experiencing

severe hypomagnesemia. The normal serum magnesium level is 1.6 to 2.6 mg/dL (1.3 to 2.1 mEq/L).

12. **Serum calcium of 7.8 mg/dL:** Hypocalcemia is a classic sign of severe hypomagnesemia (less than 1.2 mg/dL). The normal total serum calcium level is 8.2 to 10.2 mg/dL for adults.
13. **Serum potassium of 3.1 mEq/L:** Hypokalemia is common in clients with hypomagnesemia, occurring in 40% to 60% of cases. Diuretic therapy and diarrhea also result in the loss of magnesium and potassium. The normal reference range for serum potassium in an adult client is 3.5 to 5.0 mEq/L.
14. **Blood alcohol level of 0.11:** This means that the client's blood alcohol concentration is 11%, indicating intoxication. A blood alcohol level of 0.08 to 0.10 is considered legally drunk. Alcohol stimulates the renal excretion of magnesium, which is also increased in diabetic ketoacidosis (DKA), hypophosphatemia, and hyperaldosteronism resulting from liver disease.
15. **Liver function tests (LFTs):** LFTs are used to identify acute or chronic tissue damage; elevated levels may be seen in alcoholism, liver disease, and many other disorders. This client's liver enzymes are elevated, most likely due to alcoholism:
    - **Lactate dehydrogenase (LDH) of 262 units/L:** Normal reference range is 90 to 250 units/L.
    - **Serum alkaline phosphatase (ALP) of 190 units/L:** Normal reference range is 25 to 142 units/L.
    - **Serum aspartate aminotransferase (AST or SGOT) of 52 units/L:** Normal reference range is 13 to 40 units/L.
    - **Serum alanine aminotransferase (ALT or SGPT) of 64 units/L:** Normal reference range is 7 to 40 units/L.
16. **ECG showing sinus tachycardia with occasional multifocal PVCs :** About half of all adults experience occasional premature ventricular contractions (PVCs) throughout the day that are of no significance. This client, however, has an increased heart rate (tachycardia) with occasional multifocal PVCs, which means that the PVCs are originating at two or more points anywhere in the left or right ventricle. Multifocal PVCs can occur sporadically, and each PVC has its own shape. The fact that the client is experiencing multifocal PVCs is of great concern because worsening of the client's hypomagnesemia and accompanying hypokalemia may precipitate a life-threatening torsades de pointes rhythm. Close observation of this client's ECG rhythm is required.

C. After analyzing the client's data, the nurse should assign a **primary** nursing diagnosis of **Risk for Injury Secondary to Muscle Weakness Related to Hypomagnesemia.** Other appropriate nursing diagnoses include, but are not limited to, Risk for Electrolyte Imbalance, Risk for Deficient Fluid Volume, Decreased Cardiac Output, Diarrhea, Risk for Impaired Liver Function, Acute Confusion, Risk-Prone Health Behavior, Risk for Falls, and Risk for Decreased Cardiac Tissue Perfusion.

D. The nurse should plan to implement the following interventions to meet the client's needs:

1. **Assess vital signs every 15 minutes × 4, hourly × 2, then every 4 hours:** This monitors the client's status and response to interventions.
2. **Administer oxygen 2 L/min via nasal cannula:** This increases perfusion to the tissues and organs.
3. **Start telemetry:** The cardiac rhythm must be monitored for dysrhythmias caused by hypomagnesemia, hypocalcemia, and hypokalemia. Magnesium deficiency affects the electrical activity and myocardial contractility of the heart. Clients with magnesium deficiency are particularly susceptible to digoxin-related arrhythmia; there is also an association between magnesium deficiency and coronary artery disease.
4. **Implement seizure precautions:** Low serum magnesium levels increase the excitability of muscles and nerves, placing the client at risk for seizure activity.
5. **Initiate an alcohol withdrawal protocol:** This helps the client withdraw from alcohol and prevents side effects, such as delirium tremens.
6. **Perform neurological checks every hour × 4, then every 4 hours:** This monitors for changes in level of consciousness.
7. **Administer magnesium sulfate 2 gm IV push now:** IV magnesium sulfate begins to correct the magnesium deficit immediately. It should be noted that with an abrupt elevation in serum magnesium levels, up to 50% of the infused magnesium will be excreted in the urine, so additional replacement therapy will be needed.
8. **Add 2 gm magnesium sulfate to 1,000 mL normal (0.9%) saline solution at 100 mL/hr daily:** This continues to increase the serum magnesium level. Clients with concomitant hypokalemia or hypocalcemia should also receive potassium and calcium replacement because these deficits may take several days to correct when treated with magnesium alone.
9. **Start magnesium chloride (Slow-Mag) 2 tablets PO daily:** This drug provides sustained-release oral replacement of magnesium to increase serum levels and prevent diarrhea, which can be caused by magnesium replacement; moderate to severe magnesium depletion requires sustained correction.

10. **Administer IV metoprolol (Lopressor) now; increase the PO dose to 50 mg twice a day:** This drug decreases the client's blood pressure, reducing the heart's workload.
11. **Initiate fall precautions:** This client is at increased risk for falls due to generalized muscle weakness.
12. **Monitor intake and output:** This monitors the client's fluid status and assists in evaluating renal function; the minimum urine output for an adult is 30 mL/hr.
13. **Reevaluate clinical signs and symptoms; repeat ECG and serum magnesium, calcium, and potassium levels in 6 hours:** These assessments monitor the client's status and response to interventions. Magnesium is slow to level out between the serum and the intracellular spaces and tissues, so the serum magnesium level may appear artificially high if it is measured too soon after a magnesium dose is administered.
14. **Initiate alcohol cessation counseling when the client is stable:** Educating the client about the negative effects of alcohol can help decrease the client's dependence on alcohol as a coping mechanism.

E. The following outcomes should indicate to the nurse that the client's hypomagnesemia has resolved:
1. **Increase in oxygen saturation levels:** The client's oxygen saturation level should be greater than 95% as measured by pulse oximetry.
2. **Increase in the serum magnesium level to the normal reference range:** The normal serum magnesium level is 1.6 to 2.6 mg/dL (1.3 to 2.1 mEq/L).
3. **Decrease in blood pressure:** In an adult client, a safe blood pressure is between 90/60 and 140/90 mm Hg. The ideal blood pressure is less than 120/80 mm Hg.
4. **Decreased heart rate; increased pulse volume:** The client's heart rate should be less than 100 bpm, and the peripheral pulses should be palpable and regular.
5. **Resolution of abnormal neuromuscular findings:** The client should be oriented to person, place, and time. Lethargy, generalized weakness, and muscle twitching should also be resolved.
6. **Resolution of abnormal ECG rhythm:** The heart rhythm should return to baseline; optimally, the client should achieve a normal sinus rhythm.

Chapter 7

A. The following *subjective* assessment findings indicate that the client is experiencing a health alteration:
1. **History of chronic kidney disease and diagnosis of end-stage renal disease:** End-stage renal disease (ESRD) occurs when kidney function is less than 10% of normal. ESRD almost always follows chronic kidney disease. Clients who have reached this stage need dialysis or a kidney transplant. The most common causes of ESRD in the United States are diabetes and high blood pressure.
2. **History of congestive heart failure (CHF):** CHF is a condition in which the heart can no longer pump enough oxygen-rich blood to the rest of the body. CHF may affect either the right side (right-sided heart failure) or the left side (left-sided heart failure) of the heart, but usually both sides are involved. As the heart loses pumping action, blood may back up into the lungs, liver, gastrointestinal tract, arms, and legs. The most common cause of CHF is coronary artery disease (CAD), a narrowing of the small blood vessels that supply blood and oxygen to the heart.
3. **History of hypertension:** High blood pressure is a primary cause of CHF. Hypertension caused by another medical condition or by a medication is called secondary hypertension. This client's secondary hypertension is most likely due to chronic kidney disease.
4. **Missed dialysis appointment 2 days ago:** Clients diagnosed with ESRD develop metabolic acidosis when they are noncompliant with dialysis treatments. In the presence of acidosis, the client may experience hyperkalemia, hyponatremia, hypocalcemia, hyperphosphatemia, and hypermagnesemia.
5. **Fatigue and itching:** Manifestations of hyperphosphatemia are usually related to its underlying cause and may include joint pain, pruritus (itching), fatigue, shortness of breath, anorexia, nausea, vomiting, and sleep disturbances.
6. **Muscle aches, weakness, and severe cramping for 1 day:** The client is experiencing muscle aches, weakness, and severe cramping secondary to the hypocalcemia that accompanies hyperphosphatemia.
7. **Sevelamer hydrochloride (Renagel) 2 800-mg tablets PO three times per day with meals:** The client is taking oral sevelamer hydrochloride to decrease the serum phosphorus level, but this medication is ineffective because of the client's ESRD and missed dialysis appointment.

B. The following *objective* assessment findings indicate that the client is experiencing a health alteration:
1. **Presence of crackles in the lungs, increased respiratory rate of 24 breaths per minute, and oxygen saturation of 91%:** Common respiratory signs of heart failure are tachypnea (increased rate of breathing) and increased work of breathing (nonspecific signs of respiratory distress). Rales or crackles, heard initially in the lung bases and, when severe, throughout the lung fields, suggest the development of pulmonary edema.
2. **Increased blood pressure of 142/98 mm Hg:** The client's blood pressure is elevated because of fluid

volume excess (FVE) secondary to decreased renal function. The client is experiencing CHF.

3. **Decreased heart rate of 58 bpm:** CHF can cause either bradycardia or tachycardia, depending on the underlying cause and severity.
4. **Jugular venous distention:** JVD is a sign of FVE caused by the client's failing kidneys.
5. **Bounding, irregular peripheral pulses:** The client's pulses are bounding because the heart has to work harder to maintain perfusion to the tissues due to CHF.
6. **Hyperactive DTRs and bowel sounds:** These are signs of hypocalcemia related to hyperphosphatemia. Calcium is a membrane stabilizer; the lack of calcium results in neuromuscular irritability.
7. **Increased serum phosphorus level of 8.2 mg/dL:** The most common cause of hyperphosphatemia is renal failure. The normal reference range for serum phosphorus in adults is 2.5 to 4.5 mg/dL (3.0 to 4.5 mEq/L).
8. **Decreased serum calcium level of 6.2 mg/dL:** Hyperphosphatemia leads to decreased levels of ionized calcium. The client is also taking a subtherapeutic dose of oral calcium. For adults, the normal reference range for total serum calcium is 8.2 to 10.2 mg/dL; for ionized serum calcium, it is 4.6 to 5.3 mg/dL.
9. **Increased serum potassium level of 6.7 mEq/L:** Renal insufficiency or failure is a primary cause of hyperkalemia because the kidneys cannot excrete excess amounts of potassium; potassium also shifts out of cells and into the extracellular fluid in the presence of acidosis.
10. **Increased serum BUN level of 68 mg/dL and serum creatinine level of 15.4 mg/dL:** The client's BUN and creatinine levels are extremely high, indicating inadequate renal function secondary to ESRD. The normal reference range for serum BUN is about 8 to 21 mg/dL; for serum creatinine, it is about 0.5 to 1.2 mg/dL.
11. **Abnormal ECG (sinus bradycardia with prolonged Q-T interval, prolonged ST segment, and PVCs):** The client is exhibiting changes in cardiac rhythm secondary to hypocalcemia.
12. **Positive Chvostek's and Trousseau's signs:** These are clinical signs of hypocalcemia related to hyperphosphatemia.

C. After analyzing the client's data, the nurse should assign a **primary** nursing diagnosis of **Excess Fluid Volume Related to Congestive Heart Failure Secondary to End-Stage Renal Disease.** Other appropriate nursing diagnoses include, but are not limited to, Risk for Electrolyte Imbalance, Impaired Gas Exchange, Decreased Cardiac Output, Fatigue, Risk for Falls, Risk for Decreased Cardiac Tissue Perfusion, and Activity Intolerance.

D. The nurse should plan to implement the following interventions to meet the client's needs:

1. **Oxygen 2 L/min per nasal cannula:** This increases perfusion to the tissues and organs and decreases the heart's workload.
2. **Place the client on telemetry:** Monitoring is required to detect cardiac dysrhythmias and observe for dysrhythmias associated with hypocalcemia.
3. **Check the patency of the dialysis site:** Prepare for emergent hemodialysis because the client must undergo dialysis immediately to correct FVE, acidosis, and electrolyte imbalances. Dialysis can be used to remove waste and water from the blood until a renal transplant can be performed, but it may be the only supportive measure available when a transplant would be inappropriate.
4. **Vital signs every 15 minutes × 2 hours, every 30 minutes × 2 hours, every 1 hour × 2 hours, then every 4 hours × 24 hours:** Establish a baseline before administering medications or performing dialysis, and monitor the client's fluid status and response to interventions.
5. **Administer Renagel after dialysis:** This drug lowers the client's serum phosphorus level to correct hyperphosphatemia.
6. **Hold furosemide:** Although furosemide is used to correct FVE and decrease hypertension, toxicity may occur in clients with renal impairment because the drug is excreted by the kidneys. Excess furosemide may result in worsening of the client's hypocalcemia and hypomagnesemia and may cause tinnitus, reversible or irreversible hearing impairment, and deafness.
7. **Monitor the client:** Strictly monitor intake and output to assess for FVE; perform neurological checks for changes in level of consciousness.
8. **Check parathyroid hormone (PTH), thyroid-stimulating hormone (TSH), and vitamin D levels:** These hormones help regulate calcium levels.
9. **Check the digoxin level:** Deteriorating renal function, dehydration, electrolyte disturbances, and drug interactions can precipitate chronic digoxin toxicity. Hyperkalemia, which is associated with renal failure, increases the client's risk for digoxin toxicity; chronic digoxin toxicity does not usually cause hyperkalemia.
10. **Recheck the serum sodium, potassium, phosphorus, calcium, glucose, creatinine, and bicarbonate levels after dialysis:** These values are used to evaluate the client's response to interventions.
11. **Low-phosphorus diet:** Restricting dietary phosphorus prevents a further increase in the serum phosphorus level.

12. **Increase Caltrate to 500 mg PO with each meal:** This drug increases the client's serum calcium level to correct hypocalcemia.
13. **Senna-S tablets at bedtime:** This drug treats constipation related to the presence of hypoactive bowel motility and calcium supplementation.
14. **Palliative care consultation:** It is important to establish the goals of care and determine the client's code status; the client will need ongoing dialysis or a kidney transplant in order to live.

E. The following outcomes should indicate to the nurse that the client's FVE has resolved:
1. All laboratory values should return to the client's baseline level or to within the normal reference ranges.
2. The client should experience a decrease in respiratory rate and blood pressure.
3. The client's heart rate and oxygen saturation level should increase.
4. ECG, JVD, DTRs, bowel sounds, and pulse volume should be within normal limits.
5. The client should test negatively for Chvostek's and Trousseau's signs.
6. The client should express an understanding of the disease process and the plan for ongoing dialysis and palliative care; the client should be educated regarding the need for a living will and health-care power of attorney.

Chapter 8

A. The following subjective assessment findings indicate that the client is experiencing a health alteration:
1. **A 4-day history of weakness, fever, nausea, vomiting, and abdominal pain**: Considering the client's history of type 2 diabetes mellitus, these manifestations are most likely related to diabetic ketoacidosis (DKA); nausea, vomiting, abdominal pain, decreased appetite, and anorexia may be present.
2. **History of type 2 diabetes mellitus (DM):** DKA, an acute, life-threatening complication of diabetes, occurs primarily in clients with type 1 diabetes, but it may occur in some clients with type 2 diabetes.
3. **Confusion:** Clients diagnosed with DKA often present with mild disorientation or confusion.
4. **Thirst and polyuria:** Increased thirst (polydipsia) and urination (polyuria) are the most common early symptoms of DKA.
5. **Metformin (Glucophage) 500 mg PO bid:** Metformin is used to treat type 2 diabetes (a condition in which the body does not use insulin normally and therefore cannot control the amount of sugar in the blood) by decreasing the amount of glucose absorbed from food and the amount of glucose made by the liver; it also increases the body's response to insulin. The client is taking a standard dose but may not be compliant with the medication regimen.
6. **History of hypertension:** The client is taking lisinopril/hydrochlorothiazide (Zestoretic) 20/12.5 mg PO once a day for the treatment of hypertension; taking this medication when dehydrated may result in hypotension.

B. The following *objective* assessment findings indicate that the client is experiencing a health alteration:
1. **Increased temperature of 101.2°F (38.4°C):** Fever is a sign of an underlying infection; it is not a sign of DKA itself.
2. **Decreased blood pressure of 86/54 mm Hg and increased heart rate of 138 bpm:** The extreme dehydration and hypovolemia that result from DKA cause hypotension and tachycardia. The client's blood pressure should be greater than 90/60 mm Hg, and the heart rate should be less than 100 bpm.
3. **Increased respiratory rate of 38 breaths per minute (Kussmaul respirations):** The client's body is attempting to compensate for the acidotic state by increasing the respiratory rate to "blow off" excess carbonic acid ions; this results in rapid, shallow breathing (Kussmaul respirations). The normal respiratory rate is 12 to 20 breaths per minute.
4. **Strong odor of ketones ("fruity" breath odor):** The fruity odor occurs when the client begins exhaling acetone; this is a definitive sign of DKA.
5. **Flushed, warm, dry skin; pink, dry mucous membranes:** The extreme dehydration and hypovolemia that result from DKA cause dry mucous membranes, poor skin turgor, and flushed, dry skin.
6. **ABG values: pH 7.16, $PaCO_2$ 20 mm Hg, HCO_3^- 6.2 mEq/L, PaO_2 90 mm Hg:** The client's blood pH is decreased to 7.16, indicating acidosis (normal pH is 7.35 to 7.45). The client's serum bicarbonate (HCO_3^-) level is 6.2 mEq/L, indicating that the acidosis is metabolic in origin (normal reference range for bicarbonate is 18 to 23 mEq/L in adults). The client's arterial carbon dioxide ($PaCO_2$) level is decreased because the lungs are compensating for the metabolic acidosis by increasing the respiratory rate. DKA is diagnosed by an arterial pH less than 7.30 with an anion gap greater than 12 mEq/L.
7. **Increased anion gap of 20.8 mEq/L:** An increased anion gap confirms the presence of metabolic acidosis. In DKA, the anion gap is usually greater than 12 mEq/L; the normal reference range in adults is 8 to 16 mEq/L.
8. **Increased serum glucose of 440 mg/dL:** The serum glucose is elevated because the client's type 2 DM is poorly controlled. In type 2 DM, insulin secretion is inadequate; peripheral insulin resistance and increased production of glucose by the liver increase plasma glucose levels (hyperglycemia). The normal

reference range for fasting blood glucose is 66 to 99 mg/dL; clients with serum glucose levels of 100 to 125 mg/dL are considered "prediabetic."

9. **Decreased serum potassium of 3.0 mEq/L:** Electrolytes, including potassium, are lost along with fluids. The client may initially experience general malaise, fatigue, and muscle weakness as a result of hypokalemia; as the potassium level continues to decrease, the client may develop flaccid muscle paralysis and arrhythmias.
10. **Increased BUN of 22 mg/dL and increased creatinine of 1.8 mg/dL:** Blood urea nitrogen (BUN) and creatinine levels are used to evaluate and measure kidney function. Elevated BUN levels may indicate acute or chronic kidney disease, damage, or failure due to an underlying condition such as diabetes mellitus, congestive heart failure, severe burns, heart attack, or dehydration; elevated creatinine levels can indicate damage to the kidney's blood vessels caused by reduced blood flow to the kidneys due to dehydration, shock, diabetes, atherosclerosis or congestive heart failure. The normal reference range for BUN is about 8 to 21 mg/dL; the normal reference range for creatinine is approximately 0.5 to 1.2 mg/dL.
11. **White blood cell (WBC) count of 20 (× 10^3/mm^3), with 60% neutrophils, 12% bands, 25% lymphocytes, and 3% monocytes:** The WBC differential count determines how many of each cell type are present in the blood. Immature forms of neutrophils, called "band" cells, form in response to infection; the presence of these immature cells is called a "shift to the left," or bandemia, and it can be the earliest sign of infection, even before the WBC count becomes elevated. The normal reference range for bands is 0% to 3%.
12. **Urinalysis positive for glucose, ketones, protein, and WBCs:** The client's urinalysis indicates that metabolic acidosis was most likely precipitated by a urinary tract infection. *Acute infection is the most common cause of DKA.*
13. **ECG showing sinus tachycardia with left ventricular hypertrophy:** Left ventricular hypertrophy is thickening of the myocardium of the left ventricle, most likely caused by the client's chronic hypertension; sinus tachycardia (heart rate greater than 100 bpm) may be attributed to the client's dehydration, infection, or both.

C. After analyzing the client's data, the nurse should assign a **primary** nursing diagnosis of **Deficient Fluid Volume [Hypertonic] Related to Osmotic Diuresis Secondary to DKA.** Other appropriate nursing diagnoses include, but are not limited to, Risk for Electrolyte Imbalance, Decreased Cardiac Output, Dysfunctional Gastrointestinal Motility, Fatigue, Nausea, Acute Confusion, Impaired Gas Exchange, Ineffective Peripheral Tissue Perfusion, Risk for Shock, Risk for Unstable Blood Glucose, Risk for Imbalanced Body Temperature, and Risk for Falls.

D. The nurse should plan to implement the following interventions to meet the client's needs:

1. **Monitor oxygen saturation continuously; administer O_2 at 2 L/min via nasal cannula as needed to maintain O_2 saturation greater than 95%:** Oxygen increases perfusion to the tissues and organs. The head of the bed should be elevated 45 degrees (semi-Fowler's position) to ease the client's respiratory effort.
2. **Assess vital signs every 15 minutes × 2 hours, then hourly until stable, then every 4 hours:** During rehydration and the administration of IV regular insulin, it is especially important to monitor the client's overall status until the client is stabilized.
3. **Start telemetry and repeat the ECG in 4 hours:** The client's cardiac rhythm must be monitored for dysrhythmias that may be caused by electrolyte imbalances. This client is at high risk for hypokalemia because the administration of insulin causes potassium to move back into the cells.
4. **Monitor strict intake and output hourly:** This assesses the client's fluid volume status and kidney function. This intervention is especially important because the client is dehydrated secondary to osmotic diuresis, and kidney function may be impaired due to renal damage secondary to diabetes.
5. **Hold oral medications until instructed to resume:** Withholding oral medications reduces nausea and vomiting and prevents a further decrease in blood pressure secondary to the administration of lisinopril/hydrochlorothiazide (Zestoretic).
6. **Monitor the blood glucose level per insulin protocol (every 15 to 60 minutes):** This assesses the client's blood glucose level and response to insulin therapy.
7. **Administer 10 to 20 units of regular insulin (as ordered), and begin an insulin drip per insulin protocol:** Regular insulin is the only insulin that can be administered intravenously for the treatment of DKA. Insulin is a high-risk medication, especially when using the IV route, and it should be administered by an experienced registered nurse or health-care provider. Most institutions have an insulin protocol in place to help the nurse adjust the amount of insulin infused based on the client's blood glucose level.
8. **Administer IV 0.9% normal saline solution 1,000 mL over 30 minutes, then a second 1,000 mL over 60 minutes, while monitoring blood pressure**

tolerance, and monitor for fluid volume excess (FVE): Most clients with DKA are profoundly dehydrated, and IV saline provides rapid rehydration, enabling the kidneys to eliminate excess glucose, electrolytes, and toxins. The client should be monitored for signs of FVE, such as peripheral edema and crackles in the lungs on auscultation (pulmonary edema), and the blood pressure must be closely monitored to prevent fluid overload.

9. **Change the IV fluid to dextrose 5% in normal saline when the blood glucose level reaches 250 mg/dL:** Providing dextrose prevents hypoglycemia when the blood glucose level decreases to 250 mg/dL or less.
10. **Discontinue the insulin drip and administer subcutaneous regular insulin per sliding scale when the acidosis or ketosis is corrected and the client can tolerate oral intake:** This provides the client with ongoing insulin coverage after serum glucose levels have returned to baseline and the client is taking fluids orally.
11. **Provide a clear liquid diet as tolerated:** A clear liquid diet prevents nausea and vomiting.
12. **Obtain laboratory values hourly × 4, then every 4 hours: glucose, sodium, potassium, creatinine, and BUN.** These assessments are used to evaluate the client's response to therapy and can assist in planning further treatment.
13. **Obtain ABGs 2 hours after the initiation of insulin therapy:** ABGs evaluate the status of the client's acid-base balance.
14. **Obtain urine for culture and sensitivity, and report the results to the health-care provider:** This identifies the organism causing the client's urinary tract infection (UTI), which is the underlying cause of the DKA.
15. **Administer IV ciprofloxacin (Cipro) 400 mg every 12 hours:** Ciprofloxacin is in a class of antibiotics called fluoroquinolones and is used to treat certain types of UTI.
16. **Implement fall precautions:** The client is at increased risk for falls related to weakness secondary to dehydration and electrolyte imbalance.
17. **Provide client education when the client is stable:** Educate the client about the etiology, treatment, and prevention of DKA and associated fluid and electrolyte imbalances; the goal is to help the client manage serum glucose levels and prevent the development of DKA.

E. The following outcomes should indicate to the nurse that the client's metabolic acidosis has resolved:

1. **Gradual decrease in blood glucose to within normal limits for this client:** The client's blood glucose level should be less than 200 mg/dL following acute treatment for DKA; the normal reference range for blood glucose is 66 to 99 mg/dL.
2. **Increase in blood pressure and pulse volume:** The client's blood pressure should be greater than 90/60 mm Hg, and the peripheral pulses should be palpable and regular bilaterally.
3. **Decrease in heart rate and respiratory rate:** The client's heart rate should be 60 to 100 bpm, and the respiratory rate should be 12 to 20 breaths per minute.
4. **Return of all laboratory values to within the normal reference ranges:** The client's WBC count should be improving; the serum potassium level should be within the normal reference range of 3.5 to 5.0 mEq/L; the client's serum BUN and creatinine levels should be within normal limits; and the urinalysis should reveal a specific gravity within normal limits and should be negative for glucose and ketones.
5. **Resolution of metabolic acidosis:** The client's serum pH should increase to the normal reference range, the ABGs and anion gap should be within normal limits, and the ketone odor of the client's breath should have dissipated.
6. **Toleration of a clear liquid diet:** Nausea and vomiting should be resolved, and the client should be able to tolerate the oral intake of clear liquids.
7. **Level of consciousness improved to alert and oriented × 3:** The client should no longer exhibit signs of confusion and should be oriented to person, place, and time.
8. **Evaluation of client education:** The client should be able to verbalize and demonstrate methods to prevent DKA and manage diabetes.

References

American Heart Association. (2010). Sodium (salt or sodium chloride): reducing sodium in your diet. http://www.americanheart.org/presenter.jhtml?identifier=4708.

Beaman, N. (2008). *Pharmacology Clear and Simple: A Drug Classifications and Dosage Calculations Approach*. Philadelphia, PA: F. A. Davis.

Berman, A., Snyder, S., Kozier, B., and Erb, G. (2012). *Kozier & Erb's Fundamentals of Nursing: Concepts, Process, and Practice* (9th ed.). Upper Saddle River, NJ: Pearson.

Braun, B. (2012). Water-electrolyte balance, acid-base balance. In *Basics of I.V. Therapy*. Retrieved from http://www.iv-partner.com/.

Carson, J., Grossman, B., Kleinman, S., Tinmouth, A., Marques, M., Fung, M., . . . Djulbegovic, B. (2012). Red blood cell transfusion: a clinical practice guideline from the AABB. *Ann Intern Med.* 157(1):49–58.

Deglin, J. H., Vallerand, A. H., and Sanoski, C. A. (2013). *Davis's Drug Guide for Nurses* (13th ed.). Philadelphia, PA: F. A. Davis.

Diabetes Education Online, Diabetes Teaching Center at the University of California, San Francisco. (2010). Type 1 diabetes: diabetes treatment: calculating insulin dose. Retrieved from http://www.deo.ucsf.edu/type1/diabetes-treatment/medications-and-therapies/type-1-insulin-rx/calculating-insuliin-dose.html.

Diehl-Oplinger, L., and Kaminski, M. (2004). Choosing the right fluid to counter hypovolemic shock. *Nursing.* 34(3):52–54.

Dugdale, D. C. (2009). Digitalis toxicity. In *Medline Plus Medical Encyclopedia.* Retrieved from http://www.nlm.nih.gov/medlineplus/ency/article/000165.htm.

Holte, K., Sharrock, N. E., and Kehlet, H. (2002). Pathophysiology and clinical implications of perioperative fluid excess. *Br J Anaesth.* 89(4):622–632. Retrieved from http://bja.oxfordjournals.org/cgi/reprint/89/4/622.

Ignatavicius, D., and Workman, M. (2012). *Medical-Surgical Nursing: Patient-Centered Collaborative Care* (7th ed.). St. Louis, MO: Saunders.

Institute for Safe Medicine Practices. (2012). ISMP's list of high alert medications. *Institute for Safe Medicine Practices Tools.* Retrieved from http://www.ismp.org/tools/highalertmedications.pdf.

Institute for Safe Medicine Practices. (2009). Plain D5W or hypotonic saline solutions post-op could result in acute hyponatremia and death in healthy children. *Institute for Safe Medicine Practices Newsletter.* Retrieved from http://www.ismp.org/Newsletters/acutecare/articles/20090813.asp.

Jones, S. (2010). *ECG Notes: Interpretation and Management Guide* (2nd ed.). Philadelphia, PA: F. A. Davis.

Lemone, P., and Burke, K. (2010). *Medical-Surgical Nursing: Critical Thinking in Client Care* (5th ed.). Upper Saddle River, NJ: Pearson Prentice Hall.

Lewis, J. L., III (Reviewer). (2009). Disorders of potassium concentration. In *The Merck Manuals Online Library.* Retrieved from http://www.merckmanuals.com/professional/endocrine_and_metabolic_disorders/electrolyte_disorders/disorders_of_potassium_concentration.html?qt=&sc=&alt=.

Lowdermilk, D. L., Perry, S. E., Cashion, K., and Alden, K. R. (2010). *Maternity and Women's Health Care* (10th ed.). St. Louis, MO: Mosby.

Mayo Clinic Staff. (2011). Potassium supplement (oral route, parenteral route). *MayoClinic.com Health Information.* Retrieved from http://www.mayoclinic.com/health/drug-information/DR602373.

Mayo Clinic Staff. (2010). High blood pressure (hypertension). *MayoClinic.com Health Information.* http://www.mayoclinic.com/health/diuretics/hi00030.

Moses, S. (Revised 2010). Magnesium sulfate aka: magnesium replacement. *Family Practice Notebook, LLC.* Retrieved from http://www.fpnotebook.com/Renal/Pharm/MgnsmSlft.htm.

National Institutes of Health, Office of Dietary Supplements. (Reviewed 2012). Dietary supplement fact sheet: calcium. Retrieved from http://ods.od.nih.gov/factsheets/Calcium-HealthProfessional/.

National Institutes of Health, Office of Dietary Supplements. (Reviewed 2010). Dietary supplement fact sheet: magnesium. Retrieved from http://ods.od.nih.gov/factsheets/Magnesium-HealthProfessional/.

Nix, C. (2012). *Williams' Basic Nutrition and Diet Therapy* (14th ed.). St. Louis, MO: Mosby.

Novello, N. P., and Blumstein, H. A. (2010). Hypermagnesemia: treatment and medication. Retrieved from http://emedicine.medscape.com/article/766604-treatment.

Perkin, R. M., Swift, J. D., Newton, D. A., and Anas, N. (2012). *Pediatric Hospital Medicine: Textbook of Inpatient Management* (2nd ed.). Philadelphia, PA: Wolters Kluwer Health/Lippincott Williams & Wilkins.

Perry, S., Hockenberry, M., Lowdermilk, D., and Wilson, D. (2010). *Maternal Child Nursing Care* (4th ed.). St. Louis, MO: Mosby.

Phillips, B. J. (2004). Electrolyte replacement: a review. *Internet Journal of Internal Medicine.* 5(1). DOI: 10.5580/1cf4.

Potter, P., Perry, A., Stockert, P., and Hall, A. (2012). *Fundamentals of Nursing* (8th ed.). St. Louis, MO: Mosby.

Quraishy, N., Bachowski, G., Benjamin, R., Eastvold, P., et al. (2010). A compendium of transfusion practice guidelines. Retrieved from http://www.redcrossblood.org/sites/arc/files/pdf/Practice-Guidelines-Nov2010-Final.pdf.

Roberts, K. B. (2007). Dehydration. In *The Merck Manuals Online Medical Library*. http://www.merck.com/mmpe/sec19/ch276/ch276b.html.

Strunden, M., Heckel, K., Goetz, A., and Reuter, D. (2011). Perioperative fluid and volume management: physiological basis, tools and strategies. *Ann Intensive Care.* 1:2. Retrieved from http://www.annalsofintensivecare.com/content/pdf/2110-5820-1-2.pdf.

Townsend, M. C. (2011). *Psychiatric Mental Health Nursing* (7th ed.). Philadelphia, PA: F. A. Davis.

U.S. Department of Agriculture, Agricultural Research Service. (2009). *USDA National Nutrient Database for Standard Reference.* Release 22. Nutrient Data Laboratory Home Page. Retrieved from http://www.ars.usda.gov/ba/bhnrc/ndl.

Van Leeuwen, A. M., Poelhuis-Leth, D., and Bladh, M. (2011). *Davis's Comprehensive Handbook of Laboratory and Diagnostic Tests With Nursing Implications* (4th ed.). Philadelphia, PA: F. A. Davis.

Venes, D., et al (Eds.). (2013). *Taber's Cyclopedic Medical Dictionary* (22nd ed.). Philadelphia, PA: F. A. Davis.

Ward, S. L., and Hisley, S. M. (2011). *Maternal-Child Nursing Care: Optimizing Outcomes for Mothers, Children and Families.* Philadelphia, PA: F. A. Davis.

Wilkinson, J., and Treas, L. (2011). *Fundamentals of Nursing: Theory, Concepts & Applications* (2nd ed.). Philadelphia, PA: F. A. Davis.

Williams, L., and Hopper, P. (2011). *Understanding Medical-Surgical Nursing* (4th ed.). Philadelphia, PA: F. A. Davis.

Index

Note: Illustrations are indicated by *(f)*; tables by *(t)*; boxes by *(b)*.

A

D

I

J

K

L

Q

R

T

U

V